RA

The AIDS pandemic

The AIDS Pandemic: Impact on Science and Society

The AIDS Pandemic: Impact on Science and Society

Edited by
Kenneth H Mayer and HF Pizer

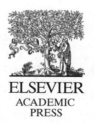

ELSEVIER
ACADEMIC
PRESS

AMSTERDAM BOSTON HEIDELBERG LONDON NEW YORK OXFORD
PARIS SAN DIEGO SAN FRANCISCO SINGAPORE SYDNEY TOKYO

Elsevier Academic Press
525 B Street, Suite 1900, San Diego, California 92101-4495, USA
http://www.elsevier.com

Elsevier Academic Press
84 Theobakl's Road, London WC1X 8RR, UK
http://www.elsevier.com

Library of Congress Control Number: 2004116779

British Library Cataloguing in Publication Data
A catalogue record for this book is available from the British Library

ISBN 0-12-465271-9

Printed and bound in Great Britain
05 06 07 08 9 8 7 6 5 4 3 2 1

Contents

v

Contributors

Frederick L Altice
Associate Professor and Director of Clinical Research, AIDS Program, Section of Infectious Diseases, Yale University School of Medicine, New Haven, USA

Deborah Anderson
Professor, Obstetrics and Gynaecology, Boston University School of Medicine, Boston, USA

John-Manuel Andriote
Washington, DC, USA

Priya Bery
Director of Policy & Research, Global Business Coalition on HIV/AIDS, New York, USA

Chris Beyrer
Director, Fogarty AIDS International Training & Research Program, Johns Hopkins University, Bloomberg School of Public Health, Baltimore, USA

Samuel A Bozzette
Department of Medicine, University of California San Diego, La Jolla, USA

Susan Buchbinder
Director, HIV Research Section, San Francisco Department of Health, San Francisco, USA

Patricia Case
Program in Urban Health, Department of Social Medicine, Harvard Medical School, Boston, USA

Sreekanth K Chaguturu
Resident in Internal Medicine, Massachusetts General Hospital/Harvard Medical School, Boston, USA

Myron S Cohen
Professor of Medicine, Microbiology and Immunology, University of North Carolina-Chapel Hill, Bioinformatics Building, Chapel Hill, USA

Contributors

Myron E Essex
AIDS Prevention Initiative in Nigeria, Harvard School of Public Health, Boston, USA

Paul Farmer
Brigham and Women's Hospital, Division of Social Medicine & Health Inequalities, Boston, USA

Jennifer Furin
Brigham and Women's Hospital, Division of Social Medicine & Health Inequalities, Boston, USA

Polly F Harrison
Director, Alliance for Microbicide Development, Silver Spring, Maryland, USA

Mina C Hosseinipour
Assistant Professor, Division of Infectious Diseases, School of Medicine, University of North Carolina, Chapel Hill, North Carolina, USA

Phyllis J Kanki
Director, AIDS Prevention Initiative in Nigeria, Harvard School of Public Health, Boston, USA

Salim S Abdool Karim
Deputy Vice Chancellor, University of Natal, South Africa

Mitchell H Katz
Director, San Francisco Public Health Department, Epidemiology and Biostatistics, University of California, San Francisco, USA

Jeffrey D Klausner
San Francisco Department of Health, San Francisco, USA

N Kumarasamy
Chief Medical Officer, YRG Centre for AIDS Research and Education, Principal Investigator-ACTU/HPTN052-Chennai site, Voluntary Health Services, Tharamani, India

Trisha L Lamphear
The Alliance for Microbicide Development, Silver Spring, Maryland, USA

Zita Lazzarini
Director, Division of Medical Humanities, University of Connecticut Health Center, Farmington, USA

Kenneth H Mayer
Professor of Medicine and Community Health, Brown University/Miriam Hospital, Providence, USA; Fenway Community Health

James D Neaton
Professor of Biostatistics, School of Public Health, University of Minnesota, Minneapolis, USA

Laurence Peiperl
Department of Medicine, University of California, San Francisco, USA

Willo Pequegnat
Associate Director, Structural and International HIV/STD Prevention Programs, Center for Mental Health Research on AIDS, National Institute of Mental Health, Bethesda, USA

H F Pizer
Founder and Principal, Health Care Strategies, Harvard Street, Cambridge, MA, USA

Michael R Reich
Harvard University Center for Population and Development Studies, Cambridge, USA

Sandra A Springer
Clinical Instructor, AIDS Program, Section of Infectious Diseases, Yale University School of Medicine, New Haven, USA

Steffanie A Strathdee
Division of International Health and Cross-Cultural Medicine, Department of Family Health Sciences, University of California San Diego School of Medicine, USA

Jonathan E Von Kohorn
Halloran & Sage LLP, Westport, USA

David Walton
Partners In Health, Boston, USA

Preface

Dr. Rieux resolved to compile this chronicle ... to state quite simply what we learned in a time of pestilence: That there are more things to admire in men than to despise.

Albert Camus, *The Plague*, Part V

The premise of this book, *The AIDS Pandemic: Impact on Science and Society*, is that the AIDS epidemic has transformed the multiple disciplines it has touched from molecular virology to the conduct of clinical trials to bioethics and macro-economics. I developed this perspective because I have been fortunate to work over the last two decades with remarkable people, who have taught me many unique lessons about the ways in which health care professionals, academic researchers, and community activists can mobilize to understand, and to address, a newly emerging public health crisis.

I initially became aware that there was going to be a burgeoning public health problem with what came to be known as AIDS while doing an Infectious Disease fellowship at Brigham and Women's Hospital and Harvard Medical School in Boston, while also working at Fenway Community Health in Boston. My affiliation with Fenway is ongoing, sustained, and ever changing because of the superb working environment and colleagues that I have been fortunate to know over more than two decades. The executive directors of Fenway have been a talented group of individuals, particularly Sally Deane, Dale Orlando, Michael Savage and most notably Dr Stephen Boswell, who has led the agency to develop programs of international renown in developing a paradigm for community-based responses to the AIDS epidemic. I am fortunate to have several stellar intellectual colleagues at Fenway, including Dr Steven Safran, Dr Judy Bradford, as well as administrative directors including, Louise Rice and Rodney VanDerwarker. It has been edifying to watch successive generations of Fenway research team members go on and develop their careers, going back to school to become physicians, clinical psychologists, and public health researchers, or making other contributions to community health defined as broadly as possible. It is a unique environment, given its roots in the gay and lesbian communities, while at the same time creating a new model of community-based research.

When I first came to Brown University in 1983, there was virtually no organized community-based response to dealing with the rapidly emerging AIDS epidemic in Providence and south-eastern New England. My academic chief, the Director of the Division of Infectious Diseases, Dr Stephen Zinner (whose own research did not focus on AIDS), created a very supportive environment which allowed me to develop my clinical work, as well as a program of community-based research in Rhode Island. Within two years of my arrival at Brown, Dr Charles Carpenter assumed the position of Physician-in-Chief at The Miriam Hospital, and was committed to creating a center of excellence for HIV care and clinical research. Chuck was one of the first people to recognize that the emerging epidemic would severely impact America's underclass, particularly the most vulnerable populations, e.g. women of color; and he set about to create a program that was culturally sensitive and distinctive in its ability to address the manifold concerns of people living with HIV and, at the same time, to do excellent clinical research. Chuck soon was joined by Dr Timothy Flanigan, now the Director of the Division of Infectious Disease at Brown. Tim's dynamism expanded the programs at The Miriam Hospital Immunology Center and led to the attraction of whole cadre of talented, younger clinical investigators who have made an impact on developing community-based programs that address the real world needs of people living with HIV, while developing important clinical and laboratory information. Dr Susan Cu-Uvin, who oversees the clinic, has contributed enormously to our understanding of the gynecological manifestations of HIV disease and the effects of antiretroviral therapy on HIV acquisition and transmission. Dr Jody Rich has reframed the model of harm reduction for injecting drug users in creative ways that range from creating a drop-in center which deals with the panoply of needs that drug users may have, ranging from de-addiction services, to access to sterile syringes, to vaccination against hepatitis A and B and screening for sexually transmitted infections.

I am also fortunate to have interacted with a number of outstanding junior colleagues, including Drs Michelle Lally, Jennifer Mitty, Karen Tashima, Herb Harwell, David Pugatch, Mark Lurie, Kate Morrow, and Grace Macalino. Our Chief of Medicine, Dr Edward Wing, has integrated the clinical and research environments through his unqualified support of best practices.

In addition to excellent medical research colleagues, I have been privileged to work with some outstanding public health researchers and practitioners, including Drs Sally Zierler, Vincent Mor, Stephen McGarvey, and Terri Wetle. The deans at Brown's Medical School have been uniformly supportive, starting with Dr David Greer, succeeded by Dr Donald Marsh, and most recently, Dr Richard Besdine. In summary, the environment at Brown has been extremely conducive to trans-disciplinary thinking, resulting in unique research studies and the generation of new data that has direct impact on the lives of people living with HIV and those at most risk for AIDS. One of the most wonderful parts of being a faculty member at Brown University is the access to stellar students, whose intellectual capabilities are astounding, and whose idealism and commitment to international public health continue to inspire the faculty to redouble our efforts and think creatively about our research endeavors.

Although my initial work in the AIDS epidemic focused on the burgeoning epidemic in New England among men who have sex with men and women at risk for HIV, it became clear very early on that the largest impact of the epidemic would be outside the United States. About 10 years ago I took over responsibility for a program set up at Brown, in conjunction with Tufts University, to coordinate a training program to develop international research infrastructure for clinical, laboratory, and behavioral investigators from five countries in Southern and Eastern Asia. I have been particularly fortunate to develop an on-going and every-growing relationship with several remarkable Asian organizations, most notably YRG Care, a community-based organization in Chennai (Madras), Southern India. My colleagues there, Drs Suniti Solomon, and Balakrishnan, N Kumarasamy, as well as the administrative leadership, Mr AK Ganesh and Mr AK Srikrishnan have taught me an immeasurable amount about how a community-based organization can scale-up, one program at a time, to develop multifaceted responses to a burgeoning local epidemic, and in the process, create a model of community-based research that offers lessons for colleagues in other parts of Asia, as well as Africa and other developing nations, in addition to clinical researchers and students in resource-rich environments.

The AIDS epidemic has led to some distinctive relationships and partnerships. One of my other full-time jobs has been to serve as a member of the Board of Directors of the American Foundation for AIDS Research, an organization that helped to jumpstart many important AIDS-related research and public policy issues. I continue to be in awe of the dynamic moral leadership of Dr Mathilde Krim, the founder of amFAR, as well as her talented staff, including the CEO, Jerry Radwin, the Vice Presidents for Public Policy, Jane Silver and now Judith Auerbach, and the Vice President for Clinical Research, Kevin Frost. The impressive volunteerism of the Board, ranging from successful people in the world of business and the media to distinguished research scientists and public health officials, also serves to remind me of the unique civil society response to AIDS that has helped us accomplish so much in the fact of this daunting epidemic.

Because of the many domains that the epidemic touches, and the need for large commitments of public resources to support AIDS-related initiatives, the role of public officials needs to be acknowledged. I have been fortunate to work in two states in New England that have had enlightened responses to the AIDS epidemic, and have learned a great deal from some very dedicated public health officials, including Jean McGuire, John Auerbach, Kevin Cranston, Dr Al DeMaria, Dr Patricia Nolan, Paul Loberti, and Tom Bertrand. Without the insight and cooperation of these officials, none of our community-based research and care programs could have moved forward. In addition, the local environment that began with Fenway Community Health has been augmented by several wonderful community-based organizations, ranging from the AIDS Action Committee of Massachusetts, to the Community Research Initiative of New England, to AIDS Project Rhode Island and AIDS Care Ocean State, to the Multi-cultural AIDS

Coalition and Latino-American Health Institute. The partnerships of these organizations with Fenway Community Health and Brown University researchers have served as a reality check for the development of community-focused research and clinical programs that are addressing the needs of the populations most affected by the epidemic.

Last, but not least, this book could not have happened without the support of administrative colleagues, particularly Lola Wright who enables me to spend so much time on the road and still be able to maintain my focus on ongoing responsibilities and commitments. In addition, my efforts at Fenway have been greatly supported by Susan Johnson, and our Fogarty International Training Grant has been wonderfully supported by Eileen Caffrey and Jennifer Hyde. I would like to acknowledge Irma Rodriguez, my colleague of 11 years, who has helped us develop new laboratory techniques to better assess the spread of HIV in New England, and throughout the world.

While thinking about this book, I have been extremely fortunate to have the loyal support and enthusiasm of my family, including my mother, Betty Mayer, as well as my sister and brother-in-law, Arlene and Stuart Shainker, and a large coterie of devoted friends. Watching my niece Haley and my nephew Danny growing, and marking birthdays and other celebrations with close friends over the past two decades has put many of my AIDS-related activities in perspective; i.e. there is an urgency to do as much as we can, as quickly as we can, to ameliorate the ravages of AIDS. But at the same time, knowing that we are all finite, it's important to step back and to celebrate the happy times that we are privileged to enjoy. I was fortunate to have two superlative role models from infancy through middle age: my father, Paul Mayer, a mechanical and civil engineer, who taught me the need to undertake any new venture with thorough planning and meticulous commitment to doing the best job possible, particularly if others were depending on the effort, and my uncle, Dr Norbert Freinkel, who taught me multiple lessons about the art and science of medical research.

This book would not be possible without the seamless collaboration with Hank Pizer, a talented medical writer, health care consultant, and dear friend of more than two decades. In the earliest days of the AIDS epidemic, because of my role as a community-based researcher and clinician, the Boston Mayor's Office asked me to help draft educational materials for at-risk individuals. I could think of no better colleague to develop these fact sheets than Hank, who had already written several excellent books about health care issues for the lay audience. Our initial collaboration led us to write the first book on AIDS for the general public, *The AIDS Fact Book* (Bantam Press, 1983) and more recently we edited *The Emergence of AIDS: The Impact on Immunology, Microbiology and Public Health* (APHA Press, 2000). The current volume builds on its predecessor, since the AIDS epidemic continues to evolve, further affecting a wider range of clinical and public health concerns, with new and more profound effects on research, care and humanity.

We hope that this book, with its remarkable cast of talented authors, will help synthesize the lessons of AIDS in ways that will inspire readers to think of new ideas to end this scourge, which already has had such a catastrophic and personal toll on tens of millions of people. We would be remiss at this juncture not to step back and remember the many friends and colleagues no longer with us because of AIDS, to celebrate their lives, to reflect on how their loss has diminished our experiences, and to resolve to do whatever we can to mitigate the further depredations of this global pandemic.

May 2004   Kenneth H Mayer

About the Editors

Kenneth H Mayer, MD, is Professor of Medicine and Community Health at Brown University, Director of the Brown University AIDS Program, and Attending Physician in the Infectious Disease Division of the Miriam Hospital in Providence, Rhode Island. In addition, he is Adjunct Professor at Harvard University's School of Public Health and Medical Research Director at Boston's Fenway Community Health Center, where since 1983 he has conducted studies of HIV's natural history and transmission. In the early 1980s, as a research fellow studying infectious diseases at Brigham and Women's Hospital, Dr. Mayer was one of the first clinical researchers in New England to care for patients living with AIDS.

In 1983, Dr. Mayer co-authored (with H.F. Pizer) The AIDS Fact Book the first book about AIDS written for the general public. In 1984, he began one of the first studies of the natural history of HIV infection, and was subsequently funded by the federal government to study biological and behavioral factors associated with male-to-male HIV transmission. Starting in 1987, he and his colleagues have been supported by the NIH and CDC to study the dynamics of heterosexual HIV transmission and the natural history of HIV in women, and to study HIV prevention interventions, ranging from vaccines (HIVNET, HVTN) to microbicides, behavioral and other strategies (HPTN). He has collaborated with basic virologists and immunologists to more accurately characterize the natural history of HIV disease. In the late 1980's, he initiated the first community-based clinical trials for people living with HIV/AIDS in New England, and helped amFAR develop its national Community-Based Clinical Trials Network (CBCTN). He subsequently was named to the Board of Directors of amFAR and is co-chair of its Clinical Research and Education Committee and a member of the Executive Committee.

Dr. Mayer is the Director of the Brown and Tufts Universities' Fogarty (NIH) AIDS International Research and Training Program, which has trained more than 50 laboratory and clinical investigators from East Asia. Dr. Mayer has worked increasingly in India and participated in many regional conferences on biological and behavioral approaches to prevention research, and the development of community-based clinical research activities in Asia. Dr. Mayer also co-edited (with H.F. Pizer) The Emergence of AIDS: Impact on Immunology, Microbiology, and Public Health, published in November 2000 by the American Public Health Association Press.

Dr. Mayer has served on the Data Safety and Monitoring Board of the NIH's AIDS Clinical Trials Group and sits on several editorial boards of scientific publications, including Clinical Infectious Diseases. He has co-authored more than 300 articles, chapters and other publications on AIDS and related infectious disease topics, and is a frequent lecturer and presenter at national and international conferences and symposia. He is currently on the national board of the HIV Medicine Association and is a former board member of the Gay and Lesbian Medical Association. He has received awards of recognition from the Governor of Massachusetts, the Rhode Island Department of Health and the Greater Boston Business Council. In 2001, he and Dr. Judith Bradford were named Co-Directors of The Fenway Institute, which is designed to conduct population-based research, develop professional and community educational programs and disseminate information related to best practices and model clinical programs relevant to the global health needs of lesbian, gay, bisexual and transgendered individuals and communities.

Dr. Mayer received his B.A. in Psychology from the University of Pennsylvania and his M.D. from Northwestern University Medical School. He completed his residency and internship in Internal Medicine at Boston's Beth Israel Hospital, while also holding clinical fellowships in medicine at Harvard Medical School. From 1980 to 1983 he completed an Infectious Diseases Fellowship at Brigham and Women's Hospital and Harvard Medical School.

H F Pizer, BA, PA is a medical writer, health care consultant and physician assistant. He has written and edited 13 books and numerous articles about health and medicine. With Kenneth Mayer he coauthored the first book about AIDS for the general public, The AIDS Fact Book (Bantam Books, 1983) and co-edited The Emergence of AIDS: Impact on Immunology, Microbiology, and Public Health (American Public Health Association Press, 2000). His other works cover a variety of subjects in health and medicine including the first books for the general public on organ transplants (Organ Transplants: A Patient's Guide with the Massachusetts General Organ Transplant Teams, Harvard University Press, 1991) and stroke (The Stroke Fact Book, with Conn Foley, Bantam Books, 1985, and the American Heart Association), and in women's health on family planning (The New Birth Control Program, with Christine Garfink, RN, Bolder Books, New York, 1977, Bantam Books, New York, 1979), parenting (The Post Partum Book, with Christine Garfink, RN, Grove Press, New York, 1979), miscarriage (Coping With A Miscarriage, with Christine O'Brien Palinski, The Dial Press, 1980), and artificial insemination (Having a Baby Without A Man with Susan Robinson, MD, Simon & Schuster, 1985). He also coauthored Confronting Breast Cancer (with Sigmund Weitzman and Irene Kuter, Random House, 1987). From 1984–1994 he was founder and President of New England Medical Claims Analysts, a health care consultancy and during that time wrote and lectured on health care cost containment. Presently he is cofounder and Principal of Health Care Strategies, Inc a consulting firm in Cambridge, Massachusetts that provides program evaluation and management consulting services to community health care providers, health care systems, and social service organizations. He is former President of the Massachusetts Association of Physician Assistants. His books have been published in English and in translation for overseas distribution by trade, mass market and academic publishers.

Dedications

Ken Mayer

In memory of my father, Paul Mayer, and uncle, Norbert Freinkel, who taught me so much, and my mother, Betty Mayer, and sister, Arlene Shainker, who continue to be great sources of support and wisdom.

Hank Pizer

For Chris, Katie and Bruce.

Introduction

Chris Beyrer

Director, Fogarty AIDS International Training & Research Program, Johns Hopkins University, Bloomberg School of Public Health, Baltimore, USA

Chris Beyrer MD, MPH, is Associate Professor in the Departments of Epidemiology and International Health and founder of the Center for Public Health and Human Rights at the Johns Hopkins Bloomberg School of Public Health. He serves as Director of Johns Hopkins Fogarty AIDS International Training and Research Program and as Faculty for the JHU Fogarty Bioethics International Training Program. Dr. Beyrer is author of the 1998 book *War in the Blood: Sex, Politics and AIDS in Southeast Asia* (Zed Books, London, St. Martins Press, New York). He has worked extensively in developing nations including Thailand, China, India, Laos, Ethiopia, South Africa, Brazil, Russia, and Tajikistan. His numerous activities include HIV/AIDS professional training, HIV vaccine testing, and studying the health risks of sex workers opiate users. From 1992–1997 he was Field Director of the Thai PAVE and HIVNET studies based in northern Thailand.

We are now well into the third decade of the HIV/AIDS pandemic, and we have seen it become the most severe infectious disease threat to humanity since the Black Death of the fourteenth century. AIDS has quite literally changed the modern world: in 1983 it was an affliction that dared not speak its name, in 2003 the subject of a US State of the Union address, the first disease to warrant its own UN Security Council resolution, now the center of passionate global ethical and moral debate. The AIDS pandemic has had impacts on an astonishingly wide range of disciplines, endeavors, cultures, and human behaviors. By bringing affected communities into the decision-making process, AIDS changed the way scientific research is conducted. By demanding, and achieving, more equitable pricing for treatment in developing countries, the global AIDS advocacy movement changed pharmaceutical industry practices worldwide. And unlike so many

1

persistent scourges of Africa or of Asia's poor, old killers like malaria, cholera, or typhoid, AIDS has been a developed and a developing country disaster – perhaps the first pandemic of our now truly interconnected world. It has already killed over 25 million human beings and orphaned 14 million more.

The dark news at the start of this new century is that far from being contained, this protean virus continues to find new populations amenable to its spread. Whole new regions of the globe seemingly spared in the first years of AIDS have proven unable or unwilling to respond to its challenges. The enormous populations now threatened – in China, Russia, Indonesia, South Asia, and Central Asia are sharply lacking in the basic tools of prevention. They have found themselves as wide open to HIV/AIDS and its wasting embrace as New York City or Port au Prince were when the virus entered their citizen's bloodstreams decades ago. The leadership failures of that early time are being replicated with terrible familiarity, despite how much more we know. As Peter Piot, Executive Director of UNAIDS, remarked on the twentieth anniversary of AIDS in 2001 'We know the epidemic is still in its early stages, that effective responses are possible, but only when they are politically backed and full-scale, and that unless more is done today and tomorrow, the epidemic will continue to grow' (UNAIDS, 2002). Viruses are parasites, obligate intracellular parasites – they require their hosts (in the case of HIV, this means people) to do the work of viral spread. The ongoing agony of the HIV pandemic is that despite all we have learned, all the tools we have developed, the treatments we can bring to bear on this infection, human beings continue to spread and to acquire HIV with awful frequency. Why are we still so far from control, much less cure?

Here is a simpler, but related, question: Of what country is Dushanbe the capital? Tajikistan is one of the five Central Asian Republics of the former Soviet Union, and the poorest of any of them. Most of the country is high mountains, the Pamirs, the Hindu Kush. It is a remote place, and an ancient one, and in the first and second decades of AIDS it was about as far from the zones of HIV spread as anywhere could be. But Tajikistan has hundreds of miles of mountain border with Afghanistan (as well as borders with China, Kyrgyzstan, and Uzbekistan). Afghanistan in 2003 was the world's leading producer of opium and heroin, exporting over 400 tonnes of refined heroin (US Department of State, 2003), making Tajikistan not remote, but utterly central to a heroin use epidemic, which now may be driving the fastest growing HIV epidemics of our time (Hamers *et al.*, 2003). Injection use of Central Asian heroin has led to explosive epidemics of HIV in Russia, Ukraine, and Belarus (Beyrer, 2002).

In August of 2003, in an effort to start an HIV research project in Dushanbe, I met with the Minister of Health of Tajikistan. He was a busy man, and a gracious one, and gave our little group close to 2 hours of his afternoon. He was eager to participate in our work, and open to the idea of prevention – but there were limits he had to respect. Methadone is illegal in Tajikistan, as was any substitution therapy, so drug treatment was not an option for our prevention efforts. Needle and syringe exchange were underway, quietly, supported by the Soros Foundation (*they* are everywhere), but again, this was not something he could too openly endorse (as a US investigator, and citizen, I could only commiserate). We were free to visit the National AIDS Program, but we should be prepared: it was 'in a primitive condition', as the translator delicately put it. We found it, some hours later, in an outlying post-industrial zone of the city. A long dank unlit hallway, some sewage problem affecting the air, a few offices with bolted doors. One woman, who seemed to be a janitor, let us into the main office: a phone, one non-functioning PC, some Russian Ministry of Health pamphlets on how HIV was not spread by mosquitoes or toilets. No staff that day, no running water either. Welcome to AIDS prevention in the twenty-first century – at least, in some parts of the developing world.

As so often in the past, in Central Asia the virus is still running ahead of us, spreading more quickly in new zones than the best pace of response we seem to be able to muster. And again, laws stand in the way of evidence-based prevention. Poverty stands in the way of the well intentioned. And harsh realities as diverse as the state of civil society in Afghanistan, the intensely addictive nature of heroin, and the efficiency of viral spread though needle sharing, stand in the way.

Should it surprise us that we have yet to turn the corner on this pandemic? Perhaps not. But we have seen extraordinary changes and advances. The authors you are about to encounter are thinking about the ways AIDS has changed the world. It is an extraordinary story.

New Century, New World: Scientific Advances in AIDS

The scientific advances that have come out of HIV/AIDS research have been nothing short of spectacular. Since HIV specifically attacks the immune system, and AIDS is a complex clinical outcome of what is fundamentally immune system failure, it is only logical that we have learned the most from this pathogen in the fields of virology and immunology. Phyllis Kanki and Myron Essex detail some of the central viral lessons HIV and its retroviral relatives have taught us. Dr Kanki herself exemplifies one critical lesson; a virologist with a strong laboratory focus, she has nevertheless done much of her work with communities in Senegal, West Africa, where both HIV-1 and its cousin, the much less common HIV-2 virus, co-circulate. The global spread of HIV is marked by ever increasing genetic and functional variation of the virus. And it is only in the 'real world' setting of human populations facing HIV spread, that many key virologic questions can be effectively addressed. Drs Kanki and Essex highlight a particular concern for the future of the pandemic, and for those researchers working on HIV vaccines – the ability of HIV to generate new forms through genetic recombination of parent viruses. Our understanding of this variation has been heavily dependent

3

on the rapidly advancing technology of genetic analysis. Only a few years ago, fully sequencing one HIV virus generally took a skilled technician about a month. Robotic genetic sequencers can now generate a full-length genome in about an hour, allowing us for the first time to generate enough sequence data to begin to understand just how quickly HIV is evolving, changing, and recombining. These advances have had benefits for other viral epidemics, most notably SARS, where the authors, sagely, conclude their review. Compared with the years it took to identify the virus causing AIDS, the SARS agent was identified, and its genome fully sequenced, in a matter of months. This would not have been possible without the genetics revolution of our time, to which HIV virology has made a substantial contribution.

A virus without a cell is an inert blueprint for disease – viruses depend on the vitality of the cells they infect for all functions that demand energy. For HIV, many of these human cells are part of the immune system, the complex highly integrated system which allows our bodies to know what is 'us,' what is foreign, what has become cancerous, what requires a vigorous response, and what we have seen, and fought off, before. Deborah Anderson takes us through this remarkable system, and the advances HIV/AIDS research has led to in our still incomplete understanding of immunity. Since the acquired immunodeficiency syndrome is the manifestation of the collapse of the exquisite harmony of immunity, AIDS treatment advances have inevitably led to work on immune reconstitution. Dr Anderson describes these, and the critical role of new assays, which can measure immune responses and interactions in living cells. She shares with us the potential for a new use of immunization, therapeutic vaccination, which may prove to play important roles in restoring immune functions hampered by HIV infection.

The truly amazing advances in AIDS treatments emerged not from any single silver bullet, but rather from a large and costly step-wide progression of clinical trials involving many thousands of human beings. Barriers between participants and researchers have been broken down. Community Advisory Boards have had real power and input into trial design and implementation. Randomized trials continue to be necessary for advancing AIDS treatments, for studying novel HIV preventive interventions and technologies, and for evaluating HIV vaccines. James Neaton describes lessons learned from the conduct of clinical trials and challenges ahead. He helps us navigate the thorny questions of appropriate endpoints for trials and appropriate trial designs for studying different strategic approaches to treatment of HIV, that have changed as HIV/AIDS care has so dramatically improved.

Ponder for a moment what the HIV/AIDS pandemic would be like if we could eradicate the virus from the body with a single dose of a cheap generic drug. And further, that the virus remained fully susceptible to that single drug, without resistant strains emerging after years of use. HIV would be eradicated in a matter of a few years, if not months, would it not? One of the painful lessons of syphilis control is that the answer to this question is ... *not*. Syphilis remains totally susceptible to plain old penicillin – it is curable for pennies. But syphilis has not been eradicated, and it remains highly associated with HIV infection from Addis Ababa to Moscow, Sao Paulo to San Francisco. As Jeffery Klausner tells us that is because it is spread primarily through sex. Sexually transmitted diseases (STDs) have always been difficult to control, for all the reasons that sexual matters, of which sexual health are a subset, have been difficult for an array of societies, the United States particularly, since sexuality for Americans has been so confounded with notions of license, class, race, gender, and power. Should we be surprised that for many African Americans the history of syphilis programs and research has so profoundly colored the HIV/AIDS epidemic? Or that despite our best efforts, HIV/AIDS is increasingly and disproportionately an African American disease? And yet there are lessons from STD control that are crucial for HIV programs, and for the behavioral changes, like increasing condom use, that are so essential to both STD and HIV prevention and control.

Advances in science and public policy eventually lead to an encounter between a patient and a provider. In the beginning, AIDS forced providers to relearn the skills of compassionate and palliative care. The care continuum had to include management of death and dying. A First World HIV/AIDS clinic is a new world now. Ken Mayer, who moves between Boston, Chennai, and Manila, and his coauthor, Sreekanth K Chaguturu, take us into this radically changed environment. It is a place where clinicians have a wide array of treatment options to offer, and where HIV infection, while still incurable, is reaching the point where we have to worry about AIDS treatment interactions with the garden-variety diseases of aging, the effects of highly active antiretroviral therapy (HAART) on fat metabolism, and the central issue of adherence.

Prevention Works

All politics is local, goes the maxim. In disease prevention this old saw roughly translates into the primary mission of local, municipal, and state health authorities to control disease. From the start of the AIDS era in the US, San Francisco has been a model and a measure of public health responses to AIDS. Dr Mitchell Katz, Director of Health for the City and County of San Francisco, shows us how prevention in the public sector changed as the US epidemic changed. Now that we have treatments, albeit complex ones – how do we support adherence to regimens, prevention for those returning to health and vitality, and improve outreach to marginalized communities that continue to lose out on the benefits of improved care? San Francisco is justly loved for her spirit of diversity and tolerance – but the community also been marked by the resurgence of risk behavior among her gay and bisexual men, rising STD rates, and polarizing debates of personal freedoms versus public goods. These changes too are part of the new face of the AIDS epidemic, and they will require new prevention approaches. Is there public sector support for innovative interventions? For prevention strategies for young men who have sex with men, or drug users, or sex workers? Dr Katz concludes his chapter with sobering questions about the future. The funding needs for life-saving AIDS drug treatment continue to grow, but will future government spending meet the demand? Will there be rationing of needed medical treatment for the poor and vulnerable? Will an end to 'AIDS exceptionalism' mean reduced efforts by government to provide needed services in other areas of health and medicine to vulnerable populations?

Recent advances in prevention have made clear the central role of HIV viral load in transmission of infection. Viral load in the pregnant mother predicts transmission to the infant; viral load in Ugandan men and women strongly determined whether their sex partners became infected, an effect more potent than gender (Quinn *et al.*, 2000). And of course, as AIDS treatments have improved, we have learned that viral load is a crucial measure of effective treatment. Myron Cohen has been a leader in the convergence of prevention and treatment, and he tells us how viral load has become something of a final common pathway both for treating HIV and, potentially, reducing infectiousness. He and Mina Hosseinipour explore a new domain: antiviral *treatment as prevention*, with a special focus on Africa. Drs Cohen and Hosseinipour's African experience is especially relevant here as one argument for the terribly high HIV prevalence rates in much of sub-Saharan Africa is that until recently, this has been an epidemic among an essentially untreated population, where only the lucky few with innate immune responses potent enough to keep their viral loads low were unlikely to transmit.

There are other key intersections between prevention and treatment and as treatment in developing countries rolls out in the coming years, these intersections will likely be of increasing importance. We have seen the emergence of what behaviorists call 'treatment optimism,' the sense that HIV is less of a concern since it has become so treatable. These authors explore the biological and public health implications of these behavioral trends – and the potentially tremendous impact such trends might have as antiretrovirals (ARVs) become more widely available globally. They raise the critical question of ARV drug resistance, and the potential for the generation and transmission of multidrug-resistant strains of HIV-1. This is not science fiction, as the recent history of multidrug-resistant tuberculosis and malaria illustrate, and it is all the more reason why prevention matters more than ever, as the majority of people living with HIV, or at risk for it, are increasingly likely to live in communities where at least some ARVs are available.

Laurence Peiperl and Susan Buchbinder remind us that a preventive HIV vaccine remains one of our best hopes to control the global pandemic. But they are cautious. The challenges that remain are enormous, and after many years of effort, with multiple Phase I and II trials in human volunteers and two Phase III efficacy trials completed, we still do not have a correlate of protection, or any empirical evidence of efficacy. The development pipeline is richer and more

6

varied then at any time in the past, and the next several years will almost certainly see a wide range of candidate antigens entering human trials. Nevertheless, the road ahead will likely be long and difficult. They have been tireless leaders in preparing both clinical trial sites and appropriate populations to participate in the global HIV vaccine research effort. Their insights here into the kinds of prevention programs needed for vaccine trial participants, and the tough questions of breakthrough infections in trials are only likely to grow in relevance as the many partners in the vaccine effort scale-up for the large trials we are going to need to get to an effective vaccine.

As with HIV vaccines, it is difficult to argue with the logic of topical microbicides as HIV prevention tools. So many of those most at risk worldwide for HIV are women, at risk for infection from men. And the few proven prevention technologies we have for heterosexual transmission, male and female condoms and behavioral risk reduction approaches, are largely under male control, or at least require male assent for use. A topical microbicide could give women something to protect themselves that they might control. Polly Harrison, a longtime researcher and advocate in the effort to develop a microbicide, and her coauthor, Trisha Lamphear, bring us up to date on this important research and development area and lead us through some of the challenging issues facing the next generation of microbicide trials in human beings.

If efficacy trials of HIV vaccines and topical microbicides appear beset with tough challenges, trials to measure the impact of behavior change strategies can make vaccines look relatively straightforward. A preponderance of these studies can and should be conducted where HIV/AIDS is most severe, in hard-hit developing countries. But the bulk of research dollars are First World investments, and must, however awkwardly, meet First World regulatory requirements. While meeting international standards of research ethics has long been a central concern in collaborative HIV/AIDS research, it is nevertheless the case that HIV trials have led to some of the most explosive and wounding ethical battles in medicine in our time. Willo Pequegnat, a behaviorist in US Government service who has been a part of prevention trials in Asia, Africa, Latin America, and the former Soviet Union, helps us negotiate the tricky terrain where ethics, politics, and the public funding of science interact. She shows us how HIV/AIDS research has changed how international collaborative research is reviewed and conducted. These changes will doubtless impact HIV vaccine trials, microbicide research, AIDS drug programs, and the novel behavioral approaches we are likely to need to contain HIV.

Globalization

At the World AIDS Conference in Durban, South Africa, in 2000 a judgment of sorts was handed down on the state of the global response to AIDS. Justice Edwin

Cameron, a South African judge and acting member of that country's highest court, delivered the Jonathan Mann Memorial Lecture. He made a simple, profoundly moving observation. He was living with AIDS and standing before us that morning thanks to antiviral therapy. And it was morally and ethically wrong that so many of his fellow citizens, and fellow Africans, were dead or dying because they could not access the same treatments. He likened the premature death of millions of people and the indifference of the privileged of the world to those deaths to the horrors of the holocaust. Gathered together in Africa for the first time, and in a place (Durban is the capital of KwaZulu Natal, the Province with the highest HIV rate of any in South Africa, at roughly a third of adults) ravaged by AIDS, the conference audience was stunned by Justice Cameron's message. Whatever one's position on social justice, public versus private goods, intellectual property rights, or the scientific soundness of the use of complex drug regimens in resource-limited settings, Cameron's moral argument that countless lives were being lost, millions of children orphaned, due to drug costs set and supported by the industrialized world, was compelling. If AIDS has changed anything, it may be the thinking that it is acceptable that the poor should die for lack of treatments the wealthy take for granted. It has been true for decades that the benefits of modern medicine continue to elude much of humanity – but it took AIDS to make us *feel* it.

Michael Reich of Harvard's Center for Population and Development Studies, and his colleague, Priya Bery of the Global Business Coalition on HIV/AIDS describe the patent laws and policies at the center of the battle over the inequities of AIDS. They begin with the market forces and pricing policies prior to the struggle over AIDS drugs that shaped drug availability in the developing world. They explore the way AIDS has altered these existing systems, and generated new tools for purchase and manufacture. They assess the role generic drug manufacturers have played, particularly in India and Brazil, which have both become significant exporters of generic AIDS drugs. And they discuss the current policy options for manufacturers, countries, and regulatory bodies as the global community struggles to make AIDS treatments a reality for those who need them, while keeping market incentives in place to continue needed HIV/AIDS research.

Despite the great geographic extent of HIV spread and the decades it has now been circulating in human populations, the zones where truly generalized high prevalence epidemics exist have remained quite limited. Every country with a population prevalence of HIV infection over 20 per cent or higher in adult men and women is in sub-Saharan Africa – indeed, all are within the southern region of sub-Saharan Africa (UNAIDS, 2002). When we speak of decade or more declines in life expectancy, of population structures distorted by young adult deaths, of villages of orphans and the elderly, of AIDS leading to famine because of lack of women farmers, we are talking about these parts of Africa, and, for now, almost nowhere else on Earth. It is Africa where we see the epidemic in its full-blown state. And it is in Africa where we are seeing, at last, a unique level of mobilization and global partnership underway. Dr Salim Abdool Karim, from the University of Natal in Durban, is one of the African researchers who helped make these partnerships happen. With the special perspective only someone living and working in the midst of the struggle can bring to it, he describes the African epidemic and the efforts underway to control, mitigate, and heal it. As Southern Africa embarks on widespread rollout of antiviral therapy, it may well be that there are lessons all of us need to hear from this most affected part of the world. Dr Abdool Karim is known across the scientific world for his eloquence and insight – we will not find a better guide to these lessons, however painful they may be.

With over one billion citizens, more than twice the population of all of Africa, the potential spread of HIV in India poses an enormous public health threat, as it does in other areas of Asia where bias and denial have abetted the epidemic. Dr N Kumarasamy, Hank Pizer and I write about links between human rights and public health. There is growing awareness among public health professionals that government negligence and corruption, the subordination of women, and the mistreatment of vulnerable populations are fundamental causes of the AIDS pandemic, as well as other major health problems of our time. With its enormous population at stake, the Asian HIV epidemic is not so much about what already has happened but what could happen if appropriate measures are not swiftly taken. We have enough evidence of success in prevention in states as diverse as Australia and Senegal to know that major epidemics of HIV are preventable. Thailand is a model for how for government and society can deal with the socially uncomfortable realities that serve to spread the virus. When HIV first appeared in Asia too many believed, or pretended to believe, that it would not be a widespread health issue. Asian 'values' would protect the populace. Denial is now out of the question. To date, compared with its enormous population HIV in Asia remains relatively contained. Prevention and care programs are being adapted to the region's kaleidoscope of cultures, languages, and development levels. So there is reason to both fear the future but also be optimistic. There even is hope that AIDS-related programs in Asia will provide a basis for expanding other public health efforts.

Social and Ethical Dimensions

In the global debate around HIV/AIDS, social justice, and human rights, few voices have spoken with the clarity and moral rigor of Paul Farmer. Drs Jennifer Furin, David Walton, and Farmer bring us up to date on the worldwide epidemiology and its implications for clinical care. Dr Farmer is a medical anthropologist with a longstanding commitment to provision of care among the rural poor in Haiti. His colleagues, Drs Furin and Walton, share with him in the mission of providing services and programs for vulnerable populations. In this chapter they look at the central issues of economic and gender inequity that continue to drive the pandemic. As he has done so eloquently for Haiti, Dr Farmer and colleagues explore the role of disenfranchisement and poverty, and how 'pathologies of power,' to use his term, lead to failures of political will to respond. As they point out, a 'majority of the world's AIDS cases are found in nations plagued by poverty, hunger, and underdevelopment.' These are the darker political and social realms, where conflict, gender-based violence, and marginality interact so powerfully with HIV. They propose innovative strategies to provide HIV prevention and care services to people living in these difficult circumstances, and suggests ways we might better coordinate international advocacy, research, and programs where they are needed most.

We have the dismal science – the economics of AIDS. Dr Sam Bozzette looks at who pays for AIDS care, and how. As with the law, AIDS funding priorities have shifted as we have moved from a catastrophic illness to a chronic disease model, from hospice care to outpatient visits and the need for long-term monitoring of adherence. Dr Bozzette draws on community clinic models to ask if the evolution of AIDS care financing might be generalized to other medical conditions.

AIDS was first known and understood as a disease of gay and bisexual men in San Francisco and New York. The association of the virus with perceived sexual deviance, stigmatized behaviors and marginalized minority groups has never left it – despite the very limited role male-to-male sexual transmission has played in the epidemics of Africa and parts of Asia. Indeed, the events responsible for most HIV infections worldwide – heterosexual intercourse, childbirth, breast-feeding – are among the most fundamental and highly valued of human acts. Nevertheless, the stigma of AIDS as something inherently shameful remains. The personal impact of AIDS on gay people in the US has been huge. But there have been social and cultural impacts as well, and some have been empowering for gays and lesbians. John-Manuel Andriote explores the interplay of sexual orientation and community responses to HIV/AIDS, as well as the impact the epidemic has had on the movement for sexual minority rights. He explores questions of identity and the power of representation in the media. He also brings us up to date on how AIDS brought gay and lesbian issues, lives, personalities, into the US mainstream. While gay and lesbian Americans continue to struggle for civil rights and social tolerance, the heroic responses of the gay community in caring for the sick did not go unnoticed. AIDS and gay people eventually became synonymous with something else in the popular imagination: courage.

It is hard to think of an evidence-based prevention tool for disease spread that has been more controversial (and less used) than harm reduction for prevention of blood-borne pathogen spread among injecting drug users. By harm reduction we mean a set of interventions which include needle and syringe exchange programs, drug treatment on demand, and non-judgmental outreach and education. Dr Patricia Case reviews the evidence for and against harm reduction as a public health strategy, and looks at why these programs have been so controversial and so politically charged. She also asks us to think about other substance use, including alcohol, and its impact on sexual spread of HIV/AIDS. Harm reduction is in some ways a philosophy of intervention – working with people where they are rather than where we wish they would be – and accepting that despite their and our best intentions, some people cannot or will not eliminate their risk taking, but can be helped to reduce it. Dr Case thinks through the value of harm reduction approaches for other public health problems.

Legalistic approaches, including incarceration, are virtually polar opposites to harm reduction. And unlike harm reduction, they have proven popular with politicians and with voters in the US, by any measure the most world's most imprisoned and imprisoning society. US prison populations have long had substantially higher HIV prevalence than the general population, and our prisons continue to be zones of high transmission risk. Drs Frederick Altice and Sandra Springer of the Yale School of Medicine look at prison health in light of AIDS, and the contentious questions that have arisen around HIV/AIDS in the prison system. They discuss such difficult areas as HIV testing in prisons, stigma among the incarcerated, health education, and the special challenges that face prison prevention and treatment efforts.

It is perhaps inevitable that a disease with as many social and ethical ramifications as HIV/AIDS should lead to matters of the law. Zita Lazzarini and Jonathan Von Kohorn's work is on the fascinating and problematic interface of law and public health. They chart the changes in legal concerns that have followed the changing course of HIV/AIDS. From an initial focus on protection of privacy, to a need to insure full access to available tools, AIDS has forced evolutions and revolutions in legal thinking in the US and abroad and, as they point out, the debates are far from over.

So, in many ways the AIDS epidemic is still in its early stages. A huge number of people have given their best ideas, energy, passion, and commitment, to an emerging global response. We have seen terrible human failures, remarkable advances, and an array of social changes – broad and deep and lasting. It is impossible to know how far we are from an HIV vaccine, or from a cure. But we can safely say this: HIV will be with us for decades to come, it will continue to challenge individuals, communities, and countries. And it will continue to demand that all of those who care about human health, social justice, and the development work needed for a more equitable human family continue to care about AIDS.

References

Beyrer C (2002) HIV infection and heroin trafficking in Eastern Europe and Central Asia. *Int J Harm Reduction* 4: 4–6.

Chris Beyrer

Hamers FF, Infuso A, Alix J, Downs AM (2003) Current situation and regional perspective on HIV/AIDS surveillance in Europe. *J Acquir Immune Defic Syndr* 32: S39–S48.

Quinn TC, Wawer MJ, Sewankambo N *et al.* (2000) Viral load and heterosexual transmission of human immunodeficiency virus type 1. Rakai Project Study Group. *N Engl J Med* 342: 921–9.

UNAIDS (United Nations Joint Programme on AIDS) (2002) *Report on the Global HIV/AIDS Epidemic*. Geneva: UNAIDS Publications.

US Department of State (2003) *International Narcotics Control Strategy Report, 2003*. Washington, DC: US State Department.

Virology

1

Phyllis J Kanki
Director, AIDS Prevention Initiative in Nigeria, Harvard School of Public Health, Boston, USA

Myron E Essex
AIDS Prevention Initiative in Nigeria, Harvard School of Public Health, Boston, USA

Phyllis J Kanki, DVM, ScD is Professor of Immunology and Infectious Disease at the Harvard School of Public Health. She received her DVM degree from the University of Minnesota and D.Sc. degree in virology from the Harvard School of Public Health. She has directed the collaborative AIDS research program between scientists at Harvard and University Cheikh Anta Diop in Dakar, Senegal for over 18 years, leading a prospective study of commercial sex workers in one of the longest studied cohorts of HIV infected women worldwide. In 2000 she initiated the AIDS Prevention Initiative in Nigeria, a multi-site collaborative and evidence based prevention program, and directs the Rapid Expansion of anti-HIV Treatment in Botswana, Nigeria and Tanzania. She has published widely and received numerous awards worldwide. Her research interests include HIV pathogenesis, molecular epidemiology, and intervention studies. Her work has described major biological differences and interactions between HIV-1 and HIV-2.

Myron E Essex, PhD is Chairman of the Harvard AIDS Institute, the Mary Woodard Lasker Professor of Health Sciences at Harvard University and Chairman of the Department of Immunology and Infectious Diseases at the Harvard School of Public Health. He holds doctorates in veterinary medicine and microbiology. He has received numerous awards, including in 1986 the Albert Lasker Medical Research Award (with Drs. Gallo and Montagnier) the highest medical research award given in the United States. Dr. Essex has authored or co-authored more than 450 scientific articles and edited seven books. He was one of the first to link animal and human retroviruses to immunosuppressive disease, suspect that a retrovirus was the agent cause in AIDS, and determine that HIV could be transmitted through blood and blood products. Since 1985, Dr. Essex and colleagues have worked with collaborators in Africa and Asia, where they conduct biological, clinical, and epidemiological studies.

In the early 1980s, our laboratory was involved in the study of retroviruses and their association with cancer. Max Essex had been involved in years of investigation on the biology of feline leukemia virus (FeLV), a retrovirus of cats that was not only associated with cancer but also immunosuppressive disorders. FeLV was only one of many known and well-studied animal retroviruses at the time. Viruses in mice, chickens, cows, sheep, and horses had been studied for years in an effort to better understand and investigate possible viral causes of human cancer. Therefore in 1982, the discovery of human T-cell leukemia virus (HTLV) seemed to be the 'holy grail' that had been searched for. However, within a few years, descriptions of a new disease or syndrome in young male homosexual populations prompted the search for the causative agent. Infectious disease specialists involved with these populations, epidemiologists, and virologists were drawn into the investigation of this new disease. In the Boston area in the mid-1980s, investigators from the Harvard School of Public Health combined expertise with clinical investigators at Mass General Hospital, Beth Israel, and the New England Deaconess hospitals to conduct studies of suspect cases and controls in a search for the etiologic agent. Small scientific meetings were held at increasing frequency to stay ahead of the new data that were being generated. These meetings brought together investigators from many different disciplines, which in retrospect promoted the public health perspective of the field. New funding opportunities also encouraged multidisciplinary groups that would study this new disease entity.

Once human immunodeficiency virus (HIV) was recognized as the etiologic agent of the acquired immune deficiency syndrome (AIDS), the field recognized some of the technical challenges of further characterizing the viral infection and therefore implementing clinical care. Retrovirus infection had only been relatively recently described in humans with HTLV-I and HTLV-II, and methods for diagnosis through antibodies or virus isolation were relatively new and distinct from other viral systems. Therefore the need for new technologies to address this virus infection was recognized early in the epidemic. In later years, the use of polymerase chain reaction (PCR) technology to detect and quantitate virus provided the foundation for clinical management of this disease. As epidemiologists recognized the alarming increase of HIV/AIDS cases across the globe, the use of PCR-based sequencing techniques allowed the realization of the tremendous diversity of HIV viral strains that compose what we now recognize as the global HIV/AIDS pandemic.

History of the Discovery of HIV

AIDS was first recognized as a new and distinct clinical entity in 1981 (Gottlieb *et al.*, 1981; Masur *et al.*, 1981; Siegal *et al.*, 1981). The first cases were recognized because of an unusual clustering of diseases such as Kaposi sarcoma and *Pneumocystis carinii* pneumonia (PCP) in young homosexual men. Although such unusual diseases had previously been observed in distinct subgroups of the population – such as older men of Mediterranean origin in the case of Kaposi sarcoma or severely immunosuppressed cancer patients in the case of PCP – the occurrence of these diseases in previously healthy young people was unprecedented. Since most of the first cases of this newly defined clinical syndrome involved homosexual men, lifestyle practices were first implicated and intensively investigated. These included the exposure to amyl or butyl nitrate 'poppers' or the frequent contact with sperm through rectal sex, which might have acted as immunostimulatory doses of foreign proteins or antigens.

However, AIDS cases were soon reported in other populations as well, including injection drug users (IDUs) (Anonymous, 1982) and hemophiliacs (Davis *et al.*, 1983; Poon *et al.*, 1983; Elliott *et al.*, 1983). Similar to investigations of male homosexual populations, these new risk groups were exposed to doses of foreign proteins and antigens but through the blood. In the case of IDUs, this would occur through intravenous injection of drugs and needle sharing, and in the case of hemophiliacs through the therapeutic infusion of Factor VIII. Asymptomatic hemophiliacs and IDUs were often found to have unusual immunological tests, such as the inverted T lymphocyte helper:suppressor ratios (i.e. less than the normal 1:1 ratio of helper to suppressor cells). These abnormal tests suggested a problem with the cellular immune system, with low numbers of helper T lymphocytes, also referred to as CD4+ lymphocytes, a finding similar to that observed in many AIDS patients.

Three new categories of AIDS patients were soon observed, including blood transfusion recipients (Curran *et al.*, 1984; Jaffe *et al.*, 1984), adults from Central Africa (Clumeck *et al.*, 1983; Piot *et al.*, 1984; Van de Perre *et al.*, 1984), and infants born to mothers who had AIDS or were IDUs (Rubinstein *et al.*, 1983; Oleske *et al.*, 1983; Scott *et al.*, 1984). The transfusion-associated cases had received blood donated from an AIDS patient at least three years before they began showing symptoms (Curran *et al.*, 1984; Jaffe *et al.*, 1984). Based on the disparate populations afflicted with this new malady and the emerging epidemiology of the disease, the possible infectious etiology for AIDS was considered (Francis *et al.*, 1983).

Multiple studies were initiated to determine the possible role of various microorganisms, especially viruses, in causing AIDS. These studies measured and compared seroprevalence rates for suspect viruses in AIDS patients and controls. The shortlist of candidate viruses included: cytomegalovirus, which was already associated with immunosuppression in kidney transplant patients; Epstein–Barr virus, which was a lymphotropic virus; and hepatitis B virus, which was known to occur at elevated rates in both homosexual men and recipients of blood or blood products. However, based on the unique clinical syndrome and unusual epidemiology of AIDS, if one of these viruses was to be etiologically involved, it would presumably have been a newly mutated or recombinant genetic variant.

At the same time, our group (Essex *et al.*, 1983), Gallo and his colleagues (Gelmann *et al.*, 1983), and Montagnier and his colleagues (Barre-Sinoussi *et al.*, 1983) postulated that a variant T lymphotropic retrovirus (HTLV) might be the etiologic agent of AIDS. Indeed, HTLV, discovered by Gallo and his colleagues in 1980, was the only human virus known to infect T helper (CD4+) lymphocytes at that time (Poiesz *et al.*, 1980). This seemed reasonable since it was already clear that T helper lymphocytes were selectively depleted by the causative agent in clinical AIDS (Rubinstein *et al.*, 1983; Ammann *et al.*, 1983; Fahey *et al.*, 1984; Lane *et al.*, 1985). In addition, HTLV was known to transmit through the same routes as the etiologic agent of AIDS: sexual contact (with transmission apparently more efficient from males), by blood, and from mother to baby (Essex, 1982). Finally, HTLV-I was also known to induce immunosuppression (Essex *et al.*, 1984), as we had previously recognized in animal retrovirus systems (Essex *et al.*, 1985).

AIDS patient blood samples were repeatedly cultured in an attempt to find a virus related to HTLV-I or HTLV-II (Kalyanaraman *et al.*, 1982). Although antibodies cross-reactive with HTLV-I and HTLV-related genomic sequences were found in a minority of AIDS patients (Gelmann *et al.*, 1981; Barre-Sinoussi *et al.*, 1983; Essex *et al.*, 1983), the reactivity was weak, suggesting either AIDS patients were also infected with an HTLV, or that a distant, weakly reactive virus was the causative agent. Soon after, Gallo and his colleagues obtained proof that AIDS was linked to an HTLV (Popovic *et al.*, 1984; Gallo *et al.*, 1984; Schupbach *et al.*, 1984). Further characterization of the agent – now termed HIV-1 – revealed that it was the same as the isolate detected earlier by Montagnier and his colleagues (Barre-Sinoussi *et al.*, 1983). Despite controversy over the names and identity of certain isolates, this new and unique human pathogen was clearly not only a distant genetic relative of the known HTLV virus but may have been recently introduced to humans from a primate reservoir (Essex and Kanki, 1988).

After HIV-1 was recognized as the cause of AIDS, it was also recognized that this virus was new, at least to inhabitants of the Western Hemisphere. This raised the question of whether HIV-1 was also new to Old World human populations, such as Africa, or whether it recently entered humans from another species. Reports of diseases such as AIDS had not been reported in these populations. It is conceivable that if HIV-1 had been present in Africa for some time, the interplay between pathogen and host would have led to a less virulent virus and people with genetic resistance to the lethal properties of the virus. However, early clinical studies did not indicate differences in the pathogenicity of the virus–host interactions in Africa compared with the United States or Europe.

HIV-1 or a related virus was likely present in human populations in Central Africa at the same time or even before AIDS was diagnosed in the United States.

In the early 1980s, Africans residing in Europe were presenting with similar clinical signs and symptoms of AIDS (Clumeck *et al.*, 1983). Serum samples collected from Africans at earlier periods were also examined for the presence of antibodies reactive with HIV-1. In some cases, the examination of stored samples suggested elevated rates of infection in Africa during the mid-1960s to 1970s (Saxinger *et al.*, 1985). Subsequently, it was revealed that most of those surveys were conducted with first-stage tests that were imperfect. In addition, the reactors were mostly false positives, due either to contamination of the HIV antigen or to 'sticky sera' containing antibodies that reacted non-specifically because the sera had been repeatedly frozen and thawed and maintained under poor conditions.

While examining sera taken from Africa in the period 1955 to 1965, we found one antibody-positive sample that was clearly positive in a specific manner (Nahmias *et al.*, 1986). When tested with the highly specific test radioimmuno-precipitation, this sample contained high titers of antibodies that were reactive with virtually all the major antigens of HIV-1. This sample represented only a rare positive reactor in a high-risk group of individuals suffering from tuberculosis and AIDS-like illness in a region that subsequently had high rates of infection with HIV-1. However, only 1 per cent or fewer of the individuals who tested positive were from what is now classified as a region of moderate to high prevalence (Kinshasa, Zaire), which suggests that the virus was then only rarely present in places that would now be classified as within the 'AIDS Belt of Africa.'

AIDS Denial

The recognition that AIDS is caused by HIV was not easy for some to accept. A small group of scientists have persisted in denial of the overwhelming evidence for causation. Additionally, various conspiracy theories have emerged suggesting that HIV-1 was deliberately created by germ warfare scientists. While such proclamations seem silly or irrational to informed medical scientists, they interfere with constructive attempts to educate appropriate population groups.

One reason why some have been reluctant to accept that AIDS is an infectious disease caused by HIV-1 is the very prolonged induction period combined with a very high mortality rate. Most infectious diseases occur after a short induction period. Even for the small number of infectious diseases with a very long induction period caused by viruses, such as tropical spastic paraparesis, adult T cell leukemia or shingles, only a small fraction of infected people experience that clinical outcome. The definition of AIDS as an amalgamation of clinical outcomes ranging from tuberculosis to chronic diarrhea to cancer (e.g. lymphoma and Kaposi sarcoma) also may cause confusion for those trying to accept HIV-1 as the single etiologic cause. This only becomes logical when it is recognized that AIDS disease is fundamentally an irreversible destruction of the immune system. All of the other outcomes are secondary to the immune destruction.

Another problem in understanding AIDS etiology may be a lack of appreciation of the discipline of epidemiology and dissension about the proper definition of cause. For epidemiologists, a very high-risk association, such as for tobacco and lung cancer, is sufficient to ascribe cause. Using analogous logic, the causal association between HIV-1 infection and subsequent destruction of the immune system is overwhelming. In prospective cohort studies, almost all HIV-1-infected people eventually develop immune depletion. This association is much higher than for such viral infections as polio or flu. Concerning time and spatial geographic associations, clinical AIDS rates have exactly paralleled HIV infection rates, whether in Bombay, San Francisco or Nairobi, allowing for the 5- to 15-year induction period.

Until recently, a lack of understanding about how HIV-1 caused immune depletion helped those who reject epidemiology to deny causation. This situation has changed dramatically, however, with the recognition that HIVs-1 can be highly lytic for T4 lymphocytes (Yu *et al.*, 1994), and that very large numbers of T4 cells are killed by the virus *in vivo* (Wei *et al.*, 1995; Ho *et al.*, 1995). Further, while the very low rate of infected circulating lymphocytes was interpreted by some as incompatible with the destruction of large numbers of cells, recent studies reveal that most HIV-1 is in lymph nodes rather than blood, and up to 25–50 per cent of lymph node T cells may be infected (Pantaleo *et al.*, 1993). HIV-1 is also highly unusual as a virus that targets T4 lymphocytes and macrophages, both essential components of the immune system. Finally, HIV-1 is transmitted in exactly the same way as clinical AIDS: by blood, by sex, and from mother to infant. When taken together, these various correlations provide inescapable evidence that HIV-1 must be the cause of AIDS.

HIV-related Retroviruses of Monkeys

Soon after the recognition of clinical AIDS in people, several clinical reports described outbreaks of severe infections, wasting disease, and death in several colonies of Asian macaque monkeys housed at primate centers in the United States (Letvin *et al.*, 1983; Henrickson *et al.*, 1983). Due to their similarity to the human syndrome, these diseases were designated simian AIDS or SAIDS. As in the case of human AIDS, many possible causes were considered. Following the recognition that SAIDS appeared to be of infectious origin, cytomegalovirus of monkeys was also considered as a possible etiologic agent.

However, seroepidemiological screening revealed that a proportion of the SAIDS monkeys had antibodies that cross-reacted with HIV (Kanki *et al.*, 1985a,b) while healthy monkeys had no such antibodies. Although the antibodies cross-reacted with core antigens of HIV-1, they showed only very weak cross-reactivity with the envelope antigens. Further characterization of the cultures revealed the presence of HIV-like particles and antigens detectable with antibodies from either SAIDS monkeys or people with AIDS. The sizes of the protein antigens detected by radioimmunoprecipitation analysis were similar to those of HIV-1. When these antigens were tested with sera from people with AIDS or healthy carriers, virtually all sera had antibodies cross-reactive to core antigens. This primate virus was named STLV-III due to its relationship to HIV-1 (which was then called HTLV-III and/or LAV), and later termed simian immunodeficiency virus or SIV (Biberfeld *et al.*, 1987).

An animal model for AIDS was an important advance at the time, particularly given the close similarities of both the disease and the animal host. However, the origin of the virus remained a puzzle. Although cases of AIDS had been reported in Africa, at the time AIDS cases in Asia were considered quite rare. We tested the hypothesis that the natural primate host for SIV would be able to sustain infection without significant disease, and that this primate would most likely reside in Africa. At least half of the healthy wild-caught African green monkeys showed evidence of exposure to SIV on the basis of antibodies (Kanki *et al.*, 1985a, 1986a). Although it was possible that SIV caused some type of disease that had not been recognized, it was clear that the disease did not resemble the lethal immunosuppressive syndrome found in Asian macaque monkeys. Similarly, captive African mangabey monkeys infected with SIV revealed no disease symptoms. The pathogenic effects of SIV appeared to be species-specific. Further studies of wild-caught Asian monkeys demonstrated that SIV was not a natural infection of these primates. It is generally believed that SIV was introduced to Asian macaques in captivity, explaining in part the unusual and high mortality induced by SIV.

More recent studies reveal that several African monkey species are infected with different SIVs. These include several species commonly described as African greens, such as vervet, grivet, sabaeus, and tantalus, as well as mona, diana, Sykes', mandrill, and sooty mangabey species (Tsujimoto *et al.*, 1988; Johnson *et al.*, 1989; Allan *et al.*, 1991). Thus far, SIVs have not been described in Asian species or in baboons, though these species can be infected in captivity with some primate lentiviruses. As a group, the SIVs are more closely related to HIV-2s than to HIV-1s, although some, such as the mandrill SIV, are evolutionarily distant (Tsujimoto *et al.*, 1988). The sooty mangabey monkey virus and the Senegalese human HIV-2, on the other hand, are essentially the same at the genetic level (Peeters *et al.*, 1989; Essex, 1994; Kirchhoff *et al.*, 1997). It is this virus that also apparently accidentally infected the Asian macaques in captivity (Essex and Kanki, 1988).

The possibility that SIV might cause disease rarely in African monkeys in advanced age could not be ruled out. The high prevalence of infection in wild-caught monkeys supported the notion that these African species of primates had evolved to a more benign coexistence with the virus in which infection did not affect survival. This was clearly different from the case of SIV in Asian primates or HIV-1 in people. Because wild macaques do not appear to be infected with

SIV, and because the virus is limited to African primates, it appears likely that the virus accidentally infected captive rhesus monkeys in recent times. New SIVs are still being described and it is possible that species specificity may play a role in the level of host–virus adaptation and therefore levels of population infection (Georges-Courbot *et al.*, 1998). Currently it appears that natural SIV infection of African primates does not result in significant disease, supported by the high seroprevalence rates in most species evaluated. It thus appears that virus–host interaction has resulted in a non-pathogenic infection and the genetic, immunological and virus determinants of this relationship are worthy of further study.

We could speculate that the virus had either moved from subhuman primates to people prior to the mid-1950s or had been introduced to the cities through the migration of a few resistant carriers from a previously isolated group of people. However if HIV-1 had been present in rural areas, we might expect to find that Africans demonstrate greater resistance to infection and disease development, owing to genetic selection and evolution of the human species. In prospective studies conducted to date, Africans infected with HIV-1 appear to develop clinical AIDS and other signs and symptoms of HIV disease as rapidly as individuals in the United States or Europe (Mann *et al.*, 1986; Marlink *et al.*, 1994). Furthermore, the degree of genomic variation seen in African isolates of HIV-1 was greater than that seen for viruses from Europe or the United States.

A virus that could be a progenitor of HIV-1 was isolated from a chimpanzee in Central Africa (Huet *et al.*, 1990). This finding, combined with the knowledge that all HIV-1 viruses tested appear to be avirulent when inoculated into chimpanzees, is also compatible with a subhuman primate origin for HIV-1. Some African isolates of HIV-1 appear to be as close to the chimpanzee isolate as to other prototype strains of HIV-1 (De Leys *et al.*, 1990; Zekeng *et al.*, 1994). These findings appear to have been confirmed by more detailed genetic analysis of a virus from a chimpanzee housed in the United States, although the exact history and pedigree of this animal is unclear (Gao *et al.*, 1999).

HIV-2 – HIV Closely Related to SIV

Because a relative of HIV-1 – SIV – had been found in wild African monkeys and was only about 50 per cent related to HIV-1 at the genomic level, it seemed logical that viruses more highly related to SIV might also be present in human populations. Serum samples from West African prostitutes were examined to determine if they had antibodies that were more highly cross-reactive with SIV than with HIV-1 (Barin *et al.*, 1985). Through Western blot and radioimmunoprecipitation methods, it became clear that a significant proportion of Senegalese prostitutes had antibodies that were highly reactive with all the major antigens of SIV detected by this technique. When the same SIV antigens were reacted with sera from HIV-1-infected individuals of either European or Central African origin with classic disease manifestations of AIDS, little or no reaction was seen with the envelope antigens. The class of reactivity seen with serum samples from West African prostitutes was in fact virtually indistinguishable from that seen with serum samples from African monkeys or captive rhesus macaques (Kanki *et al.*, 1986b; Hirsch *et al.*, 1989; Essex, 1994).

HIV-1 Subtypes

The HIV virus lifecycle requires transcription of the viral RNA into a DNA copy that becomes randomly integrated into the host cellular DNA. The transcription process is performed by the virus enzyme reverse transcriptase, which is error-prone. As a result, each round of replication results in at least one mutation per genome copy. The genetic variation of HIV is hierarchical, as depicted in the simplified schematic of subtype variation, interpatient variation, and intrapatient variation (Figure 1.1). HIV-1 virus isolates from North Americans and Europeans showed distinct genetic variability compared with the variability in viruses from African patients (McCutchan *et al.*, 1996; Burke and McCutchan, 1997). This variability was more dramatic than the recognized genetic variability between viral isolates

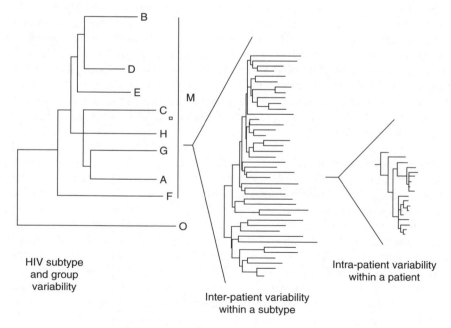

Fig. 1.1   Levels of HIV genetic diversity. Courtesy of Phyllis J Kanki.

from a single geographic region (i.e. inter-isolate variability) (Myers and Pavlakis, 1992; Korber *et al.*, 1995). In turn, this was also distinguishable from the genetic variation that was seen at the level of an individual patient (i.e. intrapatient variability). At the level of the individual patient, a swarm or quasi-species of highly related but distinguishable viral variants has been demonstrated throughout the course of HIV infection (Goodenow *et al.*, 1989; Balfe *et al.*, 1990; Delassus *et al.*, 1991). Genetic diversity is therefore a major characteristic of the HIV viruses and provides a major obstacle to drug and vaccine development.

Remarkably, all the HIVs-1 isolated from the United States and Western Europe through 1994 have been of a single subtype, B. Most of the diverse subtypes of HIV-1 have been found in sub-Saharan Africa. Subtypes A, C, and D in particular have been found more frequently than other subtypes in Africa. A high rate of spread of HIV-1 for Africa appeared during the 1980s, at about the same time the epidemic spread in the United States and Europe. The movement of populations and extensive international travel makes the likelihood of mixing subtypes inevitable, and non-B subtypes have already been identified, and are increasing in the United States and Europe.

In Asia, the introduction and spread of HIV-1 appeared about a decade later than in the West (see Chapter 15 for details). In Thailand, HIV-1 subtype B was detected in intravenous drug users during the mid-1980s. During the late 1980s, subtype E was first detected. By the early to mid-1990s, HIV-1 subtype E had spread very rapidly throughout heterosexuals in Thailand, with the highest rates in the northern regions of the country (Weniger *et al.*, 1994). Although apparently present earlier in the region, HIV-1 subtype B never spread to cause a major heterosexual epidemic as did HIV-1 subtype E. In China, the epidemic in IDUs is a unique recombinant virus of C and B. In heterosexual populations, subtype E appears to be the predominant subtype, similar to that of much of South-East Asia. This complex mixture of HIV-1 subtypes in Asia has challenged vaccine development efforts, since distinct subtype epidemics are being observed in different high-risk populations.

A similar situation occurred in India with HIV-1 subtypes B and C. While subtype B appeared to be introduced earlier among IDUs, this subtype did not spread as rapidly among heterosexuals as did subtype C. Previously associated with the massive heterosexual epidemic in southeastern Africa, subtype C also caused a rapid heterosexual epidemic in western India, initially spreading from the Bombay region (Jain *et al.*, 1994; Weniger *et al.*, 1994). In the past 7–8 years, it is clear that subtype C is the sole viral subtype responsible for the newest and perhaps most frightening of HIV epidemics, worldwide. In most countries of southern Africa, rapid dissemination of HIV infection has been described with rates ranging from 10 to 40 per cent in pregnant women in most countries of the region. As a result of these significant increases in subtype C infection in Africa, and its predominance in places such as India and perhaps China, this viral subtype is responsible for over half of all HIV infections worldwide (UNAIDS, 2002).

An even more distant subtype, designated HIV-O, has been detected in Cameroon (Nkengasong *et al.*, 1994). The viruses isolated from this subtype are even less related to HIV-1 subtypes A through H than either of the other subtypes are related to each other, yet HIV-O is more related to HIV-1 than to HIV-2 (Gurtler *et al.*, 1994). To emphasize this distance, HIV-1 subtypes A through H are designated the major group (M), and HIV-O is designated the outgroup (O) (Charneau *et al.*, 1994). Despite extensive serosurveys, the distribution of HIV-O appears to be quite restricted (Peeters *et al.*, 1997). While HIV-1 subtypes A through H probably had a common human progenitor ancestor, HIV-O no doubt entered independently from a chimpanzee host. HIV-2 almost certainly entered independently from monkey species native to West Africa (Essex and Kanki, 1988; Hirsch *et al.*, 1989).

The movement and distribution of HIV-1 subtypes throughout the world is often perplexing, particularly when subtypes such as E to H appear to be isolated more frequently in such places as Asia, South America, or eastern Europe than in Africa, where they presumably originated (Louwagie *et al.*, 1993; Bobkov *et al.*, 1994). However, the viruses that have been isolated and characterized were acquired for analysis from convenience samples and therefore may suffer from extensive regional selection bias and inadvertent clustering. In the future, it will be important to develop more consistent surveillance methods and full-length sequence analysis to generate a true global map of HIV subtypes.

Emergence of HIV-1 Disease Phenotypes

Our understanding of the epidemiology and biology of different HIV-1 subtypes is critical to future intervention efforts, and further studies are clearly needed (Anderson *et al.*, 1996). Studies have demonstrated differences in the ability of non-B and B subtype viruses to infect Langerhans' cells, a critical cell in hetero-sexual transmission of HIV. This suggests that the viral properties of non-B subtype viruses would facilitate heterosexual transmission and may have contributed to the dramatic epidemic spread in Asia and Africa (Soto-Ramirez *et al.*, 1996). A cross-sectional study of heterosexual couples in Thailand suggests a higher risk of heterosexual transmission of subtype E compared with subtype B (Kunanusont *et al.*, 1995). Studies in many African countries have described multiple HIV-1 subtypes, but it is not known if subtypes enter populations at different time points, or if the distribution of subtypes reflects the dynamics of different sub-type-specific transmission potentials. Studies in South Africa demonstrate the association of certain subtypes with different modes of HIV transmission: sub-type B viruses are associated with homosexual transmission, and non-B subtypes are associated with heterosexual transmission (Vanharmelen *et al.*, 1997). Future detailed studies of prospectively followed cohorts will be necessary to determine differences in pathogenicity and transmissibility of different subtypes.

Phyllis J Kanki and Myron E Essex

Host selection of HIVs-1 for efficiency of heterosexual transmission may partially explain the high rates of heterosexual transmission seen with subtypes C and E (Soto-Ramirez *et al.*, 1996). HIV-1 subtype B, the major subtype in the developed world, appears to have undergone counterselection (i.e. less likely to be selected for compared with more virulent or transmissible viruses) to lose the phenotypic property of efficient heterosexual transmission. If efficient heterosexual transmission requires a particular genotype for vaginal infection, such sequences may have been partially lost by these HIV-1 B 'strains' that have been repeatedly passaged by blood exposure or rectal intercourse. Many of the non-B subtypes, on the other hand, could theoretically maintain vaginal phenotypic properties through regular heterosexual transmission in Africa and Asia (Kunanusont *et al.*, 1995; Soto-Ramirez *et al.*, 1996).

Based on prospective studies of female sex workers in Dakar, Senegal, we have recently reported on disease progression in non-B subtype infections with known time of infection. In evaluating AIDS-free survival curves of women with incident subtype A, C, D, and G infection, we have shown distinct differences in AIDS-free survival (Kanki *et al.*, 1999). The comparison of non-A subtypes with subtype A demonstrated a significantly longer AIDS-free survival for women infected with subtype A. Due to the small sample size per subtype, our estimate of AIDS incidence should be considered imprecise, and further study is clearly warranted. Cross-sectional studies indicate a significant proportion of AIDS cases with subtype A infection in West and East Africa (PJ Kanki, unpublished data, 1998). Further study of HIV-1 subtype natural history and progression from different geographic regions is clearly needed to better evaluate the role of viral subtype differences and AIDS pathogenesis.

Viral Load and HIV Pathogenesis

Human immunodeficiency virus infection results in progressive loss of immune function marked by depletion of the CD4+ T lymphocytes, leading to opportunistic infections and malignancies characteristic of the syndrome termed AIDS. A number of host and viral factors influence the rate of disease progression. Studies in the West prior to the implementation of antiretroviral therapy suggested a median time to AIDS ranging from 8 to 10 years. Historically, CD4+ T lymphocyte counts provided the most reliable prognostic marker of HIV progression (Fahey *et al.*, 1984). In addition, other prognostic markers of progression to AIDS included immunologic markers of immune dysfunction which included cutaneous anergy (Redfield *et al.*, 1986; Blatt *et al.*, 1993), serum β2-microglobulin, and neopterin levels (Fahey *et al.*, 1990). In the past, quantitation of viral infection was performed with imperfect and/or laborious methods. The serologic quantitation of the viral core antigen, p24 was frequently considered as a surrogate marker of high viral burdens (Allain *et al.*, 1987; Dewolf *et al.*, 1997).

Quantitative viral culture was difficult to perform and not cost effective for clinical monitoring on a regular basis (Coombs *et al.*, 1989; Ho *et al.*, 1989). HIV viral expression as measured by mRNA was also considered an important marker that preceded immunologic compromise (Gupta *et al.*, 1993; Saksela *et al.*, 1994). More qualitative characteristics of the HIV virus infection included the syncytium-inducing properties of the virus, which were often coupled with viral burden; the syncytium-inducing viruses were associated with high viral loads and rapid progression and non-syncytium-inducing viruses associated with lower virus loads and slow progression (Tersmette *et al.*, 1988; Fenyo *et al.*, 1989).

The development of the sensitive PCR-based technology to reliably quantitate RNA levels of virus in the plasma revolutionized our abilities to track viral infection. PCR technology is based on the use of a temperature-sensitive DNA polymerase. A target sequence is identified in the DNA sequence and appropriate primers are designed to span the sequence of interest. The primers need to be as similar to the original target sequence as possible. Once the primers anneal to the target sequence the temperature-sensitive polymerase begins to transcribe sequences, matching the sequence that it has found in the sample. When the temperature increases, the strands of DNA separate and the primer binding and polymerase reaction occurs again. In this way, a large number of exact DNA copies can be made given the cycles of temperature and the availability of primer, nucleotides, and polymerase.

Minute copies of DNA can be detected in large volumes of DNA with this very sensitive technology.

Mellors and colleagues provided important new evidence that such quantitation of plasma levels of RNA virus, or viral load, were important predictors of disease progression (Mellors *et al.*, 1997). Based on the large US cohort studies of homosexual men, the risk of developing AIDS and death was significantly associated with baseline plasma viral loads, independent of CD4+ lymphocyte counts (Mellors *et al.*, 1995, 1996). It is worth noting that these studies and many of the ensuing viral load studies were conducted in the US and Europe, where subtype B HIV-1 infection is predominant. In viral load studies, as we will discuss further, it is critical to consider the populations studied, HIV viral subtypes, and methodologies employed.

Many studies that have followed the natural history of HIV infection over time have now reported on the utility of viral load determinations to track and predict disease progression. Since a variety of other markers, most notably lymphocyte subset data, were frequently available the relationship of viral load with CD4+ lymphocytes counts has been regularly evaluated. It has been important to evaluate the viral load's predictive value over the full course of HIV's natural history, and this has required analysis from long-standing cohort studies, where time of infection has been known and where observation times predated the use of antiretroviral therapy.

The large US Multi-center AIDS Cohort Study (MACS) has demonstrated a strong correlation in initial HIV RNA loads with declines in CD4 lymphocyte counts. Both initial HIV RNA levels and slopes were associated with AIDS-free times. HIV RNA load at the first seropositive visit, similar to three months after seroconversion, was highly predictive of AIDS, and subsequent HIV RNA measurements showed even better prognostic discrimination. However, HIV RNA slopes in the three years preceding AIDS and HIV RNA levels at AIDS diagnosis showed little variation according to total AIDS-free time (Lyles *et al.*, 2000). The MACS study population is largely a white homosexual male cohort, and it may not be possible to generalize all of these findings to other population groups with different modes of transmission and different viral subtypes.

Sabin and colleagues have reported a similar predictive value of plasma viral loads in the large European hemophilia cohorts where their results confirm the importance of the HIV RNA level in assessing the long-term prognosis in individuals infected with HIV (Sabin *et al.*, 1998). The risk of developing AIDS and death remained low when the HIV-1 RNA level was below 4 log 10 copies/ml, but increased rapidly thereafter, supporting current guidelines for the initiation of antiretroviral therapy after the viral load has exceeded this level (Sabin *et al.*, 2000). In the French SEROCO study of HIV seroconverters ($n = 330$), patients who remained AIDS-free had lower early viral loads and, on average, a longer period of viral load decline after infection (36 versus 18 months), followed by a slower viral load increase compared with those who progressed to AIDS (Hubert *et al.*, 2000). A true plateau-phase after the seroconversion period was observed, lasting approximately four years, identified only in patients who remained AIDS-free for at least 90 months. In multivariate analysis, both early viral load and later changes were significant predictors of progression to AIDS (Hubert *et al.*, 2000).

Primary HIV Infection and Viral Setpoint

In recent years, through the study of primary HIV infection, we have learned that some degree of virus containment occurs in the very early phases of HIV infection *in vivo*. During this critical period, a complex dynamic of infecting virus and responding host and immune factors leads to the establishment of a level of viremia, or viral setpoint, that appears predictive of subsequent HIV progression rates and survival (Mellors *et al.*, 1995, 1996). The incubation period from initial infection to onset of symptoms is an average of 21.4 days (SD = 9.6 days, range: 10–55 days) and the self-limited illness resolves within 1–3 weeks. Current data suggest that HIV viral load in the blood reaches a peak in the first 15–30 days, concurrent with a precipitous drop in CD4+ T cell count and increase in absolute number of CD8+ lymphocytes (Clark *et al.*, 1991; Clark and Shaw, 1993; Clark and Wolthers, 2000). Subsequent to these early events and tied to the resolution of the acute clinical syndrome is the lowering of HIV load and rebound of CD4+ T lymphocyte levels.

Corey and colleagues have reported considerable variability in the viral burden during these early phases of HIV infection, after 120 days after acquisition, followed by a rapid decrease in plasma HIV RNA levels to an inflection point, after which they gradually increase (Schacker *et al.*, 1998). The early infection phase continues over the next 6–12 months, with seeding and establishment of HIV viral load in blood and lymphoreticular tissues (Fauci, 1993, 1996; Haynes *et al.*, 1996). The establishment of 'steady-state viremia' or viral setpoint is attained during this phase of infection and remains relatively invariant throughout much of the long incubation period.

It is now well established that the level of HIV-1 plasma viremia early in infection is highly predictive of future clinical course (Mellors *et al.*, 1995, 1996; Stein *et al.*, 1997). Cross-sectional studies of long-term non-progressors (LTNPs) as a group have demonstrated a significantly lower cell and plasma viral burden when compared with rapid progressors (Cao *et al.*, 1995; Rinaldo *et al.*, 1995; Pantaleo *et al.*, 1995). Increases in plasma viremia are correlated with increase in proviral burden, quantitative virus isolation, and quantity of virus in lymphoreticular tissue (Haynes *et al.*, 1996). The stability of virion-associated HIV-1 RNA levels suggests that an equilibrium between HIV-1 replication rate and efficacy of immunologic response is established shortly after infection and persists throughout the asymptomatic period of the disease. Thus, defective immunologic control of HIV-1 infection may be as important as the viral replication rate for determining AIDS-free survival.

HIV Therapy and Viral Load

In HIV-1 infection, treatment with highly active antiretroviral therapy (HAART) has been shown to drastically lower plasma viremia, and this is currently used as an indicator of the effectiveness of treatment (Obrien *et al.*, 1998; Panther *et al.*, 2000). After discontinuing HAART, individuals had rebounds in their viral burdens approximating pre-HAART levels, even after a significant lapse of time approaching five years (Hatano *et al.*, 2000). In addition, the viral load at baseline is predictive of the rate of HIV-1 decline following antiretroviral therapy (Notermans *et al.*, 1998). Multiple studies have shown that the current repertoire of antiretroviral drugs is insufficient to completely eradicate HIV-1 from infected individuals (Wong *et al.*, 1997; Finzi *et al.*, 1997; Dornadula *et al.*, 1999).

In the era of HIV treatment, the use of sequential HIV RNA measurements may be more meaningful than any single measurement. The pre-treatment slopes of HIV-1 RNA decline in the acutely infected individuals increased significantly ($p = 0.0001$) after initiation of antiretroviral therapy. However, these post-treatment slopes were lower than those found in the chronically infected individuals ($p = 0.012$). Slopes were inversely correlated ($p = 0.012$) with baseline HIV-1 RNA (Putter *et al.*, 2000).

The combination of multiple adverse side-effects associated with HAART and the stringent demands for regimen adherence have prompted the design of new treatment strategies. Several studies have examined the longitudinal effects of multiple scheduled treatment interruptions where the long-term safety of this experimental protocol is largely unknown, particularly with respect to the generation of resistant viruses. However, such a treatment strategy would improve the likelihood of long-term adherence; the use of individual viral load plateaus will serve as an important guide in the aggressiveness and timing of treatment interruptions (Hatano *et al.*, 2000).

What the Future Holds

In just over two decades, the world has come to recognize a uniquely pathogenic new virus. The early epidemiologic pattern of the HIV/AIDS epidemic presented unique challenges to virologists, epidemiologists, clinicians, and public health officials. Throughout its 20-year history the epidemic continues to challenge us within our respective disciplines and in many ways has promoted an integration of these fields in an effort to curb its spread. Although the discovery of this new pathogen occurred relatively quickly after the first cases, there are still many questions as to how such a chronic virus infection can be so uniformly virulent 8–10 years post infection.

Many mysteries still surround the origin of the HIV virus and its relatives. The prevalence of the related simian viruses in African primates is so high that it suggests an ancient and stable virus–host relationship, and one that has developed into a virtually innocuous virus infection. As an intermediate, the HIV-2 virus is significantly less pathogenic than HIV-1, taking 20–30 years to develop AIDS, although the end-stage disease appears similar. We are still trying to discover the viral and host mechanisms by which this virus is able to persist for such a long period of time in an asymptomatic phase and yet somehow be triggered to cause fatal immunosuppression decades later.

Through molecular techniques such as PCR diagnostics and high-throughput sequencing we can now further appreciate the genetic diversity of HIV and SIVs. A decade ago it would take months to generate and analyze the sequence of a single HIV virus, a feat that this now readily achieved in a few days. We have also seen these technologies brought to bear on other epidemics of infectious diseases such as the recent severe acute respiratory syndrome (SARS) epidemic in Asia. There is no doubt that such new techniques will expedite our characterization of the ever-changing HIV epidemic and assist researchers in predicting the viral genotype that is relevant for targeting.

The genetic diversity of the virus at the level of the infected individual is now appreciated as a quasi-species rather than a single genotype that continues to challenge the immune system and clearly plays a role in the pathogenicity of the virus. It also presents a significant barrier to the current armamentarium of anti-retroviral drugs that we can provide to our patients with the emergence of viral resistant variants that may continue to require better and different therapies to control virus infection over the long term. At present, we do not have such therapies to affect a cure and the various viral reservoirs and significant viral replication rate suggest that this will be nearly impossible in the near future. Genetic diversity in HIV evidenced by different strains or subtypes has yielded a complex global map of variant viruses, affecting our ability to diagnose, treat, and ultimately vaccinate against an ever-changing set of viruses. We already recognize that these subtypes infecting a single population can generate recombinant viruses at an incredible rate which might predict that vaccine development may never keep pace to provide sterilizing immunity.

New technologies have made significant advances in our research to better understand and control this virus. The ability to measure HIV-1 viral load has revolutionized our ability to track virus infection and replication in the patient. The advent of viral load assays has been both a technological as well as pragmatic feat, supplying a sturdy clinical measure for the management of AIDS patients. Formerly, clinicians and scientists relied on difficult and cumbersome plasma and peripheral blood mononuclear cell cultures for virus isolation or p24 antigen quantitation to monitor infection in the individual patient. The development of PCR-based methods to measure viral RNA has been particularly useful in following patients and their therapeutic management. Importantly the measurement of viral burden has provided new insights into the mechanisms of HIV transmission and pathogenesis.

The twenty-first century will no doubt bring new technologies and research advances to HIV/AIDS research. In the past few years we have seen the global community at least acknowledge the inequalities of the HIV/AIDS global epidemic, and renewed interest and support for prevention, treatment and vaccines are being directed to the developing world. This is where the HIV/AIDS epidemic is most complex from a virological point of view, with multiple subtypes and types of HIV viruses and the ever-growing proportion of complex recombinants. The need to test HIV interventions and vaccines in these parts of the world is therefore critical, since their effects on the HIV/AIDS epidemic in these populations will have the largest impact. As scientists we need to continue our efforts to insure that good science, public health, and effective health policy will end the HIV/AIDS epidemic in the next century.

References

Allain J, Laurian Y, Paul D *et al.* (1987) Long-term evaluation of HIV antigen and antibodies to p24 and gp41 in patients with hemophilia. Potential clinical importance. *N Engl J Med* 317: 1114–21.

Allan JS, Short M, Taylor ME *et al.* (1991) Species-specific diversity among simian immunodeficiency viruses from African green monkeys. *J Virol* 65: 2816–28.

Ammann AJ, Abrams D, Conant M *et al.* (1983) Acquired immune dysfunction in homosexual men: immunologic profiles. *Clin Immunol Immunopathol* 27: 315–25.

Anderson RM, Schwartlander B, McCutchan F, Hu D (1996) Implications of genetic variability in HIV for epidemiology and public health. *Lancet* 347: 1778–9.

Anonymous (1982) Epidemiologic aspects of the current outbreak of Kaposi's sarcoma and opportunistic infections. *N Engl J Med* 306: 248–52.

Balfe P, Simmonds P, Ludlam CA, Bishop JO, Brown AJ (1990) Concurrent evolution of human immunodeficiency virus type 1 in patients infected from the same source: rate of sequence change and low frequency of inactivating mutations. *J Virol* 64: 6221–33.

Barin F, M'Boup S, Denis F *et al.* (1985) Serological evidence for virus related to simian T-lymphotropic retrovirus III in residents of West Africa. *Lancet* ii: 1387–90.

Barre-Sinoussi F, Chermann J-C, Rey F *et al.* (1983) Isolation of T-lymphotropic retrovirus from a patient at risk for acquired immune deficiency syndrome (AIDS). *Science* 220: 868–70.

Biberfeld G, Brown F, Esparza J *et al.* (1987) Meeting report: WHO working group on characterization of HIV-related retroviruses: Criteria for characterization and proposal for a nomenclature system. *AIDS* 1: 189–90.

Blatt S, Hendrix C, Butzin C *et al.* (1993) Delayed-type hypersensitivity skin testing predicts progression to AIDS in HIV-infected patients. *Ann Intern Med* 119: 177–84.

Bobkov A, Cheingsong-Popov R, Garaev M *et al.* (1994) Identification of an env G subtype and heterogeneity of HIV-1 strains in the Russian Federation and Belarus. *AIDS* 8: 1649–55.

Burke DS, McCutchan FE (1997) Global Distribution of Human Immunodeficiency Virus-1 Clades in: Rosenberg SA, ed. *AIDS: Biology, Diagnosis, Treatment and Prevention*. Philadelphia, PA: Lippincott-Raven Publishers, pp. 119–26.

Cao Y, Qin L, Zhang L, Safrit J, Ho DD (1995) Virologic and immunologic characterization of long-term survivors of human immunodeficiency virus type 1 infection. *N Engl J Med* 332: 201–8.

Charneau P, Borman AM, Quillent C *et al.* (1994) Isolation and envelope sequence of a highly divergent HIV-1 isolate: definition of a new HIV-1 group. *Virology* 205: 247–53.

Clark DR, Wolthers KC (2000) T-cell dynamics and renewal in HIV-1 infection. *Aids Pathog* 28: 55–64.

Clark SJ, Shaw GM (1993) The acute retroviral syndrome and the pathogenesis of HIV-1 infection. *Immunology* 5: 149–55.

Clark S, Saag M, Decker W *et al.* (1991) High titers of cytopathic virus in plasma of patients with symptomatic primary HIV-1 infection. *N Engl J Med* 324: 954–60.

Clumeck N, Mascart-Lemone F, de Maubeuge J, Brenez D, Marcelis L (1983) Acquired immune deficiency syndrome in Black Africans [letter]. *Lancet* 1: 642.

Coombs RW, Collier AC, Allain J *et al.* (1989) Plasma viremia in human immunodeficiency virus infection. *N Engl J Med* 321: 1621–31.

Curran JW, Lawrence DN, Jaffe H *et al.* (1984) Acquired immunodeficiency syndrome (AIDS) associated with transfusions. *N Engl J Med* 310: 69–75.

Davis KC, Horsburgh CR, Jr, Hasiba U, Schocket AL, Kirkpatrick CH (1983) Acquired immunodeficiency syndrome in a patient with hemophilia. *Ann Intern Med* 98: 284–6.

De Leys R, Vanderborght B, Vanden Haesevelde M *et al.* (1990) Isolation and partial characterization of an unusual human immunodeficiency retrovirus from two persons of west-central African origin. *J Virol* 64: 1207–16.

Delassus S, Cheynier R, Wain-Hobson S (1991) Evolution of human immunodeficiency virus type 1 nef and long terminal repeat sequences over 4 years in vivo and in vitro. *J Virol* 65: 225–31.

Dewolf F, Spijkerman I, Schellekens PT *et al.* (1997) Aids prognosis based on HIV-1 RNA, CD4+ T-cell count and function – markers with reciprocal predictive value over time after seroconversion. *AIDS* 11: 1799–806.

Dornadula G, Zhang H, VanUitert B *et al.* (1999) Residual HIV-1 RNA in blood plasma of patients taking suppressive highly active antiretroviral therapy. *JAMA* 282: 1627–32.

Elliott JL, Hoppes WL, Platt MS, Thomas JG, Patel IP, Gansar A (1983) The acquired immunodeficiency syndrome and Mycobacterium avium-intracellulare bacteremia in a patient with hemophilia. *Ann Intern Med* 98: 290–3.

Essex M (1982) Adult T-cell leukemia/lymphoma: Role of a human retrovirus. *J Natl Cancer Inst* 69: 981–5.

Essex M (1994) Simian immunodeficiency virus in people [editorial; comment]. *N Engl J Med* 330: 209–10.

Essex M, Kanki P (1988) The origins of the AIDS virus. *Sci Am* 259: 64–71.

Essex M, McLane MF, Lee TH *et al.* (1983) Antibodies to cell membrane antigens associated with human T-cell leukemia virus in patients with AIDS. *Science* 220: 859–62.

Essex M, McLane MF, Tachibana N, Francis DP, Lee TH (1984) Distribution of antibodies to HTLV-MA in patients with AIDS and related control groups in: Gross L, ed. *Human T-cell Leukemia Viruses*. New York: Cold Spring Harbor Press, pp. 355–62.

Essex M, McLane MF, Kanki PJ, Allan JS, Kitchen LW, Lee TH (1985) Retroviruses associated with leukemia and ablative syndromes in animals and in human beings. *Cancer Res* 45: 4534s–4538s.

Fahey JL, Prince H, Weaver M *et al.* (1984) Quantitative changes in T helper or T suppressor/cytotoxic lymphocyte subsets that distinguish acquired immune deficiency syndrome from other immune subset disorders. *Am J Med* 76: 95–100.

Fahey JL, Taylor JM, Detels R *et al.* (1990) The prognostic value of cellular and serologic markers in infection with human immunodeficiency virus type 1. *N Engl J Med* 322: 166–72.

Fauci AS (1993) Immunopathogenesis of HIV infection. *J Acquir Immune Defic Syndr* 6: 655–62.

Fauci AS (1996) Host factors and the pathogenesis of HIV-induced disease. *Nature* 384: 529–34.

Fenyo EM, Albert J, Asjo B (1989) Replicative capacity, cytopathic effect and cell tropism of HIV. *AIDS* 3: 5S–12S.

Finzi D, Hermankova M, Pierson T *et al.* (1997) Identification of a reservoir for HIV-1 in patients on highly active antiretroviral therapy. *Science* 278: 1295–300.

Francis DP, Curran JW, Essex M (1983) Epidemic acquired immune deficiency syndrome (AIDS): Epidemiologic evidence for a transmitted agent. *J Natl Cancer Inst* 71: 1–6.

Gallo RC, Salahuddin SZ, Popovic M *et al.* (1984) Frequent detection and isolation of cytopathic retroviruses (HTLV-III) from patients with AIDS and at risk for AIDS. *Science* 224: 500–3.

Gao F, Bailes E, Robertson DL *et al.* (1999) Origin of HIV-1 in the chimpanzee *Pan troglodytes troglodytes*. *Nature* 397: 436–41.

Gelmann EP, Wong-Staal F, Kramer RA, Gallo RC (1981) Molecular cloning and comparative analyses of the genomes of simian sarcoma virus and its associated helper virus. *Proc Natl Acad Sci USA* 78: 3373–7.

Gelmann EP, Popovic M, Blayney D *et al.* (1983) Proviral DNA of a retrovirus, human T-cell leukemia virus, in two patients with AIDS. *Science* 220: 862–5.

Georges-Courbot MC, Lu CY, Makuwa M *et al.* (1998) Natural infection of a household pet red-capped mangabey (*Cercocebus torquatus torquatus*) with a new simian immunodeficiency virus. *J Virol* 72: 600–8.

Goodenow M, Huet T, Saurin W, Kwok S, Sninsky J, Wain-Hobson S (1989) HIV-1 isolates are rapidly evolving quasispecies: evidence for viral mixtures and preferred nucleotide substitutions. *J Acquir Immune Defic Syndr* 2: 344–52.

Gottlieb MS, Schroff R, Schanker HM, Weisman JD, Fan PT, Wolf RA (1981) *Pneumocystis carinii* pneumonia and mucosal candidiasis in previously healthy homosexual men: evidence of a new acquired cellular immunodeficiency. *N Engl J Med* 305: 1425–31.

Gupta P, Kingsley L, Armstrong J, Ding M, Cottrill M, Rinaldo CR (1993) Enhanced expression of human immunodeficiency type 1 correlates with development of AIDS. *Virology* 196: 586–95.

Gurtler LG, Hauser PH, Eberle J *et al.* (1994) A new subtype of human immunodeficiency virus type 1 (MVP-5180) from Cameroon. *J Virol* 68: 1581–5.

Hatano H, Vogel S, Yoder C *et al.* (2000) Pre-HAART HIV burden approximates post-HAART viral levels following interruption of therapy in patients with sustained viral suppression. *AIDS* 14: 1357–63.

Haynes BF, Pantaleo G, Fauci AS (1996) Toward an understanding of the correlates of protective immunity to HIV infection. *Science* 271: 324–8.

Henrickson RV, Maul DH, Osborn KG *et al.* (1983) Epidemic of acquired immunodeficiency in rhesus monkeys. *Lancet* 1: 388–90.

Hirsch VM, Olmsted RA, Murphey-Corb M, Purcell RH, Johnson PR (1989) An African primate lentivirus (SIVsm) closely related to HIV-2. *Nature* 339: 389–92.

Ho DD, Moudgil T, Alam M (1989) Quantitation of human immunodeficiency virus in the blood of infected persons. *N Engl J Med* 321: 1621–5.

Ho DD, Neumann AU, Perelson AS, Chen W, Leonard JM, Markowitz M (1995) Rapid turnover of plasma virions and CD4 lymphocytes in HIV-1 infection. *Nature* 373: 123–6.

Hubert JB, Burgard M, Dussaix E *et al.* (2000) Natural history of serum HIV-1 RNA levels in 330 patients with a known date of infection. *AIDS* 14: 123–31.

Huet T, Cheynier R, Meyerhans A, Roelants G, Wain Hobson S (1990) Genetic organization of a chimpanzee lentivirus related to HIV-1. *Nature* 345: 356–9.

Jaffe HW, Francis DP, McLane MF *et al.* (1984) Transfusion-associated AIDS: serologic evidence of human T-cell leukemia virus infection of donors. *Science* 223: 1309–12.

Jain MK, John TJ, Keusch GT (1994) Epidemiology of HIV and AIDS in India. *AIDS* 8: S61–75.

Johnson PR, Gravell M, Allan J *et al.* (1989) Genetic diversity among simian immunodeficiency virus isolates from African green monkeys. *J Med Primatol* 18: 271–7.

Kalyanaraman VS, Sarngadharan MG, Robert-Guroff M, Miyoshi I, Golde D, Gallo RC (1982) A new subtype of human T-cell leukemia virus (HTLV-II) associated with a T-cell variant of hairy cell leukemia. *Science* 218: 571–3.

Kanki PJ, Kurth R, Becker W, Dreesman G, McLane MF, Essex M (1985a) Antibodies to simian T-lymphotropic retrovirus type III in African Green monkeys and recognition of STLV-III viral proteins by AIDS and related sera. *Lancet* i: 1330–2.

Kanki PJ, McLane MF, King NWJ *et al.* (1985b) Serologic identification and characterization of a macaque T-lymphotropic retrovirus (HTLV) type III. *Science* 228: 1199–201.

Kanki P, Hunt RD, Essex M (1986a) The Pathobiology of Macaque Retroviruses closely related to Human T-cell Lymphotropic Viruses in: Salzman, LA, ed. *Animal Models of Retrovirus Infection and Their Relationship to AIDS*. Orlando, FL: Academic Press, pp. 223–32.

Kanki PJ, Barin F, M'Boup, S *et al.* (1986b) New human T-lymphotropic retrovirus related to simian T-lymphotropic virus type IIIAGM (STLV-IIIAGM). *Science* 232: 238–43.

Kanki PJ, Hamel DJ, Sankalé J-L *et al.* (1999) Human immunodeficiency virus type 1 subtypes differ in disease progression. *J Infect Dis* 179: 68–73.

Kirchhoff F, Pohlmann S, Hamacher M *et al.* (1997) Simian immunodeficiency virus variants with differential T-cell and macrophage tropism use CCR5 and an unidentified cofactor expressed in CEMX174 cells for efficient entry. *J Virol* 71: 6509–16.

Korber BT, Allen EE, Farmer AD, Myers GL (1995) Heterogeneity of HIV-1 and HIV-2. *AIDS* 9: S5–18.

Kunanusont C, Foy HM, Kreiss JK *et al.* (1995) HIV-1 subtypes and male-to-female transmission in Thailand. *Lancet* 345: 1078–83.

Lane HC, Masur H, Gelmann EP *et al.* (1985) Correlation between immunologic function and clinical subpopulations of patients with the acquired immune deficiency syndrome. *Am J Med* 78: 417–22.

Letvin NL, Eaton KA, Aldrich WR *et al.* (1983) Acquired immunodeficiency syndrome in a colony of macaque monkeys. *Proc Natl Acad Sci USA* 80: 2718–22.

Louwagie J, McCutchan F, Mascola J (1993) Genetic subtypes of HIV-1. *AIDS Res Hum Retroviruses* 9 (Suppl 1): 147s–150s.

Lyles RH, Munoz A, Yamashita TE *et al.* (2000) Natural history of human immunodeficiency virus type 1 viremia after seroconversion and proximal to AIDS in a large cohort of homosexual men. *J Infect Dis* 181: 872–80.

Mann JM, Bila K, Colebunders RL *et al.* (1986) Natural history of human immunodeficiency virus infection in Zaire. *Lancet* 2: 707–9.

Marlink R, Kanki P, Thior I *et al.* (1994) Reduced rate of disease development after HIV-2 infection as compared to HIV-1. *Science* 265: 1587–90.

Masur H, Michelis MA, Greene JB *et al.* (1981) An outbreak of community-acquired Pneumocystis carinii pneumonia: initial manifestation of cellular immune dysfunction. *N Engl J Med* 305: 1431–8.

McCutchan F, Salimen MO, Carr JK, Burke DS (1996) HIV-1 genetic diversity. *AIDS* 10: S13–S20.

Mellors J, Kingsley L, Rinaldo C, Jr *et al.* (1995) Quantitation of HIV-1 RNA in plasma predicts outcome after seroconversion. *Ann Intern Med* 122: 573–9.

Mellors JW, Rinaldo CR Jr, Gupta, P, White RM, Todd JA, Kingsley LA (1996) Prognosis in HIV-1 infection predicted by the quantity of virus in plasma. *Science* 272: 1167–70.

Mellors JW, Munoz A, Giorgi JV *et al.* (1997) Plasma viral load and CD4(+) lymphocytes as prognostic markers of HIV-1 infection. *Ann Intern Med* 126: 946–54.

Myers G, Pavlakis GN (1992) In: Levy JA, ed. *The Retroviridae*. New York: Plenum Press, pp. 1–37.

Nahmias AJ, Weiss J, Yao X *et al.* (1986) Evidence for human infection with an HTLV-III/LAV-like virus in Central Africa. *Lancet* 1: 1279–80.

Nkengasong JN, Janssens W, Heyndrickx L *et al.* (1994) Genotypic subtypes of HIV-1 in Cameroon. *AIDS* 8: 1405–12.

Notermans DW, Goudsmit J, Danner SA, Dewolf F, Perelson AS, Mittler J (1998) Rate of HIV-1 decline following antiretroviral therapy is related to viral load at baseline and drug regimen. *AIDS* 12: 1483–90.

Obrien TR, Rosenberg PS, Yellin F, Goedert JJ (1998) Longitudinal HIV-1 RNA levels in a cohort of homosexual men. *J Acquir Immune Defic Syndr* 18: 155–61.

Oleske J, Minnefor A, Cooper R *et al.* (1983) Immune deficiency syndrome in children. *JAMA* 249: 2345–9.

Pantaleo G, Graziosi C, Demarest JF *et al.* (1993) HIV infection is active and progressive in lymphoid tissue during the clinically latent stage of disease. *Nature* 362: 355–8.

Pantaleo G, Menzo S, Vaccarezza M *et al.* (1995) Studies in subjects with long-term non-progressive human immunodeficiency virus infection. *N Engl J Med* 332: 209–16.

Panther LA, Tucker L, Xu C, Tuomala RE, Mullins JI, Anderson DJ (2000) Genital tract human immunodeficiency virus type 1 (HIV-1) shedding and inflammation and HIV-1 env diversity in perinatal HIV-1 transmission. *J Infect Dis* 181: 555–63.

Peeters M, Honore C, Huet T *et al.* (1989) Isolation and partial characterization of an HIV-related virus occurring naturally in chimpanzees in Gabon. *AIDS* 3: 625–30.

Piot P, Quinn TC, Taelman H *et al.* (1984) Acquired immunodeficiency syndrome in a heterosexual population in Zaire. *Lancet* 2: 65–9.

Poiesz BJ, Ruscetti FW, Gazdar AF, Bunn PA, Minna JD, Gallo RC (1980) Detection and isolation of type C retrovirus particles from fresh and cultured lymphocytes of a patient with cutaneous T-cell lymphoma. *Proc Natl Acad Sci USA* 77: 7415–19.

Poon MC, Landay A, Prasthofer EF, Stagno S (1983) Acquired immunodeficiency syndrome with *Pneumocystis carinii* pneumonia and *Mycobacterium avium-intracellulare* infection in a previously healthy patient with classic hemophilia. Clinical, immunologic, and virologic findings. *Ann Intern Med* 98: 287–90.

Popovic M, Sarngadharan MG, Read E, Gallo RC (1984) Detection, isolation, and continuous production of cytopathic retroviruses (HTLV-III) from patients with AIDS and pre-AIDS. *Science* 224: 497–500.

Putter H, Prins JM, Jurriaans S *et al.* (2000) Slower decline of plasma HIV-1 RNA following highly suppressive antiretroviral therapy in primary compared with chronic infection. *AIDS* 14: 2831–9.

Redfield R, Wright D, Tramont E (1986) The Walter Reed staging classification for HTLV-IIILAV infection. *N Engl J Med* 314: 131–2.

Rinaldo C, Huang X-L, Fan Z *et al.* (1995) High levels of anti-human immunodeficiency virus type 1 (HIV-1) memory cytotoxic T-lymphocyte activity and low viral load are associated with lack of disease in HIV-1-infected long-term nonprogressors. *J Virol* 69: 5838–42.

Rubinstein A, Sicklick M, Gupta A *et al.* (1983) Acquired immunodeficiency with reversed T4/T8 ratios in infants born to promiscuous and drug-addicted mothers. *JAMA* 249: 2350–6.

Sabin CA, Devereux H, Phillips AN, Janossy G, Loveday C, Lee CA (1998) Immune markers and viral load after HIV-1 seroconversion as predictors of disease progression in a cohort of haemophilic men. *AIDS* 12: 1347–52.

Sabin CA, Devereux H, Phillips AN *et al.* (2000) Course of viral load throughout HIV-1 infection. *J Acquir Immune Defic Syndr* 23: 172–7.

Saksela K, Steven C, Ribinstein P, Baltimore D (1994) Human immunodeficiency virus type 1 mRNA expression in peripheral blood cells predicts disease progression independently of the numbers of CD4+ lymphocytes. Proc Natl Acad Sci USA 91: 1104–8.

Saxinger WC, Levine PH, Dean AG *et al.* (1985) Evidence for exposure to HTLV-III in Uganda before 1973. *Science* 227: 1036–8.

Schacker TW, Hughes JP, Shea T, Coombs RW, Corey L (1998) Biological and virologic characteristics of primary HIV infection. *Ann Intern Med* 128.

Schupbach J, Popovic M, Gilden RV, Gonda MA, Sarngadharan MG, Gallo RC (1984) Serological analysis of a subgroup of human T-lymphotropic retroviruses (HTLV-III) associated with AIDS. *Science* 224: 503–5.

Scott GB, Buck BE, Leterman JG *et al.* (1984) Acquired immunodeficiency syndrome in infants. *N Engl J Med* 310: 76–81.

Siegal FP, Lopez C, Hammer GS *et al.* (1981) Severe acquired immunodeficiency in male homosexuals, manifested by chronic perianal ulcerative herpes simplex lesions. *N Engl J Med* 305: 1439–44.

Soto-Ramirez L, Renjifo B, McLane MF *et al.* (1996) HIV-1 Langerhan's cell tropism associated with heterosexual transmission of HIV. *Science* 271: 1291–3.

Stein D, Lyles R, Graham N *et al.* (1997) Predicting clinical progression or death in subjects with early-stage human immunodeficiency virus (HIV) infection – a comparative analysis of quantification of HIV RNA, soluble tumor necrosis factor type i receptors, neopterin, and beta(2)-microglobulin. *J Infect Dis* 176: 1161–7.

Tersmette M, De Goede R, Al B *et al.* (1988) Differential syncytium-inducing capacity of human immunodeficiency virus isolates: frequent detection of syncytium-inducing isolates in patients with acquired immunodeficiency syndrome (AIDS) and AIDS-related complex. *J Virol* 62: 2026–32.

Tsujimoto H, Cooper RW, Kodama T *et al.* (1988) Isolation and characterization of simian immunodeficiency virus from mandrills in Africa and its relationship to other human and simian immunodeficiency viruses. *J Virol* 62: 4044–50.

UNAIDS (2002) *UNAIDS Report on the Global HIV/AIDS Epidemic 2002*. Geneva: Joint United Nations Programme on HIV/AIDS (UNAIDS).

Van de Perre P, Rouvroy D, Lepage P *et al.* (1984) Acquired immunodeficiency syndrome in Rwanda. *Lancet* 2: 62–5.

Vanharmelen J, Wood R, Lambrick M, Rybicki EP, Williamson AL, Williamson C (1997) An association between HIV-1 subtypes and mode of transmission in Cape Town, South Africa. *AIDS* 11: 81–7.

Wei X, Ghosh SK, Taylor ME *et al.* (1995) Viral dynamics in human immunodeficiency virus type 1 infection. *Nature* 373: 117–22.

Weniger BG, Takebe Y, Ou C-Y, Yamazaki S (1994) The molecular epidemiology of HIV in Asia. *AIDS* 8: 13s–28s.

Wong JK, Xignacio CC, Torriani F, Havlir D, Fitch NFS, Richman DS (1997) In vivo compartmentalization of human immunodeficiency virus: evidence from the examination of pol sequences from autopsy tissues. *J Virol* 71: 2059–71.

Yu X, McLane MF, Ratner L, O'Brien W, Collman R, Essex M, Lee TH (1994) Killing of primary CD4+ T cells by non-syncytium-inducing macrophage-tropic human immunodeficiency virus type 1. *Proc Natl Acad Sci USA* 91: 10237–41.

Zekeng L, Gurtler L, Alaneze A *et al.* (1994) Prevalence of HIV-1 subtype O infection in Cameroon: preliminary results. *AIDS* 8: 1628–9.

Immunology in the Era of HIV/AIDS

2

Deborah J Anderson
Professor, Obstetrics and Gynecology, Boston University School of Medicine, Boston, MA, USA

Deborah J Anderson, PhD is presently Professor of Obstetrics and Gynecology and Director of the Division of Reproductive Biology at Boston University School of Medicine, Boston, MA. She served as Director of the Fearing Laboratory at Harvard Medical School from 1984–2004 and remains a member of the Harvard Center for AIDS Research. Her primary research interests are mechanisms of immune defense and infection of genital tract tissues. She has published widely and received numerous awards for her research. Dr. Anderson has served on a number of professional committees and in professional organizations including the World Health Organization Human Reproduction Programme, Family Health International Technical Advisory Board, numerous National Institutes of Health (NIH) Study Sections, and the Scientific Advisory Board of the American Foundation for AIDS Research (AmFar).

Introduction

Worldwide, over 17 million people die each year from infectious diseases, with HIV/AIDS claiming an incrementally increasing share. In 2003, over 3 million people died of HIV/AIDS, and 5 million more became newly infected (www.unaids.org). Unfortunately, we can expect these numbers to increase. The AIDS epidemic is raging out of control in many regions of the world, and the majority of the 42 million people currently living with HIV/AIDS have no access to antiretroviral drugs, and a life expectancy under 10 years from the time of infection. The new antiretroviral drugs that are available to infected individuals in industrialized nations do not eliminate HIV infection, and may promote dangerous HIV mutations. Furthermore, since HIV/AIDS causes profound immunosuppression, infected people often become incubators for other infectious diseases such as drug-resistant tuberculosis, chronic cryptosporidiosis, herpes simplex disease and many others. New emerging human pathogens, be they natural or synthetic recombinant varieties, pose unforeseen and unfathomable threats to humanity. How, in this age of scientific enlightenment, has our species arrived at such a precarious point?

Although immunologists for over 200 years have succeeded in developing vaccines to control several of the most deadly infectious diseases including smallpox, poliomyelitis, diphtheria, mumps, measles and others, the continued spread of HIV, drug-resistant malaria and tuberculosis into the twenty-first century highlights the continuing threat posed by infectious diseases. Old diseases continue to pose problems, and new diseases are emerging with alarming rapidity. Since HIV/AIDS is an infectious disease that primarily targets cells of the immune system, many believe that the ultimate solution rests on an immunologic approach consisting of a preventative vaccine, coupled with therapeutic vaccines and immunotherapy for infected individuals to bolster the immune system and counter the immuno-suppressive effects of HIV. Unfortunately, this task has not been easy. The human immune system is complex and HIV is a clever adversary.

Despite huge funding initiatives and focused research mandates, the scientific community has been unable to produce effective vaccines to control *Human immunodeficiency virus type 1* (HIV-1) because of the ability of the virus to mutate very rapidly, and its capacity to subvert the immune system. Immunotherapy, likewise, has proven elusive due to the complexity of immune responses and their regulation, and the specter of autoimmunity. Yet, this is no time for complacency. This chapter will celebrate recent technical breakthroughs in the field of immunology and HIV/ AIDS, highlight the groundbreaking conceptual advances that have followed, and forecast eminent clinical applications that may yet turn the tide in humanity's epic battle against HIV/AIDS and other infectious diseases.

A Brief History of Immunology (from Silverstein, 1989)

Records dating back to the fifth century BC recognize that those who survived certain diseases became resistant to future attacks. Plague survivors were used to attend the needs of the sick and bury the dead in Ancient Greece.

In the tenth century the Chinese developed a ritual to ward off the dreaded scourge, smallpox (a disease later determined to be caused by the variola virus). The scabs of healed pustules were ground up and used as an inhalant. This earliest form of nasal immunization worked so well that the practice made its way into India and later to Turkey where Lady Mary Wortley Montagu learned of it and brought the practice (called variolation) back to England. Her adaptation was highly successful and became known to Dr Edward Jenner, who is generally considered, along with Louis Pasteur, to be the father of immunology. Jenner used the technique but was worried about its inherent danger; a small but significant number of treated individuals went on to develop full-blown smallpox. In 1796 he introduced a modified version of this early immunization technique that utilized scabs from cowpox, a disease caused by the closely related vaccinia virus, to confer immunity to smallpox.

From Jenner's introduction of smallpox vaccination in 1798 to Louis Pasteur's discovery of immunization with attenuated pathogens in 1880, nothing was known of the factors that might mediate the resulting protection. Then in 1884 a Russian zoologist Ilya Metchnikoff observed that starfish and other invertebrates were able to mobilize phagocytic cells in response to insult. He proposed that the phagocyte played a central role in both natural and acquired immunity, and founded the cellularist movement in the young field of immunology. In 1890, however, Paul Ehrlich and Richard Pfeiffer at the Koch Institute introduced a new theory. They demonstrated that humoral substances in serum from immunized animals could lyse typhoid and cholera organisms, giving rise to the humoralist movement in immunology. Ehrlich envisioned that humoral factors (antibodies) might some day be used in clinical medicine as 'magic bullets' to cure diseases.

For a quarter of a century after Pasteur, the immune response continued to be studied by medical professionals in the context of infectious diseases and vaccines. But it gradually became apparent that effective vaccines could not be produced to protect from many of the most serious diseases including tuberculosis, syphilis, most tropical diseases, and Gram-positive bacterial infections. There was a dawning realization that vaccines and immunology would not eradicate all infectious diseases, as originally hoped.

In the early 1900s medical immunology gave way to immunochemistry, and in particular the study of the fine specificity of antibodies. Serologic studies led to the discovery of blood group antigens, the major histocompatibility complex, and diagnostic tests such as the RPR (rapid plasma reagin) cardiolipin antibody test for the detection of syphilis infection. The study of antibody structure and specificity and the thermodynamics of antibody interactions became the chief preoccupations of the leaders of the field, shifting the emphasis from medical to chemical investigations.

After World War II medical applications of immunology once again came to the fore. The demonstration of clinical immunodeficiencies, the experimental effects of thymecotomy and bursecotomy, and developments in transplantation immunology cast a new light on the field of immunology. Immunological tolerance was discovered. MacFarland Burnet's clonal selection theory placed a new emphasis on the cellular dynamics of the immune response, and cellular immunology came to dominate the field. This was the cellular immunology of lymphocytes: T cells and B cells, and of their immunoregulation and functions in allograft rejection, autoimmune diseases and cancer immunosurveillance.

In the 1970s the field of immunology entered the molecular era. Advances in cell culture techniques, the discovery of monoclonal antibodies, immunochemistry, recombinant DNA methodologies, X-ray crystallography, and the creation of genetically altered animals (i.e. transgenic and gene knockout mice) have changed immunology from a largely descriptive science into one in which diverse immune phenomena can be explained in structural and molecular terms. The urgent need by the scientific community to understand the immunological effects of HIV infection has provided a major impetus to more fully understand lymphocyte phenotypes and functions. Lymphocyte cell surface receptors and intracellular signaling pathways have been described in exquisite detail. New high-throughput single cell assays have facilitated studies of immune population dynamics. In addition, the mystery of immunological diversity has been solved; lymphocyte genes coding for immunoglobulins and T cell receptors undergo somatic recombination, enabling these classes of molecules to assume a nearly infinite array of configurations capable of recognizing over 10^7 different antigens. Peptide sequencing and synthesis capabilities have enabled the mapping of antigenic epitopes and functional domains. Over 200 cytokines and chemokines, soluble mediators of immune responses, have been identified, cloned and characterized. Comparative genetics studies have revealed a phylogenetically conserved program of defense against microbes, termed innate immunity. This ancient form of immune defense is present in all multicellular organisms, including plants and insects, and plays a fundamentally important role in preventing the sexual transmission of pathogens such as HIV-1 in humans.

Molecular advances in microbiology are also contributing to immunological research. Many of the major pathogenic bacterial and viral organisms, including HIV-1, have been sequenced, and a variety of methods including proteomics, transcriptional profiling, and *in vivo* expression technology are providing new insights into the physiology of infections at the level of both the pathogen and host.

The field of immunology is coming full circle with a renewed interest in the macrophage, which had been the primary cell of focus in the initial cellular immunology revolution, but was relegated to a secondary supporting role during the lymphocyte revolution. Innate immunity (once called natural immunity) is increasingly recognized as fundamentally important in immune defense. The macrophage plays a central role in innate immunity by discriminating self from infectious nonself, and initiating a programed immune defense. Thus the macrophage has a degree of specificity heretofore unrecognized and thus a more active and significant role in immune defense. In addition, new cells have entered the immune response arena. These include natural killer cells, which specialize in recognizing and killing virus-infected and cancerous cells, the dendritic cell, a mobile and very potent antigen-presenting cell, and the epithelial cell, which provides the first line of defense against many infections and is capable of directing immune responses through the production of cytokines (promote and regulate immune responses) and chemokines and adhesion molecules (determine the types and numbers of immune cells recruited to sites of infection). Thus, the reductionist approaches of the genomics and proteomics revolutions are being surplanted by a new kind of systems biology fueled by bioinformatics that embraces the complexity and power of an integrated multicomponent immune system.

Contributions of Modern Immunology to the Understanding and Treatment of HIV/AIDS

Technological Advances

Molecular immunology

Many of the advances in immunology during the past two decades have been a direct result of the advent of powerful techniques for characterizing the structure and expression of genes, synthesizing genes at will, and manipulating genes in cells and animals. There is an extensive literature on molecular techniques used in research (comprehensively covered in Alberts *et al.*, 2002). Included here are the high-lights of some of the techniques most commonly used in immunology research.

In the late 1970s methods were developed that allowed the nucleotide sequence of any purified DNA fragment to be determined simply and quickly. DNA sequencing is now completely automated, making it possible to determine the complete DNA sequences of thousands of genes. The human genome and the genomes of many organisms including HIV-1 have been fully sequenced. A new research field, bioinformatics, has been developed to handle the enormous amount of information created by genetic sequencing. Nucleotide sequences are used to predict the amino acid sequences of proteins, and to construct DNA probes and peptides that are used in many immunological studies.

Early studies of genomic DNA utilized restriction endonucleases to cleave genomic DNA into manageable-sized fragments. There are many types of restriction endonucleases; each one cleaves DNA at a specific location corresponding to a distinct nucleic acid sequence, producing different arrays of restriction fragments. These fragments can be separated according to size by electrophoresis in an agarose gel; genes of interest can be identified using molecular probes in a hybridization technique called Southern blot hybridization, and selected for sequencing or use in expression systems. A classical technique for studying gene expression is the Northern blot technique. Messenger RNA is separated according to size by elec-trophoresis and blotted onto filter paper; labeled DNA probes reveal specific mes-senger RNAs (mRNAs) in the blot.

These techniques are still in use, but are being superseded by the polymerase chain reaction (PCR), which enables the *in vitro* cloning of selected DNA segments, and by genomic microarray technology which allows for the simultaneous detection of thousands of gene products, providing detailed comprehensive snapshots of the dynamic patterns of gene expression that underlie complex cellular processes. These techniques are widely used today to study genetic structure and to character-ize gene expression in immune cells undergoing specific types of activation.

Two important methods for studying the functional effects of specific gene prod-ucts *in vivo* are the creation of transgenic mice that overexpress a particular gene in a defined tissue, and the creation of gene knockout mice in which a targeted disruption is used to ablate the function of a particular gene. Both techniques have been widely used to analyse many biologic phenomena, including the role of cytokines and other specific gene products in immune responses and pathogenesis.

The monoclonal antibody revolution

The invention of monoclonal antibodies is heralded as one of the most important advances in the field of immunology. The basic technique, as invented by Cesar Milstein and Georges Kohler in 1975, entailed the fusion of antigen-primed spleen cells with mouse myeloma cells to make mouse hybridoma cell lines capable of producing monoclonal antibodies, antibodies of a single type and specificity (reviewed in Milstein, 1980). Mouse monoclonal antibodies are easy to produce in large quantities, and have proven over the past 25 years to be extremely useful as tools to define molecular structure and function not only of antibodies themselves, but also of other molecules that can be purified through use of monoclonal antibody capture techniques. Monoclonal antibodies, which can be mass produced as highly purified and reproducible reagents, have become key elements in highly sophisticated diagnostic tests. For example, many commercial immunoassays (i.e. radioimmunoassays and enzyme-linked immunoassays) developed for clinical diagnosis of infectious and systemic diseases rely on the detection of particular antigens in the circulation or tissues by labeled monoclonal antibodies. Tumor-specific monoclonal antibodies are used for detection of tumors *in vivo* by imaging techniques.

Monoclonal antibody technology has proven invaluable in the definition of immune cell populations and functions. In 1985 the World Health Organization established a nomenclature system for the various cell types of the immune system, based on 'cluster of differentiation' or CD numbers. The clusters are defined by monoclonal antibody binding patterns to leukocyte surface antigens. At the time of the last CD workshop in 2002, 247 CD numbers had been assigned, each representing a unique leukocyte phenotype. Phenotypic differentiation of human helper and cytotoxic T lymphocyte populations was defined by the CD nomenclature system. For a compete listing of CD molecules, see Mason (2002) or http://www.ncbi.nlm.nih.gov/prow/.

A large part of CD research was fuelled by the efforts of scientists studying AIDS to understand the effects of HIV-1 on cells of the immune system. A cornerstone for monitoring disease progression in HIV/AIDS patients is the CD4/CD8 ratio, reflecting relative proportions of CD4+ (helper) and CD8+ (cytotoxic) T lymphocytes circulating in the blood. A decrease in CD4+ lymphocyte counts to less than 200/mm^3 indicates severe immunosuppression. Similar lymphocyte profiling techniques using monoclonal antibodies are being used to monitor disease progression in patients with leukemia, autoimmune diseases and other types of infections.

Monoclonal antibodies, exemplifying Ehrlich's 'magic bullets' for the cure of human diseases, also hold great promise as therapeutic agents. In principle, specific monoclonal antibodies could be administered to patients to neutralize soluble molecules involved in pathological reactions, and toxin-conjugated antibodies could be administered to selectively kill unwanted cells such as tumor or infected cells. However, clinical research has shown that mouse monoclonal antibodies cannot be used therapeutically in humans because they elicit a heterospecific immune response in human recipients. Human hybridoma cell lines have been made, but are difficult to prepare, are unstable, and usually secrete low levels of immunoglobulin M (IgM) class antibodies of low specificity. Recently, scientists have used techniques from molecular biology to design and engineer humanized monoclonal antibodies. As a first step, chimeric antibodies were made where mouse variable and human constant regions were constructed by linking together the genes encoding them and expressing the engineered, recombinant antibodies in myeloma cells. However, when these antibodies were used therapeutically in humans, some still generated human antimouse antibody responses directed against the variable region. Another approach has been to make humanized monoclonal antibodies where only the antigen binding site was replaced with rodent binding site sequence. Humanization is now a well-established technique for reducing the immunogenicity of monoclonal antibodies from rodent sources, and for improving their activity in the human system.

The clinical application of monoclonal antibodies has been given a big boost by genetic engineering technology. It is now possible to mass produce monoclonal antibodies without relying on laborious hybridoma technology. One approach is to use complementary DNAs (cDNAs) generated from RNA isolated from spleens of immunized mice. The immunoglobulin cDNAs are expressed as fusion proteins in bacteriophage display libraries, which can readily be screened for their ability to bind to a specific antigenic sequence. The cDNA isolated from the reactive bacteriophage is linked with DNA encoding the non-antigen binding part of the human IgG molecule and the final construct is transfected into a suitable cell type for mass production, purification and use. Increasingly, plant crops are being used to produce genetically engineered human monoclonal antibodies, called 'plantibodies' (reviewed in Ma *et al.*, 1998, and Hammond *et al.*, 1999). A kilogram of pure reagent-grade plantibodies can be produced for less than US $1000, making this an inexpensive and commercially viable approach, although the mass-scale genetic engineering of plant crops for medical purposes also poses ethical and scientific challenges (Union of Concerned Scientists, 2003).

High-throughput single-cell assays

AIDS research has also promoted the development and use of high-throughput cell-based assays, enabling the measurement of multiple parameters in a single experiment. These information-rich assays provide vital information on gene expression in individual cells and cell populations, and have accelerated the functional characterization of cellular constituents involved in host defense mechanisms, effects of disease on immune cell function, and effects of vaccines and immunotherapy on cell populations.

The high-throughput assay most often used in HIV/AIDS research and clinical care is multichannel flow cytometry. The tissue lineage, maturation stage, and activation status of a cell can be determined by analyzing the cell surface and intracellular expression of different molecules. This is most often accomplished by staining the cell with fluorescently labeled probes, usually monoclonal antibodies that are specific for those molecules, and measuring the quantity of fluorescence emitted by each cell by passing the cells one at a time through a fluorimeter with a laser beam. Use of different fluorescent probes and laser wavelengths enables the simultaneous detection of several different gene products on a single cell. Investigators commonly use up to five-channel flow cytometry to enumerate peripheral blood lymphocytes that express different combinations of CD4, CD8, CD3, and activation markers. This approach is widely used to study changes in the immune system as a result of autoimmune and immunosuppressive disease states (reviewed by Cram, 2002; Valet, 2003). Flow cytometry is used clinically to monitor the depletion of CD4 T lymphocytes in HIV-1-infected patients, which is the primary measure of immunosuppression and HIV disease progression (reviewed by Mandy *et al.*, 2002).

A related assay widely used by HIV vaccine developers to monitor vaccine humoral and cellular immune responses is the ELISPOT assay. Lymphocytes from a variety of sources can be studied by this technique to determine the percentage of cells expressing specific gene products such as antibodies (e.g. IgG, IgA, and IgM) or cytokines (e.g. interferon γ, IL-4, and IL-10). The lymphocytes are seeded onto filter paper, and gene products are detected by labeled secondary antibodies that recognize these gene products. Positive cells (e.g. interferon γ-producing cells) are enumerated by counting spots made by labeled antibodies on the filter paper. When lymphocytes from vaccine recipients are stimulated with vaccine antigens and subsequently examined for gene expression in the ELISPOT assay, it is possible to enumerate and characterize lymphocytes that are responsive to vaccine antigens. In this way vaccine efficacy and T cell epitope responses can be evaluated (Mashishi and Gray, 2002; Addo *et al.*, 2003; Anthony and Lehman, 2003).

Conceptual Advances

HIV adaptive immunity

In most people infected by HIV, both humoral and cell-mediated HIV-specific immune responses develop within days of initial infection. The early response is usually robust and serves to clear most of the virus present in the blood and in circulating T cells. However, these immune responses fail to eradicate all of the virus, and the infection gradually overwhelms the immune system in most individuals (Walker and Korber, 2001). HIV infects immune cells via CD4, the primary

43

receptor molecule for HIV. HIV's primary target cell is the CD4+ helper T cell, which plays a critical regulatory role in both humoral and cellular immunity. Recent evidence indicates that HIV-1-specific CD4+ T cells are preferentially targeted and killed by HIV-1 (Douek *et al.*, 2002). Other CD4+ cells infected by HIV are macrophages and dendritic cells, antigen-presenting cells that initiate immune responses. By targeting these cells, HIV eliminates the very cells that would otherwise help maintain effective immunity against the virus itself.

Once HIV infection is established, the ongoing antigenic stimulation leads to a massive expansion of CD8+ cytotoxic T cells (CTLs) specific for HIV antigens. Ultimately, however, CTLs fail to control an established HIV infection for several reasons, including viral latency, epitope escape selection, and decreased longevity as a result of CTL death after target cell recognition (reviewed by McMichael and Rowland-Jones, 2001).

The humoral immune response to HIV infection is also robust but ineffectual. HIV infection stimulates polyclonal B cell activation and the production of massive amounts of diverse antibodies with varying affinities for HIV epitopes. High titers of anti-gp120 and anti-gp41 (HIV envelope glycoproteins) are present in most HIV-infected individuals. Neutralizing antibodies with strong affinity for HIV envelope antigens may initially control HIV replication, but eventually fail due to the generation of escape mutants (virions that express less reactive forms of the target antigen). Therefore, antibodies appear to have a minimal effect on the clinical course of disease progression (Parren *et al.*, 1999).

Some HIV-infected individuals that remain healthy with normal CD4 counts for decades (called long-term non-progressors), and highly exposed uninfected individuals (e.g. sex workers and partners of HIV-infected individuals) exhibit strong humoral and cellular immune responses that include virus-specific responses that are lacking in the immune repertoires of people with progressive infection. It has been hypothesized that these immune responses control HIV in the long-term non-progressors, and protect highly exposed individuals from HIV infection (reviewed in Chinen and Shearer, 2002). Therefore, these immune responses are being intensively studied. It is possible that the antigenic epitopes and/or the types of immune responses that underlie controlling or protective responses in these individuals will lead the way to effective HIV therapeutic or preventative vaccines.

HIV research has not only advanced knowledge of lymphocyte populations and their roles in immune defense, it has also helped uncover a network of soluble mediators of immune mechanisms called cytokines. Originally, the nomenclature of cytokines was based on their cellular source: those produced by monocytes and macrophages were called monokines, those produced by lymphocytes were called lymphokines, and those produced by one type of leukocyte population acting upon another were called interleukins. However, it soon became apparent that this nomenclature system was problematic because the same cytokine can be produced by lymphocytes, monocytes, and a variety of other cell types including endothelial and epithelial cells, and that cytokines can have wide-ranging effects on cells other than leukocytes. However, the interleukin (IL) nomenclature is still in use. Cytokines are now often grouped according to function and receptor usage (Abbas and Lichtman, 2003).

Cytokines are soluble effectors of immune function and are therefore attractive candidates for immunotherapy. Several have been used for the treatment of HIV-infected patients:

- Interleukin 2 (IL-2), a key cytokine produced by CD4 cells to boost cytotoxic T cell responses in CD8+ T cells, could help overcome immunosuppression in AIDS due to CD4 depletion. IL-2 has been administered to AIDS patients with varying results, and is also being administered in clinical trials along with HIV vaccines to boost HIV immunity in infected individuals with viral suppression following antiretroviral therapy (Miller *et al.*, 2001).
- The colony-stimulating factor (CSF) cytokines G-CSF and GM-CSF have been administered to HIV-infected patients to reduce leukocytopenia, enhance phagocytic function, and decrease opportunistic infections (Hartung *et al.*, 2001).
- IL-10, a pleiotropic cytokine which enhances CTL and natural killer (NK) cell activity in certain systems and inhibits proinflammatory cytokine secretion, was administered to HIV-infected subjects in a Phase 1 clinical trial. Decreased proinflammatory cytokine secretion and CD3 cell counts were observed. HIV-1 viral load was suppressed in the low dose group by >50 per cent, but this result was not confirmed in a subsequent study (Weissman, 2001).
- IL-12, a cytokine that plays a major role in regulating immunity to pathogens, is decreased in HIV-infection. (The HIV protein Tat directly inhibits IL-12 production from stimulated peripheral blood mononuclear cells (PBMCs).) Therefore, IL-12 has been administered to chronically SIV-infected monkeys, and to HIV-infected humans in Phase 1 clinical trials to determine if this cytokine is tolerated and can restore immune function. The simian studies showed an increase in NK activity and interferon γ (IFNγ)-producing capabilities after IL-12 administration, but no decrease in SIV viral load. The clinical study in humans did not show any effect on HIV viral load or CD4 cell count. Therefore, IL-12 may not be useful as a single therapeutic agent, but is still being considered as a means to enhance the immune response in patients on HAART, and as an adjuvant with a prophylactic or therapeutic vaccine to enhance cellular immunity (McDyer *et al.*, 2001).
- Interferon α (IFNα) is a cytokine produced by a variety of cells that has anti-viral as well as antiproliferative and immunomodulating effects. IFNα is currently approved for the treatment of AIDS-related Kaposi sarcoma and hepatitis B and C. However, none of the studies thus far have demonstrated that IFNα therapy has any effect on clinical HIV disease progression (Kovacs, 2003).

A number of HIV therapies are also envisaged for the chemokine system. HIV uses chemokine receptors, especially CCR5 and CXCR4, as entry co-receptors to penetrate cell membranes. Chemokines such as RANTES, MIP-1α, MIP-1β, and SDF-1 can block HIV interaction with these co-receptors and block HIV infection. A variety of chemically modified chemokines, chemokine derivatives, and chemokine receptor antagonists are being developed for potential use in HIV prophylaxis and therapy. The sites of interaction between chemokine co-receptors and the HIV-envelope gp120–CD4 complex are being pursued as immunization targets (Tarr and Lucey, 2001).

Innate immunity

HIV-1 preferentially infects immune cells that coexpress the CD4 receptor and chemokine receptors CXCR4 or CCR5. Evidence from simian SIV transmission studies and *in vitro* HIV infection models indicate that sexual transmission of HIV occurs via macrophages and T lymphocytes that express these receptors in genital tract and rectal mucosae; Langerhans' cells, a specific type of highly motile dendritic cell found in skin, may deliver intact HIV to T cells and macrophages by trapping HIV on its surface through binding to mannose receptors (reviewed by Pope and Haase, 2003). Sexually transmitted diseases (STDs) such as chancroids and chlamydia are associated with increased HIV transmission because they increase the numbers of HIV target cells in the genital tract mucosa, and can cause epithelial abrasions, facilitating the passage of HIV into target-cell-rich stromal tissues and blood vessels. Even so, the sexual transmission of HIV-1 occurs at a far lower rate (about 1 in 1000 acts of heterosexual intercourse on average) than many other STDs (reviewed in Politch and Anderson, 2002). This suggests that the epithelial barriers and innate immune responses in mucosal tissues may provide important protection against HIV-1 infection.

Innate immunity provides the first line of defense against infections (for a detailed review see Abbas and Lichtman, 2003). The innate immune system consists of epithelial barriers and circulating cells and proteins that recognize microbes or substances produced during infections and initiate antimicrobial responses. The principal effector cells of innate immunity are epithelial cells, macrophages, neutrophils, and natural killer cells. The mechanisms of innate immunity are present before encounter with microbes, and are rapidly activated by infection. One of the most important mechanisms of innate immunity is the generation of antimicrobial substances, including small inorganic molecules (e.g. hydrogen peroxide, nitric oxide), small antimicrobial proteins (e.g. defensins and cathelicidins), and large proteins (e.g. lysozyme, azurocidin, cathepsin G, phospholipase A2, and lactoferrin). By producing these antimicrobial factors, innate immunity rapidly limits the expansion of invading pathogens and provides time for more effective host adaptive immunity to be generated.

The best known of the innate immunity peptides are defensins, cysteine-rich peptides made up of only 29–34 amino acids, that are present at epithelial surfaces in many species including humans. Some types of defensins are also present in neutrophil granules. Defensins are broad-spectrum antibiotics that kill a wide variety of bacteria and fungi. There is also some evidence that certain members of the defensin family have antiviral effects, including activity against HIV. The synthesis of defensins is upregulated in response to inflammatory cytokines such as IL-1 and tumor necrosis factor (TNF) (defensin biology is reviewed in Yang *et al.*, 2002).

Innate and adaptive immunity work together. Innate immunity provides signals for the adaptive immune system to mount a protective host immune response. The molecules produced during innate immune reactions that function as second signals for lymphocyte activation include co-stimulators, cytokines, and complement breakdown products.

When phagocytic antigen-presenting cells such as macrophages encounter microbial products, they respond by expressing high levels of B7-1 and B7-2, endowing them with the ability to stimulate T cell responses. They also produce cytokines that promote the growth and differentiation of T cells. One such cytokine is IL-12, which stimulates naïve T cells to develop into T helper type 1 (TH1) effector cells that mediate cellular cytotoxic immunity. The best-defined innate immunity signal for B cell activation is a breakdown product of the complement component C3, called C3d. Microbes, including HIV-1, can activate complement through interaction with immunoglobulins, or directly through the alternate pathway, giving rise to complement breakdown products including C3d. When B lymphocytes recognize a microbial antigen through binding to their antigen receptors, and simultaneously recognize bound C3d via surface complement receptors, they become activated to produce antibodies against the antigen. In addition, some of the mediators of innate immunity, such as B-defensins, are chemotactic for T lymphocytes.

Adaptive immune responses also serve to enhance innate immunity. For example, in cell-mediated adaptive immune responses, antigen-specific T lymphocytes produce cytokines that activate phagocytes, important effectors of innate immunity. B lymphocytes produce antibodies that use two effector mechanisms of innate immunity, phagocytes and the complement system, to eliminate microbes.

One of the most exciting stories in contemporary immunology has been the discovery of recognition mechanisms of innate immunity. Cells involved in innate immune defense must be able to recognize microbes as distinct from self. Innate immunity is triggered immediately after microbial invasion in response to highly conserved structures present on microorganisms. These include nucleic acids that are unique to microbes, such as double-stranded RNA found in replicating viruses or unmethylated CpG DNA sequences found in bacteria; features of proteins that are found in microbes, such as initiation by *N*-formylmethionine, which is typical of bacterial proteins; and complex lipids and carbohydrates that are synthesized by microbes but not by mammalian cells such as lipopolysaccharides produced by Gram-negative bacteria, teichoic acids in Gram-positive bacteria, and mannose-rich oligosaccharides found in bacterial but not mammalian glycoproteins. The receptors of the innate immune system are encoded in the germline and therefore have a much more limited repertoire than receptors on cells participating in adaptive immunity, which undergo somatic recombination to attain their diversity. It is estimated that the innate immune system can recognize about 10^3 molecular patterns whereas the adaptive immune system can recognize 10^7 or more distinct antigens.

There are several classes of receptors on phagocytes that mediate innate immunity. Mannose receptors enable phagocytes to bind and ingest microbes via recognition of terminal mannose and fucose residues of glycoproteins and glycolipids found on microbial cell walls. Receptors for opsonins promote phagocytosis of microbes coated with antibodies and complement proteins. This mechanism may be activated by HIV-1. G protein-coupled receptors are also expressed on leukocytes and function to stimulate migration of leukocytes to sites of infection. The toll-like receptors (TLRs) are a family of membrane proteins that serve as pattern recognition receptors for a variety of microbe-derived molecules and stimulate innate immune responses. Five primary members have been identified: TLR2, which recognizes various structures on a wide variety of microbes including bacteria, fungi, and mycobacteria; TLR3, which recognizes double-stranded RNA present in many viruses; TLR4, which recognizes lipopolysaccharide (LPS) and heat shock protein 60 expressed on Gram-negative bacteria and chlamydia; TLR5, which recognizes flagellin of flagellated bacteria; and TLR9, which recognizes CpG DNA in bacteria and protozoans. The genes that are expressed in response to TLR signaling encode proteins important in many different components of innate immune responses. The predominant signaling pathway used by TLRs results in the activation of NF-κB, which results in the upregulated expression of inflammatory cytokines (TNFα, IL-1, and IL-12), endothelial adhesion molecules, and antimicrobial molecules. NF-κB activation is a double-edged sword because it can also induce the expression of HIV-1 in latently infected cells via binding to and activating long terminal repeat DNA sequences in the HIV genome (Griffin *et al.*, 1989). This could be a mechanism promoting HIV replication and viremia in HIV-infected cells activated by opportunistic infections.

Mucosal immunology

The majority of human pathogens, including HIV, infect across mucus membranes which are protected by an integrated network of specialized cells and tissues, called the mucosal immune system, that employs both innate and acquired immune defense mechanisms. The surface area of mucosal tissues in the lungs, mammary glands, gastrointestinal and genital tracts collectively cover approximately $300–400\,m^2$ (about the area of a football field!), and daily production of IgA, the major antibody isotype in external secretions, at $40\,mg/kg$ per day, exceeds that of the daily production of all other immunoglobulins in the body combined. The number of T cells residing in mucosal tissues, estimated to be in the order of 10^9, also far exceeds the number of T cells normally found in the bloodstream (only 2 per cent of total), lymph nodes and spleen (reviewed in Staats and McGhee, 1996). Yet much less is known about mucosal immunology than systemic, or 'mainstream' immunology. It has been far easier to study lympho-cytes and other molecular mediators in blood and lymphoid tissues than in mucosal secretions and tissues. This disparity is reminiscent of the story of the man found searching for his keys under a street lamp on a dark night, not because he lost them there, but because the lighting was better.

Interest in mucosal immunology has increased due to the realization that mucosal responses may be key to preventing mucosal HIV transmission and adverse effects of HIV disease on mucosal tissues. However, to date none of the leading HIV vaccines in clinical trials has been designed to specifically induce mucosal immunity. The mucosal immune system has discrete immune induction sites, pri-marily in the Peyer's patches in the intestine, which give rise to mucosal humoral and cellular responses that are distinct from peripheral responses. Nonetheless, mucosal immunity also employs some components of systemic immunity: serum antibodies are found in mucosal secretions at much reduced concentrations, and recent studies indicate that many but not all T cells in mucosal tissue have char-acteristics, such as distinct VB gene sequences, that are similar to those found in T cells in the periphery, indicating a common derivation. Some vaccine research groups are exploring ways to deliver HIV vaccines to the mucosal immune system via oral, genitorectal, or nasal routes, but most of the large commercial efforts are

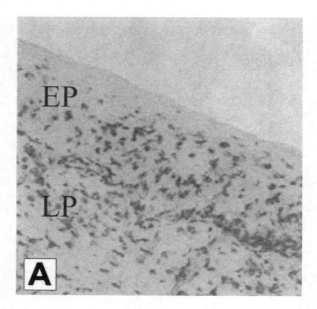

Fig. 2.1 (A) Microscopic cross-section of the human vaginal wall, processed by immunohistochemistry to reveal white blood cells (stained dark). HIV is sexually trans-mitted from men to women by binding to dendritic cells and infecting CD4+ T cells which can be found in the vaginal and cervical epithelium (EP) and lamina propria (LP).

still using systemic immunization protocols (for detailed information on many different aspects of mucosal immunity see Ogra *et al.*, 2004).

Mechanisms of immune evasion by viruses

Over the millions of years that viruses have coexisted with their hosts, they have evolved various clever strategies to manipulate host immunity to avoid elimination. This fascinating research area has been extensively reviewed (Abbas and Lichtman, 2003; Hewitt, 2003). HIV-1 utilizes several generic and other unique evasion mechanisms to exploit the immune system and avoid immune defense mechanisms (reviewed in Johnson and Desrosiers, 2002; Klenerman *et al.*, 2002). These strategies provide formidable challenges to the development of effective HIV-1 vaccines.

- HIV-1 utilizes key receptors on lymphocytes, CD4, and chemokine receptors CCR5 and CXCR4 to target, infect, and destroy a critical cell population for anti-HIV defense.
- HIV-1 mutates extremely rapidly because of error-prone reverse transcription coupled with a very high replication rate. It is likely that the host immune

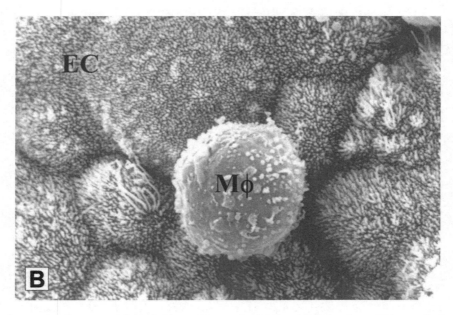

Fig. 2.1 (B) A scanning electron micrograph showing binding of an HIV+ seminal macrophage (Mφ) to vaginal epithelial cells (Ep). HIV+ cells can cross the vaginal epithelium to infect cells below thus acting as Trojan Horse vectors of HIV transmission.

response exerts selective pressure to produce viral variants that are antigenically mutated to escape detection by antibodies and T cells.

- HIV-1 infection leads to the downregulation of major histocompatibility complex (MHC) class I antigens, a mechanism that may help infected cells evade cytotoxic T cell recognition.
- HIV infection inhibits cell-mediated immunity through expansion of HIV-specific TH2 cells, which produce cytokines that can inhibit cell-mediated immunity.
- HIV-1 infection can be latent, a state characterized by infection of cells in the absence of viral protein production. This allows HIV-1 to persist while stealthily avoiding detection by cytotoxic T cells.
- HIV-1 disguises itself with glycoproteins taken from the host cell membrane during budding which can mask neutralizing antibody sites on the viral envelope.

Applications of New Discoveries to HIV/AIDS Prevention and Treatment

Vaccines

HIV-1 vaccine development faces a number of challenges. The first and most formidable are the biological challenges posed by the HIV virion. After infection, viral antigens are processed and presented to the immune system. Innate immunity is initiated, followed by adaptive immunity, mediated by cytotoxic T cells and specific antibodies. However, HIV nimbly escapes this immune response through rapid mutation, immunosuppression, and hiding. It is likely that HIV will employ these same mechanisms to avoid elimination by similar vaccine-driven immune responses. Furthermore, important infection sites for HIV-1 are the genital tract and intestinal mucosal epithelia, sites governed by different immunological principles than the peripheral immune system, which has been more extensively studied and is better understood. Mucosal sites contain a combination of peripherally derived and mucosally derived immune cell populations. Since mucosal surfaces are highly exposed to endogenous organisms and other antigenic stimuli (e.g. food in the intestinal mucosa, sperm in the genital tract), immune cells at these sites often respond to antigenic challenge with energy (i.e. oral tolerance) instead of immune activation. Most of the research on mucosal immunity has focused on the gut and lungs, and important information has been gleaned concerning induction of immune responses via Peyer's patches and other organized inductive sites in these regions. Precious little is known about eliciting immunity in the genital tract, a key target site for HIV prevention. Furthermore, there is a growing appreciation of gender differences in mucosal and systemic immune responses, which must be considered when delivering vaccines.

Recent vaccine research has come up with some innovative approaches:

1. DNA-based vaccines are being developed against many diseases including HIV, but so far have been poor inducers of antigen-specific immunity. Scientists are now working to solve this problem by combining DNA vaccines with 'molecular adjuvants' (reviewed in Ahlers *et al.*, 2003). Early data from macaque experiments to determine the effect of adding genes for the cytokines IL-12 and IL-15 to a DNA vaccine against SIV indicate that these cytokines enhance both cellular and humoral immunity (Kim *et al.*, 2001).
2. Monoclonal antibodies can be used to reverse engineer immunogens used in vaccine development. Natural HIV infection elicits poorly cross-reactive neutralizing antibodies which quickly drive escape mutant HIV evolution. A few monoclonal antibodies have been made that exhibit broad cross-neutralization, and are being used to reverse engineer immunogens that can elicit the corresponding antibody specificities *in vivo* and form a component of an effective HIV vaccine. One such monoclonal antibody, 2G12, derived from a genetic sequence of an HIV-positive patient, recognizes a dense cluster of mannose sugars on one region of the surface glycoprotein of HIV. This region is conserved (invariant) in many strains of HIV, and the monoclonal antibody is capable of neutralizing over half of the world's HIV strains. An international team of scientists have teamed up to design and test synthetic constructs that mimic the cluster of sugars recognized by 2G12, and which could constitute a potential vaccine lead. This antibody is also being mass produced by genetic engineering in tissue culture and plants for use in passive immunization protocols. Clinical trials are being planned to determine if passive immunization with HIV-specific monoclonal antibodies decreases mucosal HIV transmission through breast milk (Ruprecht *et al.*, 2003).
3. Bacterial DNA contains immunostimulatory CpG motifs that trigger an innate immune response via TLR9, characterized by the production of polyreactive immunoglobulin, chemokines, and cytokines. Synthetic CpG motif constructs mimic this activity, and are being tested as vaccine adjuvants as well as a means to enhance innate immunity to boost host resistance to infection (Verthelyi *et al.*, 2002).
4. Dendritic cells are being used to deliver therapeutic SIV vaccines for the treatment of simian AIDS (Lu *et al.*, 2003).

Topical microbicides

Topical microbicides are being developed to reduce the sexual transmission of HIV-1 and other STD pathogens. Many active formulations do not advance into clinical trials because the same properties that make them toxic to pathogens, such as dissolution of the cell membrane, also render them toxic or irritating to lymphocytes and epithelial cells, running the risk of damaging the epithelial barrier, suppressing natural innate and adaptive immune defense mechanisms and enhancing pathogen transmission. This was true for the vaginal spermicide Nonoxynol-9 which, as a detergent, stripped virus membranes and rapidly inactivated HIV and other sexually transmitted viruses, but also damaged the vaginal epithelium and caused a local inflammatory response which may actually have increased HIV transmission (Fichorova *et al.*, 2001).

An exciting new development is the incorporation of natural mediators of innate and adaptive immunity into topical formulations for use as vaginal and rectal creams to prevent HIV-1 sexual transmission. These products include:

- Low pH buffers to maintain the naturally low pH conditions of the vagina after intercourse. The acidic pH of the vagina, produced in part by lactic acid released from lactobacilli organisms, has broad-spectrum antimicrobial effects, but is neutralized after intercourse due to the alkalinity of semen.
- Lactic acid- and H_2O_2-producing lactobacilli to enhance innate immunity in the vagina.
- Genetically engineered monoclonal antibodies with specificity against HIV-1 and other STD organisms.
- Chemokines and chemokine receptor antagonists.

Since these types of antimicrobial mediators are found in the normal vaginal and rectal environments they will probably be well tolerated when applied in topical formulations. This subject is presented in more detail in Chapter 8.

Immunotherapy

Because the most serious complications of HIV infection are due to its immunosuppressive effects, immunotherapy has been considered for HIV-infected individuals to expand immune function, prevent further immunological deterioration, and improve host immune responses to HIV (reviewed in Kovacs, 2003). A variety of immune-based approaches to the management of HIV infection have been evaluated, but to date none have been documented to have a consistent clinical benefit in controlled trials. As discussed above, approaches to immune restoration have included therapy with a variety of cytokines including IFNα, IFNγ, IL-2, IL-10, IL-12, and GM-CSF. Interferon alpha appeared to have a positive effect in Kaposi sarcoma patients (treated individuals had a higher tumor regression rate), but there was no effect on CD4 cell counts. ACTG 328 examined the effect of IL-2 in a randomized trial of patients with a baseline CD4 count between 50 and 350 receiving 12 weeks of HAART. Median CD4 counts were significantly higher in the IL-2-treated group. In other studies of patients with low CD4 counts on HAART therapy, intermittent IL-2 therapy induced a significant increase in CD4+ cell counts. Therefore, some of the data from these clinical trials are encouraging, but the clinical benefit of immunotherapy has not been clearly shown. Further

53

studies are warranted, but several of the immunotherapeutic reagents cause side-effects, and therefore close management of toxicity is essential.

In the pre-HAART era, at least nine large-scale therapeutic immunization trials were conducted. HIV viral envelope proteins (gp120 and gp160) were used to immunize asymptomatic patients with high CD4 cell counts, and a variety of immunological and disease stage endpoints were monitored. Immunization with several candidate HIV vaccines stimulated HIV-specific cell-mediated immunity but did not result in changes in viral load or disease progression (reviewed by Bucy, 2003).

Another approach, called structured therapy interruption, has been tried to improve HIV immunity in infected individuals (reviewed by Allen *et al.*, 2002). The principal concept behind this approach is that a short withdrawal from therapy allows rebound of viral replication and thereby stimulates the immune system as a form of endogenous immunization. Initial small exploratory studies seemed to indicate that this approach did result in T cell activation and maintenance of low viral replication in some individuals. However larger studies have not been able to replicate these effects. The therapeutic vaccination approach should be revisited as more effective vaccines and adjuvants become available.

What the Future Holds

AIDS research over the past 20 years has garnered an astounding amount of information about the human immune system. Through the use of molecular tools, immunologists have identified and characterized the molecular signatures and functions of a wide array of immune cell types. Gene array technology has identified hundreds of molecules expressed by diverse immune cells undergoing various immunological functions. Improved tests of immune function, utilizing sophisticated techniques such as ELISPOT and flow cytometry, have enabled immunologists to monitor and understand immune responses at the level of the single cell. New molecular sequencing and synthesis methodologies have enabled scientists to construct precise antigenic epitope maps which have been used to study the fine specificity of immune responses; the most effective of the epitopes are being incorporated into molecularly defined vaccines intended to elicit precise and maximally effective immune responses.

Yet the more we discover, the greater our appreciation and wonder for the complexities of biology and the immune response: the many ways infectious organisms subvert cellular mechanisms to infect and avoid detection in their host organisms; the intricate evolutionary dance between HIV and the immune response; the fine line between protective immunity, immunopathology, and autoimmunity; the redundancy of molecular effectors of immune responses; the unexpected complexity provided by the genotypic, phenotypic, and functional polymorphism of many molecules involved in immune responses; the elegance and importance of evolutionarily conserved genetic programs governing innate immune defenses.

Much has been learned in the field of immunology over the past 20+ years, but has anything been accomplished? Has the expenditure of billions of dollars in immunology research since the beginning of the AIDS era paid off? After all these years of intensive effort we still have not produced preventative or therapeutic vaccines for HIV/AIDS, or effective immunotherapy to reverse HIV immunodeficiency. Is the rush to understand molecular details sidetracking us from more pragmatic pursuits? In the search for perfect molecularly defined vaccines and drugs, has excellence become the enemy of good?

We can be cautiously optimistic. Much has been learned about HIV immunology in a very short time. The vaccine effort is pushing forward through a combination of new-age molecular modeling technology and classical trial-and-error approaches. Consequently, a number of second-generation HIV vaccine candidates are entering clinical trials. Hopefully one of these will show efficacy and put us on the right track. Cytokines are being used as immunotherapeutic drugs in a number of diseases, and may yet prove useful in HIV/AIDS. Bioengineered anti-HIV monoclonal antibodies may someday be used to passively immunize babies to prevent vertical HIV transmission through breast milk, and in vaginal and rectal creams to protect women and men from the sexual transmission of HIV. Knowledge about strategies used by HIV-1 to evade immune defense mechanisms may someday produce novel approaches to therapy and vaccination. Importantly, the immunological community is working together with unprecedented determination and urgency to address this problem, and lessons learned in the HIV/AIDS arena can be applied to other threatening infectious diseases. Many immunologists today feel that their field is on the verge of a new unifying paradigm, much like the field of physics in the mid twentieth century. An eloquent passage in the preface of the classical textbook *The Molecular Biology of the Cell* (Alberts *et al.*, 2002) sums this up: 'as information accumulates in ever more intimidating quantities, disconnected facts and impenetrable mysteries give way to rational explanations, and simplicity emerges from chaos'. Microbes have experimented with the human immune system for millions of years. Humans have only just begun. Let's hope we can catch up before it's too late!

References

Abbas AK, Lichtman AH (2003) *Cellular and Molecular Immunology*. New York: Elsevier.

Addo MM, Yu XG, Rathod A *et al.* (2003) Comprehensive epitope analysis of human immunodeficiency virus type 1 specific T-cell responses directed against the entire expressed HIV-1 genome demonstrate broadly directed responses but no correlation to viral load. *J Virol* 77: 2081–92.

Ahlers JD, Belyakov IM, Berzofsky JA (2003) Cytokine, chemokine, and costimulatory molecule modulation to enhance efficacy of HIV vaccines. *Curr Mol Med* 3: 285–301.

Alberts B, Johnson A, Lewis J, Raff M, Roberts K, Walter P (2002) *The Molecular Biology of the Cell*, 4th edn. New York: Garland Science.

Allen TM, Kelleher AD, Zaunders J, Walker BD (2002) STI and beyond: the prospects of boosting anti-HIV immune responses. *Trends Immunol* 23: 456–60.

Anthony DD, Lehmann PV (2003) T-cell epitope mapping using the ELISPOT approach. *Methods* 29: 260–9.

Bucy RP (2003) Approach to HIV-antigen specific immune enhancement. In: Dolin R, Masur H, and Saag M, eds. *AIDS Therapy*. New York: Churchill Livingstone, pp. 284–94.

Chinen J, Shearer WT (2002) Molecular virology and immunology of HIV infection. *J Allergy Clin Immunol* 110: 189–98.

Cram LS (2002) Flow cytometry, an overview. *Methods Cell Sci* 24: 1–9.

Douek DC, Brenchley JM, Betts MR *et al*. (2002) HIV preferentially infects HIV-specific CD4+ T cells. *Nature* 417: 95–8.

Fichorova R, Tucker L, Anderson DJ (2001) The molecular basis of nonoxynol-9 induced vaginal inflammation and its possible relevance to human immunodeficiency virus-1 transmission. *J Infect Dis* 184: 418–28.

Griffin GE, Leung K, Folks TM, Kunkel S, Nabel GJ (1989) Activation of HIV gene expression during monocyte differentiation by induction of NF-kappa B. *Nature* 339: 70–3.

Hammond J, McGarvey P, Yusibov V, eds (1999) Plant biotechnology: new products and applications. *Curr Top Microbiol Immunol* 240: 1–196.

Hartung T, Gaviria JM, Garrido SM, Root RK (2001) G-CSF and GM-CSF. In: Holland SM, ed. *Cytokine Therapeutics in Infectious Disease*. Philadelphia: Lippincott, Williams & Wilkins, pp. 185–219.

Hewitt EW (2003) The MHC class I antigen presentation pathway: strategies for viral immune evasion. *Immunology* 110: 163–9.

Johnson WE, Desrosiers RC (2002) Viral persistance: HIV's strategies of immune system evasion. *Annu Rev Med* 53: 499–518.

Kim JJ, Yang JS, Manson KH, Weiner DB (2001) Modulation of antigen-specific cellular immune responses to DNA vaccination through use of Il-2, INF-gamma or Il-4 gene adjuvants. *Vaccine* 19: 2496–505.

Klenerman P, Wu Y, Phillips R (2002) HIV: current opinion in escapology. *Curr Opin Microbiol* 5: 408–13.

Kovacs JA (2003) General immune-based therapies in the management of HIV-infected patients. In: Dolin R, Masur H, Saag M, eds. *AIDS Therapy*. New York: Churchill Livingstone, pp. 275–93.

Lu W, Wu X, Lu Y, Guo W, Andrieu JM (2003) Therapeutic dendritic-cell vaccine for simian AIDS. *Nat Med* 9: 27–32. Epub 23 Dec 2002.

Ma JK, Hikmat BY, Wycoff K *et al*. (1998) Characterization of a recombinant plant monoclonal secretory antibody and preventive immunotherapy in humans. *Nat Med* 4: 601–6.

Mandy F, Nicholson J, Autran B, Janossy G (2002) T-cell subset counting and the fight against AIDS: reflections over a 20-year struggle. *Cytometry* 50: 39–45.

Mashishi T, Gray CM (2002) The ELISPOT assay: an easily transferable method for measuring cellular responses and identifying T cell epitopes. *Clin Chem Lab Med* 40: 903–10.

Mason D, ed. (2002) *Leukocyte Typing VII*. Oxford: Oxford University Press.

McDyer JF, Chang-You Wu, Kelsall BL, Seder RA (2001) Interleukin 12. In: Holland SM, ed. *Cytokine Therapeutics in Infectious Disease*. Philadelphia: Lippincott, Williams & Wilkins, pp. 85–104.

McMichael AJ, Rowland-Jones SL (2001) Cellular immune responses to HIV. *Nature* 410: 980–7.

Miller KD, Kuruppu JC, Kovacs JA (2001) Interleukin 2. In: Holland SM, ed. *Cytokine Therapeutics in Infectious Disease*. Philadelphia: Lippincott, Williams & Wilkins, pp. 85–104.

Milstein C (1980) Monoclonal antibodies. *Sci Am* 243: 66–74.

Ogra PL, Mestecky J, Lamm ME, Strober W, Bienenstock J, McGhee JR, eds (2004) *Mucosal Immunology*, 3rd edn. New York: Academic Press.

Parren PW, Moore JP, Burton DR, Sattentau QJ (1999) The neutralizing antibody response to HIV-1: viral evasion and escape from humoral immunity. *AIDS* 13(Suppl A): S137–62.

Pope M, Haase AT (2003) Transmission, acute HIV-1 infection and the quest for strategies to prevent infection. *Nat Med* 9: 847–52.

Politch JA, Anderson DJ (2002) Preventing HIV-1 infection in women. *Infert Reprod Med Clin North Am* 13: 249–61.

Ruprecht RM, Ferrantelli F, Kitabwalla M, Xu W, McClure HM (2003) Antibody protection: passive immunization of neonates against oral AIDS virus challenge. *Vaccine* 21: 3370–3.

Silverstein AM (1989) *A History of Immunology*. San Diego: Academic Press.

Staats, HF, McGhee JR (1996) Application of basic principles of mucosal immunity to vaccine development. In: Kiyono H, Ogra PL, McGhee JR, eds. *Mucosal Vaccines*. New York: Academic Press, pp. 17–39.

Tarr PE, Lucey DR (2001) Chemokines in infectious disease. In: Holland SM, ed. *Cytokine Therapeutics in Infectious Disease*. Philadelphia: Lippincott, Williams & Wilkins, pp. 145–84.

Union of Concerned Scientists Report (2003) Gone to seed. May Newsletter.

Valet G (2003) Past and present concepts in flow cytometry: a European perspective. *J Biol Regul Homeost Agents* 17: 213–22.

Verthelyi D, Kenney RT, Seder RA, Gam AA, Friedag B, Klinman DM (2002) CpG oligodeoxynucleotides as vaccine adjuvants in primates. *J Immunol* 168: 1659–63.

Walker BD, Korber BT (2001) Immune control of HIV: the obstacles of HLA and viral diversity. *Nat Immunol* 2: 473–5.

Weissman D (2001) Interleukin 10. In: Holland SM, ed. *Cytokine Therapeutics in Infectious Disease*. Philadelphia: Lippincott, Williams & Wilkins, pp. 65–84.

Yang D, Biragyn A, Kwak LW, Oppenheim JJ (2002) Mammalian defensins in immunity: more than just microbicidal. *Trends Immunol.* 23: 291–6.

Quantitative Science

3

James D Neaton
Professor of Biostatistics, School of Public Health, University of Minnesota, Minneapolis, USA

James D Neaton, PhD is Professor of Biostatistics at the University of Minnesota School of Public Health. He received undergraduate, Masters and PhD degrees in Biometry from the University of Minnesota. Since 1990, he has been Principal Investigator of the Statistical Center and Data Management Center for the Community Programs for Clinical Research on AIDS, is Principal Investigator of the ESPRIT study, a large international trial of IL-2, has participated in cardiovascular clinical trials and continues to direct the coordinating center for the NHLBI Multiple Risk Factor Intervention Trial (MRFIT). He is a former Editor-in-Chief of Controlled Clinical Trials, participates in the U.S. Public Health Service Infectious Disease Society Joint Task Force on Prevention of Opportunistic Infection in Patients with HIV-Infection, and the U.S. Public Health Service Panel on Clinical Practices for the Treatment of HIV Infection. He has published extensively in HIV/AIDS medicine and other areas in public health.

I became involved in AIDS research in 1990 as the Director of the Statistical Center for the newly funded network called the Community Programs for Clinical Research on AIDS (CPCRA). It was an exciting time to become involved in AIDS research. A few years earlier the efficacy of zidovudine (AZT) for patients with advanced HIV disease had been established (Fischl *et al.*, 1987), and in the spring of 1990, two important studies carried out by the AIDS Clinical Trials Group (ACTG) – ACTG 016 and ACTG 019 – were published (Fischl *et al.*, 1990; Volberding *et al.*, 1990). An editorial accompanying ACTG 019, titled 'Early treatment for HIV: the time has come', concluded 'The results of this study strongly support a recommendation to institute zidovudine therapy at a dose of 500 mg per day in persons with asymptomatic HIV infection and CD4+ cell counts below 500 per cubic millimeter' (Friedland, 1990).

That was 1990. In 2003, the treatment guidelines prepared by a group convened by the US Department of Health and Human Services state 'Although randomized clinical trials provide strong evidence for treating patients with <200 CD4+ T cells/mm^3, the optimal time to initiate antiretroviral therapy among asymptomatic patients with CD4+ T cell counts >200 cells/mm^3 is unknown' (Panel on Clinical Practices for Treatment of HIV Infection, 2003).

So what happened between 1990 and 2003? A great deal happened. Along with extraordinary advances in our understanding of disease pathogenesis through basic research, we learned from hundreds of clinical trials and observational studies about the efficacy and safety of new treatments for HIV, treatments substantially more effective than AZT monotherapy. In 1990, we had one approved antiretroviral drug, AZT. In 2003, there are 19 approved antiretroviral agents that are typically used in three-drug combinations referred to as highly active antiretroviral therapy (HAART). Many HAART regimens work extremely well in suppressing HIV viral load and increasing CD4+ count, resulting in a substantial reduction in the risk of the opportunistic conditions we call the acquired immune deficiency syndrome (AIDS).

We also learned that treatment efficacy was time-limited due the development of resistance, that HAART could not eradicate HIV, and that HAART was associated with unexpected toxicities. These factors resulted in more conservative recommendations about when to begin treatment with HAART by groups preparing treatment guidelines.

While the treatment advances have been significant, information is lacking to guide when to start antiretroviral therapy, how to sequence the individual drugs or classes of drugs that are available, and how to minimize the known and suspected toxicities of the drugs. Studies related to these questions are a major focus of research in the 'developed world' because treatment strategies that prolong disease-free survival by even a modest amount are significant from a public health point of view given that millions of individuals are infected. Today's research agenda includes studies which involve head-to-head comparisons of different treatment combinations; studies of new therapies that increase CD4+ count but do not affect HIV viral load; studies aiming to better understand how the effects of treatments should be monitored; and studies of treatment interruptions designed either to modify the patient's viral population to make it more susceptible to treatment, or to minimize the toxicities associated with treatment. In many respects the clinical research agenda for HIV is not too different from other chronic diseases for which there is a large body of natural history data and many treatments, but no cure.

In the 'developing world,' where morbidity and mortality rates due to HIV are the greatest, and the numbers infected are measured in tens of millions instead of millions, treatments are slowly becoming available in many locations. In this setting, the judicious uses of treatments, and use of simple tests for monitoring treatment, are important not only for prolonging disease-free survival, but also for minimizing costs. The developed and developing world share interest in many scientific questions.

The aim of this chapter is to describe some lessons learned from the design and conduct of HIV treatment trials and observational studies. The focus is on the treatment of HIV because of my limited experience in HIV prevention studies. Hopefully, some of the lessons will be relevant to HIV prevention research and also to HIV treatment research agendas that are being discussed for the developing world. Along the way, with a description of lessons learned, parallels are drawn to research on HIV prevention and research in other disease areas, and some challenges that impact the conduct of clinical research in the US and elsewhere are discussed.

Lessons

Large, multicenter randomized trials have been considered the 'gold standard' for evaluating treatments and preventive strategies in cardiovascular disease and cancer since the 1970s. Not surprisingly, many of the biostatisticians who became involved in AIDS research were experienced clinical trialists in these areas. Thus, they were able to help to define an AIDS research agenda by building on methodological expertise acquired in another disease area while learning about infectious diseases, virology and immunology. In contrast, many HIV clinical researchers had not been previously involved in multicentre clinical trials; they were working to define a research agenda that built on their knowledge of the disease, which was growing exponentially, and what they saw in their clinical practice. Sometimes these different experiences produced tension. Most of the time, it resulted in healthy partnerships in the fight against what was already the worst public health problem of the century, if not all time.

Is AIDS research different? There are many challenges to the design and conduct of AIDS clinical trials, but are these unique to AIDS? I think most of the challenges to study design and conduct are more similar than different to other areas of clinical research. However, early on, before HAART was available, the high mortality of the young people affected created pressure for fast answers. The social context of HIV is also different from that in most other disease areas, and the stigmatized nature of the individuals resulted in recruitment and retention challenges. Some notable challenges faced by AIDS researchers were: (1) learning how to effectively include large numbers of the affected community in the development of the research agenda; (2) the enrollment of minority and disenfranchised populations in research studies; (3) designing studies in the presence of a parallel track, a government-developed system for making available to patients a treatment that is considered safe before it is licensed for sale (Marshall, 1989); (4) appropriate use of surrogate outcomes like CD4+ cell count and HIV viral load (De Gruttola *et al.*, 1997; Pozniak, 1998; Hughes, 2002), and a composite endpoint, AIDS, that included 20 or more opportunistic conditions of various severity for evaluating different treatments (Neaton *et al.*, 1994); and (5) the time-limited efficacy of treatments due to antiretroviral resistance that results from inadequate adherence, use of regimens that are not potent, and infection with drug-resistant virus. Some of these challenges are discussed in later sections of this chapter.

In the early 1990s, many of the study design challenges for AIDS treatment trials were eloquently discussed in two articles, one in the medical literature and the other in the statistical literature (Byar *et al.*, 1990; Ellenberg *et al.*, 1992). Issues mentioned in these papers included: (1) the difficulty in defining or even using control groups; (2) the use of surrogate endpoints; (3) the feasibility of blinding of patients and clinicians; (4) enrollment of patients in multiple studies; and (5) non-adherence to assigned treatment or protocol procedures. Many of these challenges persist today in AIDS treatment research, and also in prevention research, as evidenced from a recent article (Gilbert *et al.*, 2003).

A commentator of one of the papers on AIDS study design issues noted that the design challenges were not unique to AIDS research (Green, 1992). As noted earlier, this is a view that I share in large part. The commentator experienced similar challenges in cancer research. I faced many of the same challenges in the cardio-vascular area before becoming involved in AIDS research. As a consequence of this belief, I feel many of the advances in clinical trial methodology resulting from work in AIDS are applicable to other clinical research areas, and vice versa. Interestingly, for epidemiology, a discipline often linked with biostatistics, Barrett-Connor noted before AIDS was recognized that infectious disease and chronic disease epidemiologist were not 'separate and unrelated species' and had important lessons to offer each other (Barrett-Conor, 1979).

Here are three lessons that I learned or that were reinforced by involvement in AIDS research:

1. Long-term, excellent follow-up is important.
2. Pragmatic and explanatory trials are needed.
3. Randomized trials and observational studies are both important.

The lessons are of a general methodological nature and I believe all may be relevant to future HIV research and to other disease areas. Following the lessons, I discuss some challenges and then summarize.

Lesson No. 1: Long-term, Excellent Follow-up is Important

If the importance of long-term follow-up was not widely appreciated among HIV researchers, the results of the Concorde study changed that (Concorde Coordinating Committee, 1994). This study indicated that the clinical benefit associated with zidovudine was transient. The authors concluded that that deferral of zidovudine until symptoms developed would be a better policy than early use among

Table 3.1 Rate ratios (immediate versus deferred zidovudine) for progression to AIDS or death during each separate year of follow-up[a].

Year of follow-up	Events/participants		Rate ratio	95 per cent CI
	Immediate	Deferred		
0–	78/4431	131/3291	0.52	0.39–0.68
1–	197/4077	160/2968	0.94	0.76–1.16
2–	251/3632	189/2586	1.05	0.87–1.27
3–	212/2763	157/2105	1.12	0.91–1.38
4–	164/1952	143/1535	0.98	0.78–1.22
≥5	124/1300	102/1028	1.10	0.84–1.43
Total	1026/4431	882/3291	0.96	0.87–1.05

[a] Taken from *Lancet* 353: 2018, figure 4, 1999.

asymptomatic patients. Not only did the results of Concorde, which had a median follow-up of 40 months, indicate that efficacy was time-limited, but when the results were combined with other completed studies with follow-up ranging from 11 to 28 months, a similar conclusion was reached (Egger *et al.*, 1994). A later meta-analysis involving 7722 patients confirmed this and documented a clear transient effect of zidovudine on progression to AIDS or death (Table 3.1) (HIV Trialists' Collaborative Group, 1999). During the first year, the rate ratio (obtained by summing the observed and expected number of events over trials) was 0.52 (95 per cent confidence interval (CI) 0.36–0.68) for immediate versus deferred zidovudine. In subsequent years, there was no further delay of progression to AIDS with use of zidovudine. Findings for mortality were consistent – at no point during follow-up was there a difference in mortality between immediate and deferred zidovudine. With early use of zidovudine, opportunistic illnesses that occur early in the disease were more likely to be delayed than those that occurred at advanced stages of HIV disease and death.

By the time Concorde finished, trials of combination nucleoside therapy were already started. When completed, the largest three of these trials (Delta, ACTG 175 and CPCRA NuCombo) had median follow-up times ranging from 27 to 34 months (Hammer *et al.*, 1996; Delta Coordinating Committee, 1996; Saravolatz *et al.*, 1996). These trials showed that use of another nucleoside reverse transcriptase inhibitor (didanosine or zalcitabine) along with AZT was superior to AZT alone in delaying progression to AIDS or death. These studies are also summarized in the paper by the HIV Trialists Collaborative Group (1999).

The planned follow-up period of these trials was largely determined by the number of primary endpoints required – they were event-driven, i.e. they required a specific number of patients to develop a primary event in order to maintain the

Table 3.2   Required number of patients with a primary endpoint for 80 per cent power to detect specified hazard ratios at the 0.05 level of significance (2-sided) for comparing two equally sized treatment groups.

Hazard ratio	Required no. of primary endpoints
0.50 (very large treatment effect, e.g. protease inhibitor versus combination nucleoside treatment)	65
0.75 (moderate effect, e.g. combination nucleoside versus monotherapy)	380
0.15 (modest effect; strategic trials in the twenty-first century)	1200

power specified for detecting the hypothesized treatment difference (Table 3.2). It is important that trials be adequately powered, that design assumptions be monitored while trials are ongoing, and that sample size and/or trial duration be modified to maintain the desired power. Power is the probability of rejecting the hypothesis of no difference when it is false. It refers to the ability of the trial to identify true differences of the size hypothesized. An inadequately powered trial for which the treatments do not differ on completion is inconclusive. Null results should be informative and if they are not resources have been wasted. The problem of interpreting poorly powered trials has been reviewed (Freiman *et al.*, 1978; Moher *et al.*, 1994).

Adequately powered event-driven trials require many events. Consider a few examples. A trial designed to detect a 50 per cent reduction in the hazard of progression to AIDS or death (a very large hypothesized treatment effect) with 80 per cent power (0.80 probability) at the 0.05 level of significance has to follow a group of patients long enough to observe 65 patients with a primary event. To detect a more modest 15 per cent difference between two groups with 80 per cent power, about 1200 patients with a primary event are needed. All of the studies mentioned above used progression to AIDS or death as part of the primary endpoint (ACTG 175 also incorporated a CD4+ decline into their composite endpoint). Trials of asymptomatic patients required longer follow-up to observe the necessary number of endpoints. Likewise, trials with active control groups instead of placebo control groups required longer follow-up because hypothesized treatment differences were smaller and event rates were generally lower. These study design considerations indicate that any study today in which treatment groups are assigned HAART and clinical endpoints are of interest will require very large numbers of patients followed for several years.

In part for this reason, nowadays, trials of new combination therapies use HIV viral load as the primary endpoint. With this endpoint, trials are typically of 6 or 12 months' duration. The arithmetic for sample size is similar, but virologic failure (failure to suppress viral load below the lower level of detection of the viral load assay being used, or suppression followed by a rebound) is a much more common event than progression to AIDS. Clinical endpoint trials to establish the efficacy of new antiretroviral drugs in the US ended with two protease inhibitor trials, both of which were stopped early (after about six months) due to overwhelming efficacy of the protease inhibitor regimens compared with the regimens which used only combination nucleoside regimens (Hammer *et al.*, 1997; Cameron *et al.*, 1998). As a consequence, combining different classes of drugs, i.e. HAART, has become standard of care.

The striking superiority of the protease inhibitor-containing regimens (the initial HAART regimens) compared with combination nucleoside therapy, coupled with the recognition that virologic control would require regimen changes or intensification of regimens, made it difficult to conduct trials with clinical endpoints (sample size considerations as discussed above aside). If the results were analyzed by intent-to-treat (all patients counted in the groups to which they were randomly assigned irrespective of adherence or changes in treatment), it might appear that an inferior control regimen was more similar to the new regimen than it really was if more patients assigned the control regimen had treatment modifications with regimens similar in potency to the new regimen. Of course given the results of Concorde, some argued that an immediate versus deferred study design for a new regimen was precisely the question that should be asked. An immediate versus deferred trial of combination nucleoside therapy was planned, but never implemented (Neaton and Wentworth, 1993). While such a trial might be of greater ultimate benefit to patients, it is not the type of trial likely to be planned for regulatory approval. On the other hand, restricting changes in therapy as new more potent agents became available was also not practical. In fact, some argued that it was unethical (Lange, 1997; Cohen, 1997). The difficulty of conducting long-term trials created a conundrum. How do you evaluate the long-term safety and efficacy of a new treatment or regimen if only short-term randomized studies are performed? A different type of study was needed. This is discussed in more detail in the next section – lesson no. 2.

Before leaving this section on follow-up, however, consider the following thoughts on the phrase 'excellent follow-up'. The validity of prospective studies is threatened by incomplete follow-up data collection for the study participants. The consequence of bias resulting from missing data is greatest for randomized clinical trials of medical and public health interventions because the results from such studies are the basis for approval for new treatments. Randomized trials are also the basis of policy statements and treatment guidelines developed by professional societies and governments. Sometimes, incomplete follow-up is a result of the study design or protocol. Trials that terminate follow-up of patients after study treatment is discontinued, due to a lack of efficacy, side-effects, or other reasons, cannot carry out a proper intent-to-treat analysis for all outcomes. As a consequence, such trials may yield biased estimates of relative efficacy and/or relative safety of the treatment under study. Such trials may only be able to assess composite end-points that combine safety and efficacy in an unbiased manner. This is, in fact, what current FDA guidance to sponsors for antiretroviral trials entails. Sponsors are advised to combine efficacy (virologic control), safety (discontinuation of treatment), and poor follow-up into a single composite outcome (Guidance for Industry, 2002). The problem is that when studies use this endpoint, follow-up is often not continued after treatment ends, so that an intent-to-treat analysis of virologic failure or other outcomes cannot be carried out.

The pros and cons of this composite endpoint have been discussed (Gilbert *et al.*, 2001; Kirk *et al.*, 2002). The point of mentioning this here is to draw attention to the fact that incomplete follow-up is sometimes by design. Stopping follow-up after one of many events that might comprise a composite endpoint occurs is a bad practice and should not be done. A similar problem with the collection of multiple events and reporting progression to AIDS in clinical endpoint studies was pointed out several years ago (Neaton *et al.*, 1994).

In most situations, incomplete follow-up results from a poor implementation plan for the protocol, not the protocol itself. Sloppily conducted trials may yield biased estimates of efficacy and safety and compromise power. A recent commentator noted that bias resulting from poor follow-up cannot be corrected in the analysis, and that widely used analytic procedures depend on assumptions that are usually not defensible (Ware, 2003). A study with poor follow-up is not likely to be salvaged by the biostatistician.

Enrollment of minorities and those in lower socioeconomic groups has been a major challenge to HIV researchers. Stigmatization, distrust of the research process, and poor access to medical care made this difficult. Many of the obstacles to enrollment are also obstacles to follow-up of such patients (El-Sadr and Capps, 1992). These are obstacles, which have to be overcome. The solution is neither to avoid enrolling such patients because of concerns about adherence to the protocol and poor follow-up, nor to enroll such patients and use a lower standard for judging the results of studies in which they participate. These obstacles have to be overcome by including clinical sites in trials that are readily accessible to these populations, ensuring that these sites have sufficient support staff to tend to the social as well as medical needs of the participants, and then holding these sites to high research standards. The experience of the CPCRA, which largely includes sites that provide primary HIV care, in following patients in clinical endpoint studies is notable. For example, for the three combination nucleoside studies previously mentioned, lost-to follow-up rates for the CPCRA NuCOMBO trial were the lowest (2.5 per cent with unknown vital status), yet they included a greater percentage of minority patients than the other US trial (ACTG 175) (43 per cent versus 29 per cent), and they included more patients with an injecting drug use history than either the ACTG 175 or the Delta study (23 per cent versus 14 per cent versus 12 per cent).

The lessons here are that long follow-up is essential. Even if this is not practical for trials done for regulatory approval, such trials are eventually necessary. The need for long follow-up in trials is not unique to HIV treatments. Gilbert *et al.* recently discussed the importance of long-term follow-up in HIV vaccine trials because the main benefits (or risks) of the vaccine may be on post-infection outcomes like disease progression and transmission (Gilbert *et al.*, 2003). The importance of long-term follow-up studies has also been emphasized for other disease areas (Machin *et al.*, 1997; Califf and Kramer, 1998). In addition, more thought and resources should be devoted to the prevention of losses – by choosing endpoints that are easily ascertainable; by educating trial participants on the importance of excellent follow-up as part of the informed consent process and throughout the trial; by investing in staffing at clinical sites to carry out this education and to assist patients with some of their social needs; by regularly discussing the importance of good follow-up with trial investigators; and by insisting on high standards. With respect to the latter point, this demand for quality must begin with the participating investigators and must carry over to regulators, editors, and those who set policy on the basis of study results. Trial reports have been improved with flow diagrams depicting exclusions from the analysis and losses (Begg *et al.*, 1996). However, in many trial reports there remains an inadequate discussion of the reasons for losses and of the potential impact of the losses on the results. Reports of observational studies would also benefit from flow diagrams similar to those shown for most published trials.

Lesson No. 2: Pragmatic and Explanatory Trials are Needed

What is a pragmatic trial? In general, a pragmatic trial is characterized by minimal inclusion and exclusion criteria, a flexible definition of 'treatment,' and outcomes suitably chosen to assess risks versus benefits. Broad generalization is a goal of pragmatic trials.

Several decades ago Schwartz and Lellouch described two ways of thinking about clinical trials: a pragmatic viewpoint and an explanatory one (Schwartz and Lellouch, 1967). With the explanatory approach, the goal was a specific research question and 'laboratory-like' conditions prevailed; with the pragmatic approach, 'normal' conditions prevailed. Buyse used these same terms to differentiate regulatory and public health trials. He noted that the former tended to be explanatory and the latter tended to be pragmatic (Buyse, 1993). The public health trials described by Buyse are essentially the large, simple trials advocated by Peto and others (Yusuf *et al.*, 1984). If you want reliable evidence, then you need to observe a large number of patients with endpoints. For some trials you have to have long follow-up to obtain the required number of patients with outcomes.

Table 3.3   Practical (pragmatic) trials versus explanatory trials.

	Practical (pragmatic)	Explanatory
Treatment	Mimics practice to determine if it *does* work	Optimized to determine if it *can* work
Trial participants	Diverse; minimal exclusions	Highly selected to show desired effect
Trial setting	Heterogeneous practice settings	Specialized research centers
Outcomes	Multiple health outcomes	Biologic marker of activity

Recently, Tunis coined another phrase to describe pragmatic trials – 'practical' clinical trials (Table 3.3) (Tunis *et al.*, 2003). He noted that the characteristic features of such trials were that they: '1) select clinically relevant alternative interventions to compare; 2) include a diverse population of study participants; 3) recruit patients from heterogeneous practice settings; and 4) collect data on a broad range of health outcomes'. In a slightly different context, Cochrane used the terms 'effectiveness' and 'efficiency' to describe two related ideas. He noted that the effectiveness of treatments was established in randomized trials, but that often different strategies of management were needed to achieve levels of effectiveness seen in trials, and that the latter included studies of the optimum use of personnel and materials (efficiency) (Cochrane, 1989). The latter is what many are now calling operational research. Cochrane was ahead of his time.

Tunis *et al.* noted that too few practical clinical trials are carried out and that, as a consequence, health care decision makers do not have adequate quality information to make well-informed decisions. Califf and Kramer make a similar point in raising the question of why hypertension trials, based on surrogate markers (blood pressure lowering) used for regulatory purposes, are not followed by trials with morbidity and mortality outcomes. They point out two misconceptions:

> The first is that government funding will be available through the National Institutes of Health (NIH) or Agency for Health Care Policy and Research to ensure that the therapy is beneficial. The second is that physicians and patients will be able to discern that a treatment is detrimental from their experience with its use in their personal practices (Califf and Kramer, 1998).

This first misconception can be dealt with by a critical evaluation of how treatments are evaluated. The NIH is already doing some work along this line in efforts to re-engineer the clinical research enterprise (Zerhouni, 2003). We cannot, in the words of a recent commentator, allow clinical trials to become 'instruments for marketing and registration', rather 'than tools for innovative care of patients' (Staessen and Bianchi, 2003).

In HIV research, like other areas of research, too few pragmatic trials have been done, and some that have been carried out have been misinterpreted. When the Concorde results were announced, many had difficulty with its pragmatic design – a comparison of immediate versus deferred zidovudine. The use of open-label (unblinded) zidovudine by the control group was considered a deficiency; it interfered with ability to understand the effects of zidovudine. One reader noted that the distinction between the immediate and deferred groups had become blurred and there was a loss of power for studying efficacy (Graham, 1994). Concorde may not have been the best design to determine whether zidovudine should be licensed, but that was not its intent. Instead, it addressed a very relevant question for clinicians and patients, and its design and results should not be confused with that of a trial that is strictly explanatory.

What types of pragmatic trials are needed today? As noted earlier, information is lacking on when to start therapy and how to sequence different regimens. The latter question of sequencing regimens is being addressed by three different trials that are more pragmatic than explanatory (MacArthur *et al.*, 2001; Smeaton *et al.*, 2001; The INITIO Co-ordinating Committee, 2001; Robbins *et al.*, 2003; Shafer *et al.*, 2003). Each trial includes three treatment groups that are initially defined by two or three classes of drugs: nucleoside reverse transcriptase inhibitors (NRTIs) plus a protease inhibitor (PI); NRTIs plus a non-nucleoside reverse transcriptase inhibitor (NNRTI); or all three classes (NRTI, PI, and NNRTI). In each protocol, there is a provision for changing therapy (e.g. switching to another class) upon virologic failure. Thus, the trials address the strategic question of whether initial antiretroviral therapy should begin with a PI, an NNRTI, or both classes along with NRTIs. The trials use drugs with established short-term efficacy (agents approved by the FDA) to address a pragmatic question: when antiretroviral therapy is begun, what HAART regimen should be used? This is an important practical question because failure on the initial regimen may limit some future drug options (e.g. due to cross-resistance). When these three trials are all completed (one has so far), collectively they will provide an important database for use in weighing the risks and benefits of each starting strategy. Not only will the relative virologic efficacy of the initial regimens be available, as in many trials carried out for drug development, but failure rates on subsequent regimens, long-term toxicities (trials are planned to run from two to five years), and clinical outcomes will also be available (a broad range of health outcomes). The multiple outcomes should make possible a 'Consumer Reports' summary with which clinicians and patients can rank order the different strategies (Califf *et al.*, 1990). However, as noted under lesson no. 1, the validity of this summary may be jeopardized if there is not excellent follow-up for all outcomes for the entire study.

Perhaps the most important pragmatic study to be done is a trial on when to initiate therapy. The principal arguments against doing such a trial are the large sample size requirements and the concern that by the time the trial has been completed, it will be obsolete. This is because there will be new treatments available which, if used, might have resulted in a different answer. This is a little like the arguments cited earlier against Concorde. Implicit in the definition of 'study treatments' for such a trial (immediate versus deferred treatment) is the possibility of using more effective treatments later in follow-up that are not available at the beginning of the study for the group assigned immediate treatment. This is a strength of the design, not a weakness. With regard to the large sample size requirements for such a trial, this becomes a moot point as we aim to deliver antiretroviral treatment to millions of people in the developing world. Hopefully, individuals infected with HIV in the developing world will join patients in the developed world as trial participants to obtain an answer to this and other pragmatic questions.

Another related, pragmatic question is 'when to stop' treatment. Based on a recent clinical trial that was terminated early, it now appears that stopping treatment among patients with multidrug-resistant virus, with a goal of producing a viral population more sensitive to antiretroviral drugs, is not a good strategy (Lawrence *et al.*, 2003). However, nearly four years elapsed between an early report of an observational study involving 39 patients (Miller *et al.*, 1999) and the results of this clinical trial. We have to do a better job of convincing clinicians and patients to be skeptical of small uncontrolled studies and to enroll in randomized trials.

Among patients with higher CD4+ cell counts, treatment interruptions are also being considered, primarily as a means of reducing drug toxicities and preserving treatment options for later in the course of the disease. The SMART study, which was initiated in 2002, is an example of a pragmatic, strategic trial. It aims to determine whether episodic use of antiretroviral therapy is as effective as continuous antiretroviral therapy in prolonging disease-free survival among patients with CD4+ cell counts of 350 cells/mm^3 or higher (SMART trial begins, 2002). In the experimental, episodic treatment group, patients discontinue therapy (or do not initiate it if it was not prescribed at entry) until their CD4+ counts decline below 250 cells/mm^3. At that time, they initiate HAART until their CD4+ increases to above 350 cells/mm^3 again, and then stop again. Inclusion criteria are minimal – essentially all HIV-infected patients meeting the CD4+ cell count entry criteria are eligible, irrespective of treatment history. Many clinical outcomes are being assessed, including not only AIDS events, but also major cardiovascular and metabolic events. Data on morbidity and mortality, together with information on drug resistance, adverse events, and quality of life, will be used to rank order the different strategies after five to seven years of follow-up, or earlier if one intervention is determined to be superior based on planned interim analyses.

Other examples of pragmatic trials are those that come under the heading of operational research – 'efficiency' studies as described by Cochrane. These are particularly important in the developing world where cost-efficiency is critical, but many are also relevant to the developed world. These investigations should include studies of different approaches to optimize patient adherence, studies on the frequency of laboratory monitoring, and studies on co-management of HIV and other infections.

These are only a few examples of pragmatic studies that might be carried out in HIV. A common feature shared by pragmatic trials is that a number of morbidity outcomes and mortality are used to evaluate the different treatment strategies as well as laboratory markers. It is not possible to completely evaluate the risks and benefits of different treatment approaches that are to be used over the long term with short-term surrogate marker studies. In a different context, Albert Einstein once said 'Some things you can count don't matter; some things that matter, you can't count'. In short-term studies such as those carried out for licensure, many things that matter cannot be counted because the follow-up is too short.

For example, consider the study carried out to evaluate the efficacy of lopinavir and ritonavir versus nelfinavir as first-line treatment for participants with HIV (Walmsley *et al.*, 2002). This well-done 48-week study included 686 patients. The study established the superiority of lopinavir – ritonavir over nelfinavir with respect to virologic response and also provided important data on short-term tolerability compared with nelfinavir. However, in the short follow-up period only eight deaths occurred and only 2 per cent of patients developed a new AIDS-defining event. Ultimately, these are the events that matter. Even the long-term effects of the regimens on CD4+ cell count (no difference was found at 48 weeks) and on the consequences of the higher rate of resistance that developed for patients assigned nelfinavir could not be evaluated in this study.

It is too strong to state that what was counted does not matter in this study, because it did. Based on the results of this and other similar trials, lopinavir – ritonavir was listed as the preferred PI regimen for initial therapy in the 2003 DHHS guidelines (Panel on Clinical Practices for Treatment of HIV Infection, 2003). However, this guidance is based on the best of an incomplete set of data. There are many examples (including HIV studies) of the use of surrogate markers in place of outcomes that are more clinically relevant that have led to incorrect decisions about the treatment's clinical benefit. Fleming and DeMets have eloquently outlined the requirements for a surrogate endpoint to substitute for a clinical outcome and cite several examples where we have been misled (Fleming and DeMets, 1996). While virologic response is a logical outcome to consider for assessing the biologic activity of an antiviral drug and perhaps licensure, other studies are needed subsequent to licensure that evaluate the long-term effects of treatment on the endpoints that matter. Does it make sense to use different treatment regimens over decades for which the impact on long-term immunologic recovery, loss of treatment options due to the development of resistance, life-threatening adverse events, and morbidity and mortality due to HIV is uncertain? Many do not think so. Groups developing treatment guidelines, HIV clinicians, and patients need information to guide treatment choices from not only randomized studies of 48 weeks' duration but also from large, longer term controlled studies.

Surrogate markers will continue to be important for early phase studies of new treatments. More research is needed on the evaluation of surrogate outcomes and this has been nicely outlined in a report of an NIH workshop (De Gruttola *et al.*, 2001). Critical to our understanding on the role of surrogates and their evaluation are studies in which both surrogates and clinical endpoints are measured.

Further research on the appropriate clinical endpoints to assess are also needed. As noted above, AIDS represents more than 20 opportunistic conditions, and all of them are not equally important in terms of severity (Neaton *et al.*, 1994). Likewise, serious adverse events are more common now than AIDS events, and it is not clear whether the events are related to specific treatments, HIV disease, or other patient characteristics (Reisler *et al.*, 2003). Thus, multiple clinical events need to be collected and evaluated to obtain a complete picture of risks and benefits.

In summary, the lesson learned is that both explanatory and pragmatic trials are needed. Trials like when to start, SMART or the three studies of sequences of initial therapy are pragmatic or practical trials that are unlikely to be funded by the pharmaceutical industry. Likewise, operational questions will require public funding. The NIH must make pragmatic trials a higher priority on their research agenda. The need for pragmatic or practical trials is not limited to HIV treatment studies. It pertains to HIV prevention research and to other disease areas as well. With respect to the former, Gilbert *et al.* have argued for 'phase 4' HIV vaccine studies after licensure to gather more data on resistance and susceptibility of vaccines and on clinical benefit (Gilbert *et al.*, 2003). Like HIV treatments, efficacy of vaccines could wane with time. More generally, like HIV treatments a variety of studies are needed to establish the public health impact of a vaccine program. This is emphasized by Halloran *et al.* (1999), who describe different study designs for estimating the effectiveness of vaccines, and who emphasize how the comparison groups, unit of observation (e.g. individual or community), and the endpoint chosen define the research question.

Lesson No. 3: Randomized Trials and Observational Studies are Both Important

Bradford Hill, considered by many to be the father of the modern clinical trial, recognized the importance of both randomized trials (the experimental approach) and observational studies. He noted wisely that 'observation in the field suggests experiment; the experiment leads back to more, and better defined, observations' (Hill, 1953). In the same paper he noted that 'observations be made in such a way as to fulfill, as far as possible, experimental requirements'. An interpretation of this latter statement is that observational studies should be done rigorously, with a protocol, and with attention to issues such as power, confounding, and high-quality data collection.

One only has to review the abstracts from AIDS scientific meetings to observe that a large number of observational studies have been carried out in HIV. Some have had a major impact on the field. One example in the United States is the Multicenter AIDS Cohort Study (MACS) (Kaslow *et al.*, 1987). Many contributions have emerged from this collaborative group of four centers. The most widely known and discussed reports are those on the prognostic importance of viral load for progression to AIDS and death over a follow-up period of about 10 years (Mellors *et al.*, 1996, 1997). The initial report, based on men in the Pittsburgh cohort (Mellors *et al.*, 1996), and the subsequent report using data for men in all four cohorts (Mellors *et al.*, 1997) had a substantial effect on how patients with HIV were monitored, how treatments were evaluated, and when therapy was initiated. Using stored blood samples, these investigators were able to show a striking relationship between a single baseline measurement of HIV RNA viral load and the rate of CD4+ decline and subsequent progression to AIDS and death. A commentator likened the findings to a speeding locomotive headed toward a ravine where the bridge had collapsed: 'The CD4+ cell count, which has been the best marker of the immediate risk for disease progression, represents the mile marker along the track that indicates the relative distance to the ravine. The HIV viral load represents the speed at which the train is moving down the track' (Saag, 1997). The findings from this study helped form a set of principles about HIV and HIV therapies that were used to guide therapeutic decisions (Report of the NIH Panel, 1998).

The work of the EuroSIDA group has also had a major impact on our understanding of HIV. Their collaborative observational study was initiated in 1994 in several European countries (Lundgren *et al.*, 1997). Over the last decade, numerous reports have been published describing the types of antiretroviral treatments and prophylaxis for opportunistic infections used for patients infected with HIV, the incidence of different opportunistic conditions, rates of virologic failure on HAART, prognostic factors for disease progression, and time trends in morbidity and mortality (Mocroft *et al.*, 2000, 2002, 2003; Phillips *et al.*, 2001; Lundgren *et al.*, 2002). Along with the results from trials and other observational studies, data from EuroSIDA helped establish that use of prophylaxis for opportunistic infections need not be lifelong, as a result of immune function restoration with HAART (Weverling *et al.*, 1999).

Both EuroSIDA and MACS have also provided useful information on the effects of HAART on progression to AIDS and survival at the 'population' level over several years of follow-up (Tarwater *et al.*, 2001; Mocroft *et al.*, 2003). This was important because the two trials that established the efficacy of HAART on clinical outcomes were terminated early, after about six months of follow-up, when approximately a 50 per cent reduction in the hazard for both progression to AIDS and for mortality were found (Hammer *et al.*, 1997; Cameron *et al.*, 1998). Both of these epidemiologic investigations indicated that the effect of HAART compared with combination nucleoside therapy was greater than that observed in the two trials when longer follow-up was obtained. Similar conclusions were reached when rates of progression to AIDS or death were compared in two CPCRA studies – one comparing two protease inhibitors (two different HAART regimens) (Perez *et al.*, 2004) and one comparing combination nucleoside therapy with AZT monotherapy (Saravolatz *et al.*, 1996). Use of the combination nucleoside data from the NuCOMBO study as an historical control for the combined results for the two PI groups in the later trial indicated that the hazard was reduced by 50 per cent in the first six months, consistent with two trials that were terminated early, but that it declined further to a 75 per cent reduction in the hazard after 2–3 years of further follow-up.

Few would argue with the importance of observational studies for describing treatment and disease patterns and for identifying predictors of progression in treated and untreated individuals. A more controversial matter is the role that observational studies should play in understanding the effectiveness of different treatments, e.g. analyses like those mentioned above on the effectiveness of HAART (Sabin and Phillips, 2001). This controversy concerning the use of observational studies, more broadly non-randomized studies, is not unique to HIV research (Green and Byar, 1984; Temple, 1990; Benson and Hartz, 2000; Concato *et al.*, 2000; Pocock and Elbourne, 2000; Ioannidis *et al.*, 2001; Collins and MacMahon, 2001; MacMahon and Collins, 2001).

MacMahon and Collins make the important point that because of the potential for bias, observational studies are best suited for detecting large effects of treatment, not moderate or small effects (MacMahon and Collins, 2001). Byar *et al.* (1990) also identified this as one of five requirements that had to be met before an uncontrolled study of a new drug was carried out instead of a randomized study. Thus, while observational data (non-randomized comparisons) might correctly identify the large effects of PI therapy compared with combination nucleoside regimens, as cited in the examples above, the relative effectiveness of different HAART regimens as starting therapy on progression to AIDS would not be reliably estimated because the differences are likely modest and could be obscured by bias. This is an important principle, which is not widely appreciated – you need a precision instrument (i.e. a randomized trial) to detect small to moderate effects, but a sledge hammer (i.e. an observational study) might do for large effects. Related to this, the impact that even modest treatment effects can have on public health is often either not recognized or ignored. With that recognition, studies that require large numbers of participants followed for many years become a priority. However, not everyone has the energy and patience for such studies. Also, such studies can be, but do not necessarily have to be (see lesson no. 2), expensive. Because we are at a stage of HIV research where incremental improvements in morbidity and mortality are likely to be modest, one should be skeptical of attempts to use observational data to determine the effectiveness of treatments and to address questions about when antiretroviral therapy should be initiated (more on this topic later). Moderate differences in survival over 10 years between a policy of early treatment versus one of deferral could have a major public health impact.

MacMahon and Collins also note that observational studies can play an important role in identifying adverse effects of treatment. The Data Collection on Adverse Events of anti-HIV Drugs (D:A:D) collaboration is a good example of such a study (Friis-Moller *et al.*, 2003). This prospective collaboration of 11 cohort studies, which was part of an initiative by European regulators to better understand and quantify the adverse effects of HAART, was designed to study the relationship of duration of antiretroviral therapy on risk of myocardial infarction. Important features include: (1) a planned sample size and power estimates; (2) procedures for review of outcome measures using standardized procedures; (3) training of study personnel on data collection procedures; and (4) a pre-specified analysis plan. The study had a protocol! It typifies what Bradford Hill was referring to when he proposed that 'observations be made in such a way as to fulfill, as far as possible, experimental requirements' (Hill, 1953).

Currently, the best set of data on the 'when to start' question comes from a pooling of 13 cohort studies (Egger *et al.*, 2002). By pooling several studies, the investigators were able to examine the prognosis of 12 574 patients who were started on HAART at different levels of CD4+ cell count and viral load. Over an average of about two years of follow-up, 1094 patients developed AIDS or died and 344 died. This collaboration is more powerful (has many more events) than other studies from a statistical point of view (Hogg *et al.*, 2001; Opravil *et al.*, 2002; Anastos *et al.*, 2002; Pallela *et al.*, 2003; Ahdieh-Grant *et al.*, 2003; Kaplan *et al.*, 2003). Recall from lesson no. 1, if only modest differences in two treatment strategies are considered plausible, but nevertheless you feel it is important to know if they exist, a large number of events are required to reliably compare them. Only one of the other studies cited had more than 100 events among patients in the groups who initiated therapy with CD4+ counts >200 cells/mm^3 (Kaplan *et al.*, 2003); the others had less than 50 events. However, even in the large ART Collaboration, for the CD4+ cell count strata of most interest – those starting between 200 and 349 cells/mm^3 and those starting when the CD4+ cell count was 350 cells/mm^3 or greater – there was a combined 262 AIDS or death events and 84 deaths.

A few years ago at an NIH workshop on the 'when to start' question, a design that required about 1200 primary events (a trial powered to detect a modest, but important, difference in progression to AIDS or death) was proposed (National Institute of Allergy and Infectious Diseases, 2000). It involved enrolling patients with CD4+ cell counts above 350 cells/mm^3 and beginning treatment immediately in one-half of the patients and deferring treatment in the other half until the CD4+ count dropped to 200 cells/mm^3. In order to obtain 1200 events, it was estimated that about 14 000 patients would have to be enrolled and followed for at least eight years. One reason for mentioning this is to contrast two important statistics between the work of the ART Collaboration and the proposed trial: (1) 262 versus 1200 patients with events; and (2) two versus eight years of follow-up. Quite apart from other concerns about confounding factors and lead-time bias that are present in observational studies like this (more about this later), the largest of the studies so far is too small (there are too few events to rule out important differences in progression between the two CD4+ cell count strata) and follow-up is too short. The number of events can be increased by adding more patients to the collaboration or by extending follow-up. The latter is more important. Because of the concerns about time-limited efficacy due to the accumulation of drug resistant mutations (maybe 5–10 years now instead of 1–2 years with AZT monotherapy) and long-term toxicities, longer follow-up is critical. It is possible that the preferred strategy (starting HAART when the CD4+ count is high versus lower) after 2–3 years of follow-up may be different from the preferred strategy based on 5–10 years of follow-up. Phillips *et al.* (2003) made this same point when discussing this question. In general, the rationale for longer follow-up in observational studies is the same as that for clinical trials that was mentioned in lesson no. 1.

While observational studies have lacked power, some have developed innovative methods for coping with lead-time bias (Pallela *et al.*, 2003; Ahdieh-Grant *et al.*, 2003). These approaches have attempted to deal with the problem that analyses, such as those in the ART Collaboration, are not directly addressing – the question about when to start therapy. A better analysis would identify individuals above 350 cells/mm^3 who are starting treatment and a comparable group above 350 cells/mm^3 who are not, and follow both groups for several years for important outcomes. Outcomes of interest would be counted during the deferral period before starting treatment as well as after starting HAART at a lower CD4+ cell count. 'Lead-time' refers to the time it takes a person to progress to a later stage of disease (from a high CD4+ count to a lower one). That time needs to be considered. As noted under lesson no. 2, with this approach, the analysis is more likely to also partially account for the possibility that deferral may result in better treatments being available at the time treatment is initiated. This is an important part of the 'when to start' question. The availability of more potent treatments and improved skills for using available treatments seems very plausible given the rate at which new treatments have been approved and the rate at which these complex treatments have been introduced into practice. Data from one observational study indicate that the rate of virologic failure associated with HAART has declined between 1996 and 2001, supporting this assumption (Phillips *et al.*, 2003).

If a randomized trial of 'when to start' was to be conducted, multiple outcomes would be identified for comparing the different treatment strategies defined. These would include all-cause mortality, cause-specific mortality, progression to AIDS, specific AIDS-defining events, especially those that are more life threatening (Neaton *et al.*, 1994), and major metabolic and cardiovascular events thought to be associated with HAART. It would also be important to assess quality of life and cost. While such a study might be powered to detect modest differences in all-cause mortality, it would be important to be able to compare groups for both

75

AIDS-related morbidity and mortality and non-AIDS-related morbidity and mortality. One would probably advise a Data Monitoring Committee overseeing the trial not to stop the trial in the first 4–5 years of follow-up because early trends favoring one group might reverse. These design features are mentioned because, to the extent possible, observational studies aiming to address this question should try to mimic the design of the trial. However, a suggestion to carry out an observational study on this question with eight years of follow-up, to carry out interim analyses with attention to control of type I error, and to not report the results until there was proof beyond a reasonable doubt of a difference, might be a hard sell.

In summary, the lesson here is that both randomized trials and observational studies are needed. Because of the interest in low-incidence events, both randomized and observational studies will have to be large. Because long-term effects are of interest, both will also have to be carried out over several years.

Observational studies may be best used to identify uncommon adverse effects of treatment. A cohort study like D:A:D is an excellent prototype. In addition, if data collection were better standardized across HIV research groups, it might be possible to rapidly implement case–control studies to understand factors related to rare adverse events that were systematically collected. Similarly, the case–control approach can be a useful and efficient approach to study the association of measurements made on stored specimens with clinical outcomes.

Like Bradford Hill, the well-known biostatistician Jerry Cornfield appreciated the value of both observational and experimental evidence. He noted: 'If important alternative hypotheses are compatible with available evidence, then the question is unsettled, even if the evidence is experimental. But, if only one hypothesis can explain all the evidence, then the question is settled, even if the evidence is observational' (Cornfield, 1959). Perhaps with larger observational studies with longer follow-up some of the controversies about 'when to start' will be resolved. Presently, there are too many alternatives so the question is unsettled.

Challenges

There is a Gary Larson cartoon that features five guys in a car, one in a clown suit, with a caption that reads 'Deep inside, Brian wondered if the other guys really listened to his ideas or regarded him only as comic relief'. It is not always easy to convince colleagues and funding agencies that randomized studies are needed, especially large, long-term ones. Even when study ideas have been accepted, there are many challenges to overcome. For example,

1. To create lasting, cost-effective infrastructures for conducting trials.
2. To achieve simplicity and cost-effectiveness without jeopardizing trial conduct and patient safety.
3. To recruit and train investigators to participate in collaborative trials.

Challenge No. 1: Creating Lasting, Cost-effective Infrastructures

Creating cost-effective infrastructures to do large trials is a major challenge. Networks like the CPCRA and the Adult AIDS Clinical Trials Network (AACTG) do not have a sufficient number of sites to carry out trials like SMART. Also, because of competing priorities, they might not want to invest heavily in one study, as it might have to be done at the expense of others. It is notable that, of the 10 largest treatment trials conducted to date with sample sizes that range from 1583 to 4150, two were carried out by the AACTG, two by the CPCRA, two largely by pharmaceutical sponsors, and the remaining four by collaborative groups formed to do the study (and not anything else) (Emery *et al.*, 2002; Delta Coordinating Committee, 1996; Volberding *et al.*, 1990; El-Sadr *et al.*, 1999; Hammer *et al.*, 1996; Tambussi *et al.*, 2003; CAESAR Coordinating Committee, 1997; Alpha Coordinating Committee, 1996; Concorde Coordinating Committee, 1994; Gordin *et al.*, 2000). (Trials are listed in order of sample size.)

It was for the reasons mentioned above that a different type of organization was established to conduct the Evaluation of Subcutaneous Proleukin® in a Randomized International Trial (ESPRIT), which is the largest HIV treatment trial to date (Emery *et al.*, 2002). In order to enroll the required 4000 patients quickly, sites were identified in 25 countries for participation – 248 sites eventually enrolled patients. Only investigators interested in the trial question were included. Funding for sites is primarily based on patient enrollment and follow-up. There was less investment in site infrastructure in ESPRIT than there has been for sites in the established networks. To help sites get established to carry out the study, to facilitate local and regional coordination, and to assist with data collection and monitoring, 25 National Trial Coordinating Centers and four Regional Coordinating Centers were established. Models similar to ESPRIT are used for large trials conducted by the pharmaceutical industry; a similar model was also used effectively in the Antihypertensive and Lipid-Lowering Treatment to Prevent Heart Attack Trial (ALLHAT) that was sponsored in large part by the National Heart, Lung and Blood Institute (Wright *et al.*, 2001).

The problem with this approach is that once the trial has been completed, the investigators are no longer funded to carry out further related research. Thus, while this approach to conducting large studies is efficient in the short term, it may not be efficient in the long term if site recruitment and coordinating center establishment have to be repeated again and again. At a meeting in January 2003 organized by the Director of the NIH, the general problem of how clinical research in the US is conducted was a major focus of discussion (Zerhouni, 2003). In the US, there is a need to establish an integrated clinical research system. One suggestion was to create a certified clinical research corps that could collect data on outcomes and quality of care and conduct large clinical trials. For the conduct of large strategic trials, the goal should be to create highly visible mega-networks that hundreds of clinicians, academic-based and otherwise, would want to participate in. Some minimal infrastructure costs should be provided. However, this cannot be too much because as one commentator noted you would be paying for lots of staff that are 'dressed up but with no place to go'.

Some guidance on how to approach the development of cost-effective infra-structures can be obtained from other health care systems. Tognini *et al.* described the framework they used for the GISSI trial of thrombolytic and anticoagulant therapy that they conducted in Italy in patients with a myocardial infarction (Tognini and Bonati, 1986; Tognini *et al.*, 1990). They adopted their whole national health system as their 'research laboratory'. They noted that the frame-work for conducting GISSI was perhaps more interesting than the results of the study. They recognized that scientific investigation within a national health system was a reasonable and cost-efficient approach for obtaining answers to important public health questions. Some features of their organization that are relevant to the establishment of a corps of HIV researchers to perform clinical trials are: (1) provision of education and field training to participating physicians; (2) provision of technical support to sites; and (3) provision of a network of monitors to help with data collection, which was simple by comparison to most HIV studies. Their goal was to change the culture of routine care: 'A trial is no longer perceived as a "foreign" body searching for a place in a busy routine, but is recognized as part of the general framework in which all patients without contraindications belong naturally'.

In order to permit more large HIV studies to be done in a cost-efficient manner, something similar to the model described by Tognini *et al.* is needed. Even though there is not a national health system in the United States, such a model might work if physicians were offered the opportunity to participate in a 'research laboratory' where they could discuss study designs and research strat-egies for addressing important practical questions about HIV care, and where they could enroll their patients in trials considered to be of national and inter-national importance. To be cost-effective, most funding for investigators would come through their enrollment of participants in specific studies. To enable par-ticipation by many physicians, studies would be relatively simple. Key data elem-ents would be standardized and quality assurance efforts would be focused on these key data items. Sites would receive assistance with data collection. Participating clinicians would be able to look to the network not only as place for enrolling patients in protocols but for discussing research methodology. These study characteristics, simplicity and focused standardization and quality assur-ance efforts, would permit participation in HIV research by clinicians in both academic and non-academic settings. It would also permit collaboration with clinicians in other 'research laboratories' in other countries. It could provide a model for how future 'research laboratories' are established in developing countries.

Challenge No. 2: Achieving Simplicity and Cost-effectiveness Without Jeopardizing Trial Conduct and Patient Safety

Simplicity is difficult to achieve in large part of because of regulatory require-ments, oversight mechanisms, and a belief by some that a study should be judged by how much data are collected. The reaction to cases of fraud and lapses in the protection of research participants has generally been more layers of administra-tive oversight, and more data collection and more on-site monitoring. All of these result in more complicated and expensive studies. Some of this is necessary, but much is probably not. It is fair to say that researchers have created the problems but researchers have not been effective in defining efficient systems to prevent fraud and improve safety monitoring and reporting.

Richard Horton, Editor of *The Lancet* summarized public perception of clinical trials in a paper titled 'The clinical trial: deceitful, disputable, unbelievable, unhelpful, and shameful – what next?' (Horton, 2001). In this paper Horton argued for five propositions that he felt undermined the validity of trials. He argued that trials were deceitful because of fraudulent behavior by investigators. Many trials were disputable because of the way they were designed and conducted and, in many cases, because of the way they were reported in journals and in the press (e.g. trial reports emphasized efficacy more than safety and costs). Horton also argued that many trials are unbelievable because of commercial interests and because of the way they were conducted and reported, i.e. the Consolidated Standards of Reporting Trials (CONSORT) guidelines (Begg *et al.*, 1996) were not being followed. The latter concern is related to the discussion under lesson no. 2 – industry sponsors are more likely to design a 'can it work' trial than a 'does it really work' trial. Many trials were considered unhelpful by Horton for related reasons – the authors failed to properly integrate the results of the trial with what was already known about the treatment or disease in the discussion section of their paper and because trial results were communicated to the public in a confusing way.

His fifth proposition was that trials were shameful for taking advantage of popu-lations in resource-poor countries, for using inadequate control groups, for not fully explaining the risk and benefits of treatment to trial participants, and for not adhering to standards of good clinical practice.

Horton concluded his rather depressing review by describing some ways to move forward. One of his recommendations was to encourage trial participants to be more powerful advocates for trials. For this, AIDS research is ahead of the game. As noted in the Introduction, the inclusion of AIDS activists in the devel-opment of the research agenda was perhaps a unique challenge that AIDS researchers faced and largely succeeded at. What better way to influence the public perception of trials than to involve the public in design and evaluation of studies as well as participants. The involvement of the affected community as advocates for clinical trials is probably more evident in AIDS research than in any other area. Activists insisted on being part of the research process in the 1980s. After some initial skepticism and fears, they were embraced. They now are not only powerful advocates for funding of trials by government and industry, but they are also part of protocol teams designing studies and writing summaries of studies as well as trial participants. They are doing their part to make trials less disputable.

Another of his recommendations was to think more critically about the practical methodology of the studies we undertake. Large, long-term trials do not have to be expensive. The simplicity and cost-savings achieved by stripping trials of unnecessary regulatory requirements and ancillary data could result in more studies being done. More research on the practical methodology for conducting studies is needed.

Two areas in need of research are the amount of data collection and extent of on-site monitoring carried out in trials. How does one go about convincing investigators in a trial that too many data are to be collected? Peto suggests that 'the statistician should, at the design stage, cross out most of things that the trial organizer thinks he wants to ask!' (Peto, 1978). This might not work for everyone! However, if completed trials were summarized on how many data were collected and how many were actually used, this may be helpful in arguments to reduce the amount of information collected.

Sampling methods should also be considered for large clinical endpoint trials as many outcomes can be compared between groups with a smaller sample size than that required for the clinical outcomes. In addition, clinical endpoint studies provide an opportunity to perform measurements on those with events and a sample of those who did not experience an event to understand predictors of outcomes. The enhanced efficiency in the use of major endpoints with case–cohort sampling methods has been reviewed (Prentice, 1990).

In general, a trial should not be judged by how much data it collects and the sophistication of the measurements performed. It should be judged by the impact the results have on medical practice and scientific thinking. It is very easy to fall into the bad habit of collecting data because it might be a missed opportunity, or collecting data just in case something unexpected occurs – the 'what if game'. We need to resist that vigorously. Ederer provides a thoughtful discussion of this point and notes that while the prevailing view is often that extra data collection comes with little extra cost, 'the cost may be heavy' (Ederer, 1975).

Horton's observation that trial reports and communications pay more attention to efficacy than safety has been noted by others (Ioannidis and Lau, 2001). We expend extraordinary resources on the collection of safety data and do not report the data adequately. In some cases this is due to how the data were collected. In other cases, data collected under the heading of 'safety' are unnecessary. For example, adverse events of low-grade severity may be important to document in initial studies of antiretroviral drugs. However, in large, strategic trials in which a number of drug combinations may be used over several years of follow-up, collection of such data may be difficult to interpret and may jeopardize the quality of other more important data on morbidity. Improved and more efficient safety monitoring could also be achieved by reviewing and coordinating the efforts by the various groups who assume some of this responsibility. Califf *et al.* made several recommendations for improving safety monitoring and for avoiding duplication of efforts (Califf *et al.*, 2003).

In many trials an independent organization is funded to carry out on-site audits of the data collected by each clinical center. The extent of on-site auditing varies widely in government and industry sponsored trials (Cohen, 1994). While a number of authors have described monitoring and auditing procedures employed and the results of them (Mauer *et al.*, 1985; Weiss *et al.*, 1993; Shapiro and Charrow, 1989), few have considered the cost-effectiveness of independent audits (George, 1998), and none have experimentally evaluated the merits of more versus less data auditing on trial results. Such an experiment was proposed for ESPRIT, but there was reluctance by the NIH to reduce on-site audits to the extent that were proposed. Equipoise on this issue needs to be stimulated. Högel and Gaus (1999) made a strong case that resources might be better targeted at an independent trial instead of independent auditing. Their paper highlights the importance of considering on-site audits as one of many factors in study design and quality assurance to consider for ensuring that the results of trials are accurate.

Challenge No. 3: Recruiting and Training Investigators to Participate in Collaborative Trials

Arthur Kornberg, who won the Nobel Prize for the laboratory synthesis of DNA, speculated that if he had gone into clinical practice he would have collected and analyzed data on one of numerous puzzling questions that clinicians face. He observed 'what a wonderful difference it would make if tens of thousands of physicians could report once in their lifetime how they had reshaped a fact of medical science' (Kornberg, 1989). In order to ensure that thousands do participate in research, we have to do things differently. As noted above, we need to create trial infrastructures which involve more clinicians. We also need improved training programs and better reward systems for clinical researchers who contribute to large clinical trials.

There is a shortage of people to work on clinical trials. More clinical research training programs that emphasize multidisciplinary teams are needed. The training needs to be more than didactic. Training programs must include a strong practical component where individuals with different training (medical specialists, biostatisticians, pharmacists, ethicists) prepare research protocols together. The goal should be to strengthen skills in both research methodology and in collaboration. This might be accomplished by creating infrastructures at research universities that mimic, on a smaller scale, what is done in the trial networks. In a similar vein, DeMets called for a systematic plan for training that would ensure the next generation of clinical trialists are available in adequate numbers to meet the challenges. He noted that adequate curriculum and incentives for delivering the training do not currently exist (DeMets, 2002).

It is difficult to attract young physician-scientists as investigators in large, long-term clinical trials. Donald Fredrickson, former Director of the NIH, expressed it well over 30 years ago: 'Clinical trials lack glamour, they strain our resources and patience, and they protract to excruciating limits the moment of truth' (Fredrickson, 1968). This is not the way you would want to start your conversation with a potential clinical researcher. Of course, Fredrickson realized trials were indispensable. Nevertheless, building a workforce to carry out the trials will be difficult. Many academic promotion systems require strong evidence of scholarly achievement, which may be difficult to achieve as an investigator in a large trial (Remington, 1979).

Summary

Substantial advances have been made in our understanding of HIV and treatments for it. There are many potent treatment combinations that significantly prolong disease-free survival for individuals with advanced HIV (CD4+ <200 cells/mm^3 or AIDS). Optimizing this treatment through more head-to-head trials of potent regimens and providing it to eligible individuals must be a priority in the developing and developed world. Our knowledge base about treatment of participants with earlier HIV disease is expanding. However, given the known toxicities associated with treatment and the cost, further research is needed on when to treat. In the coming years, research on methods for sparing treatment to avoid toxicities without increasing risk of AIDS events or permanent immune system damage must also be a priority.

Given the millions infected with HIV around the world, even modest improvements in our treatment success will have a substantial public health impact. Large randomized trials will be required to identify these modest improvements. To rapidly carry out these trials and to bring state of the art treatments to the developing world, the global research effort on HIV has to expand. This expansion has already occurred in areas of HIV prevention. With the expanding availability of antiretroviral treatment, it should be possible to expand it for HIV treatment research.

Several years ago Richard Remington, a well-known biostatistician and health administrator, commenting on cardiovascular research, noted that both basic science and applied research were needed; both research on prevention and treatment were needed; and that research on the 'need to know (research on mechanisms of disease) and the need to take action (intervention in the individual and community to control disease' were important (Remington, 1982). He felt that arguing for one type of research at the expense of another would defeat the goal of controlling cardiovascular disease. This is true today in HIV research. A case can be made both for short-term and long-term studies, both pragmatic and explanatory trials, and both observational and randomized studies. All are needed, in resource-rich and resource-poor countries, to control HIV disease.

There are many challenges to overcome in order to more efficiently carry out large, international trials. Of course, the challenges cited in this chapter are minor compared to the challenges of providing effective treatment and prevention programs to the millions who are infected and who are at risk for infection in resource-poor countries. Many of the pragmatic research questions mentioned in lesson no. 2 can be addressed by collaborations between research-rich and resource-poor countries. Joint participation in research would be an excellent way of training much needed HIV researchers in the developing world. Furthermore, research in other areas has shown that familiarization and personal experience with treatments in trials is likely to result in more rapid adoption in routine practice if the treatment is found to be effective (Ketley and Woods, 1993).

Participation in research studies is considered good by most patients, and not just because of access to new and better treatments. One study carried out among patients who had survived a myocardial infarction found that the additional medical monitoring and personal awareness/reassurance received were considered more important than physical improvement (Mattson *et al.*, 1985). Likewise, one of the reasons Gifford *et al.* (2002) argued that it was important to eliminate the disparities by race and ethnic group for access to HIV research was because participating patients often received case management and other resources as well as primary care by participating in research. Thus, there are many reasons for participating in HIV research besides access to new treatments.

In summary, substantial advances were made in our knowledge of HIV pathogenesis and in HIV treatments during the last decade of the twentieth century. During the first decade of the twenty-first century we should see the results of a number of studies aimed at optimizing the use of the available treatments that will further advance our knowledge base. With this information and the efforts, which have begun to build the capacity to do research in many more places around the world, many more individuals will be able to participate in the next generation of research studies. This will be good for those trial participants for the reasons mentioned above. Since the participation by many more in research will result in more rapid answers to research questions, future participants will also benefit.

References

Ahdieh-Grant L, Yamashita TE, Phair JP, Detels R *et al.* (2003) When to initiate highly active antiretroviral therapy: a cohort approach. *Am J Epidemiol* 157: 738–46.

Alpha Coordinating Committee (1996) European/Australian randomised double-blind trial of two doses of didanosine in zidovudine-intolerant patients with symptomatic disease. *AIDS* 10: 867–80.

Anastos K, Barron Y, Miotti P, Weiser B *et al.* (2002) Risk of progression to AIDS or death in women infected with HIV-1 initiating highly active antiretroviral treatment at different stages of disease. *Arch Intern Med* 162: 1973–80.

Barrett-Conor E (1979) Infectious and chronic diseases epidemiology: separate and unequal? *Am J Epidemiol* 109: 245–9.

Begg C, Cho M, Eastwood S, Horton R *et al.* (1996) Improving the quality of reporting of randomized controlled trials. The Consort Statement. *JAMA* 276: 637–9.

Benson K, Hartz AJ (2000) A comparison of observational studies and randomized controlled trials. *New Engl J Med* 342: 1878–86.

Buyse M (1993) Regulatory versus public health requirements in clinical trials. *Drug Infect J* 27: 977–84.

Byar DP, Schoenfeld DA, Green SB, Amato DA *et al.* (1990) Design considerations for AIDS trials. *N Engl J Med* 323: 1343–8.

CAESAR Coordinating Committee (1997) Randomised trial of addition of lamivudine or lamivudine plus loviride to zidovudine-containing regimens for patients with HIV-1 infection: the CAESAR trial. *Lancet* 349: 1413–21.

Califf RM, Kramer JM (1998) What have we learned from the calcium channel blocker controversy? *Circulation* 97: 1529–31.

Califf RM, Harrelson-Woodlief L, Topol EJ (1990) Left ventricular ejection fraction may not be useful as an endpoint of thrombolytic therapy comparative trials. *Circulation* 82: 1847–53.

Califf RM, Morse MA, Wittes J, Goodman SN *et al.* (2003) Toward protecting the safety of participants in clinical trials. *Controlled Clin Trials* 24: 256–71.

Cameron DW, Heath-Chiozzi M, Danner S *et al.* (1998) Randomized placebo-controlled trial of ritonavir in advanced disease. *Lancet* 351: 543–9.

Cochrane AL (1989) *Effectiveness and Efficiency. Random Reflections on Health Services.* Cambridge: The Nuffield Provincial Hospitals Trust, Cambridge University Press.

Cohen J (1994) Clinical trial monitoring: hit or miss? *Science* 264: 1534–7.

Cohen J (1997) AIDS trials ethics questioned. *Science* 276: 520–3.

Collins R, MacMahon S (2001) Reliable assessment of the effects of treatment on mortality and major morbidity, I: clinical trials. *Lancet* 357: 373–80.

Concato J, Shah N, Horwitz RI (2000) Randomized, controlled trials, observational studies, and the hierarchy of evidence. *N Engl J Med* 342: 1887–92.

Concorde Coordinating Committee (1994) Concorde: MRC/ANRS randomised double-blind controlled trial of immediate and deferred zidovudine in symptom-free HIV infection. *Lancet* 343: 871–81.

Cornfield J (1959) Principles of research. *Am J Ment Defic* 64: 240–52.

De Gruttola V, Fleming T, Lin DY, Coombs R (1997) Perspective: Validating surrogate markers – are we being naïve? *J Infect Dis* 175: 237–46.

De Gruttola VG, Clax P, DeMets DL *et al.* (2001) Considerations in the evaluation of surrogate endpoints in clinical trials: summary of a National Institutes of Health workshop. *Controlled Clin Trials* 22: 485–502.

Delta Coordinating Committee (1996) Delta: a randomised double-blind controlled trial comparing combinations of zidovudine plus didanosine or zalciabine with zidovudine alone in HIV-infected individuals. *Lancet* 348: 283–91.

DeMets DL (2002) Clinical trials in the new millennium. *Stat Med* 21: 2779–87.

Ederer F (1975) Practical problems in collaborative clinical trials. *Am J Epidemiol* 102: 111–18.

Egger M, Neaton JD, Phillips AN, Davey Smith G (1994) (Letter to the Editor) Concorde trial of immediate versus deferred zidovudine. *Lancet* 353: 1355.

Egger M, May M, Chene G, Phillips AN *et al.* (2002) and the ART Collaboration. Prognosis of HIV-1 infected patients starting highly active antiretroviral therapy: a collaborative analysis of prospective studies. *Lancet* 360: 119–29.

Ellenberg SS, Finkelstein DM, Schoenfeld DA (1992) Statistical issues arising in AIDS clinical trials (with Discussion). *J Am Stat Assoc* 87: 562–83.

El-Sadr W, Capps L (1992) The challenge of minority recruitment in clinical trials for AIDS. *JAMA* 267: 954–7.

El-Sadr WM, Luskin-Hawk R, Yurik TM, Walker J *et al.* (1999) A randomized trial of daily and thrice-weekly trimethoprim-sulfamethoxazole for the prevention of Pneumocystis carinii pneumonia in human immunodeficiency virus-infected persons. *Clin Infect Dis* 29: 775–83.

Emery S, Abrams DI, Cooper DA, Darbyshire JH *et al.* (2002) The evaluation of subcutaneous Proleukin® (interleukin-2) in a randomized international trial: rationale, design, and methods of ESPRIT. *Controlled Clin Trials* 23: 198–220.

Fischl MA, Richman DD, Grieco MH *et al.* (1987) The efficacy of azidothymidine (AZT) in the treatment of patients with AIDS and AIDS-related complex: a double-blind, placebo-controlled trial. *N Engl J Med* 317: 185–91.

Fischl MA, Richman DD, Hansen N *et al.* (1990) The safety and efficacy of zidovudine (AZT) in the treatment of subjects with mildly symptomatic human immunodeficiency virus type I (HIV) infection: a double-blind, placebo-controlled trial. *Ann Intern Med* 112: 727–37.

Fleming TR, DeMets DL (1996) Surrogate end points in clinical trials: are we being misled? *Ann Intern Med* 125: 605–13.

Fredrickson DS (1968) The field trial: some thoughts on the indispensable ordeal. *Bull NY Acad Med* 44: 985–93.

Freiman JA, Chalmers TC, Smith H, Jr, Kuebler RR (1978) The importance of beta, the type II error and sample size in the design and interpretation of the randomized control trial. *N Engl J Med* 299: 690–4.

Friedland GH (1990) Early treatment for HIV: The time has come. *N Engl J Med* 322: 1000–2.

Friis-Moller N, Sabin CA, Weber R *et al.* for the Data Collection on Adverse Events of Anti-HIV Drugs (DAD) Study Group (2003) Combination antiretroviral therapy and the risk of myocardial infarction. *N Engl J Med* 349: 1993–2003.

George SL (1998) Clinical trials audit and quality control. In: Armitage P, Colton T, eds. *Encyclopedia of Biostatistics*. Chichester: John Wiley & Sons.

Gifford AL, Cunnningham WE, Heslin KC *et al.* (2002) Participation in research and access to experimental treatments by HIV-infected patients. *N Engl J Med* 346: 1373–82.

Gilbert PB, DeGruttola V, Hammer SM, Kuritzkes DR (2001) Virologic and regimen termination surrogate end points in AIDS clinical trials. *JAMA* 285: 777–84.

Gilbert PB, DeGruttola VG, Hudgens MG *et al.* (2003) What constitutes efficacy for a human immunodeficiency virus vaccine that ameliorates viremia: issues involving surrogate end points in phase 3 trials. *J Infect Dis* 188: 179–93.

Gordin F, Chaisson RE, Matts JP, Miller C *et al.* (2000) Rifampin and pyrazinamide vs isoniazid for prevention of tuberculosis in HIV-infected persons. *JAMA* 283: 1445–50.

Graham NMH (1994) Letter to the editor. *Lancet* 343: 1355–6.

Green S (1992) Comment on statistical issues arising in AIDS clinical trials. *J Am Stat Assoc* 87: 571–2.

Green S, Byar DP (1984) Using observational data from registries to compare treatments: the fallacy of omnimetrics. *Stat Med* 3: 361–70.

Guidance for Industry (2002) Antiretroviral drugs using plasma HIV RNA measurements – clinical considerations for accelerated and traditional approval. US Department of

Health and Human Services. Food and Drug Administration. Center for Drug Evaluation and Research (CDER), October, www.fda.gov/cder/guidance/

Halloran ME, Longini IM, Jr., Struchiner CJ (1999) Design and interpretation of vaccine field studies. *Epidemiol Rev* 21: 73–88.

Hammer SM, Katzenstein DA, Hughes MD, Gundacker H *et al.* (1996) A trial comparing nucleoside monotherapy with combination therapy in HIV-infected adults with CD4 cell counts from 200 to 500 per cubic millimeter. *N Engl J Med* 335: 1081–90.

Hammer SM, Squires KE, Hughes MD *et al.* (1997) A controlled trial of two nucleoside analogues plus indinavir in persons with human immunodeficiency virus infection and CD4 cell counts of 200 per cubic millimeter or less. *N Engl J Med* 337: 725–33.

Hill AB (1953) Observation and experiment. *N Engl J Med* 248: 995–1001.

HIV Trialists' Collaborative Group (1999) Zidovudine, didanosine, and zalcitabine in the treatment of HIV infection: meta-analyses of the randomised evidence. *Lancet* 353: 2014–25.

Högel J, Gaus W (1999) The procedure of new drug application and the philosophy of critical rationalism or the limits of quality of assurance with good clinical practice. *Controlled Clin Trials* 20: 511–18.

Hogg RS, Yip B, Chan KJ, Wood E *et al.* (2001) Rates of disease progression by baseline CD4 cell count and viral load after initiating triple-drug therapy. *JAMA* 286: 2568–77,

Horton R (2001) The clinical trial: deceitful, disputable, unbelievable, unhelpful, and shameful – what next? *Controlled Clin Trials* 22: 593–604.

Hughes MD (2002) Evaluating surrogate endpoints. *Controlled Clin Trials* 23: 703–7.

Ioannidis JP, Lau J (2001) Completeness of safety reporting in randomized trials: an evaluation of 7 medical areas. *JAMA* 285: 437–43.

Ioannidis JPA, Haidich A, Pappa M, Pantazis N *et al.* (2001) Comparison of evidence of treatment effects in randomized and non-randomized studies. *JAMA* 286: 821–30.

Kaplan JE, Hanson DL, Cohn DL, Karon J *et al.* (2003) When to begin highly active anti-retroviral therapy? Evidence supporting initiation of therapy at CD4+ lymphocyte counts <350 cells/μL. *Clin Infec Dis* 37: 951–8.

Kaslow RA, Ostrow DG, Detels R, Phair JP, Polk BF, Rinaldo CR (1987) The Multicenter AIDS Cohort Study: rationale, organization, and selected characteristics of the participants. *Am J Epidemiol* 126: 310–18.

Ketley D, Woods KL (1993) Impact of clinical trials on clinical practice: example of thrombolysis for acute myocardial infarction. *Lancet* 342: 891–4.

Kirk O, Pedersen C, Law M *et al.* (2002) Analysis of virological efficacy in trials of anti-retroviral regimens: drawbacks of not including viral load measurements after premature discontinuation of therapy. *Antiviral Ther* 7: 39–48.

Kornberg AR (1989) *For Love of Enzymes. The Odyssey of a Biochemist.* Cambridge, MA: Harvard University Press.

Lange J (1997) Current problems and the future of antiretroviral drug trials. *Science* 276: 548–50.

Lawrence J, Mayers DL, Huppler-Hullsiek K, Collins G *et al.* (2003) Structured treatment interruption in patients with multidrug-resistant human immunodeficiency virus. *N Engl J Med* 349: 837–46.

Lundgren JD, Phillips AN, Vella S, Katlama C *et al.* (1997) Regional differences in use of antiretroviral agents and primary prophylaxis in 3122 European HIV-infected patients. *J Acquir Immune Defic Syndr Hum Retrovirol* 16: 1534–600.

Lundgren JD, Mocroft A, Gatell JM, Lederberger B *et al.* (2002) EuroSIDA Study Group. A clinically prognostic scoring system for patients receiving highly active antiretroviral therapy: results from the EuroSIDA study. *J Infect Dis* 185: 178–87.

MacArthur RD, Chen L, Mayers DL, Besch CL *et al.* (2001) The rationale and design of the CPCRA (Terry Beirn Community Programs for Clinical Research on AIDS) 058 FIRST (Flexible Initial Retrovirus Suppressive Therapies) Trial. *Controlled Clin Trials* 22: 176–90.

Machin D, Stenning SP, Parmar MKB *et al.* (1997) Thirty years of Medical Research Council randomized trials in solid tumours. *Clin Oncol* 9: 100–14.

MacMahon S, Collins R (2001) Reliable assessment of the effects of treatment on mortality and major morbidity, II. Observational studies. *Lancet* 357: 455–62.

Marshall E (1989) Quick release of AIDS drugs. *Science* 245: 345–7.

Mattson ME, Curb JD, McArdle R (1985) Participation in a clinical trial: the patient's point of view. *Controlled Clin Trials* 6: 156–67.

Mauer JK, Hoth DF, Macfarlane DK *et al.* (1985) Site visit monitoring program of the clinical cooperative groups: results of the first 3 years. *Cancer Treat Rep* 69: 1180–7.

Mellors JW, Rinaldo CR, Gupta P, White RM, Todd JA, Kingsley LA (1996) Prognosis in HIV-1 infection predicted by the quantity of virus in plasma. *Science* 272: 1167–70.

Mellors JW, Munoz A, Giorgi JV, Margolick JB *et al.* (1997) Plasma viral load and CD4+ lymphocytes as prognostic markers of HIV-1 infection. *Ann Intern Med* 126: 946–54.

Miller V, Rottmann C, Hertogs K, Larder BA *et al.* (1999) Mega-HAART, resistance and drug holidays (Abstract 30). Program and Abstracts for the 2nd International Workshop on Salvage Therapy for HIV infection, Toronto. *Antivir Ther* 4: 223–31.

Mocroft A, Katlama C, Johnson AM, Pradier C *et al.* (2000) for the EuroSIDA Study Group. AIDS across Europe, 1994–98: the EuroSIDA study. *Lancet* 356: 291–6.

Mocroft A, Brettle R, Kirk O, Blaxhult A *et al.* (2002) EuroSIDA study group. Changes in the cause of death among HIV positive subjects across Europe: results from the EuroSIDA study. *AIDS* 16: 163–71.

Mocroft A, Lederberger B, Katlama C, Kirk O *et al.* for the EuroSIDA Study Group (2003) Decline in AIDS and death rates in the EuroSIDA study: an observational study. *Lancet* 362: 22–9.

Moher D, Dullberg CS, Well GA (1994) Statistical power, sample size, and their reporting in randomized controlled trials. *JAMA* 272: 122–4.

National Institute of Allergy and Infectious Diseases (2000) Division of Acquired Immunodeficiency Syndrome (DAIDS). *Summary: When-to-Start Antiretroviral Therapy Workshop*, September. www.niaid.nih.gov/daids/therapeutics/news/antiretroviral.htm

Neaton JD, Wentworth DN (1993) Statistical design considerations for a large, simple trial (LST) on timing of combination nucleoside treatment. *Joint Statistical Meetings*, August, San Francisco, CA.

Neaton JD, Wentworth DN, Rhame F, Hogan C, Abrams DI, Deyton L (1994) Considerations in choice of a clinical endpoint for AIDS clinical trials. *Stat Med* 13: 2107–25.

Opravil M, Lederberger B, Furrer H, Hirschel B *et al.* (2002) Clinical efficacy of early initiation of HAART in patients with asymptomatic HIV infection and CD4 cell count >350 × 106/l. *AIDS* 16: 1371–81.

Pallela FJ, Deloria-Knoll M, Chiel JS, Moorman AC *et al.* (2003) Survival benefit of initiating antiretroviral therapy in HIV-infected persons in different CD4+ cell strata. *Ann Intern Med* 138: 620–6.

Panel on Clinical Practices for Treatment of HIV Infection (2003) http://AIDSinfo.nih.gov (accessed July 2003).

Perez G, MacArthur R, Walmsley S *et al.* (2004) A randomized clinical trial comparing nelfinavir and ritonavir in patients with advanced HIV disease (CPCRA 042/CTN 102). *HIV Clin Trials* 5: 7–18.

Peto R (1978) Clinical trial methodology. *Biomedicine* 28: 24–36.

Phillips AN, Staszewski S, Weber R, Kirk O *et al.* (2001) for the Swiss HIV Cohort Study, the Frankfurt HIV Clinic Cohort, and the EuroSIDA Study Group. HIV viral load response to antiretroviral therapy according to the baseline CD4 cell count and viral load. *JAMA* 286: 2560–97.

Phillips AN, Lepri AC, Lampe F, Johnson M, Sabin CA (2003) When should antiretroviral therapy be started for HIV infection? Interpreting the evidence from observational studies. *AIDS* 17: 1863–9.

Pocock SJ, Elbourne DR (2000) Randomized trials or observational tribulations? *N Engl J Med* 342: 1907–9.

Pozniak A (1998) Surrogacy in HIV-1 clinical trials. *Lancet* 351: 536–7.

Prentice RL (1990) Opportunities for enhancing efficiency and reducing cost in large scale disease prevention trials: a statistical perspective. *Stat Med* 9: 161–72.

Reisler RB, Han C, Burman WJ *et al.* (2003) Grade 4 events are as important as AIDS events in the era of HAART. *J Acquir Immune Defic Syndr* 34: 379–86.

Remington RD (1979) Problems of university-based scientists associated with clinical trials. *Clin Pharmacol Ther* 25: 662–5.

Remington RD (1982) Lewis A. Connor Memorial Lecture. Choices that must not be made. *Circulation* 66: 481–6.

Report of the NIH Panel to define principles of therapy of HIV infection (1998) *Ann Intern Med* 128: 1057–78.

Robbins GK, De Gruttola V, Shafer RW *et al.* (2003) Comparison of sequential three-drug regimens as initial therapy for HIV-1 infections. *N Engl J Med* 349: 2293–303.

Saag MS (1997) Use of viral load in clinical practice: Back to the future. *Ann Intern Med* 126: 983–5.

Sabin CA, Phillips AN (2001) Treatment comparisons in HIV infection: the benefits and limitations of observational cohort studies. *J Antimicrobial Chemother* 47: 371–5.

Saravolatz LD, Winslow DL, Collins G, Hodges JS *et al.* (1996) Zidovudine alone or in combination with didanosine or zalcitabine in HIV-infected patients with the acquired immunodeficiency syndrome or fewer than 200 CD4 cells per cubic millimeter. *N Engl J Med* 335: 1099–106.

Schwartz D, Lellouch J (1967) Explanatory and pragmatic attitudes in therapeutical trials. *J Chronic Dis* 20: 637–48.

Shafer RW, Smeaton LM, Robbins GK *et al.* (2003) Comparison of four-drug regimens and pairs of sequential three-drug regimens as initial therapy for HIV-1 infection. *N Engl J Med* 349: 2304–15.

Shapiro MF, Charrow RP (1989) The role of data audits in detecting scientific misconduct. *JAMA* 261: 2505–11.

SMART trial begins (2002) AIDS Patient Care STDS. www.smart-trial.org (accessed 1 September 2004).

Smeaton LM, Degruttola V, Robbins GK, Shafer RW (2001) ACTG (AIDS Clinical Trials Group) 384: A strategy trial comparing consecutive treatments for HIV-1. *Controlled Clin Trials* 22: 142–59.

Staessen JA, Bianchi G (2003) Registration of trials and protocols. *Lancet* 362: 1009–10.

Tambussi G, Levy Y, Mitsuyasu R *et al.* (2003) CD4 count increases in patients with CD4 counts of 50–300 treated with intermittent IL-2: immunologic results from the Study of IL-2 in Combination with Active Antiretroviral Therapy (SILCAAT) Trial. Paper presented at the 8th European AIDS Conference, 25–29 October 2003, Warsaw, Poland.

Tarwater PM, Mellors J, Gore ME *et al.* (2001) Methods to assess population effectiveness of therapies in human immunodeficiency virus incident and prevalent cohorts. *Am J Epidemiol* 154: 675–81.

Temple R (1990) Problems in the use of large data sets to assess effectiveness. *Int J Techn Assess Health Care* 6: 211–19.

The D:A:D Study Group (2004) Antiretroviral combination treatment and risk of myocardial infarction. *N Engl J Med* (in press).

The INITIO Co-ordinating Committee (2001) An open-label randomized trial to evaluate different therapeutic strategies of combination therapy in HIV-1 infection: design, rationale, and methods of the Initio Trial. *Controlled Clin Trials* 22: 160–75.

Tognini G, Bonati M (1986) Second-generation clinical pharmacology. *Lancet* 2: 1028–9.

Tognini G, Franzosi MG, Garattini S, Maggioni A *et al.* (1990) The case of GISSI in changing the attitudes and practice of Italian cardiologists. *Stat Med* 9: 17–27.

Tunis SR, Stryer DB, Clancy CM (2003) Practical clinical trials. Increasing the value of clinical research for decision making in clinical and health policy. *JAMA* 290: 1624–32.

Volberding PA, Lagakos SW, Koch MA *et al.* (1990) Zidovudine in asymptomatic human immunodeficiency virus infection: a controlled trial in persons with fewer than 500 CD4-positive cells per cubic millimeter. *N Engl J Med* 322: 941–9.

Walmsley S, Bernstein B, King M *et al.* (2002) Lopinavir-ritonavir versus nelfinavir for the initial treatment of HIV infection. *N Engl J Med* 346: 2039–46.

Ware JH (2003) Interpreting incomplete data in studies of diet and weight loss. *N Engl J Med* 348: 2136–7.

Weiss RB, Vogelzand NJ, Peterson BA *et al.* (1993) A successful system of scientific data audits for clinical trials. *JAMA* 270: 459–64.

Weverling Gj, Mocroft A, Lederberger B *et al.* (1999) Discontinuation of *Pneumocystis carinii* pneumonia prophylaxis after start of highly active antiretroviral therapy in HIV-1 infection. EuroSIDA Study Group. *Lancet* 353: 1293–8.

Wright JT, Cushman WC, Davis BR, Barzilay J *et al.* (2001) The Antihypertensive and Lipid-Lowering Treatment to Prevent Heart Attack Trial (ALLHAT): clinical center recruitment experience. *Controlled Clin Trials* 22: 659–73.

Yusuf S, Collins R, Peto R (1984) Why do we need some large, simple randomized trials? *Stat Med* 3: 409–20.

Zerhouni E (2003) Medicine. The NIH roadmap. *Science* 302: 63–72.

The Public Health Response to HIV/AIDS: What Have We Learned?

4

Mitchell H Katz
Director, San Francisco Public Health Department, University of California, San Francisco, USA

Mitchell H Katz, MD is the former Chief of Research and Director of the AIDS Office for the City and County of San Francisco and former Chief of Research for its AIDS Office. He is Professor of Medicine, Epidemiology and Biostatistics at the University of California, San Francisco. Dr. Katz is a graduate of Yale University and Harvard Medical School and has published extensively in the fields of epidemiology and HIV/AIDS. He initiated a publicly funded needle exchange in San Francisco that now exchanges 2 million dirty needles for 2 million clean needles a year, and created the first county-based postexposure prophylaxis for sexual and injection drug use exposures.

When trying to resolve a difficult situation in my current role as Director of the San Francisco Department of Public Health, I often ask myself: 'How did we do it at the AIDS Office?' The fact that seven years after leaving the AIDS Office to become Director of the Department, I still draw heavily on my six years in that office says a great deal about how AIDS energized and revolutionized public health.

Building San Francisco's AIDS Program

San Francisco was hit early and hard by the AIDS epidemic. Along with New York City and Los Angeles, it was one of the first cities to diagnose AIDS cases, but compared with these other cities, it experienced a much greater burden of disease because it had a markedly smaller population with a much higher concentration of gay and bisexual men. By 1983, a disease that had been unheard of just two years earlier had already affected 469 people in San Francisco and killed 182 of them. In a city of less than 750 000 inhabitants with a population of gay and bisexual men of approximately 58 000, AIDS had become the dominant issue.

Another major way in which San Francisco was different from other cities was the markedly greater political muscle of the gay community. In 1977 San Francisco became the first American city to elect an openly gay Supervisor/City Councilperson to office, Harvey Milk. When he was fatally shot, along with pro-gay Mayor George Moscone, in 1978, it further galvanized the gay community. A Milk supporter and an openly gay man, Harry Britt, was appointed by then Mayor Dianne Feinstein. He won re-election in 1979. Since that time San Francisco has always had at least one openly gay member on its Board of Supervisors; at times there have been as many as three gay and lesbian members of the 11 member body.

The political power of the gay community led to a very proactive approach towards AIDS by the San Francisco Health Department. The community recognized how serious a threat AIDS was, and clamored for the rapid development of services. At first the Department's response to AIDS was primarily through the Bureau of Disease Control, where the epidemiology staff tracked the epidemic. But as the need for services and prevention intervention efforts became paramount, the San Francisco Department of Health created the AIDS Office in 1983 with eight staff members. The Department decided to create a separate AIDS Office primarily because the rest of the Department could not move fast enough to handle the tremendous needs of this emerging infection. By the time I became Director of the Office in 1992, the Office had grown to about 90 staff members and had a budget of US$43 million. When I left the Office in 1997, the budget was up to US$73 million and over 100 people worked there.

Staff were initially drawn to work in the AIDS Office because they believed in the dual missions of the program: to care for HIV-infected people and to prevent others from becoming infected. The *esprit de corps* of the office was to work till the job was done, even if that meant 100-hour weeks. Being told that something could not be done in the county system was seen as a challenge and not as a deterrent; achieving the bureaucratically impossible task was a rite of passage for each staff member.

Beyond the work ethic, the Office developed several principles of how to do its job, in particular the importance of not making decisions in the traditional governmental way but rather establishing methods for participatory decision-making with and within the community. This has now become the dominant paradigm in the Department as a whole. For example, when we wanted to provide a more coordinated pre-hospital care system in San Francisco for residents calling 911, we convened a series of meetings in 1995 with Health Department paramedics, firefighters, private ambulance providers, union leaders, emergency room doctors and nurses, and citizen representatives. For many of the participants, the philosophy of inclusiveness and the methods of consensus building that we had practiced regularly at the AIDS Office for several years, were new. Committee members were surprised at the willingness of the Department to let the process choose the new configuration for pre-hospital care, and even more delighted when they found they could reach consensus, despite several years of bickering, about the best way to configure services.

In addition to changing the decision-making paradigm, the AIDS epidemic broadened our view of the service continuum needed by clients. In fact, it was largely based on our success in providing supportive housing (i.e. housing with on-site supportive services such as case management, substance treatment) for people with AIDS, that our health department developed a supportive housing program for people with other medical illnesses. We have found that using a supportive housing model we have been able to take people suffering from mental illness, substance abuse, and other chronic illnesses (e.g. diabetes, chronic obstructive pulmonary disease) directly from the street and place them. Because this group has high medical costs when they are homeless, we have found supportive housing programs to be extremely cost effective: a month of housing costs less than a single day in our acute care hospital. The programs have also been able to retain two-thirds of clients in housing for two years or more.

The AIDS epidemic invigorated community mobilization and empowerment as prevention strategies. We have found these strategies helpful in a number of areas within the Department. For example, we have worked with elders and disabled people to develop ways of increasing pedestrian safely (i.e. bubble-out curbs at corners that shorten walking distances across intersections, lights that count down the time that people have to reach the sidewalk). Pushing the envelope further, our health department has mobilized injection drug users to learn how to give CPR and administer Narcan to shooting partners who overdose on heroin.

Many of the public health lessons have had national impacts on medical care for HIV/AIDS and other diseases. For example, the community mobilization around AIDS resulted in the Food and Drug Administration (FDA) speeding drug approvals for all types of drugs. The AIDS epidemic has also brought us a new type of advocacy, one that is not always polite, but often effective in influencing local and national politics.

These major changes in public health brought about by the AIDS epidemic are listed in Table 4.1 and discussed in greater detail below.

Decision-Making

The AIDS epidemic has had a major impact on how decisions are made within public health. Prior to the epidemic, the major paradigm in both public health and medicine was the 'expert/doctor' telling the 'patient/client/community member'

Table 4.1   Lessons from AIDS for public health.

Decision-making process	Share power with the community
	Involve affected people in all decision-making bodies
	Make certain that decision-making groups reflect the diversity of the problem
	Obtain and use data to make decisions
Service needs	Broad continuum of care including non-medical services and alternative medicine
	Case management for disenfranchised populations or people navigating complicated service delivery systems
	Need for cultural competency in all aspects of service delivery
	Importance of privacy
Disease prevention model	Limitations of traditional public health approach
	Importance of health education, health promotion, community mobilization, and community empowerment models
Advocacy	Affected people are the most effective advocates
	Single-issue advocacy works
	Advocacy does not have to be polite

what to do. This was not a paradigm that would have ever been successful in handling the AIDS epidemic.

The community first hit by AIDS was young gay men in urban areas. Having recently won greater acceptance on a societal level, gay men were not willing to accept, without questioning, the pronouncements of pubic health and medical leaders. Further, because AIDS was a new disease the public health and medical 'experts' really knew little more about it than members of the gay community, who were seeing first hand the devastation it caused. Some community-based non-professionals were rapidly developing their own theories, often closer to the truth than those of the scientific community, on the causes of AIDS.

Finally, because the prevention of HIV required community members to make behavioral changes voluntarily, the traditional public health approaches to handling epidemics – case finding, case treatment, vaccination, isolation – were not helpful. Instead, ways of engaging the community to support norms of safe sex were needed.

The AIDS epidemic has proven that the best way of gaining the support of a community is actively to involve them in the decision-making process. This requires 'giving up' power, something many government bureaucrats are loathed to do. But our experience has been that by giving up power, power is gained – the power to forge consensus solutions that marshal government and community forces behind the same mission.

The first step in shared decision-making is creating a panel of stakeholders. In the case of the AIDS epidemic, this meant individuals infected with the virus, their friends and family, advocates, service providers, funders, and government officials. Key to the success of these panels is including substantial (rather than token) membership of the affected community. We strove to have at least a third of individuals serving on each committee to be people living with HIV/AIDS.

Because the AIDS epidemic represents several intertwining epidemics it was equally important to make sure that all groups were represented. The needs of white gay men were different from those of gay men of color, heterosexual drug users, women who contracted HIV from their sexual partners, transgendered individuals, and youth. All needed to be included.

Once constituted, the community panel must be given a clear charge (what is it you want them to do?) and a clear understanding of what will happen to their recommendations. Our experience has been that community groups can accept that their recommendations are advisory, or subject to veto by elected officials, as long as the process is made clear and is respected. Having the group elect a chair helps to empower the group members. Often having co-chairs from distinct constituencies (one from the affected community, one from government) helps to establish the principles of collaborative decision-making.

Once you have the right people around the table and they have been given a clear charge, you must provide them with the necessary data to make good decisions. In the absence of data people will argue based on their opinions and prior experience. Conversely, providing accurate data turns contentious meetings into productive, consensus-building dialogue. This is especially true when allocation of financial resources is at stake. We have devoted a lot of effort to providing our decision-making bodies with accurate data on the number of people living with HIV/AIDS, their service needs, and the number of people at risk for HIV and their risks for seroconversion.

Not that providing relevant data was easy. HIV was not a reportable disease in California until 2003 (although AIDS was). Confidentiality concerns precluded population-based sampling. Because of the long latency period between HIV seroconversion and development of AIDS, estimated at a median of 10 years, neither AIDS reporting nor HIV antibody tests were an effective means of determining where recent infections were occurring (Rutherford, 1990). Nonetheless, these challenges led to the development of creative surveillance models. Often in collaboration with the Centers for Disease Control and Prevention (CDC), we developed a variety of surveillance tools including phone surveys, clinic-based surveys, venue-based surveys, blinded seroprevalence studies, and, in more recent years, the sensitive/less sensitive 'detuned' ELISA, to provide detailed data on the epidemic. We also did specialized studies to focus on small, hidden populations that were never represented in sufficient number in countywide surveys. For example, we conducted surveys of young men who have sex with men (Valleroy *et al.*, 2000), transgendered individuals (Clements-Nolle *et al.*, 2001), and homeless youth (Gleghorn *et al.*, 1998). As Buehler has noted, the use of multiple surveillance methods to characterize the AIDS epidemic has informed efforts on how to maintain surveillance for emerging infections as well as chronic diseases (Buehler, 2003).

The principles of community decision-making – shared power, inclusiveness, a clear charge, and a data driven process – have been interwoven into regulations concerning federal funding allocations. For example, the Health Services Resource Agency (HRSA), the funder of the Ryan White Comprehensive AIDS Resources Emergency (Care) Act of 1990, requires that each locality create a Council that includes consumers, service providers, and governmental officials, and other stakeholders to make decisions on allocation of resources to different service categories (i.e. the percentage of money going to medical care, the percentage going to housing, the percentage going to case management, etc.) (Marx, 1997). And, as testimony to the integrity of the process, allocations differ across localities and have changed over the course of the epidemic.

Similarly the CDC created a community-based planning process in 1994 to govern how federal prevention dollars are spent. The Prevention Planning Committee must include community representatives, epidemiologists, government officials, and other stakeholders. The groups are charged with identifying the best approaches for preventing infection among those groups at highest risk of becoming infected. To assure that each locality's request fulfills the priorities of its planning group, the CDC requires that the planning council issue a letter of concurrence (Valdiserri, 2003).

The San Francisco Department of Public Health has also found these principles of community engagement useful in a wide range of decision-making activities, including determining how to design a facility for people with chronic mental illness, how to decrease asthma incidence, and how to build a new hospital. We have noted that many funders, both governmental and private philanthropic groups, now require that programs create and support decision-making panels. This is a change that I expect will only increase in coming years as policy leaders recognize the value of community process.

Service Needs

As is the case for any serious disease, people with HIV/AIDS need medical services – doctors, nurses, hospital services, pharmaceuticals, and laboratory services. However, the AIDS epidemic has taught us the importance of providing a broader array of health-related services as shown in Table 4.2. Provision of supportive services was the central ingredient in what became known as the San Francisco AIDS Model. San Francisco's large, cohesive, gay community rallied to care for its own. A variety of supportive services were provided to help people with AIDS deal with the overwhelming issues of being diagnosed with a life-threatening illness. Services were provided by small, non-profit organizations working with a large cadre of volunteers (Arno, 1986).

Table 4.2   Health-related services needed for people with HIV/AIDS.

Traditional medical services	Physician visits
	Nursing visits
	Hospitalization
	Medications
	Laboratory
Alternative health services	Acupuncture
	Herbal remedies
	Megavitamins
	Massage
Supportive services	Benefits counseling/advocacy
	Housing
	Food
	Transportation
	Emotional support
	Legal services (e.g. wills)
	Day care
	Help taking care of pets
Related health services	Dentistry
Coordination	Case management

Investigators found that the San Francisco model was successful in shortening hospitalizations. Hospitalizations at the San Francisco General Hospital were significantly shorter (11.7 days) than hospitalizations for AIDS in New York (25.4 days) (Arno and Hughes, 1987). Based in large part on the success of the San Francisco model, the CARE Act provided funding to localities to provide a full continuum of services, including medical care, supportive services, alternative health services, dentistry, and case management (Marx, 1997). To recognize how radical a notion this was, remember that the federal Medicaid and Medicare programs do not pay for supportive services.

The Housing Opportunities for People with AIDS (HOPWA) program broadened the federal service continuum for people with AIDS to include housing. This appropriation from the US Department of Housing and Urban Development of US$1.7 billion between 1992 and 2003 has provided funding for housing-related expenses (e.g. capital expenses associated with acquisition of property, rental subsidies, financial assistance to prevent evictions) (www.hud.gov/offices/cpd/aidshousing/programs/index.cfm). The program recognizes that many people living with HIV/AIDS are homeless or unstably housed and that it is extremely difficult to maintain health status and provide complicated medical treatments to people who lack stable housing.

The success of housing programs for HIV-infected people has led to greater support of housing as part of the service continuum for people with chronic disease, including people with mental illness and substance abuse. Because studies have shown that localities can recoup 95 per cent of the costs of supportive housing (i.e. housing with supportive services) due to the decreased utilization of health services and lower incarceration rates (Culhane *et al.*, 2001), we are likely to see many more public health housing models in the coming years.

Early in the AIDS epidemic there were treatments for some of the opportunistic infections, but no effective treatments against the virus itself. Even when effective treatments became available (AZT was approved by the Food and Drug Administration in 1987) the treatments were highly toxic. It is therefore not surprising that many people with HIV/AIDS sought out alternative treatments. The most sought after alternative modalities have been acupuncture, herbal remedies, megavitamins, and massage.

What is especially interesting is how the use of alternative therapies by people with HIV/AIDS presaged the widespread use of alternative therapies by the general public. By 1997 42 per cent of Americans had used at least one alternative therapy in the prior year (Eisenberg, 1998). Not only has the use of alternative therapies become common in the general population, but these therapies have also been increasingly accepted and even encouraged by some Western trained physicians.

Providing coordination of care through case management has been found to decrease unmet needs for supportive services and also results in clients being more likely to receive life-saving treatment (Katz *et al.*, 2001). Based in part on the success of case management in helping people with HIV/AIDS to get the services they need, case management models have been developed for many other populations, including breast cancer patients, homeless people, and the mentally ill. Use of case management as a treatment strategy for disenfranchised people is likely to increase in the future.

Cultural Competency and Privacy

Because HIV/AIDS disproportionately affected stigmatized groups (e.g. gay men, injection drug users) and people of color, two other key principles of providing health care emerged from the AIDS epidemic: the importance of cultural competency of care providers and the importance of privacy.

The AIDS epidemic taught us the importance of understanding the cultural baggage that both providers of care and clients bring to the health encounter. For example, some people with HIV/AIDS have been reluctant to take antiretroviral therapy because of prior bad experiences with the medical system. Gay and lesbian people, drug users, people of color, and women all have reasons to be suspicious of the medical establishment given the prior practices and stated beliefs of medical professionals. Also, physicians may have preconceptions about certain types of patients (e.g. drug users will try to manipulate me to get unneeded pain medicines).

As the epidemic affected new populations, our understanding of culture needed to grow and deepen. For example, in the early 1990s a group of youth providers met with me to explain the importance of creating programs that were specific to youth. Until that moment I had never considered whether our programs were 'ageist,' i.e. whether youth would feel comfortable going to them. I just assumed that young people would choose what program to go to based on ethnicity, gender, sexual preference, and geography – the major ways that we had organized our services. I learned in discussion with youth – who expressed how uncomfortable they felt in adult-dominated clinical settings – that I was wrong; to make our system more culturally competent we devoted new resources to making our system competent for youth.

Cultural competency gives us a framework to understand and to deal with these issues. In San Francisco having a culturally competent AIDS system meant having ethnic-specific, sexual orientation-specific, and women-specific agencies, along with multicultural ones. It meant recognition that providing translators, although an important step, does not assure that people from different cultures are cared for in a competent way. Six years ago one rarely heard the term cultural competency outside of AIDS. Now several national bodies have created training manuals and advocated for cultural competency programs (Department of Health and Human Services, 2001; Linkins *et al.*, 2002). This movement is likely to increase because it is a better way of providing services.

Many people with HIV/AIDS fear disclosure of information about their health. This fear has been fueled by several cases of job discrimination, housing discrimination, domestic violence, as well as the inability of infected people to obtain life, disability, or health insurance (Institute of Medicine, 1986; Gostin and Webber, 1998). (Even having a *negative* HIV antibody test has at times been sufficient evidence for refusing coverage on the grounds that it suggests the person is in a high-risk group for HIV/AIDS.) Influenced by these lessons, as well as growing concern of the public about the increasing computerization of medical data, the Congress of the United States passed a national policy, the Health Insurance Portability and Accountability Act (HIPPA), with very strict rules governing release of medical information (Gostin, 2001).

Adapting the Disease Prevention Model

The traditional public health methods for controlling communicable diseases are case finding, case treatment, partner notification and treatment, quarantine, and vaccination. While these strategies have been helpful in eliminating and controlling a number of infectious diseases ranging from smallpox to gonorrhea, they have been much less useful in controlling the HIV epidemic.

As discussed above, HIV has a long asymptomatic latency period. Therefore, it has been difficult to identify people who are infected when they are still asymptomatic. The only way to know for certain if a person is infected is for them to take an HIV antibody test. The test was first licensed in 1985, and it was initially unknown whether healthy people who tested positive for the antibodies would become ill or were immune (i.e. were like people who test positive for hepatitis B antibody and are immune to the disease). Unfortunately, natural history studies of HIV found that the vast majority of people who were infected would become ill if they did not receive treatment.

Even once the meaning of the test became clear, it has been difficult to convince at-risk asymptomatic people to have themselves HIV tested for a variety of reasons. The stigma attached to HIV results in HIV-infected people encountering discrimination in many areas of their lives including job discrimination, social avoidance, discrimination in receipt of medical care, and the impossibility of obtaining life, disability, or health insurance (Institute of Medicine, 1986; Kass *et al.*, 1992; Gostin and Webber, 1998; Herek *et al.*, 2002; Valdiserri, 2002). These all result in people at risk for HIV being reluctant to get themselves HIV tested. Also, psychological barriers such as fear and denial played a large role in people not going for testing or not returning for the results (Catania *et al.*, 1990; Irwin *et al.*, 1996).

The end result of all of these factors is that many people do not get themselves HIV tested until they have AIDS or HIV-related symptoms (Levi, 2002). Even once a person has tested HIV positive antibody there are still a large number of obstacles to successfully using a communicable disease control model. To prevent inadvertent disclosures of HIV status and to encourage at-risk people to test for HIV, the United States and other Western countries set up anonymous testing sites. Because testing is anonymous, it cannot be reported to health departments in the way that laboratories and clinicians report other communicable diseases. Therefore, any further action depends on the willingness of the client to disclose their result. Even assuming a client is willing to come forward, because no eradication therapy is available, case identification does not have the power it has with diseases such as syphilis or gonorrhea.

Although partner notification has been used successfully with HIV in some populations (Landis *et al.*, 1992; Fenton and Peterman, 1997), a strategy that is very successful with controlling sexually transmitted diseases, is also hampered by the long latency period between HIV infection and development of AIDS (West and Stark, 1997). Especially among first time testers, it is unclear when the person became infected, making it extremely difficult to narrow down a likely set of sexual or needle-sharing partners who could then be interviewed. In San Francisco's gay community, where there is a high prevalence of infection, a high level of knowledge in the community about the likelihood that prior partners have been infected, and where many partners are anonymous, HIV partner notification has generally not been efficacious.

Quarantine, a very effective tool for infectious diseases with short latencies, such as severe acute respiratory syndrome (SARS), has no utility for HIV infection. It is neither practical nor ethical to quarantine people who are HIV infected, especially since HIV can only be transmitted via intimate contact, prenatal exposure, or blood products, as opposed to diseases such as chickenpox and SARS that are transmitted through casual human interactions.

A vaccine – the ultimate weapon in the public health arsenal against infectious diseases, the vanquisher of smallpox, polio and measles – has proven elusive. In fact, since the HIV virus was first identified in 1984, scientists have predicted that an HIV vaccine with protective immunity is five years away. Sadly, it never seems to get any closer.

Because the traditional communicable disease control model has been of limited utility in combating HIV, the HIV epidemic has forced public health to rediscover and reinvigorate health education, community mobilization, community empowerment, and other public health strategies for controlling epidemics. Ironically, these strategies may be much more effective in battling the non-infectious disease epidemics that plague Western countries in the twenty-first century: obesity, diabetes, and substance abuse.

Health education and health promotion have been among the most effective weapons we have had in the battle against HIV. To protect themselves from becoming HIV infected people must know how HIV is transmitted and how to prevent it. Throughout the epidemic a variety of health education methods have been used to educate the public about HIV, including television and radio commercials, print ads in newspapers, bus shelters and billboards, group sessions in schools, churches, community centers, and individual sessions with doctors, nurses, health educators, and HIV antibody test counselors. Along the way, health education has successfully countered a number of misconceptions about HIV, including that you can tell by looking at a person whether they are HIV infected, that HIV can be transmitted through shaking hands or sharing bathrooms, and that you can't contract HIV from sex if you are straight (heterosexual).

Health education is and will continue to be a key strategy in communicating to the public about emerging infections such as anthrax and SARS. One of the frustrations with the federal handling of the 2001 anthrax outbreak in the United States was that the information provided by the CDC was not clear, accurate, and consistent regarding how anthrax was transmitted. In comparison, the handling of the SARS outbreak in 2003 was successful and the CDC was able to correct a lot of misinformation that was being spread about SARS.

Although necessary, knowledge is not in-and-of-itself sufficient to prevent HIV infections. For example, in San Francisco's gay community, where knowledge of HIV is high, HIV incidence rates remain high as well (Katz *et al.*, 2002). The reasons why people engage in unsafe sex even when they know that it could result in HIV infection range the whole spectrum of human motivations. People have unsafe sex because it is more intimate, it feels better, they are in a power relationship where they cannot demand that a condom be used, they are depressed, they are in denial that they can become infected, they are in denial that the other person is infected, they have such significant competing life problems that they are not particularly worried that they will become infected, they are high on drugs, they believe it is inevitable that they will become infected, they believe that if they become infected they will simply take the necessary medications, the condom breaks, etc. (Penkower *et al.*, 1991; Stall *et al.*, 2003).

Although the reasons people put themselves at risk are large in number, we have learned through the AIDS epidemic a great deal about how to bring about long-lasting behavioral change. As exemplified by the response of San Francisco's gay community at the start of the epidemic, community mobilization is a very powerful health promotion strategy (Wohlfeiler, 1997). San Francisco's gay community was able to drive the new HIV infection rate down from a high of 8000 infections per year in 1983 to 5000 new infections by 1987 (Katz, 1997). What was especially remarkable about the success of this intervention is that it was done with relatively little government funding. While the government was stupefyingly slow in recognizing and funding prevention efforts (Francis, 1992), the community came together to prevent new infections (Shilts, 1987).

Starting in the early 1980s, the community made certain that no one would forget about AIDS. These activities are described in detail in Randy Shilts' book, *And the Band Played On* (1987). Informal discussions among friends and acquaintances expanded into community meetings with public officials, often heated. There were constant reminders of the need to stay safe from posters in windows of local stores and safe-sex brochures. Fundraisers were sponsored, and political work and lobbying efforts were carried out. Condom and Bleach man paraded through the streets at street fairs and festivals. (Interestingly, we have reused the concept recently to counter an increase in syphilis cases among men who have sex with men. We introduced the character the Healthy Penis along with his nemesis Phil the syphilis sore at the Gay Pride Parade to raise awareness of the growing number of cases.) The Sisters of Perpetual Indulgence (a group of men dressed in nuns' habits) dispensed safe-sex advice along with condoms. People volunteered to participate in studies like the San Francisco City Clinic Cohort and the San Francisco Men's Study so as to contribute to knowledge about HIV. The overall effect was development of a peer norm that emphasized the importance of each person protecting himself or herself against HIV.

The reason the community mobilization was so successful was that there was a clear threat to the community; the density of infection was high; the community was united in protecting itself; and it had social and political power (Katz, 1997).

Unfortunately, other communities that have been hard hit by the epidemic – injection drug users, communities of color – have not had the internal resources to mobilize. To overcome this limitation, we and other health departments have developed community empowerment models. The goal of an empowerment model is to spark the type of community mobilization that worked so well in the gay community. For example, several studies have shown that identifying, training, and supporting key community opinion leaders is successful in decreasing unsafe sex (Kelly *et al.*, 1991; Kegeles *et al.*, 1996; Valdiserri *et al.*, 2003).

Financially supporting empowerment models can be a bit of a challenge for government entities that are accustomed to tightly worded contracts that explicitly state what the 'deliverables' are. How can an agency state what services it will be providing if the point is to work with the community to determine what services they need? We handled this in the case of a gay/bisexual/queer and questioning youth empowerment model (Q action) (Wohlfeiler, 1997) by funding them to convene meetings of youth, ask the youth what type of program they wanted to do, and then use the money to implement the program. We never stated explicitly what the service was. (Getting this contract approved though our county bureaucracy was one of those 'rites of passage' accomplishments of the AIDS Office I spoke about in the introduction.)

Similar community empowerment models have been successful among low-income African American women (Sikkema *et al.*, 2000; Lauby *et al.*, 2000), among injection drug users (Rietmeijer *et al.*, 1996), and among diverse communities of high-risk people (CDC AIDS Community Demonstration Projects Research Group, 1999).

We, and others, have used community empowerment models to spark community interest in a number of non-AIDS areas over the last few years. For example, in response to the national epidemic of childhood obesity, our health department is currently working with a broad coalition to improve the nutrition of children. The coalition includes parents, youth, teachers, school officials, public health officials, physicians, nurses, and others. The coalition is taking a multipronged approach to improving nutrition, including health education, advocacy work with school officials on the importance of getting rid of junk food machines in the schools and providing instead healthful alternatives, and collaboration with local organic food producers.

Because the diseases that are of greatest risk to Western countries – cardiovascular disease, cancer – like AIDS, do not respond to traditional infectious disease control strategies it is likely that in the coming years there will be increased reliance on community empowerment models.

Advocacy

The AIDS epidemic produced the strongest single-issue advocacy that we have seen in the health field. Much has been learned from AIDS advocacy that is of use in the advocacy of people with other diseases. Because AIDS first hit highly stigmatized groups, the government was very slow to respond (Shilts, 1987; Francis, 1992). The result of this inattention was that the affected communities became much more politicized than they ever may have if the government had stepped in right from the beginning.

With only themselves to count on, the face of AIDS activism was not a professional lobbyist or advocate, but rather people with AIDS. Because they were dealing with this devastating disease, people with AIDS had a validity that other spokes-people do not typically have. For example, in 1985 when Ryan White, a 12-year-old boy with hemophilia and AIDS was denied the right to go to school with other children his age, many people came to understand how profound prejudices were against infected people. And when the Congress appropriated the first emergency financial relief to localities caring for a disproportionate number of people with HIV/AIDS, it was named after him. This program provided almost US$2 billion a year in 2002 for AIDS services in the United States (http://hab.hrsa.gov/tools/progressreport/).

The revelations that some famous people were suffering from HIV/AIDS, as was the case with Rock Hudson (announced in 1985) and Earwin 'Magic' Johnson (announced in 1991) – also had a tremendous impact on the general public. It is now widely recognized that the most effective spokesperson for any health issue – HIV/AIDS, breast cancer, substance abuse – is someone who is battling the illness.

Single-Issue Advocacy

However, the reasons HIV/AIDS activism has been successful go significantly beyond the effective use of patients as spokespersons. A second factor in the success of HIV/AIDS activism is the focus on HIV/AIDS as a single issue, rather than in the context of other health issues.

This may seem counter-intuitive. Why should focusing on HIV/AIDS exclusively, rather than using HIV/AIDS as an opportunity to highlight the broader problems with our health system be effective? The major reason is that it is much harder to provide the resources necessary to fix the health system, so that all people suffering from life-threatening diseases (AIDS in the era prior to the advent of effective antiretroviral therapy) or chronic diseases (AIDS in the era post development of effective therapy) receive the treatment they need. For example, the Ryan White (CARE) Act pays for a number of services – case management, substance abuse, transportation and housing – that people who suffer from diseases of equal severity are not able to access. Sometimes this produces ironic discrepancies in availability of care. For example, because of the success of HIV/AIDS advocacy in producing funding through the Ryan White CARE Act as well as local and state funding sources, I can arrange a residential substance treatment bed or a methadone maintenance slot within a day for one of my injection drug-using HIV-infected patients. However, for one of my uninfected injection drug-using patients, the wait for these services is several months. The irony of course is that substance treatment could potentially prevent the uninfected person from becoming infected. This discrepancy in funding availability has been referred to as 'AIDS exceptionalism' and has placed AIDS programs open to being attacked as unjust or unfair to other stigmatized populations with serious disease (e.g. mentally ill people) (Casarett and Lantos, 1998).

New Tactics

Another major reason for the success of HIV/AIDS activism is that it is not always polite. For example, many of the successes of HIV/AIDS activism can be attributed to the formation of ACT UP groups in several major cities in the United States and Europe. ACT UP stands for AIDS Coalition to Unleash Power and was formed in New York City in 1987 by activist Larry Kramer (Valdiserri, 2003). The civil disobedience tactics of these groups – closing bridges, sit-ins at governmental offices, booing speakers so that they could not be heard – while upsetting to some, unquestionably brought attention and results. This strategy was also made more successful by having other AIDS activists participate in advisory groups in more conventional ways. Agreeing to follow the recommendations of the more 'moderate' elements became a way of avoiding having to deal with the more extreme part of ACT UP. The effect of this 'good cop/bad cop' was seen in almost every facet of the struggle against AIDS. In fact, even the very definition of AIDS was heavily influenced by activism. Activists were rightly concerned that the surveillance definition used by the CDC was too narrow, with the result that many people were dying of AIDS without being counted. As a result, the 1992 expansion of the AIDS definition included three indicator diagnoses which were thought to be particularly common among disenfranchised people with HIV: recurrent bacterial pneumonia, pulmonary tuberculosis, and cervical cancer (CDC, 1992; Buehler, 2003).

HIV/AIDS activism had a tremendous effect on the federal drug approval process. Pressure by activists led the Public Health Service to approve an expanded-access program that made drugs available to affected individuals prior to the formal approval process by the Food and Drug Administration (FDA). The effort by activists also led the FDA to increase its speed in approving therapies. Both of these changes have benefited people with other diseases as well, including people with Alzheimer's disease and cancer (Wachter, 1992). Equally significant, ACT UP pushed successfully for greater inclusion of women, ethnic minorities, and injection drug users in drug trials and other research on AIDS, an initiative now strongly supported by the National Institutes of Health.

ACT UP, along with other AIDS activists also helped change the methodology of drug studies. For example, AIDS advocates called for the acceptance of surrogate markers, such as improvements in CD4 lymphocyte counts as acceptable proof of the efficacy of drug therapy rather than requiring longer survival before approving drugs. Similarly, ACT UP and other advocates of people with HIV/AIDS pushed for the development and greater use of alternative research designs rather than randomized blinded controlled trials, such as open-label randomization (patients are randomized to therapy but know what they are taking). And when investigators failed to provide these types of studies, advocates taught research subjects how to get their medications tested outside of the study so they could learn whether they were receiving placebo or active medications. While these strategies were very upsetting to investigators accustomed to performing their trials in traditional ways, researchers were spurred to develop new methods to deal with these real life situations.

What the Future Holds

Even if the AIDS/HIV epidemic ended, the lessons it has brought would continue to affect public health on a broad range of issues. The importance of community planning is well accepted among public health practitioners and is often an element required by federal and local funders. The benefits of providing a fully integrated continuum of services, beyond medical services, is equally well appreciated and is often requested by patients suffering from non-AIDS-related diseases, such as cancer and hepatitis C.

Prior to the AIDS epidemic one rarely heard about culturally competent care. If it was raised at all, it was usually in the context of caring for people who spoke a different language than the provider. But now we understand that language is only one part of cultural competency and health care institutions routinely assess themselves for cultural competency and seek to improve in those areas where they fall short. Part of the impetus for focusing on cultural competency is that it is a good business strategy (i.e. enables you to attract and keep customers) and it improves office morale and minimizes the risk for the employer of workplace harassment suits.

Passage of HIPPA has created new attention to the importance of maintaining privacy of medical information. The strength of community organization and empowerment models and the success of single-issue advocacy by people directly affected by a disease have been shown in the areas of breast and prostate cancer and hepatitis C. Overall, the greater involvement of affected individuals in their care can only improve outcomes.

What is less clear is how support for HIV/AIDS will change in the coming years. Is today's reduced community involvement an unavoidable result of prior successful community activism plus the discovery of effective drug treatment? Should it be a surprise that with patients living longer and better, the fear that motivated activists and ordinary individuals early on in the epidemic inevitably would wane? Perhaps the most telling (and disturbing) sign is how much less visible HIV/AIDS issues are in epicenters, such as San Francisco and New York. Agencies can no longer recruit as many volunteers; charitable giving to HIV/AIDS organizations is down; fewer people walk and run in organized fundraisers; several agencies have had to let go of staff or curtail their programs.

The indigenous community mobilizations around HIV/AIDS prevention in cities with large gay and bisexual male populations have fizzled out. In fact, multiple studies have shown significant increases in unsafe behavior as well as increases in sexually transmitted diseases in these cities (Kalichman *et al.*, 1997; Katz *et al.*, 1998, 2002; Van de Ven *et al.*, 1998; Ekstrand *et al.*, 1999; Dodds *et al.*, 2000).

And while experts debate whether 'barebacking' (anal intercourse without a condom) is a new phenomenon or a new spin on the small group of individuals who have consistently engaged in unsafe sex, the fact is that the peer norm in San Francisco and these other cities of consistently staying safe has dissipated.

Why has this occurred when there still is no cure or vaccine available? The reasons for the dissipation in community commitment to unsafe sex are numerous and complicated. But a very large part appears to be a product of our success: the availability of highly active antiretroviral therapy (HAART or 'drug cocktails') has had the result that people who once feared certain death if they were to become infected no longer have these worries (Chen *et al.*, 2002; Katz *et al.*, 2002). It turns out that fear of death was a very powerful spark of community mobilization.

Also, many of the behavioral changes that occurred in the early 1980s have been hard to sustain for the same reasons that many people who lose weight put it back on; the same reasons that many people who quit smoking relapse. As hard as it is to make behavioral changes it is even harder to sustain them for decades of time.

Whatever the causes, it is not surprising that as the gay community has shown less concern for preventing HIV transmission, that the general public is less interested in supporting these efforts as well.

The increased political strength of conservatives also bodes poorly for HIV/AIDS programs in the coming years in several ways. There has already been increasing pressure at the federal level to focus more resources on abstinence-only models and to not fund programs with extremely explicit materials. Although there is a place for encouraging abstinence, we know that it is not a strategy that is useful for the majority of people at risk for HIV.

We also know that for prevention programs to be maximally effective they have to appear relevant to the target audience. This is why it has been so disturbing that the federal government has ordered the San Francisco Stop AIDS agency to stop certain sexually explicit prevention workshops. Just a few months before the CDC had concluded that 'the design and delivery of Stop AIDS prevention activities was based on current and accepted behavioral science theories in the area of health promotion' (Ornstein, 2003). It was clear that conservative politics had triumphed over science. Similarly, HIV/AIDS and researchers in other areas of sexual behavior were chilled to find that their names had been compiled by a conservative group, the Traditional Values Coalition and submitted to Representative Billy Tauzin, a Louisiana Republican who chairs the House Energy and Commerce Committee. One of its subcommittees reviews grants awarded by the National Institutes of Health (Herbert, 2003).

There is also fear that HIV/AIDS programs will not fair well financially in the coming years. Already, several epicenters such as New York and San Francisco have had reductions in their total financial allocations under Ryan White (CARE) Title I. These losses have been difficult to sustain because while the incidence of AIDS (the annual number of new AIDS cases) has dropped dramatically, the number of people living with AIDS has dramatically increased. The reason is that HAART has resulted in fewer people developing AIDS but has resulted in an even greater reduction in the number of AIDS deaths.

In addition to the increase in the size of the population of people with HIV/AIDS, the costs of providing pharmaceutical care to this group continues to increase. To date, most of the costs of AIDS drugs have been covered via a combination of federal and state funding through the Medicaid program and the AIDS Drug Assistance Program (ADAP). ADAP is funded through the Ryan White Care Act. In 2003, the funding for ADAP (federal and state) was US$948 million (http://www.hab.hrsa.gov/programs/factsheets/adap1.htm), up from US$204 million in 1996, the year that protease inhibitors first became available. In addition to these increases in funding, several cost-savings methods have been applied including use of a variety of pharmaceutical discount programs. Unfortunately, despite these increases in funding and cost savings measures, ADAP funding is insufficient to cover demand for medications. The result is that many states in the United States effectively ration medications to economically poor, uninsured people with HIV/AIDS by maintaining wait lists, limiting the total number of drugs a person with HIV/AIDS can receive, or restricting the formulary (not including all effective drugs on the formulary). As these restrictions increase, we could see a greater and greater disparity by income in the percentage of HIV-infected people receiving treatment and decreased survival among low-income populations due to them being less likely to receive treatment (McFarland *et al.*, 2003).

I fear that in the next years AIDS exceptionalism will end, but not the way I had hoped. My hope has been that we would resolve the dilemma caused by AIDS exceptionalism by providing the same needed services for all people suffering from illness. For example, if the United States provided universal health insurance with drug coverage it would not be necessary to fund the medical care components of the Ryan White (CARE) program or the ADAP program. Instead all people with serious illness would have access to needed medications. Similarly, were the same support services available for disenfranchised populations or those who have to navigate a difficult treatment system, we would not need services only for people with HIV/AIDS. Instead I fear we will see AIDS exceptionalism end by no longer providing needed medical care or supportive services to people with HIV/AIDS or any of the populations struggling with poverty and serious illness.

References

Arno PS (1986) *Am J Public Health* 76: 1325–30.
Arno PS, Hughes RG (1987) *N Y State J Med* 87: 264–72.
Buehler JW (2003) In: Valdiserri RO, ed. *Dawning Answers: How the HIV/AIDS Epidemic Has Helped to Strengthen Public Health*. New York: Oxford University Press, pp, 33–55.
Casarett DJ, Lantos JD (1998) *Ann Intern Med* 128: 759–9.
Catania JA *et al.* (1990) *AIDS* 4: 261–3.

CDC (Centers for Disease Control and Prevention) (1992) *MMWR Morb Mortal Wkly Rep* 41: 1–19.

CDC AIDS Community Demonstration Projects Research Group (1999) *Am J Public Health* 89: 336–45.

Chen CY *et al.* (2002) *Am J Public Health* 92: 1387–8.

Clements-Nolle K *et al.* (2001) *Am J Public Health* 91: 915–21.

Culhane DP *et al.* (2001) *The New York/New York Agreement Cost Study: The Impact of Supportive Housing on Services Use for Homeless Mentally Ill Individuals.* New York: Corporation for Supportive Housing.

Department of Health and Human Services, Office of Minority Health (2001) *National Standards for Culturally and Linguistically Appropriate Services in Health Care: Final Report.* Washington, DC: Department of Health and Human Services.

Dodds J *et al.* (2000) *BMJ* 320: 1510–11.

Eisenberg DM *et al.* (1998) *JAMA* 280: 1569–75.

Ekstrand ML *et al.* (1999) *AIDS* 13: 1525–33.

Fenton KA, Peterman TA (1997) *AIDS* 11: 1535–46.

Francis DP (1992) *JAMA* 268: 1444–7.

Gleghorn AA *et al.* (1998) *Drug Alcohol Depend* 51: 219–27.

Gostin LO (2001) *JAMA* 285: 3015–21.

Gostin LO, Webber DW (1998) *JAMA* 279: 1108–13.

Herbert R (2003) *New York Times.*

Herek GM *et al.* (2002) *Am J Public Health* 92: 371–7.

Institute of Medicine, National Academy of Sciences (1986) *Confronting AIDS: Directions for Public Health, Health Care, and Research.* Washington, DC: National Academy Press.

Irwin KL *et al.* (1996) *AIDS* 10: 1707–17.

Kalichman SC *et al.* (1997) *Health Psychol* 16: 369–73.

Kass NE *et al.* (1992) *Am J Public Health* 82: 1277–9.

Katz HH (1997) *J Acquir Immune Defic Syndr* 14 (Suppl 2): S38–S46.

Katz MH *et al.* (1998) *J Acquir Immune Defic Syndr Hum Retrovirol* 19: 178–81.

Katz MH *et al.* (2001) *Ann Intern Med* 135: 557–65.

Katz MH *et al.* (2002) *Am J Public Health* 92: 388–94.

Kegeles SM *et al.* (1996) *Am J Public Health* 86: 1129–36.

Kelly JA *et al.* (1991) *Am J Public Health* 81: 168–71.

Landis SE *et al.* (1992) *N Engl J Med* 326: 101–6.

Lauby JL *et al.* (2000) *Am J Public Health* 90: 216–22.

Levi J (2002) *Am J Public Health* 92: 339–40.

Linkins KW *et al.* (2002) *Indicators of Cultural Competence in Health Care Delivery Organizations: An Organizational Cultural Competence Assessment Profile.* The Lewin Group, Inc.

Marx R (1997) *J Acquir Immune Defic Syndr* 14: 44–55.

McFarland W *et al.* (2003) *J Acquir Immune Defic Syndr* 33: 96–103.

Ornstein C (2003) *Los Angeles Times,* pp. B1.

Penkower L *et al.* (1991) *Am J Public Health* 81: 194–6.

Rietmeijer *et al.* (1996) *AIDS* 10: 291–8.

Rutherford GW *et al.* (1990) *BMJ* 301: 1183–8.

Shilts R (1987) *And The Band Played On.* New York: The Penguin Group.

Sikkema KJ *et al.* (2000) *Am J Public Health* 90: 57–63.

Stall R *et al.* (2003) *Am J Public Health* 96: 939–42.

Valdiserri RO (2002) *Am J Public Health* 92: 341–2.

Valdiserri RO, ed. (2003) *Dawning Answers: How the HIV/AIDS Epidemic Has Helped to Strengthen Public Health.* New York: Oxford University Press.

Valdiserri RO *et al.* (2003) *Nat Med* 9: 881–6.
Valleroy LA *et al.* (2000) *JAMA* 284: 198–204.
Van de Ven *et al.* (1998) *Aust N Z J Public Health* 22: 814–18.
Wachter RM (1992) *N Engl J Med* 326: 128–33.
West GR, Stark KA (1997) *AIDS Educ Prevent* 9 (Suppl B): 68–78.
Wohlfeiler D (1997) In: Minkler M, ed. *Community Organizing and Community Building for Health*. New Jersey: Rutgers University Press, pp. 230–43.

AIDS and Sexually Transmitted Disease Prevention and Control

5

Jeffrey D Klausner
San Francisco Department of Health, San Francisco, USA

Jeffrey D Klausner, MD, MPH is a Deputy Health Officer and Director of Sexually Transmitted Disease Prevention and Control Services in San Francisco, Medical Director of the municipal STD Clinic, Associate Clinical Professor of Medicine at University of California San Francisco, Attending Physician in Medicine, AIDS and Infectious Diseases at San Francisco General Hospital and President of the California STD Controllers' Association. Dr. Klausner received his Medical Degree from Cornell University, trained in Internal Medicine at New York University-Bellevue Hospital and was an Epidemic Intelligence Service Officer for the Centers for Disease Control and Prevention. He received his MPH from the Harvard School of Public Health and completed an Infectious Disease Fellowship at the University of Washington. He serves as a consultant, co-investigator and principal investigator on several trials utilizing biological outcomes as measures of the effectiveness of prevention interventions and has published extensively on sexually transmitted diseases and HIV/AIDS.

The AIDS epidemic has profoundly altered the prevention and control of sexually transmitted diseases (STDs). Before the advent of AIDS in the early 1980s, STD prevention and control activities were largely hierarchical, government-run, disease-oriented programs focused on syphilis and gonorrhea in high-risk populations like sex workers or urban gay men. In the general population the sentiment was that the serious sequelae of STDs were in the past and with time STDs would become nothing more than a social inconvenience. While major US cities maintained STD prevention and control programs across a broad range of funding and capacity, their efforts between 1950 and 1980 provided little more than a revolving clinic door of treatment and re-treatment.

The AIDS epidemic caused STD prevention and control programs to consider the community at risk, understand issues of sociopolitical vulnerability and research interventions aimed at primary prevention, reducing individual sexual risk behavior. STD prevention and programs took the best attributes of the new paradigm of HIV prevention – community participation, peer-to-peer education and patient-centered care – and built these on top of the foundations of STD control: case-identification, treatment, and partner notification.

The first and most basic interaction between a medical care provider and a patient is the interview, the period when relevant health information is collected and a bond of trust is forged. Prior to AIDS, this may have been a cursory assessment of medication allergies and medical conditions. A generation later, this interview has evolved into a comprehensive evaluation of sexual risk-taking behavior identifying specific sexual acts – oral, anal, and/or vaginal intercourse as a receptive or insertive partner protected with a condom or not; personal co-factors that may impact sexual risk behavior like substance use including Viagra, methamphetamine, and other drugs of abuse; mental health issues like depression, anxiety, or stress syndromes; and community co-factors like social norms and sexual networks.

While gay men were the primary socially and behaviorally defined group at risk for HIV infection in the United States with a fairly unique culture of sexual risk behavior, young heterosexual adults of color are increasingly being affected by AIDS and are the focus of STD prevention and control programs in the twenty-first century. This has resulted in translating the initial efforts in gay men's sexual health promotion and disease prevention to other populations at risk. Now in STD clinics across the country serving a range of populations, behavioral risk assessments are conducted to identify behaviors modifiable by the patient. Peer-to-peer sexual health outreach programs, community advisory boards, and effective STD/HIV prevention counseling interventions have been developed for a variety of at-risk groups.

The San Francisco Perspective

The San Francisco municipal STD clinic, City Clinic, was at ground zero at the beginning of the AIDS epidemic in the United States. Since the early 1930s men, women, children, and those who eschew even such basic labels, have come for confidential and free evaluations, diagnosis and treatment for STDs.

There are nearly 55 000 gay men or other men who have sex with men in San Francisco. In a City with a population of 800 000, this means that about 1 out of 4 men between 20 and 50 years old have sex with men and are potentially at risk for HIV infection. San Francisco was one of the first places where AIDS was recognized and studied. During the early years, however, AIDS was treated as an immunologic disorder of uncertain origin and the clinical manifestations were primarily unusual types of pneumonia and cancer. Thus, in San Francisco, the initial medical specialists involved in the epidemic were lung and cancer specialists. The AIDS epidemic continues to decimate the gay male population in San Francisco. Over 20 000 gay men have died. Currently, about 1 in 3 or 18 000 gay men are HIV-infected in San Francisco and there are 1000 new HIV infections a year (Sexually Transmitted Disease Prevention and Control Services, 2002). Recent treatment advances have changed the diagnosis of HIV infection from a death sentence to a life-long chronic infection. While treatment saves individual lives, it is also creating a greater number of infectious people capable of spreading the infection to others. HIV-infected people may be infectious for life. How STD control programs respond to HIV transmission and how the AIDS epidemic has changed STD prevention and control has an interesting history.

Origins of STD Control

STD prevention and control programs in the USA exist at the Federal level coordinated by the Division of STD Prevention at the Centers for Disease Control and Prevention and at State and local levels. Funding to local programs comes from either Federal or State grants and the county or city. Most State laws mandate that health officers control the spread of certain STDs. Some aspects of STD control are explicit in the law, such as physician or laboratory-based disease reporting, investigation, partner notification, treatment, isolation and education. While the law spells out what needs to be done, there are no defined sources of revenue or specific minimum expenditures per capita.

Table 5.1 shows the range of common strategies to control STDs. Primary prevention strategies aim to prevent people from being exposed to infection whereas secondary prevention strategies aim to prevent serious medical consequences in those already infected and prevent subsequent transmission. STD prevention and control programs use both strategies supporting community and provider education, screening and treatment efforts including specially designated STD clinics where people can access diagnosis and treatment usually at no or very low cost.

Current Federal and local STD control programs evolved with early US military efforts to control venereal diseases. In World War I, loss of active duty time due to sick days from STDs matched troop readiness losses due to combat injury and other communicable diseases (Brandt, 1987). During military training young men were stationed in remote camps surrounded by newly arising towns often inhabited by a variety of merchants seeking to capture both the recruits' limited pay and their free time. There was no shortage of brothel owners and sex workers among these merchants. The combination of youth, distance from home and numerous available sex partners fostered early epidemics of gonorrhea and syphilis among these recruits. The initial military response was to isolate men and punish them by deducting pay for sick days due to venereal disease. Eventually more

Table 5.1   Common measures to control sexually transmitted diseases.

Primary prevention	
Delay of sexual activity	To prevent exposure to possible infection
Condom use	To prevent exposure to possible infection or transmission of current infection
Behavioral risk reduction	To reduce the number of sex partners and modify type of sexual activity to reduce exposure to possible infection
Post-exposure prophylaxis	Treatment after exposure to reduce the likelihood of infection
Secondary prevention	
Case identification	Diagnosis and treatment of new infections to reduce the frequency of infection and subsequent transmission
Partner notification	Informs recent sex partners of possible exposure to infection resulting in evaluation and/or treatment to reduce the frequency of infection and subsequent transmission
Epidemiologic treatment	Treats likely exposed sexual contacts to reduce the frequency of infection and subsequent transmission based on demographic or behavioral characteristic
Mass or selective mass treatment	Treats a group of people based on possible exposure to reduce the frequency of infection and subsequent transmission
Population-based screening	Tests asymptomatic people to identify infections to reduce frequency of infection and subsequent transmission

enlightened leaders understood the need to provide alternative activity to alcohol abuse and sex. Sports, music and spiritual programs soon developed and military camps became a balance of training and recreation. But once deployed, soldiers were vulnerable to disease in theatres of war. STDs continued to incapacitate troops despite mandatory education and provision of condoms. Troops were obvious bridges of infection from groups with high levels of infection like sex workers to lower risk partners in civilian life.

During the same period, in the private sector STDs were increasingly impacting the health of women, couples and families, robbing women of their fertility and men of their sexual function. Men abandoned barren wives and families disintegrated. Society blamed women and a social hygiene movement began with social progressives trying to save the family, women and preserve the social order. Since STDs were seen as breaking society apart, these infections and those who acquired them were severely stigmatized. Physicians treating infected patients were outcast and research to diagnose and treat disease did not receive needed resources. The shadow of immorality associated with these diseases created opposing forces between those who preached personal responsibility and those who provided non-judgemental education and care; a dichotomy that would split the response to AIDS decades later.

The social progressives were ultimately successful, however, in creating a national movement with organizations that developed sex education programs and ultimately political support for a national STD control program in the US Public Health Service. One of its first leaders was Dr Thomas Parran, the former health commissioner from New York State. Dr Parran outlined the basic strategy to control STDs: identify new cases of infection, treat those infected; notify and treat recent sex partners and build local capacity – the foundations of STD control (Parran, 1937). Through massive testing efforts to identify cases of infection either voluntarily or through laws which required testing for marriage or discharge from the hospital, a high number of syphilis cases were identified. With the advent of penicillin in 1943, effective treatment became available. The Public Health Service trained investigators in partner notification to elicit the names and locations of recent sex partners and trace these contacts to assure evaluation and treatment. These efforts greatly reduced community levels of syphilis and gonorrhea. From Dr Parran's report as US Surgeon General in 1937 describing this strategy and the infrastructure required to control STDs, the next 45 years were a period of refinement, successes and transient set backs. With apparent declines in STD rates, the funding of programs would decrease, resulting in subsequent increases in case rates. Funding increases would follow with declines in new infections. The cycle of varying funding and cases would continue and is known as Brown's Law, which states that the rates of STDs are inversely correlated with the amount of funding to control infections (Brown and Blount, 1973).

While in the late 1960s and 1970s STDs were increasing as a result of decreased control efforts and new attitudes about sexual behavior in the general population, STDs were epidemic in certain populations such as gay men. By 1982 in San Francisco there were over 2000 new cases of syphilis a year compared with about 600 in 1960 (Sexually Transmitted Disease Prevention and Control Services, 2002). Gonorrhea was epidemic at over 18 000 cases a year compared with 2400 in 1960 (Sexually Transmitted Disease Prevention and Control Services, 2002). San Francisco had the dubious distinction of having the highest STD rates in the nation. Lines of patients for San Francisco City Clinic went around the block and more than 200 patients were seen a day. Clinical evaluation was minimal and injectable treatment a matter of course.

The high rate of STDs in the late 1970s set the stage for the introduction and rapid emergence of HIV infection in San Francisco in the early 1980s. During the first years of the epidemic there were an estimated 6000–8000 new HIV infections a year. Much of these infections went undetected since many new infections were without symptoms and diagnostic tests did not become available until years later. Case surveillance was limited – HIV infection was not reportable – so it is only by back calculating from rates of AIDS cases in the 1990s that we can estimate the number of new HIV infections 10–15 years earlier.

Evolution of HIV Prevention Outside of STD Control Programs

The advent of the AIDS epidemic could have strengthened STD control programs if AIDS had been responded to as a traditional STD. But nothing about AIDS was traditional and everything about the public health response was exceptional. It was not until 1984, at least three years after the first recognized cases of AIDS in 1981, that a sexually transmitted virus was confirmed as the causative agent of AIDS. Because the first reaction to a situation often defines it, not identifying HIV as a sexually transmitted pathogen immediately shaped the public health response. AIDS was affecting a disenfranchised community in the United States, gay men, and since those in the mainstream community acquired infection through blood-borne exposure, the public health response focused on securing the blood supply and providing supportive health care. The larger public ignored the disease among gay men, and local, State and the Federal government left these communities across the country to create their own responses. The stigma strongly associated with prior STDs and those infected was compounded, since AIDS affected people were already severely stigmatized because of their sexual or other risk behaviors.

Partly because of the stigmatized route of transmission, the nature of the affected populations and the resulting community-based response, the strategies for HIV prevention developed outside STD control programs. The main focus of the response was public education and changing individual risk behavior. Gay men, long stigmatized and oppressed by general society, held fierce concepts of individuality and individual rights. While demanding government intervention, the government response had to guarantee autonomy, weighing individual rights over community health. Thus, anonymous HIV testing programs became available, even protected by legislation in states like California, which greatly hampered public health efforts to identify cases and conduct partner notification. Case reporting of new HIV infections, a mainstay of traditional STD control programs, was non-existent. Partner elicitation and contact tracing, though encouraged was not mandated. While some professionals in STD control programs moved into HIV prevention programs, most STD control programs remained focused on traditional STDs. This allowed and enabled parallel and separate HIV prevention programs to develop at the local, State and Federal level. Advocates demanded a unique response to AIDS directing funding to the community beyond the reach of technocrats and public health professionals who had failed to respond to the epidemic in a culturally competent and effective manner.

Dual programs and funding developed which persisted for at least the first 15 years of the epidemic with rare communication and collaboration between professionals in HIV prevention and STD control. Only over the past five years has there been increased integration of HIV prevention and STD control programs and a public health response to HIV infection having shades of similiarity to the disease control strategy used to control other STDs (CDC, 2003). Differences in the application of public health tools still exist between the HIV prevention and STD control professionals and the communities they serve arising from attitudinal differences in beliefs of personal responsibility, trust in the government, rights to privacy and value of public versus individual health. Some view the reporting of new cases of HIV infections as intrusive and a violation of privacy while others see the lack of it as neglectful of the community health. Some see access to bath houses and sex clubs as a guaranteed personal right while others see the venues as amplifiers of disease within the population and call for their closure (Farley, 2002). So in the United States STD control as conceived by Dr Parran has never been fully applied for HIV prevention. Tools such as routine case identification through mandatory screening and case-based reporting were eschewed due to the stigma and fear of possible discrimination. Isolation was impractical for an infection with life-long infectivity and partner notification felt to be a violation of privacy and ineffectual intervention for an untreatable condition.

STDs and HIV Transmission

Meanwhile in Africa, STD control was being considered in a completely different paradigm. There had never been effective STD control programs in most countries. The spectrum of disease-reporting capacity and resources for STD diagnosis and treatment was varied. Most countries had no infrastructure or financial resources for STD prevention. Poorly trained health workers in local clinics treated most STDs with insufficient and inconsistent supplies of medications. Since the majority of AIDS cases in Africa had acquired HIV through heterosexual contact, it was imperative to understand why such a rapid and devastating epidemic took hold in Africa while at the same time seemed to be sparing much of the Western world. Kenyan research teams in the late 1980s identified that STDs, in particular, infections that cause genital ulcerations, were highly associated with HIV transmission (Cameron *et al.*, 1989). The ulcers seemed both to increase the infectiousness of someone already HIV infected and increase the susceptibility of someone exposed to an HIV-infected partner. Additional studies showed that the rates of HIV infection were significantly greater in those with more STDs than in those with fewer. In 1999, then Director of the Centers for Disease Control and Prevention, Division of STD Prevention, Dr Wasserheit reviewed over 2000 studies to demonstrate the consistency of the effect of STDs on risk for HIV transmission and calculated that the average effect of STDs on HIV transmission was

116

between 2- and 5-fold increased risk (Fleming and Wasserheit, 1999). These studies supported the idea that one of the reasons there were wide differences in the number and distribution of HIV infections in Africa versus the West was the difference in the frequency of STDs. What logically followed was that if STDs could be controlled in Africa, HIV transmission could be reduced.

The first prospective study in female sex workers in Zaire to show a temporal relationship of STDs and HIV infection demonstrated that in those women who had fewer new STDs over time there was also a reduction in the rate of new HIV infections (Laga *et al.*, 1994). Women were encouraged to use condoms and get regular STD check-ups and treatment. Those with the most frequent STD check-ups and fewest STDs had the lowest rate of new HIV infections. The number of sex partners and condom use was not correlated with HIV infection in the final analysis. This study was crucial in clarifying the role that STDs had in HIV transmission. New STDs increased an individual's risk of becoming HIV infected, demonstrating that STDs was a more important risk factor than the number of sex partners.

So now two important aspects of the interaction between STDs and HIV were well understood. STDs were more common in people with HIV and if a person acquired a new STD, he or she was at greater risk of becoming HIV infected. This set the stage for the next level of evidence and the type of evidence that public health policy makers and public health professionals use to support major changes in disease control strategies – experimental interventions.

In observational studies where researchers count the number of events without manipulating the exposure, many factors could explain the findings. In this situation cause and effect can be difficult to prove. The definitive research studies control the exposure and randomly assign different exposures to groups of individuals. These individuals are then carefully followed over time to measure the desired outcome. The rate of the outcome in each group is compared and then can be directly related to the known exposure. Giving people new STDs and following them for new HIV infection would not be ethical, but an experiment where one actively reduced the number of STDs in one group and not in another group could be ethical, at least by the standards of the time, since the group not receiving STD treatment was receiving the standard of local care, which unfortunately in most of Africa is nothing.

STD Treatment and HIV Prevention

Three studies in which STDs were treated in an effort to reduce HIV transmission have been completed. Each study treated STDs in a different way, making them not only excellent examples of different STD strategies but highlighting the complexities of interpreting the findings of population-based research. Researchers completed the first study in the Mwanza district of Tanzania (Grosskurth *et al.*, 1995). In this study researchers randomly assigned 12 villages to either enhanced STD diagnosis and treatment services where trained clinicians in STD management and adequate medications for treatment were available versus standard diagnostic services and care. In the intervention communities the rate of STDs decreased and there was a substantial 42 per cent reduction in the number of new HIV infections. As expected but rarely proven, improved STD treatment services reduced the prevalence of STDs (Mayaud *et al.*, 1997). These findings generated great excitement for health professionals in Africa who thought an effective disease control strategy for HIV prevention had been found – STD treatment (Laga, 1995).

To further evaluate and understand the impact of STD control a second group of researchers on the other side of Lake Victoria in Uganda implemented a different STD control strategy to prevent new HIV infections (Wawer *et al.*, 1999). Researchers randomly assigned 10 clusters of villages to receive mass treatment with several antibiotics effective against up to six STDs or to receive mass treatment with antibiotics effective against intestinal worm infections. The study team treated members of each village every 10 months for at least three rounds of treatment. Mass treatment as a means to control STDs had been successfully implemented in prior populations with some success. If the entire at-risk population is treated at a single time and the frequency of STDs can be reduced such that no one is infected, there can be no continued spread of infection. In one study among female sex workers in a migrant farm community, treating all the sex workers with penicillin reduced the frequency of syphilis by half (Jaffe *et al.*, 1979). In order for mass treatment to be successful, a high proportion of the population has to be treated and the community has to be relatively closed, that is, with limited migration of new people into the community. In the Uganda mass treatment study, treatment was successful in reducing the number of STDs in the villages assigned to STD treatment; however, there was no change in the number of HIV infections. Disheartening as this was, researchers had several explanations.

One explanation considered that the HIV epidemic in Tanzania was in a much earlier stage where STDs would have greater impact on transmission compared to the stage of the epidemic in Uganda, where it was of a longer duration and less impacted by STDs (Hitchcock and Fransen, 1999). Why epidemics in various stages are differentially impacted by co-factors like STDs is a complicated issue, mostly theoretical in nature, supported by little empirical evidence. A second more plausible explanation was the role of another STD that was common but not treated in the Uganda study and unusually rare in the Tanzania population, namely genital herpes.

Recent evidence increasingly demonstrates the important role that genital herpes has in the transmission of HIV infection. In Uganda, 85 per cent of genital ulcers with an identified cause were from genital herpes, yet because genital herpes is caused by a virus and these viruses cannot be cured or eradicated from infected people with a single dose of treatment, mass treatment precluded any reduction in genital herpes. In Tanzania, however, genital herpes was rare, thus the lack of STD treatment for genital herpes had little impact and the study intervention was successful.

A third explanation focused on the role of symptomatic versus asymptomatic STDs. Contrary to popular opinion, most STDs are without symptoms (Institute of Medicine, 1997). Men and women get infected from others and more often than not do not develop any symptoms. These asymptomatic carriers go on to spread the infections, unknowingly, to others. In the West, this knowledge has led to the widespread implementation of screening programs or STD testing in people without symptoms to identify and treat infections (CDC, 2002a). Screening programs to control STDs have become a mainstay of STD prevention. Data from screening programs demonstrate that not only does screening reduce the rate of infection but it also reduces complications (Scholes *et al.*, 1996). Screening relies on medical providers and health care delivery systems to test routinely sexually active adults at periodic intervals. Current recommendations for the control of chlamydia infection in the United States state that all sexually active women age 25 years and less should be screened annually. Because there are no symptoms it is often difficult to know how long someone has been infected and very difficult among those with multiple partners to know who infected whom. The relative role that asymptomatic versus symptomatic infections have in HIV transmission is largely speculative but some evidence suggests that symptomatic infections may be more important.

Symptomatic STDs are associated with significant inflammation at the site of infection. This inflammation is characterized by numerous white blood cells, including target cells for HIV infection, and intercellular chemical messengers or cytokines that serve to increase HIV viral replication and the amount of HIV in genital secretions. Treatment can reduce the amount of HIV in infectious genital fluids. Thus, there is biological evidence that STD treatment could reduce HIV transmission (Cohen *et al.*, 1997; McClelland *et al.*, 2001).

Thus, in the Tanzania study based on increasing the availability of STD diagnostic and treatment services, most people with symptomatic STDs were treated whereas in the Uganda study a much greater proportion of people with asymptomatic STDs were treated and what treatment was available to symptomatic people with STDs between mass treatment rounds was uncertain. So, in Tanzania more symptomatic people were treated – people with greater risk for transmission and acquisition of HIV infection – while in Uganda, more asymptomatic people were treated – and treatment of asymptomatic people may be less important in reducing HIV transmission since given the absence of symptoms, they are already less likely to transmit or acquire HIV infection.

A third and more recent study incorporated STD treatment and attempts to change the sexual risk behavior of people living in villages in Uganda (Kamali *et al.*, 2003). In this study researchers randomly allocated 18 villages to three study arms: (1) community-level intervention for sexual risk behavior reduction; (2) STD treatment and community-level intervention for sexual risk behavior reduction; or (3) neither. The results of this study did not support an important effect of STD treatment on the rate of new HIV infections. While rates of syphilis and gonorrhea did decline, these decreases were not associated with reduced rates of new

HIV infections. The researchers again cited similar explanations about the potential stage of the epidemic and role of genital herpes. Similar to the second study the HIV epidemic was in a more mature stage and while genital herpes was common, it was untreated.

The one consistent finding from these studies may be the role of genital herpes in HIV transmission (Wald and Link, 2002). Currently, the National Institutes of Health is supporting a study to determine whether the suppression of genital herpes with daily antiviral therapy in people with evidence of prior infection and who are at high risk for acquiring HIV infection will be effective in reducing the number of new HIV infections. It will be critical that patients enrolled in the study have a recent history of frequent symptomatic episodes of genital herpes such that suppression of these episodes in the treatment group markedly reduces their risk of HIV acquisition. Just as symptoms probably played an important role in the success or failure of the studies in Africa, if the two groups in the herpes suppression prevention study have similar infrequent episodes of symptomatic genital herpes than it may be unlikely that genital herpes suppression will have the desired effect.

Behavioral Risk Reduction and STD Prevention

So far we have discussed different effective strategies in STD control including: (1) case-identification, treatment, and partner treatment; (2) mass treatment; and (3) screening and treatment. These biomedical interventions require a common element – effective treatment. Since for many years there was no effective treatment for HIV infection, the major area for the development of HIV prevention was in behavioral interventions. Behavioral interventions for HIV prevention aimed to reduce the sexual risk behavior – namely unprotected sexual intercourse – associated with HIV transmission. There are few, if any, practical behavioral interventions that have been shown to reduce the number of new HIV infections. One intervention worth reviewing that did reduce the frequency of new STDs was Project Respect.

Project Respect was an intervention trial designed to see if client-centered risk reduction counseling could reduce an individual's sexual risk behavior and subsequent number of new STDs (Kamb *et al.*, 1998). Researchers reported that two counseling sessions as compared with two information and education sessions reduced by about 30 per cent the frequency of new STDs. Researchers also studied the effect of four counseling sessions and found no added benefit. Client-centered risk reduction counseling is an interactive process between a trained counselor and an at-risk patient. The counselor initiates the session by assessing the patient's sexual risk behavior (i.e. number and type of partners, specific type of acts of sex – oral, anal, vaginal, use of condoms, use of drugs, etc.). With the help of the counselor the patient then identifies some aspect of sexual risk behavior that he or she feels able to control and hence reduce. The counselor and patient end the discussion with an agreement where the patient intends and has skills to reduce that specific behavior. At the second counseling session, this specific risk behavior is evaluated, challenges and solutions to risk reduction maintenance are identified and successes reinforced. While some clinics have implemented client-centered risk reduction counseling as an STD prevention strategy, the necessary training for counselors, availability of counselors and commitment by both patients and providers has limited its usefulness as a widespread and effective STD control strategy.

Condom Policy and Distribution

In Thailand, one of the most effective STD control and HIV prevention strategies has been policy change. In the late 1980s Thailand was identified as country with a high number of new HIV infections, in particular among female sex workers in brothels and in young male military recruits (Nelson *et al.*, 1993). At the time it was common and socially acceptable for young men to have their first sexual experiences in brothels. While brothels and prostitution were not technically legal, the sex industry existed with little government interference and was a well-known and significant aspect of tourism. Recognizing the need to protect the health of its military and hopefully with some consideration to the health and welfare of sex workers, the Thai government developed and enforced a policy of 100 per cent condom use in all brothels. Authorities inspected venues and held owners accountable. This policy directly resulted in a dramatic decline in STDs and new HIV infections among sex workers and Thai military recruits (Nelson *et al.*, 1996). In addition, likely related to massive community-level education efforts, the frequency of brothel use among Thai military recruits for their first sexual experience also declined. Men either delayed their first sexual experiences or had first sexual experiences with partners who were not sex workers.

Condom promotion, distribution, education, and social marketing has been a key strategy in STD control and more recently in HIV prevention. When used correctly and consistently, condoms effectively reduce the transmission of STDs, including HIV. While condoms are not perfect, no prevention strategy is – even abstinence as a strategy can fail as people who avoid sex succumb to peer pressure, coercion, substance use, or fatigue. In San Francisco, condom distribution was an important part of the early response to AIDS. Community-based organizations were funded by the local government – and still are – to distribute condoms in sex clubs, bars, parks, adult bookstores, and other venues where either sex might occur or people at risk for HIV infection visit. No distribution program can be effective, however, without a social context and norm for using condoms.

After dramatic increases in condom use by gay men in San Francisco, there have been some declines in regular condom use since 1996. Either due to less fear of AIDS in HIV-uninfected men because of advances in the treatment of HIV infection, a similar decreased concern in sexually active HIV-infected men about transmitting AIDS, or what some have called 'prevention fatigue' – people tired of being safe all the time – the use of condoms among people with partners of either opposite or unknown HIV serostatus has declined (Stall *et al.*, 2000). Sex clubs in San Francisco still require condoms to be used for anal intercourse but enforcement is intermittent. Going into the third decade of the AIDS epidemic, one gay men's bath house and sex club in Berkeley still has no policy requiring condom use for sexual intercourse.

Unlike in Thailand, Americans are inconsistent in their adoption of condom use and condom use policies. Somewhat reassuring, however, has been the steady increases in condom use among adolescents in the United States (CDC, 2002b). School condom availability programs, thought by some to promote sexual behavior, have been shown to be safe and effective without any increase in associated sexual activity (Guttmacher *et al.*, 1997). Condom manufacturers lacking the profitability of major industries like alcoholic beverages, tobacco, and pharmaceuticals limit general advertising and usually target young adults in select media in the United States. In Uganda, however, condom promotion efforts are widespread, and researchers generally agree that along with the promotion of abstinence and monogamy these have been crucial to recent successes in the reduction of new HIV infections in young adults (Whitworth *et al.*, 2002).

STDs in HIV Surveillance

Other ways the AIDS epidemic has impacted STD control is the integration of STD surveillance into HIV prevention and the role of HIV counseling and testing into STD clinical care. Since both STDs and HIV are transmitted through sexual intercourse and STDs may either be precursors to HIV infection or identify those at risk, successful HIV surveillance programs have incorporated markers of sexual risk such as rectal gonorrhea in their efforts to monitor groups at risk of HIV infection. Rectal gonorrhea is a particularly useful measure of HIV risk in gay men because it is highly associated with risk for HIV infection and can routinely be reported by laboratories to local health departments (Katz *et al.*, 2002; Kim *et al.*, 2003). Health departments can track rates of rectal gonorrhea in specific age groups, racial and/or ethnic groups, and neighborhoods to target HIV prevention efforts. Rectal gonorrhea rates in HIV-uninfected men can be used to measure the success of HIV prevention programs focusing on behavioral change including condom use and partner reduction. In San Francisco, we have used rectal gonorrhea to identify risk factors for infection that would be similar to HIV infection. Since HIV infection did not become a reportable condition in San Francisco until 2001–2002, rectal gonorrhea was a surrogate marker that could readily be studied. Analyses showed that anonymous sex at commercial sex venues, meeting sex partners on the Internet, methamphetamine use, and Viagra use were risk factors for rectal gonorrhea (Kim *et al.*, 2003). Thus, interventions aimed at educating people with these behaviors or at reducing the frequency of these risk behaviors might reduce the frequency of rectal gonorrhea, and importantly new HIV infections as well.

HIV Counseling and Testing in STD Clinics

Since the discovery of the first test for HIV infection, STD clinics and control programs were among the first sites to offer HIV counseling and testing. People seeking STD care were at higher risk for HIV infection and a well-functioning testing infrastructure existed. Since 1984, the San Francisco City Clinic has administered nearly 100 000 HIV tests. HIV testing is not a quick blood test but incorporates risk assessment and risk reduction counseling. By State law, each HIV test must be administered by a certified trained counselor who educates the patient about the test, evaluates the patient's risk for HIV infection and conducts patient-centered risk reduction counseling. Just as with any medical intervention, the quality and effect of HIV counseling will vary based on the skills and experience of the counselor and unique characteristics of the patient, but HIV counseling and testing has been deemed an effective HIV prevention intervention and has been evaluated in randomized clinical trials (Voluntary HIV-1 Counseling and Testing Efficacy Study Group, 2000). The incorporation of HIV counseling and testing in STD control programs has afforded the opportunity to have trained counselors on site in many clinics and attract people at risk for HIV infection into STD care. At San Francisco City Clinic this model has allowed people identified as HIV infected to access HIV care readily and for research studies to be undertaken to develop new ways to monitor the rate and characteristics of those newly HIV infected (Schwarcz *et al.*, 2002).

HIV Prevention as STD Control

A technique pioneered by researchers in North Carolina has been the use of HIV viral RNA testing to identify HIV-infected individuals before HIV antibody can be detected (Pilcher *et al.*, 2002). This may be one of the most significant recent advances in HIV prevention as the field moves more towards adopting traditional STD control strategies and perhaps further modernizes into what may be called 'HIV control'. Since current HIV tests rely on the detection of the presence of HIV antibody, people may be infected and have undetectable antibody soon after infection. While most tests detect antibody to HIV 4–6 weeks after infection, HIV viral RNA tests detect the presence of virus as early as 10 days after infection. Closing this window period between infection and antibody detection could identify a greater number of people with infection. This is important not only because more people with infection might be detected but because people in this window period are highly infectious.

Soon after HIV infection the virus replicates reaching millions of copies of RNA per milliliter of plasma. Subsequently, through mechanisms not well understood but likely to be under immunologic control, the viral load decreases to a set point usually at about 100 000 copies of RNA per milliliter of plasma. This log reduction in viral load is a potentially critical factor in the infectiousness of an individual since the plasma viral load strongly correlates with HIV infectivity (Quinn *et al.*, 2000). The higher the plasma viral load the more infectious a person is. Thus a person with a plasma viral load in the millions of copies during this window period before detectable antibody is highly infectious relative to others with more long-standing infection. Secondly, the behavioral context during which a person is infected may be a high-risk period during which a person may have multiple sex partners or be engaging in other behaviors or have conditions that amplify sexual risk such as substance use or mental health problems. By identifying people during this period and counseling them about their infection a resultant behavior change may ensue, reducing subsequent transmissions and the risk to others. Thirdly, people recently infected with HIV may be in a particular social-sexual network where recent partners have also been recently infected. STD control strategies such as partner elicitation, contact tracing, and partner notification could be effective in identifying HIV-infected members of this network and reducing the transmission of additional infections.

A recent addition to HIV counseling and testing has been the determination of the duration of infection in those with HIV antibody positive tests. Experimental evidence demonstrates that the duration of infection correlates with the concentration of HIV antibody in the serum (Janssen *et al.*, 1998). Just as the presence or absence of HIV antibody in people with detectable plasma HIV RNA can differentiate very early from early infection, the concentration of antibody can differentiate between early and late infection. Using the Serum Testing Algorithm for Recent HIV Seroconversion (STARHS), by measuring the antibody status of an undiluted versus a diluted serum specimen, laboratorians can determine whether a person has been infected with HIV for more or less than about six months. As previously mentioned, this technique has allowed researchers to describe the rate of new infections in certain populations and is being evaluated as a means to identify social-sexual networks of recent infection. Similar to STD control strategies, HIV control strategies could be focused on those with the most recent infections and HIV prevention interventions targeted to these populations and associated risk factors for newly acquired HIV infection.

As of Fall 2003, the San Francisco City Clinic is testing people at risk for HIV infection using all three tests: HIV RNA, HIV antibody, and if HIV antibody positive, STAHRS. As a combined research and public health intervention, this strategy may increase the effectiveness by which new cases of HIV infection are identified, particularly in the most infectious individuals, and allow intervention through risk reduction counseling and partner management services to reduce the number of new HIV infections at the community level. Furthermore, studies that identify risk factors and social-sexual networks associated with recent HIV infection may be useful in targeting prevention interventions such as those studies done in STD outbreaks that have identified brand new factors like the use of the Internet and stimulated the development of Internet-based STD prevention activities (Klausner *et al.*, 2000).

Recreational Drug Use and Risk

Addressing substance abuse has become an important component of STD control and HIV prevention programs. While not characteristic of traditional infectious disease control programs that focus on case identification, reporting, treatment, and isolation, addressing behavioral risk factors for disease more closely mirrors chronic disease prevention programs. As HIV infection has evolved into a more chronic disease and STDs increasingly are understood to be related to certain co-morbid behaviors like substance abuse, there has been increased attention to addressing this co-factor. Several research studies have shown stimulant drug use like methamphetamine to be associated with the risk for HIV acquisition. Cross-sectional studies have shown that those with HIV infection are more frequent users of methamphetamine, and prospective observational studies have shown that methamphetamine users are more likely to acquire HIV infection (Stall and Purcell, 2000).

Questions remain on how to respond effectively to methamphetamine use and the risk for HIV infection – whether social marketing programs to reduce demand for methamphetamine through advertising highlighting the adverse effects of methamphetamine use similar to current tobacco control programs can be effective versus provision of individual level methamphetamine treatment services similar to opiate addiction treatment services versus increased law enforcement to abate the supply versus some combination of the above or something entirely new. This is one of the most significant challenges currently in the HIV epidemic in gay men and other men who have sex with men where stimulant drug use is common. Data show that up to 25 per cent of gay men and other men who have sex with men who have recently become HIV infected have used methamphetamine in the past three months (San Francisco Department of Public Health, 2002).

Methamphetamine use was associated with increased sexual risk behavior, both increased number of sex partners and decreased condom use. Among HIV-infected men up to one-third seen at the San Francisco City Clinic are methamphetamine users. Methamphetamine can be taken through injection, through inhalation, swallowing, and rectal insertion. Methamphetamine injection drug users are among the highest risk for HIV infection, with some studies demonstrating an annual infection rate of 10–20 per cent (Golden *et al.*, 2003). While HIV infection through the sharing of needles might seem to be the obvious route, because of the available and effective needle exchange programs, most injection drug users acquire HIV infection sexually (Kral *et al.*, 2001).

Because of the biological effects of methamphetamine use on erectile function, many methamphetamine and other stimulant users have difficulty in having or maintaining an erection. For years, this biological consequence resulted in an effect on sexual behavior in men who have sex with men where methamphetamine users were more likely to engage in receptive anal intercourse versus insertive anal intercourse. Some experts in sexual behavior believe that by limiting the sexual versatility of these high-risk men and since transmission of HIV is less efficient from the rectum to the penis compared with from the penis to rectum, the continued transmission of HIV infection by HIV-infected people practicing receptive anal intercourse was less likely. In addition, HIV-infected men may experience an increased frequency of impotence, either due to coexistent medical conditions like diabetes or vascular disease or side-effects of commonly prescribed medications. Couple the increased frequency of impotence in the risk population of methamphetamine users and in HIV-infected men who have sex with men and the increased erectile firmness required for anal penetration versus vaginal penetration, and anal intercourse was becoming less common. Had this circumstance gone untreated the trend may have resulted in less HIV transmission. At the same time, however, a new drug entered the marketplace that was widely available, relatively safe, and very effective at reversing impotence related to chemical or vascular causes, Viagra (sildenafil citrate).

Walking through a sex club in the Winter of 2001, I stepped on a plastic and foil package which would not have normally struck me had I not felt a particular pill wrapper quality to them with the characteristic hard plastic center. I bent down to pick it up and was surprised to see the characteristic Viagra label. Thinking how explosive the recreational use of Viagra in multiple partner settings might be, I quickly implemented a population-based survey at City Clinic, as a means to understand potential new sexual and drug using behaviors. Rapid surveys characteristically serve to inform and develop hypotheses for outbreak investigations in disease control activities (Kim *et al.*, 2002). The survey is a public health tool that can inform or direct public health professionals but cannot prove causation or usually intervene, in and of itself, to prevent disease transmission. Findings of the survey suggested that the recreational use of Viagra, defined as Viagra use outside of medical supervision, was common, about one-third of gay men and one in eight heterosexual men had used Viagra in the past year. More importantly Viagra users, particularly HIV-infected Viagra users, were more likely to engage in risky sexual behavior associated with HIV transmission and also more likely to be diagnosed with an STD at the time of the survey. These findings generated substantial discussion (Tuller, 2001) and also suggested a new portal for HIV prevention interventions. Viagra users could be targeted for STD/HIV prevention education and STD/HIV screening. Viagra use, especially recreational Viagra use, could be reduced in this population. Convincing the Food and Drug Administration and the manufacturer, Pfizer, Inc., however, to take effective action on the basis of the evidence continues to prove to be difficult (Chase, 2003).

The Internet and STD Transmission and HIV Prevention

Linking Viagra marketing and availability, methamphetamine distribution, and easy access to new sex partners is the Internet. The Internet as a venue for sex partnering and STD transmission was first identified and described in the Summer of 1999 (Nieves, 1999). While seeing a patient that Spring at the San Francisco City Clinic, I asked the patient how many sex partners he had had in the past two months. He said 14. I then asked how many he had in the past year. He replied 14. Being curious about this response, I asked what happened two months ago. He told me he got on line. I didn't understand what he meant until he told me how one goes to online chatrooms, sites created by Internet service providers like America Online (AOL), and finds chatrooms specific to certain sexual behaviors and geographic areas to meet new sex partners. My patient had been able to meet 14 new sex partners in the past couple of months without having to leave his living room. Similar to the public health response to Viagra, we implemented a survey at City Clinic in 1999 to learn that about 32 per cent of men were meeting partners online (Kim *et al.*, 2001). More recently this has increased, and various surveys and cities report that more than 40 per cent of gay men meet new partners online. In the current syphilis epidemic in San Francisco, a majority of new syphilis cases have met new sex partners online. Responding to this fact, health departments have partnered with community-based organizations to work together and collaborate with Internet service providers. Often the Internet service providers do have staff interested in HIV prevention. Using community leaders and organizations to approach the Internet service providers to implement prevention activities has been more fruitful than when the health department takes the lead, since legal jurisdiction in this area is poorly defined.

To address the issue of the Internet and STD and HIV prevention, the Centers for Disease Control convened a national meeting of sexual health and disease control experts in August 2003. There were over 300 participants from Europe, Australia, Canada, and the United States. Clearly, the importance of Internet-based sex partnering and the opportunity for both disease transmission and prevention was receiving international attention. As the first meeting on the topic, most presentations were descriptive in nature, that is, reporting on the frequency and characteristics of people meeting new sex partners online. There were some presentations on Internet-based prevention interventions ranging from using e-mail for partner notification (a twenty-first century strategy originally described by Dr Thomas Parran in the 1930s), websites, online advertisements called 'banner ads' about sexual health, STDs, and HIV, chatroom one-on-one outreach, expert forums, and online STD testing. Because of the need for innovation in HIV prevention and the documented impact of the Internet on STD and HIV transmission, organizations had rapidly taken to Internet-based prevention. This being very early in the new field of Internet-based STD/HIV prevention, good evaluations of different strategies were lacking.

Impact of HIV Therapy and HIV Medication Advertising

One unexpected aspect of the AIDS epidemic and its impact on STD prevention and control has been the recent medical and psychosocial effects of highly active antiretroviral therapy. Antiretroviral therapy has been an outstanding success story in modern medicine. Patients within days and months of dying have had their disease progression halted. While treatment for opportunistic infections in the past delayed mortality, effective antiretroviral therapy reversed the ongoing immunologic decline. With this 'Lazarus effect' came renewed physical energy and sexual interest. A study in AIDS patients showed that patients on antiretroviral therapy had higher rates of new STDs than those not on antiretroviral therapy (Scheer *et al.*, 2001). As the years progressed with increasing clinical success of antiretroviral therapy, there was an increase in the number of new STDs in patients on therapy. Thus, therapy was associated with increases in STDs. Adding to the clinical benefits of antiretroviral therapy were the increase in direct-to-consumer drug advertisements in communities severely affected by AIDS touting the benefits of the drugs. The advertisements, however, went beyond realistic expectations since the drugs all had serious potential side-effects, often debilitating diarrhea and neuropathy. If the drugs were causing individual benefits and increased sexual activity, there was concern that the advertisements were decreasing the concern and fear people might have about AIDS.

Once again, the survey was a useful tool for assessing the impact that HIV drug advertisements might be having on community perceptions and sexual risk behavior. In a study of gay men at the San Francisco City Clinic, men who were increasingly exposed to drug advertisements were less fearful of AIDS and most likely to engage in high-risk sexual behavior (Klausner *et al.*, 2002). So while HIV-infected men were benefiting from the drugs, HIV-uninfected men were taking more chances, thinking AIDS was a manageable disease. In order to change the negative impact of the advertising, the San Francisco Department of Public Health asked the pharmaceutical manufacturers to offer a more balanced message. The manufacturers, thinking that if they changed the advertisements they might become less competitive and less profitable, refused. Having no choice, the health department requested the FDA to mandate changes by the manufacturers. Since the liberalization of direct-to-consumer advertising in 1997, the FDA had less opportunity to review advertisements and usually only assessed the text of advertisements and not images. While the text in these advertisements may not have directly over-stated the potential benefits of the drugs, the images of men climbing mountains, sailing boats, and exuding sexuality were found to be misleading. In April 2001, the FDA Division of Drug Marketing, Advertising and Communications issued a regulatory letter to nine HIV pharmaceutical manufacturers requiring them to modify all direct-to-consumer advertisements within 90 days.

Post-exposure HIV Prophylaxis (PEP) in STD Clinics

Antibiotic treatment after exposure to treatable infections has been a mainstay of disease prevention for diseases like syphilis and tuberculosis. In syphilis control, people who have been recently exposed to syphilis are treated with penicillin by injection to prevent the development of syphilis infection. The incubation period, or time from exposure to infection, during which preventive treatment can be effective for syphilis is about one month. Preventive therapy for syphilis is highly effective and may prevent more than 95 per cent of infections in those exposed (Hook *et al.*, 1999). Treating people exposed to tuberculosis with six months of antituberculosis therapy after exposure is also highly effective and a standard of medical care and tuberculosis control.

During the early period in the AIDS epidemic, a landmark study was done that demonstrated the effectiveness of post-exposure HIV prophylaxis (PEP) for people exposed to HIV from needlestick or percutaneous exposure (Cardo *et al.*, 1997). In this study, people taking antiretroviral therapy for HIV infection were 80 per cent less likely to become HIV-infected compared with people who did not take therapy. Some caveats were that therapy had to be started within 72 hours of exposure and the duration of treatment had to be at least 28 days.

It was not long before advocates for HIV prevention for people with sexual expos-ure to HIV infection considered the use of PEP (Katz and Gerberding, 1997). Providing PEP to people with a well-defined high-risk sexual exposure, like a woman who has had vaginal intercourse and semen exposure to an HIV-infected partner, or a man who has had receptive anal intercourse and semen exposure to an HIV-infected partner, could reduce the likelihood of HIV transmission by 10-fold from an estimated chance without PEP of 1 in a 100 to 1 in 1000. Creating PEP pro-grams and making PEP available to a high-risk community, however, might disin-hibit safer sex behavior and if it did not work to prevent HIV transmission could have disastrous consequences. In order to understand the effects of the provision of PEP, initial programs were conducted under research study protocols with rigorous observation (Roland *et al.*, 2001). These studies failed to support a negative impact of PEP but were not designed to measure the effectiveness. Given the absence of the negative impact and the true potential for benefit, PEP programs have increasingly become available in public settings. San Francisco's PEP program is coordinated at the San Francisco City Clinic and the San Francisco General Hospital where people can be evaluated and, if indicated, receive PEP seven days a week. In 2002, City Clinic provided about 100 people with PEP for sexual exposure to HIV infection. Since the true risk of exposure is unknown, how well PEP works is uncertain. One public health benefit of providing PEP in an STD clinic is that people can undergo a full STD evaluation for more common infections like gonorrhea, chlamydia, syphilis, and herpes simplex virus.

Venue Notification

Since many of the sex partners in the current epidemics of STDs and HIV in gay men and other men who have sex with men are unnamed because of distrust in local health departments or because the sexual encounters are anonymous where no name or contact information is exchanged, partner notification is limited as a disease control strategy (Kent *et al.*, 2003). Unknown partners cannot be notified. Social network theory tells us, however, that people find sex partners in similar social-sexual networks, such that venues or places where people meet sexual partners may be reasonable surrogates for these networks. Similar people with similar risk tend to congregate and meet in similar places, so places like bath houses, chatrooms, or bars may identify specific sexual networks. Knowing that similar people at risk may be identified by a meeting place suggests that while a unique partner cannot be notified, people who meet at a unique venue can be and those people might be at a similar level of risk as the actual partner. To this end, health departments have increasingly asked new cases of STDs, including HIV, where they meet new sexual partners.

The reported venue can be targeted for educational efforts, outreach, STD screening and, depending on the type of venue, can notify its patrons or members of the potential increased risk for STDs (Michaud *et al.*, 2003). This strategy has been effective at adult bookstores where syphilis cases have met anonymous partners, online chatrooms, sex clubs, bars, and private parties. New cases have been identified and brought to treatment similar to successful outcomes with partner notification. Often it can be challenging to secure the cooperation of a private business to educate or inform patrons if that business believes that doing so somehow acknowledges responsibility for the transmission of disease. While businesses, particularly commercial sex venues, do have a responsibility to create environments that support safer sex, only individuals physically transmit STDs. That said, however, businesses can, as perhaps an unintended consequence of the nature of their business, facilitate the transmission of disease through either providing physical space for sex or making it easier to find new sex partners and once made aware of new cases of disease should make all possible efforts to reduce this risk through awareness and education efforts. Currently, there is little legal precedent for liability in this regard so efforts must be collaborative in spirit and often involve the community from where the cases arise.

Collaboration with Community-based Organizations

Perhaps one of the most obvious impacts of AIDS on STD control programs has been the recent shift towards increasing collaborations between community-based organizations and local public health agencies. In the early response to the AIDS epidemic, community-based organizations were key in defining how AIDS would be controlled; in fact, the creation and empowerment of community-based organizations was an HIV prevention strategy in and of itself. Now STD control programs are recognizing the value of community partnerships and Federal STD control funds include a mandatory percentage that must be used to support community-based organizations. In the context of the recent syphilis epidemic among men who have sex with men in major cities across the United States, many STD control programs have been successfully collaborating with community-based organizations. In Chicago, for example, the STD control program works closely with the Howard Brown clinic, a local gay, bisexual, lesbian, and transgender medical center, to facilitate partner notification activities. In Philadelphia, the Department of Public Health supports a community-based organization to conduct outreach on the Internet. Through this collaboration of 693 men with whom outreach was done, 292 (42 per cent) men were screened for syphilis and 69 (10 per cent) for HIV infection (Locke and Salmon, 2003).

In addition to collaborations with community groups, many STD control programs now have community advisory boards and community partners groups that advise and shape STD control policy and programs. Some programs require that community-based committees review educational and promotional materials to assure that the images and messages are appropriate for the target population. This involvement of community members on advisory boards, planning groups, and review committees in STD control programs is a direct result of similar activities in HIV prevention programs.

What the Future Holds

HIV/AIDS has transformed STD prevention and control by highlighting the importance of effective STD control programs in the prevention of HIV infection. Research studies have shown that STD control can reduce new HIV infections. The advent of AIDS has brought new experts into STD control resulting in increasing program innovation and evaluation. The continued pressing need for effective HIV control activities has forced traditional STD control programs to incorporate primary and secondary HIV prevention activities like HIV counseling and testing, post-exposure prophylaxis, HIV early care services and work with community groups most at risk not only for STDs but for HIV. STD programs are increasingly under the spotlight to demonstrate the effectiveness of interventions and justify resource allocation. By integrating the strengths of HIV prevention – community mobilization, respect for individual autonomy, patient-centered risk reduction, and frank education – STD programs can move in to the twenty-first century better positioned to improve the sexual health of the population.

What has been obviously missing for STD control in recent years has been advocacy. If we can learn anything from colleagues in HIV prevention, it is how to be effective advocates for sound, rational policy that balances individual rights and the public health and continued, if not expanded, support and resources for education in sexual health and disease control programs. How to mobilize communities around sexual health in the United States is a major challenge.

Many hold the future solutions to improved STD prevention and control, similar to other social problems, to be in technology through advances in immunization, materials science, and communication. Efficacious immunizations have been developed for genital herpes, human papillomavirus, and hepatitis B infection. While hepatitis B immunization is now recommended for all newborns and in many States is required for school entry, how these other vaccines will be deployed is a matter of great concern. Will policy makers recommend that all people receive immunizations for these STDs or only those at elevated risk? Will parents agree to immunize newborns for infectious diseases transmitted through sexual behavior? Will governments and third-party payers pay for prevention interventions in these people, and will manufacturers bring the products to market if the profits are not guaranteed? Ideally, because health is a fundamental human right, the government would purchase immunizations of public health importance and make these available at no cost to individuals and provide adequate reimbursement to those providing the immunizations. Effective immunizations are ultimately cost saving if future infections and complications are prevented.

A second area making rapid technological advances is the development of microbicide gels or chemical films that can be applied within the vagina, rectum or potentially on the penis to prevent the transmission of infection. An 'armor plate' for the genital areas susceptible to infection could enable people to continue to engage in sexual intercourse without risk or at much reduced risk of acquiring STDs. Research in this area is promising but questions of how truly effective potential agents will be, about cost and distribution, and the use or uptake by those most at risk remain.

A third and exciting area combining the social movement of increased patient autonomy and responsibility is increased access to self-diagnosis and appropriate treatment through advances in technology. With the advent of molecular DNA analysis for the diagnosis of genital infections like chlamydia or gonorrhea, people will be able to purchase specimen collection kits at convenience stores and pharmacies to use in the privacy of their own home, drop specimens off at the pharmacy, or mail them back to a laboratory (Bloomfield *et al.*, 2002). By bypassing a medical provider for screening tests, more people may get screened for infection and ultimately treated. Increasing access to screening tests and test results through the Internet may also be more common (Levine and Klausner, 2003). Obtaining treatment for self-collected laboratory-diagnosed STDs through the Internet may also become possible. Using these tools to educate and empower people at risk for infection and eliminating barriers to screening may expand population-based screening and lead to reductions in STDs.

Finally, the culture wars between STD control and HIV prevention may end. As STD control programs reliant on a medical model of disease control learn from colleagues in HIV prevention about community-capacity building and addressing community-level vulnerability in risk, and HIV prevention advocates increasingly realize the public health benefit of case identification, reporting, and partner notification, HIV prevention and STD control programs will integrate to be more effective and better serve the population.

References

Bloomfield PJ, Kent C, Campbell D *et al.* (2002) Community-based chlamydia and gonorrhea screening through the United States mail, San Francisco. *Sex Transm Dis* 29: 294–7.

Brandt AM (1987) *No Magic Bullet*. New York: Oxford University Press.

Brown WJ, Blount JH (1973) The effectiveness of the epidemiologic approach to syphilis control. *J Reprod Med* 11: 123–4.

Cameron DW, Simonson JN, D'Costa LJ *et al.* (1989) Female to male transmission of human immunodeficiency virus type 1: risk factors for seroconversion in men. *The Lancet* 2: 403–7.

Cardo DM, Culver DH, Ciesielski CA *et al.* (1997) A case-control study of HIV sero conversion in health care workers after percutaneous exposure. Centers for Disease Control and Prevention needlestick surveillance group. *N Engl J Med* 337: 1485–90.

CDC (Centers for Disease Control) (2002a) Sexually transmitted diseases treatment guidelines, 2002. *MMWR Morb Mortal Wkly Rep* 51: 1–80.

CDC (2002b) Trends in sexual risk behaviors among high school students – United States, 1991–2001. *MMWR Morb Mortal Wkly Rep* 51: 856–9.

CDC (2003) Advancing HIV prevention: new strategies for a changing epidemic – United States, 2003. *MMWR Morb Mortal Wkly Rep* 52: 329–56.

Chase M (2003) A doctor fights for new warnings on Viagra labels. *Wall Street J* Friday 7 March 2003. pp. A1, A6.

Cohen MS, Hoffman IF, Royce RA *et al.* (1997) Reduction of concentration of HIV-1 in semen after treatment of urethritis: implications for prevention of sexual transmission of HIV-1. *The Lancet* 349: 1868–73.

Farley T (2002) Cruise control – bathhouses are reigniting the AIDS crisis. It's time to shut them down. *Washington Monthly* 34: 36 (6 pages).

Fleming DT, Wasserheit J (1999) From epidemiological synergy to public health policy and practice: the contribution of other sexually transmitted diseases to sexual transmission of HIV infection. *Sex Transm Infect* 75: 3–17.

Golden MR, Brewer DD, Wood RW *et al.* (2003) Association of methamphetamine use with HIV among MSM tested for HIV in an STD clinic. *15th Biennial Congress of the International Society for Sexually Transmitted Diseases Research (ISSTDR)*. Ottawa, Ontario, p. 107.

Grosskurth H, Mosha F, Todd, J *et al.* (1995) Impact of improved treatment of sexually transmitted diseases on HIV infection in rural Tanzania: randomised controlled trial. *The Lancet* 346: 530–6.

Guttmacher S, Lieberman L, Ward D *et al.* (1997) Condom availability in New York City public high schools: relationships to condom use and sexual behavior. *Am J Public Health* 87: 1427–33.

Hitchcock P, Fransen L (1999) Preventing HIV infection: lessons from Mwanza and Rakai. *The Lancet* 353: 513–14.

Hook EW, Stephens J, Ennis DM (1999) Azithromycin compared with penicillin G benzathine for treatment of incubating syphilis. *Ann Intern Med* 131: 434–7.

Institute of Medicine (US). Committee on Prevention and Control of Sexually Transmitted Diseases (1997) *The Hidden Epidemic: Confronting Sexually Transmitted Diseases.* Washington DC: National Academy Press.

Jaffe HW, Rice D, Voigt R *et al.* (1979) Selective mass treatment in a venereal disease control program. *Am J Public Health* 69: 1181–2.

Janssen RS, Satten GA, Stramer SL *et al.* (1998) New testing strategy to detect early HIV-1 infection for use in incidence estimates and for clinical and prevention purposes. *JAMA* 281: 1893.

Kamali A, Quigley M, Nakiyingi J *et al.* (2003) Syndromic management of sexually-transmitted infections and behavior change interventions on transmission of HIV-1 in rural Uganda: a community randomised trial. *The Lancet* 361: 645–52.

Kamb ML, Fishbein M, Douglas JM *et al.* (1998) Efficacy of risk-reduction counseling to prevent human immunodeficiency virus and sexually transmitted diseases. *JAMA* 280: 1161–7.

Katz MH, Gerberding, JL (1997) Postexposure treatment of people exposed to the human immunodeficiency virus through sexual contact or injection drug use. *N Engl J Med* 336: 1097–100.

Katz MH, Schwarcz S, Kellogg TA *et al.* (2002) Impact of highly active antiretroviral treatment on HIV seroincidence among men who have sex with men: San Francisco. *Am J Public Health* 92: 388–94.

Kent C, Stockman J, Klausner JD (2003) Traditional partner management for syphilis among men who have sex with men provided little intervention: San Francisco, 2001–2002. *15th Biennial Congress of the International Society for Sexually Transmitted Diseases Research (ISSTDR)*, Ottawa, Ontario, p. 181.

Kim AA, Kent C, McFarland W, Klausner JD (2001) Cruising on the Internet Highway. *J Acquir Immune Defic Syndr* 28: 89–93.

Kim AA, Kent C, Klausner JD (2002) Increased risk of HIV and sexually transmitted disease transmission among gay or bisexual men who use Viagra, San Francisco 2000–2001. *AIDS* 16: 1425–8.

Kim AA, Kent C, Klausner JD (2003) Risk factors for rectal gonorrhea amidst a resurgence of HIV infection. *Sex Transm Dis* 30: 813–17.

Klausner JD, Wolf W, Fischer-Ponce L *et al.* (2000) Tracing a syphilis outbreak through cyberspace. *JAMA* 284: 447–9.

Klausner JD, Kim A, Kent CK. (2002) Are HIV drug advertisements contributing to increases in risk behavior among men in San Francisco, 2001? *AIDS* 16: 15–16.

Kral AH, Bluthenthal RN, Lorvick J *et al.* (2001) Sexual transmission of HIV-1 among injection drug users in San Francisco, USA: risk-factor analysis. *The Lancet* 357: 1397–401.

Laga M (1995) STD control for HIV prevention – it works! *The Lancet* 346: 518–19.

Laga M, Alary M, Nzila N *et al.* (1994) Condom promotion, sexually transmitted diseases treatment, and declining incidence of HIV-1 infection in female Zairian sex workers. *The Lancet* 344: 246–8.

Levine D, Klausner JD (2003) Syphilis screening via online lab slips. *2003 STD/HIV Prevention and the Internet.* Washington, DC: National Coalition of STD Directors, p. 55.

Locke K, Salmon M (2003) The power of collaboration: Internet outreach to MSM in Philadelphia. *2003 STD/HIV Prevention and the Internet*. Washington, DC: National Coalition of STD Directors, p. 71.

Mayaud P, Mosha F, Todd J *et al.* (1997) Treatment of cervicitis is associated with decreased cervical shedding of HIV-1. Non-ulcerative sexually transmitted diseases as risk factors for HIV-1 transmission in women: results from a cohort study. *AIDS* 11: 1873–80.

McClelland RS, Wang C, Mandaliya K *et al.* (2001) Treatment of cervicitis is associated with decreased cervical shedding of HIV-1. *AIDS* 15: 105–10.

Michaud JM, Ellen J, Johnson SM, Rompalo AM (2003) Responding to a community outbreak of syphilis by targeting sex partner meeting location: an example of a risk-space intervention. *Sex Transm Dis* 30: 533–8.

Nelson KE, Celentano DD, Suprasert S *et al.* (1993) Risk factors for HIV infection among young adult men in northern Thailand. *JAMA* 270: 955–60.

Nelson KE, Celentano DD, Eiumtrakol S *et al.* (1996) Changes in sexual behavior and a decline in HIV infection among young men in Thailand. *N Engl J Med* 335: 297–303.

Nieves E (1999) Privacy questions raised in cases of syphilis linked to chat room. *New York Times* 25 August 1999, p. A1.

Parran T (1937) *Shadow on the Land: Syphilis*. New York: The American Social Hygiene Association.

Pilcher CD, McPherson JT, Leone PA *et al.* (2002) Real-time, universal screening for acute HIV infection in a routine HIV counseling and testing population. *JAMA* 288: 216–21.

Quinn TC, Wawer MJ, Sewankambo N *et al.* (2000) Viral load and heterosexual transmission of human immunodeficiency virus type 1. Rakai Project Study Group. *N Engl J Med* 342: 921–9.

Roland ME, Martin JN, Grant RM *et al.* (2001) Postexposure prophylaxis for human immunodeficiency virus infection after sexual or injection drug use exposure: identification and characterization of the source of exposure. *J Infect Dis* 184: 1608–12.

San Francisco Department of Public Health. HIV/AIDS Statistics and Epidemiology Section (2002) *HIV/AIDS Epidemiology Annual Report*. San Francisco Department of Public Health.

Scheer S, Chu PL, Klausner JD *et al.* (2001) Effect of highly active antiretroviral therapy on diagnoses of sexually transmitted diseases in people with AIDS. *The Lancet* 357: 432–5.

Scholes D, Stergachis A, Heidrich FE *et al.* (1996) Prevention of pelvic inflammatory disease by screening for cervical chlamydial infection. *N Engl J Med* 334: 1362–6.

Schwarcz SK, Kellogg TA, McFarland W *et al.* (2002) Characterization of sexually transmitted disease clinic patients with recent human immunodeficiency virus infection. *J Infect Dis* 186: 1019–22.

Sexually Transmitted Disease Prevention and Control Services (2002) San Francisco Sexually Transmitted Disease Annual Summary, 2001. San Francisco Department of Public Health.

Stall R, Purcell D (2000) Intertwining epidemics: a review of research on substance use among men who have sex with men and its connection to the AIDS epidemic. *AIDS Behav* 4: 181–92.

Stall RD, Hays RB, Waldo CR *et al.* (2000) The Gay 90's: a review of research in the 1990s on sexual behavior and HIV risk among men who have sex with men. *AIDS* 14: S101–14.

Tuller D (2001) Experts fear a risky recipe: Viagra, drugs and HIV. *New York Times* Tuesday 16 October 2001, pp. D5, D8.

Voluntary HIV-1 Counseling and Testing Efficacy Study Group (2000) Efficacy of voluntary HIV-1 counselling and testing in individuals and couples in Kenya, Tanzania, and Trinidad: a randomised trial. *The Lancet* 356: 103–12.

Wald A, Link K (2002) Risk of human immunodeficiency virus infection in Herpes Simplex Virus Type-2 seropositive persons: A meta-analysis. *J Infect Dis* 185: 45–52.

Wawer MJ, Sewankambo NK, Serwadda D *et al.* (1999) Control of sexually transmitted diseases for AIDS prevention in Uganda: a randomised community trial. *The Lancet* 353: 525–35.

Whitworth JA, Mahe C, Mbulaiteye SM *et al.* (2002) HIV-1 epidemic trends in rural south-west Uganda over a 10-year period. *Trop Med Int Health* 7: 1047–52.

HIV Treatment Meets Prevention: Antiretroviral Therapy as Prophylaxis

6

Myron S Cohen
Professor of Medicine, Microbiology and Immunology, University of North Carolina, Chapel Hill, Bioinformatics Building, Chapel Hill, USA

Mina C Hosseinipour
Assistant Professor, Division of Infectious Diseases, School of Medicine, University of North Carolina, Chapel Hill, North Carolina, USA

Myron S Cohen, **MD** is the J. Herbert Bate Professor of Medicine, Microbiology and Immunology and Chief of the Division of Infectious Disease at the University of North Carolina School of Medicine, Chapel Hill. He directs the NIH-STD Clinical Trials Unit, the NIH Pathogenesis and Training Grant and Co-directs the NIH Fogarty Center. He graduated Phi Beta Kappa from the University of Illinois, received his medical degree from Rush Medical College and completed Fellowship training in Infectious Diseases at Yale University. Dr. Cohen has served as Chair of the NIH Special Study Section on AIDS Drug Development and the HIV Prevention Network Antiretroviral Working Group. He has published extensively in the area of sexually transmitted diseases, including HIV and worked collaboratively on projects overseas. From 1997–2002 he was UNC's Principal Investigator of an NIH/NIAID funded multiple site consortium for STD-Clinical trials and continues as Co-Investigator on a number of related projects.

Mina C Hosseinipour, **MD, MPH** is Research Assistant Professor and Infectious Diseases specialist at the University of North Carolina School of Medicine, Chapel Hill, North Carolina. She is a graduate of the Northwestern University Medical School and completed her Fellowship training in Infectious Diseases and her MPH at UNC Chapel Hill. She has worked within the UNC AIDS Clinical Trials Unit and conducts HPTN and ACTG Clinical Research Trials at UNC's Project in Lilongwe, Malawi.

There are four kinds of sexually transmitted diseases (STDs): those that produce mucosal inflammation (e.g. gonorrhea, chlamydia, trichomonas), those that cause genital ulcers (e.g. herpes, chancroid, syphilis), those that produce epithelial cell changes (human papillomavirus), and those that cause no genital tract signs or symptoms, but rather use the genital tract for systemic access (e.g. hepatitis C and B, CMV, and HIV). While syphilis was the 'shadow on the land' until development of penicillin, and chlamydia was the most important STD in the 1970s and 1980s and remains an important source of morbidity, without doubt HIV has become the most important STD (and infectious disease) in the twenty-first century. However, from the beginning of the epidemic, AIDS was treated as an exception, and never as an STD. At first the disease was only observed in gay men, and before the causative virus was discovered a variety of non-sexual causes were postulated. Indeed, the first reports of heterosexual transmission of HIV were very unwelcome news. By the time HIV was discovered, the nascent AIDS research community was already dominated by virologists and a burgeoning class of 'AIDS care givers' from several medicine specialties (infectious diseases, hematology, immunology). This infection was forever separated from the other STDs, and 'AIDS exceptionalism' had begun. AIDS and HIV were so stigmatized that HIV control measures became tied up in a political storm that led to the voluntary counseling and testing strategies that remain in place today, linked to novel pre- and post-test counseling requirements. Such separation has had tragic consequences because (not surprisingly) the biological, epidemiological, and public health principles of all STDs (including HIV) are the same.

Investigators at University of North Carolina (UNC) have been studying STDs, and in particular gonorrhea, since the late 1960s. This has included intensive study of the biology of transmission of *Neiserria gonorrhoeae* required for vaccine development. In 1989 we conducted a study designed to measure the concentration of gonococci in semen, and the time required for antibiotic to eliminate the organism from these genital secretions. Excited by these results, we reasoned that similar studies related to HIV, and connecting STDs and HIV would be important.

As late as 1989 only a handful of studies related to HIV had been undertaken, including a shockingly small number of research subjects. As it became clear that heterosexual transmission of HIV would become of great importance, our research group developed a long-range research strategy that will be apparent from the structure of this chapter and many of the results presented.

1. We worked to develop reliable assays to quantitate HIV in semen and other genital secretions (Dyer *et al.*, 1998).
2. We examined the concentration of HIV in semen in large numbers of subjects, both in the US and in developing countries. Indeed, to achieve this goal we began the UNC Project in Malawi in 1994.

3. We examined the effects of classical STDs and especially gonorrhea on excretion of HIV in semen and blood plasma (Cohen *et al.*, 1997).
4. We determined the effects of antiviral therapy on HIV in semen, and related the pharmacology of the drugs to viral replication in the genital tract.
5. With the help of the late Dr David Barry at Burroughs Wellcome Research in RTP we started studies of zidovudine in semen before the drug was commercially available.
6. We proposed to examine whether antiretroviral drugs can be used to prevent sexual transmission of HIV. The formation of the National Institutes of Health (NIH) HIV Prevention Trial Network in 1996 set the stage for such a trial (HPTN 052) scheduled to begin in 2004.

Obviously, many research groups developed similar interests and the results have unraveled the biology of the sexual transmission of HIV outlined below and elsewhere in this book. The critical importance of sexual behavior to the epidemic has led to a novel and often interesting marriage (really a *ménage à cinque*) between behavioral scientists, biologists, clinicians, epidemiologists, and public health officials. The HIV epidemic is still in its early phases. While the devastation in sub-saharan Africa has been overwhelming, the future of HIV in Eastern Europe and Russia, China, and India (where most people on the planet live) remains unknown. There is no time for complacency or wishful thinking or modestly successful prevention measures. Indeed, the vast research output from the past 23 years must be applied to innovative and novel prevention strategies. This chapter is designed to provide context to one of many potential strategies that holds great promise … antiretroviral therapy (ART) for prevention.

HIV prevention activities have now had more than 20 years of development with what can be best characterized as limited success (DeCock *et al.*, 2002). HIV prevention activities are bounded by biological, historical, social, political, economic, and public health considerations (Cohen *et al.*, 1999). A list of prevention strategies available or in development is provided in Table 6.1 (Galvin and

Table 6.1   HIV prevention strategies available or in development.

1	STD control, behavior change, condoms
2	Vaccines (trials ongoing)
3	Treatment of bacterial vaginosis
4	Topical microbicides (trials ongoing)
5	The diaphragm (trials ongoing)
6	Male circumcision (trials ongoing)
7	Antiviral therapy (an HPTN trial)
8	Societal (structural) change: incentives for safer sex?

Cohen, 2004). To date, most resources have been directed toward promotion of safer sex combined with voluntary counseling and testing (VCT) programs (DeCock *et al.*, 2002). Safer sex programs in Thailand (Nelson *et al.*, 1996; Low-Beer and Stoneburner, 2003) and Uganda (Mbuyaiteye *et al.*, 2002; Low-Beers and Stoneburner, 2003) have clearly reduced the spread of HIV. The success of these programs appears to have resulted in large part from partner number reduction and widespread condom usage (Low-Beers and Stoneburner, 2003; Shelton *et al.*, 2004).

Very little attention, however, has been paid to the behavior of HIV-infected people, mostly because of limited resources for HIV treatment in developing countries, and well-justified concerns about stigma (Bayer, 1991). Highly effective antiretroviral therapy (ART) for HIV became available in 1997, and such therapy has greatly reduced the morbidity and mortality of infection (Mocroft *et al.*, 2003). ART has also been used successfully to inhibit vertical transmission of HIV (Mofenson *et al.*, 1999; Mofenson and McIntyre, 2000; Guay *et al.*, 1999). The widespread and global use of ART anticipated in the coming years will have a major effect on the HIV epidemic, whether or not such effects are studied (Wainberg and Friedland, 1998). Strategic thinking about the use of ART requires consideration beyond personal benefit, but about the health of the public as well. This chapter addresses HIV prevention in infected subjects, or those at very high risk for infection, with emphasis on application of ART.

HIV Transmission

The biology of transmission of HIV has been addressed in detail elsewhere in this book. Briefly, HIV transmission depends on the infectiousness of the host and the susceptibility of the partner (Royce *et al.*, 1997). HIV transmission in serodiscordant couples in Uganda depended primarily on the viral burden of the index case (Quinn *et al.*, 2000). Individuals with a viral burden less than 3500 HIV RNA copies/ml serum failed to transmit HIV. Nearly half of transmission events could be traced to infected subjects with blood viral burden exceeding 35 000 copies HIV RNA/ml serum. In a study of 1022 discordant couples in Zambia (Fideli *et al.*, 2001), 162 partners acquired HIV (8.6/100 patient years). Both male and female 'transmitters' had significantly higher plasma HIV RNA than non-transmitting study subjects; each log10 increment in HIV RNA was associated with risk ratios of 2.5 for female-to-male transmission and 1.8 for male-to-female transmission. No transmission events occurred when the infected case had an HIV RNA less than 1000 copies/ml. In a study of discordant couples conducted in Thailand (Tovanabutra *et al.*, 2001), blood plasma HIV RNA concentration was also the best predictor of transmission and increased incrementally as HIV

RNA increased; no transmission events occurred if the HIV RNA was below 1000 copies/ml.

HIV in blood serves as a surrogate for the HIV in mucosal secretions to which the susceptible hosts are exposed. HIV concentrations in genital (Coombs *et al.*, 2003) and rectal secretions (Lampinen *et al.*, 2000) show a high degree of correlation with the concentration of HIV in blood. Antiviral therapy further increases the correlation of HIV in blood and semen as viral replication is inhibited in all compartments (Chakraborty *et al.*, 2003). However, local production of HIV in the genital tract has been demonstrated (Delwart *et al.*, 1998; Kiessling *et al.*, 1998) and is increased by the inflammation produced by STDs (Ping *et al.*, 2000).

Comparison of the concentration of HIV in semen with clinical trial results led to the development of a probabilistic model of male-to-female HIV transmission (Chakraborty *et al.*, 2001; Figure 6.1). The average risk of sexual transmission of HIV is about 1/1000 episodes of sexual intercourse, a rate that would be expected to occur when the concentration of HIV in semen is between 10 000 and 100 000 copies (Chakraborty *et al.*, 2001; Gray, 2001; Figure 6.1). Such concentrations of HIV are most frequently detected in the semen of untreated male subjects with established HIV disease (Coombs *et al.*, 2003; Vernazza *et al.*, 2000). Such low efficiency of transmission HIV (at least relative to other STDs) does not explain the magnitude of the HIV epidemic in so many parts of the world (Galvin and Cohen, 2004). However, epidemiologic studies have generally not been designed to capture or account for brief, hyperinfectious periods (e.g. around the time of acute HIV infection, or during periods of concomitant STDs) that might lead to much higher probability of transmission (reviewed by Chakraborty *et al.*, 2001). Factor(s) that increase the concentration of HIV in the genital tract of the infected subject or the number of receptive cells (or number of receptors per cell) in the

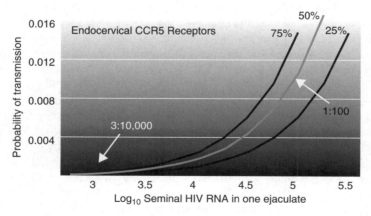

Fig. 6.1 Predictors of transmission of seminal HIV RNA. From Chakraborty *et al.* (2001).

exposed sexual partner increase the risk of HIV transmission (Figure 6.1). Classical STDs are probably the most important co-factors for HIV transmission (Fleming and Wasserheit, 1999; Galvin and Cohen, 2004). STDs that cause mucosal ulceration and/or inflammation greatly (but reversibly) increase shedding of HIV in the female (Ghys *et al.*, 1997) and male (Cohen *et al.*, 1997) genital tract. STDs also increase the number of receptive cells detected in the genital tract (Levine *et al.*, 1998).

The stage of HIV infection may also help to define the probability of transmission (Cates *et al.*, 1997). Acute HIV infection occurs within hours or days after exposure, and is characterized by detection of HIV RNA or p24 antigen in the blood of a subject who has not yet developed an HIV antibody response (Pilcher *et al.*, 2002). While patients with established HIV infection develop immune responses that can limit viral replication, such responses have not yet developed in people with acute HIV infection (Rosenberg *et al.*, 1997). Accordingly, people with acute HIV infection have very high viral burden (Pilcher *et al.*, 2001, 2004 a, b). For example, the median viral burden of 24 patients in Malawi with acute HIV infection was greater than 1 million copies/ml blood plasma. Accordingly, patients with acute HIV infection may be uniquely important in the spread of HIV (Jacquez *et al.*, 1994; Koopman *et al.*, 1997), and the probability of transmission associated with acute infection may be more than 20 times greater than during established infection (Pilcher, 2004, b).

Recent work by Wawer *et al.* (2003) strongly supports these ideas. She found that about half of all HIV transmission events observed in the Rakai study could be ascribed to patients with early HIV infection. Accordingly, detection and management of patients with acute HIV infection might provide an entirely unique HIV prevention strategy, as discussed below.

In addition, HIV and STDs are frequently co-transmitted. More than a decade ago Cameron and co-workers (1989) presented compelling evidence for co-transmission of HIV and genital ulcer pathogens. In a prospective study of 422 high-risk men in Nairobi, 8.2 per cent acquired HIV. Ninety-six per cent of the men who acquired HIV had identifiable risk factors including genital ulcer (risk ratio 4.7) or lack of circumcision (risk ratio 8.2). Among a subgroup of 73 men with a single exposure to a sex worker acquired HIV within 12 weeks of observation, and every man who acquired HIV had a genital ulcer. Bollinger *et al.* (1997) examined 3874 HIV antibody-negative serum specimens from an STD clinic in Pune, India for p24 antigen. Acute HIV was detected in 58 subjects (1.5 per cent prevalence, 51/58 men). Pilcher *et al.* (2004a) studied 1361 men in an STD clinic in Malawi. Forty-four per cent of the clients were HIV antibody positive. Among antibody-negative men presenting with ulcer and adenopathy, the risk of acute HIV was 7.5 per cent. Increasing HIV incidence has been reported in a retrospective study of serum specimens obtained from homosexual men visiting an STD clinic in Amsterdam (Dukers *et al.*, 2002); 70 per cent of men with 'early' infection (defined by detection of HIV antibodies with weak avidity) had a concurrent STD. The logical focus for detection of patients with acute HIV infection is in STD clinics, especially clinics that serve high-risk populations such as gay men or sex workers.

Antiretroviral Therapy for Prevention

Antiretroviral therapy can be used to prevent sexual transmission of HIV in two ways: (a) to reduce infectiousness or (b) as pre-exposure or post-exposure prophylaxis (PEP). The success of each strategy depends on the pharmacology and biology of the antiviral agents employed.

The Pharmacology of ART in the Genital Tract

The ability of antiretroviral agents to penetrate the genital tract is of central importance to the use of ART, and the selection of the most appropriate antiviral agents (Kashuba *et al.*, 1999). Nucleoside analogues (NRTI agents) achieve high concentrations in semen (Figure 6.2). Zidovudine, lamivudine, and stavudine

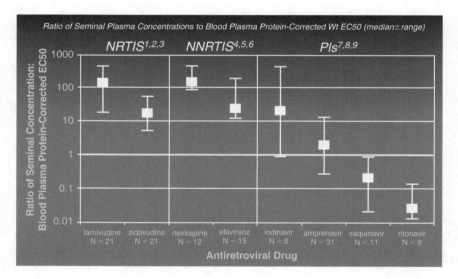

Fig. 6.2 Drug concentrations in semen. [1]Pereira *et al.* (1999); [2]Henry *et al.* (1988); [3]GlaxoWellcome, personal communication, 2000; [4]Kashuba *et al.*, unpublished data; [5]Taylor *et al.* (2000a); [6]Product Monographs (2000); [7]Taylor *et al.* (2000b); [8]Pereira *et al.* (2001); [9]Molla *et al.* (1998).

achieve seminal concentration greater than blood. These nucleoside agents also undergo the required phosphorylation in the genital tract (Reddy *et al.*, 2003).

Among the non-nucleoside reverse transcriptase inhibitors (NNRTIs), nevirapine concentration in semen is 60–100 per cent that of blood plasma levels, while efavirenz concentration in semen is 2.5–10 per cent of that of blood; these concentrations exceed the IC_{50} of wild-type HIV-1 (Figure 6.2). Protease inhibitors generally achieve the lowest concentrations in the male genital tract, although the seminal:blood ratios vary for each compound (indinavir > amprenavir > ritonavir = saquinavir > nelfinavir).

The pharmacology of antiretroviral drugs in the female genital tract has been less well studied. In the only published investigation (Si-Mohammed *et al.*, 2000), eight antiretroviral agents were examined, however only low concentrations of indinavir, didanosine, lamivudine, and zidovudine could be detected. Cervicovaginal lavage used in this study for specimen collection may have resulted in excess dilution. Using a more sensitive collection technique, Min *et al.* (2002) evaluated protease inhibitors and non-nucleoside analogue agents in female genital secretions. Cervical fluid blood ratio varied dramatically among agents in a class. Nevaripine and indinavir provided levels closest to those obtained in blood, whereas penetration of other protease inhibitors was more limited: indinavir (60 per cent) > amprenavir > lopinavir > saquinavir > ritonavir. For both male and female genital secretions, compounds with low protein binding and greater lipophilicity achieve the greatest concentrations, and such information can be used to develop new ART regimes focused on prevention.

Antiretroviral Drugs Reduce Shedding of HIV in the Genital Tract

Many studies of excretion of HIV in semen have been undertaken (reviewed by Coombs *et al.*, 2003). In general, ART (two or more antiretroviral drugs) can be expected to reduce the concentration of HIV in seminal plasma (Kashuba *et al.*, 1999, table 6.3). These benefits can often be sustained for long periods of time. For example, Pereira *et al.* (1999) studied nine men given zidovudine/lamivudine, and observed nearly complete suppression of HIV for more than 256 weeks in some subjects. However, HIV can still be detected intermittently in cell culture (Krieger *et al.*, 1995), and HIV DNA can be recovered from the cellular fraction of semen, regardless of therapy (Zhang *et al.*, 1998, 1999; Vernazza *et al.*, 2000). HIV-infected cells likely become the source of HIV in genital secretions observed in patients on suppressive antiviral therapy who acquire an STD (Taylor *et al.*, 2000a). Given that it remains unclear whether HIV is transmitted in a cell-free or cellular form, inability to eliminate HIV from infected cells remains a potential constraint for the use of ART in prevention.

ART also reduces recovery of HIV RNA from cervical secretions. Cu-Uvin and co-workers (2000) obtained samples of infected blood plasma and cervico-vaginal lavage samples from 25 HIV-infected women before and after aggressive ART. Before the initiation of therapy they were able to detect HIV in the genital secretions in 51 per cent of women with CD4 count less than 200 compared with 18 per cent of women with CD4 count greater than 200. Addition of ART reduced the detection of HIV; HIV could only be detected in 15 per cent of women provided ART. Using a more sensitive method of HIV RNA detection (<80 copies/ml), Fiore *et al.* (2003) were able to detect cervical–vaginal HIV RNA in 28 per cent of women despite the use of highly active ART (HAART). Additionally, among women with undetected plasma HIV RNA, 25 per cent had detectable cervical vaginal HIV RNA, demonstrating the potential for local replication at the genital level.

Hart *et al.* (1999) studied HIV in blood plasma, vaginal secretions and cervical mucus in 52 HIV-infected women. The cell-free and cell-associated HIV in blood plasma and vaginal secretions were greater in subjects with lower CD4 count, and the concentrations of HIV in blood and genital secretions were highly correlated. Eleven women initiating therapy were compared with seven women not receiving therapy. Subjects receiving therapy had significantly less HIV in vaginal secretions than the control group.

HIV RNA has also been evaluated in rectal specimens (Lampinen *et al.*, 2000). Among 233 homosexual men in Seattle, HIV RNA could be detected in 49 per cent of the men who were not receiving therapy, 30 per cent of men receiving therapy that did not include a protease inhibitor, and 17 per cent of men on triple drug therapy that included a protease inhibitor. HIV DNA was recovered from 58 per cent of specimens harvested from men not receiving therapy or on therapy that did not include a protease inhibitor, 43 per cent of men taking triple drug therapy including a protease inhibitor, and 58 per cent of men who were not taking a protease inhibitor.

Will ART Reduce Sexual Transmission of HIV?

While available evidence suggests that ART will suppress the sexual transmission of HIV, such an effect has not been proven. Indeed, the recognition of *de novo* viral resistance in patients with untreated HIV infection strongly suggests that they acquired infection from someone receiving ART (Little *et al.*, 1999, 2002; Brown *et al.*, 2003). These concerns not withstanding, several lines of evidence support the potential of ART. First, ART clearly suppresses vertical transmission of HIV (Guay, 1999; Mofenson and McIntyre, 1999; Mofenson *et al.*, 2000). The probability of vertical transmission of HIV (like sexual transmission) is tightly linked to the mothers' blood viral burden (Mofenson *et al.*, 2000). However, the biology of vertical and sexual transmission is entirely different, limiting greatly extrapolation of these results.

Second, Musicco and co-workers (1994) evaluated HIV transmission in 436 discordant couples. A small proportion of the subjects (15 per cent) with more advanced disease took zidovudine. HIV transmission was increased among people whose partners had lower CD4 counts or HIV antigenemia, The relative risk of HIV transmission from a man to his partner was reduced by zidovudine use (odds ratio (OR) = 0.5, 95 per cent confidence intervals (CI) 0.1–0.9) or condoms (OR = 0.2, 95 per cent CI 0.1–0.4). However, this was a retrospective analysis of data at a time when zidovudine was the only antiretroviral drug available so these results cannot be construed as compelling.

Third, the effects of the availability of ART in different communities on HIV incidence has been studied. Katz *et al.* (2002) measured the incidence of HIV, rectal gonorrhea, and risky sexual behavior in San Francisco. The results suggested that availability of ART led to increased risky sexual behavior and spread of STDs without preventing HIV. However, this report conflicts with other reports from San Francisco, Taiwan, and Europe.

Porco *et al.* (2003) examined HIV transmission probability in a cohort of gay men in San Francisco before and after the widespread availability of ART (1994–1999). The results demonstrated decreasing HIV acquisition despite increased numbers of episodes of receptive anal intercourse, and resurgent STDs in the community. The author estimated that the risk of HIV transmission decreased, a 48 per cent decline. Similar results have been observed in the gay community in Amsterdam. Couthino and co-workers have conducted a detailed study of 1062 gay men (the Amsterdam Cohort Study) since 1984. The introduction of ART in 1996 was associated with increased risky sexual behaviors (Dukers *et al.*, 2001) and STDs (Stolte *et al.*, 2001). However, a very large decrease in HIV incidence was observed between 1985 and 1993, and HIV incidence has fluctuated at low levels since that time (Dukers *et al.*, 2001).

Fang *et al.* (2004) studied the spread of HIV in Taiwan as a function of national prevention and treatment policies. Taiwan initiated a national HIV surveillance policy in 1989. This included screening of all blood donors, and extensive VCT for high-risk populations, and compulsory testing of military personnel and prisoners. From 1984 to 2002, 29 429 255 tests were conducted, in a population of 22 520 776. Four thousand three hundred and ninety HIV infected people were detected (0.019 per cent prevalence). In 1997 Taiwan initiated free antiviral therapy to all HIV-infected people, including all subjects identified by surveillance. The authors examined HIV in the population before and after the introduction of ART, and noted a 48 per cent reduction in expected transmission of HIV. Stable rates of STDs were observed, suggesting that ART and not behavior change accounted for the results.

While these epidemiologic studies are extremely informative, they are limited by the data collected and their etiologic implications. Because the methods employed do not allow HIV exposure to be characterized, people receiving ART may never have encountered the subjects included in surveillance.

Fourth, mathematical modeling has been used to examine the potential effects of ART (Blower *et al.*, 2000, 2003; Garnett *et al.*, 2000; Law *et al.*, 2001; Nagelkerke *et al.*, 2002; Blower and Farmer, 2003; Gray *et al.*, 2003). While modeling is an important tool, all models are limited by cascading assumptions about the magnitude and duration of benefit afforded by HIV, sexual risk-taking behavior, and development of HIV resistance. For example, the models assume that ART will lead to a step-wise reduction in infectiousness. Indeed, Law *et al.* (2001) extrapolated from a study in Uganda to predict that ART would reduce HIV transmission probability by a factor of 10. But ART is designed to reduce viral burden below the level of detection as rapidly as possible, and empirical data actually suggest that HIV transmission will not occur when the concentration of HIV is reduced below a critical threshold (Quinn *et al.*, 2000; Chakraborty *et al.*, 2001). Second, the degree to which people receiving ART will increase risk-taking behavior (more dangerous sex acts, more partners, more sex acts) remains unclear (see below). Third, the magnitude of HIV resistance likely to develop when ART is used to prevent transmission is unknown. Fourth, it is widely believed that patients will not remain sufficiently adherent to protect their sexual partners or limit development of resistance. Adherence data collected from patients receiving suppressive therapy has emphasized the difficulty that patients encounter, and the poor durability of most ART regimens. These data have been collected primarily from HIV-infected subjects in developed countries. However, patients in resource-constrained countries may actually do better with therapy than expected (Farmer *et al.*, 2003). Fifth, models of benefit of ART are bounded by the size of the population that receives therapy, which might have been under-estimated, especially considering the plethora of ART initiatives that have surfaced. Finally (and likely of greatest importance), no model takes into consideration brief windows of high level of HIV transmission that likely dominate the HIV epidemic. ART provided to patients at highest risk of transmission (e.g. those with acute HIV) might have disproportionate benefit. In general, we believe the importance of modeling rests in development of testable hypotheses.

In summary, the ability of ART to reduce the sexual transmission of HIV has not been proven. Accordingly, the NIH has agreed to support a clinical trial designed to address HIV transmission directly through the HIV Prevention Trials Network (www.hptn.org). HPTN 052 is a randomized trial of 1750 discordant couples in which the HIV-infected index case will be randomized to early or delayed antiviral therapy. Subjects will be enrolled with CD4 count exceeding 350, a level at which therapy would be considered optional by current US and World Health Organization (WHO) guidelines. When CD4 count falls below 200, subjects will be provided ART for the duration of the trial. All couples will receive maximal counseling for HIV prevention and free condoms. The study has 90 per cent power to detect 35 per cent difference in transmission. The study is to be conducted in six countries, including the US, for seven years. More details can be found at www.hptn.org/research_studies/hptn052.asp.

Other Considerations: New Thinking about the HIV-infected Subject

Stage of HIV Infection

As indicated above, patients with acute HIV infection likely represent a high risk for transmission. However, public health strategies to detect such patients have heretofore not been developed (Ruiz *et al.*, 2001). Since 2000 North Carolina has launched an innovative screening program designed to detect acute HIV in all subjects seeking care at STD clinics and other public HIV-testing sites (Pilcher *et al.*, 2002). This strategy uses pooling of specimens to detect serum HIV RNA in subjects who are HIV antibody negative. Case finding can lead to detection of additional subjects with either acute or established infection. This program has led to detection of many unrecognized cases of HIV in North Carolina (Pilcher *et al.*, 2002), and an HIV epidemic in African American college students (Hightow *et al.*, 2003). Similar studies are now planned for South Africa, Malawi, China, and other parts of the US. Detection of patients with acute HIV might also benefit the health of the infected subject. While the best treatment for such patients is unknown, early intervention with ART has been used to reduce viral burden and viral 'set point' (Rosenberg *et al.*, 2000). The public health benefits of prevention directed at subjects with very high viral burden and high-risk sexual behavior are likely to be substantial (Cates *et al.*, 1997).

Behavior Change

The effects of ART treatment on sexual behavior are critical, but poorly understood and conflicting. Kravcik and co-workers (1998) interviewed patients about their perceptions of ART. Twenty per cent of people believed that protease inhibitors would reduce the need for safer sexual practices. Miller and co-workers (2000) examined sexual behavior among 191 HIV-infected individuals in France. The majority of subjects (81 per cent) reported having unprotected anal or vaginal intercourse during the study period, at a time when they recognized they were HIV infected; after initiation of protease inhibitors no significant increase was found in the sexual activity of the subjects. Desquilbet *et al.* (2002) studied risky sexual behavior in 242 French patients with primary HIV infection. The majority of patients (87 per cent) had one or more sex partners, and 32 per cent reported an unprotected encounter. However, patients receiving ART (72 per cent) had less risky behavior than those who remained untreated (OR = 0.6, 95 per cent CI 0.2–1.5). Van der Straten and co-workers (2000) studied sexual behavior in 104 serodiscordant couples, two-thirds of whom reported unprotected intercourse. However, the authors found little to suggest that antiretroviral drug therapy inspired risk-taking behavior. Stolte *et al.* (2001) studied STDs in gay men in Amsterdam.

These investigators detected an increase in rectal gonorrhea and early syphilis, coincident with introduction of ART, likely due to changes in risk-taking behavior (Dukers *et al.*, 2001). Indeed, the degree of viral suppression and improvement in immunological function (CD4 count) reported to the patient may directly influence sexual behavior (Dukers *et al.*, 2001). Increased risk-taking behavior in HIV-infected patients receiving therapy has also been reported directly from several STD Clinics in the US (Brewer *et al.*, 2001; Hart *et al.*, 2001; Scheer *et al.*, 2001). Among HIV-infected patients in Côte d'Ivoire, abstinence was the most common prevention strategy reported. Patients receiving ART did not report increased sexual frequency or risky behavior (Moatti *et al.*, 2003). Prevention messages for infected people are only now being developed (Jansen *et al.*, 2001; Ruiz *et al.*, 2001). To date HIV prevention efforts directed toward clinicians providing medical care have been modest (Margolis *et al.*, 2001; Marks *et al.*, 2002).

Resistance

The success of ART for prevention may be limited by development of resistance. Recent studies demonstrate considerable HIV resistance in newly diagnosed patients (Little *et al.*, 2002). However the rates of resistant HIV may actually be lower than expected (Brown *et al.*, 2003), suggesting reduced viral fitness or other antiviral effects. In addition, resistant HIV isolates have been detected in genital secretions (Eron *et al.*, 1998; Mayer *et al.*, 1999) and sexual transmission of such resistant variants has been demonstrated (Angarano *et al.*, 1994; Conlon *et al.*, 1994; Imrie *et al.*, 1997). The antiviral combinations best suited to HIV prevention have not been determined; however, some drugs may be of greater public health benefit than others (Kashuba *et al.*, 1999). Considerations about patient adherence, regimen choice, and treatment interruption will need to assess potential effects on transmission of HIV.

Prevention Versus Treatment

Major limitation(s) of ART for prevention include (1) a belief that therapy must compete for resources with prevention activities (Marseilles *et al.*, 2002; Creese *et al.*, 2002); (2) lack of therapy in developing countries (Farmer, 1999); (3) clinical guidelines that fail to seriously consider prevention in the treatment setting (Ruiz *et al.*, 2001). Withholding therapy for the sake of prevention will not withstand moral scrutiny (Farmer *et al.*, 2001). ART will soon be available to those in need. UNAIDS, Doctors Without Borders, Family Health International, Partners in Health and many private companies and other NGOs have initiated ART programs. Perhaps most important, WHO, the Global Fund to Fight AIDS, TB and Malaria, and the US Presidential Initiative has focused on delivery of ART to 3 000 000 patients by the end of 2005 (www.globalfund.org). Current treatment guidelines must urgently reconsider prevention opportunities.

Myron S Cohen and Mina C Hosseinipour

ART for Pre- and Post-exposure Prophylaxis for HIV-negative People

Three lines of evidence suggest that ART can be used for HIV prophylaxis: animal studies, human studies of prophylaxis to prevent vertical transmission of HIV, and prophylaxis after needlestick injury (Cohen *et al.*, 2001).

Animal Studies

In the macaque model, ART given in sufficient concentration for an appropriate duration can provide protection from HIV infection. Tenofovir prevented SIV infection after intravenous challenge if it was given within 24 hours of exposure, and continued for more than 10 days (Tsai *et al.*, 1995). Tenofovir also provided protection to four animals after mucosal exposure to HIV if the drug was initiated 12 hours after exposure (4/4 animals protected) or 72 hours after exposure (3/4 animals protected). Benefits were observed in animals treated for a full 28 days (Otten *et al.*, 2000). Other animal studies using different ART drug combinations, different inoculum size, and different times of intervention have shown less reliable benefit (reviewed by Cohen *et al.*, 2001). In general, the results suggest a narrow window of opportunity for intervention; Hu and co-workers (2000) noted SIV infection of vaginal dendritic cells in the macaque only an hour after exposure.

Post-exposure Prophylaxis for Vertical Transmission

The prophylaxis provided for vertical transmission has focused primarily on the pre-exposure window, designed to reduce the mother's blood viral burden (Mofenson and MacIntyre, 2000). However, several studies have shown a benefit when the neonate is provided ART as well. In studies conducted in Uganda (Guay *et al.*, 1999) and South Africa (Moodley, 2003), HIV transmission was further reduced when the infant was provided PEP. In addition, infants provided PEP when HIV-infected mothers missed intrapartum therapy demonstrated 48 per cent reduction in HIV acquisition (Wade *et al.*, 1998). While the most cost-effective regimens utilize nevaripine alone, observed resistance to nevirapine has engendered a controversy about the most appropriate form of therapy (Beckerman, 2003).

Needlestick Injury

The potential efficacy of post-exposure prophylaxis after needlestick is limited to a retrospective case–control study by Cardo and co-workers (1997). Thirty-three cases were retrospectively identified from reports to national surveillance systems in the United States, Italy, France, and the United Kingdom. Six hundred and seventy-nine controls were selected from the US through voluntary reports to a Centers for Disease Control and Prevention (CDC) needlestick study. People who took zidovudine after percutaneous exposure had an 81 per cent reduction in risk for HIV seroconversion after adjusting for other confounding factors. Deep injury, visible blood on the device, procedures involving needles in vessels, and terminal illness in the source patient were all associated with an increased risk for HIV seroconversion. Specific CDC guidelines after needlestick injury are available (CDC, 2000; Gerberdering, 2003).

Post-exposure Prophylaxis (PEP) for Sexual Transmission of HIV

The ability of PEP to prevent sexual transmission of HIV in humans has not been studied, so the exact benefit of such therapy is not known. However, many research groups have conducted operations research on PEP, and included (statistically underpowered) estimation of protection. The feasibility of PEP for non-occupational exposure has been addressed extensively in San Francisco. In one study 401 subjects presenting within 72 hours after a sexual or intravenous drug exposure to a known or suspected HIV-infected individual were offered ART (Kahn *et al.*, 2001). Patients also received risk reduction and adherence counseling. The majority of the participants ($n = 375$) presented after a sexual exposure. Treatment was initiated at a mean of 33 hours post-exposure, and 78 per cent of the subjects completed four weeks of therapy. Three individuals seeking treatment were already HIV infected, but no seroconversions in subjects offered PEP were documented. However, the effectiveness of PEP could not be assessed by this study since there was no control group and 57 per cent of the subjects did not know the HIV status of the source partner. The study demonstrated a demand for PEP following sexual exposure, good adherence, and minimal toxicity.

Investigators in Brazil (Harrison *et al.*, 2000, 2001; Schecter *et al.*, 2002) conducted a PEP in high-risk homosexual men study focusing on self-administered initiation of therapy. Subjects were provided the initial doses (4 days) of PEP to take immediately after perceived exposure. Subjects deemed at significant risk by a clinician in follow-up exam were then offered 24 additional days of therapy. PEP was initiated by 65/202 subjects on 92 occasions over 16 months of the study and therapy was considered appropriate in 90.2 per cent of these events. While side-effects were reported by 74 per cent of subjects, 86 per cent of subjects completed a full 28-day course of therapy. Eight seroconversions were observed in the study population, but only in one subject who initiated PEP. The investigators reported reduced rather than increased risk-taking behavior in the study population.

In France, the government supports the use of antiretroviral prophylaxis and appropriate counseling for victims of rape. Benais and co-workers (2000) reported their experience in five emergency medicolegal units in Paris that have been in operation since June 1999. A total of 2550 victims of rape were offered triple-drug ART with stavudine, didanosine, and nelfinavir within 48 hours of the assault, but only 100 subjects were treated. No laboratory toxicities were recognized, but many patients discontinued therapy and 25 per cent failed to return for follow-up. No patients acquired HIV.

Another study focused on sexual assault was conducted in San Francisco where PEP has been offered to all victims of rape since April 1998 (Myles *et al.*, 2000). Subjects who present within 72 hours of potential exposure were offered a 10-day supply of zidovudine/lamivudine (Combivir) with an additional 18 days of therapy provided in a follow-up visit. A total of 376 patients were evaluated, 3 per cent of whom were found to be HIV-positive at baseline, and 213 subjects were offered PEP. Only 32.4 per cent of these subjects chose to initiate therapy, and only 12 per cent returned to complete the course of therapy. White, college-educated males with stable housing and subjects reporting anal penetration were the most likely to initiate prophylaxis. The authors concluded that PEP should be offered to all victims of a rape as part of comprehensive counseling.

South Africa has among the highest reported incidence of sexual assaults in the world (300/100 000) with an annual incidence of 4.4–7.2 per cent and a prevalence of 19.1–28.4 per cent. Wulfsohn and co-workers (2003) studied 687 rape survivors in Johannesberg, of whom 16.1 per cent were HIV infected at baseline. Four hundred and thirty-five people received PEP within 72 hours, but only 173 subjects returned for 6-week follow-up. In addition, while prescriptions to complete a 28-day course were provided, the number who followed through is unknown. One subject who received PEP within 53 hours acquired HIV. The South African government has agreed to provide free PEP to victims of sexual assault.

Limitations of PEP

The limitations of PEP include cost, toxicity, sexual disinhibition, potential for antiviral resistance, and lack of appropriate infrastructure to offer such therapy in a timely fashion. Behavioral effects of availability of PEP were included in several studies which demonstrated reductions rather than increases in self-reported risk (Martin *et al.*, 2001; Schecter *et al.*, 2002). However, in San Francisco and Boston PEP studies, 17 and 14 per cent of participants, respectively, requested a second course of PEP (Martin *et al.*, 2001).

ART has serious side-effects, even when used for a brief period of time. The US CDC has created a registry of side-effects in 492 health care workers with occupational exposure (Wang *et al.*, 2000) and 107 recipients of PEP for non-occupational exposure (n-PEP) (Grohskopf *et al.*, 2002). In addition 22 severe adverse PEP reactions were reported between 1997 and 2000 (CDC, 2000). These included 12 cases of severe liver toxicity from nevirapine, including a patient who required a liver transplant.

Cost Benefit Analysis of PEP to Prevent Sexual Transmission of HIV

Given the limitations of PEP clinical research, it will not be possible to demonstrate that antiviral therapy can prevent acquisition of HIV, nor to choose the best regimen to use, or proper dosage schedule. Nevertheless, some investigators have tried to develop policies for use of PEP in non-occupational settings (Katz and Gerberdering, 1998) which have generally favored fairly aggressive use of PEP. Available data have been used to model the costs and benefits of PEP for non-occupational exposure (Pinkerton *et al.*, 1998; Low-Beer *et al.*, 2000; Bratistein *et al.*, 2001). Using conservative assumptions, Pinkerton and co-workers (1998) concluded that PEP could only be considered cost-effective (i.e. a reasonable cost for quality-adjusted life years) if it were used after near certain exposure to HIV (a high probability of HIV infection in the index case) and through receptive anal intercourse. These authors also tried to examine the effects of selection of different treatment regimens, which served to emphasize lack of criteria for such selection.

CDC Guidelines for Non-occupational HIV Exposure (n-PEP) 2004

The US CDC has provided HIV occupational exposure guidelines for health care workers for the past five years (CDC, 1998, 2001). However, given the lack of data to support non-occupational PEP less formal 'management recommendations' were generated (CDC, 1998). More recently, the CDC formed an expert advisory committee to develop n-PEP guidelines that are likely to be available in 2004. These guidelines will likely emphasize the following points: (1) PEP should be initiated as soon as possible after exposure and within 72 hours; (2) successful therapy will likely require a complete 28-day course; (3) combination antiviral agents must be used, considering safety and adherence, and HIV resistance in the index case and/or the community. In addition these guidelines are likely to emphasize consideration of HIV risk in the source, and the probability of HIV transmission from exposure, risk of other STDs and pregnancy, and the importance of counseling for both adherence and (future) safer sex behavior. The CDC has contracted a 24 hour/day hotline for PEP advice (PEPline, hivcntr@nccc.ucsf.edu, 1-888-448-4911), linked to a PEP registry (www. hivpepregistry.org, 1-877-448-1737)

Pre-exposure Prophylaxis

ART could also be provided to very high-risk subjects (sex workers, gay men, intravenous drugs users) who are unable or unwilling to modify their behavior.

The development of potent ART drugs with long half-life has inspired consideration of this approach. Indeed, Jackson *et al.* (2003) studied the pharmacology of nevirapine for pre-exposure prophylaxis (PREP), and clinical trials with the drug tenofovir have started (www.gatesfoundation.org). The public health benefits of this approach are difficult to predict, but at least one modeling study has emphasized the importance of sex workers in HIV transmission (Nagelerke *et al.*, 2002). If infection develops in spite of prophylaxis, the risk of viral resistance could be substantial.

What the Future Holds

Antibiotics have achieved great success in prevention of transmission of infectious disease, even for tuberculosis where many months of multi-drug therapy are required. However, when it comes to ART for prevention, cynicism has outweighed common sense. First, early in the epidemic AIDS activist groups rejected prevention measures directed at infected subjects as a governmental attack on civil liberties, and because treatment options were very limited. Second, it was believed that the populations in greatest need of prevention (in resource-constrained countries) would never have access to ART. Third, HIV-infected cells detected in the genital tract during therapy suggest that ART might not work (Zhang *et al.*, 1998, 1999; Speck *et al.*, 1999). Fourth, adherence to complex regimens is a challenge, generally believed to be beyond the bounds of public health. Fifth, ART for prevention might increase risk behaviors. These arguments also serve to emphasize the different beliefs and experiences of the medical caregivers and public health professionals, as well as investigators working in domestic and international settings.

Many concerns about the use of ART for prevention have not been resolved, or will only be resolved by clinical trials and operations research. Stover and co-workers (2002) recently modeled the effects of an HIV prevention package for 126 low and middle income countries that embraces 12 essential (traditional) prevention interventions. The authors concluded that at least US$9.8 billion was required for a comprehensive response to the HIV epidemic, including both care and prevention. If US$4.8 billion was directed at traditional HIV prevention 29 000 000 new HIV infections might be averted by 2010. The effects of ART were not considered in this model.

In a planetary 'sea-change,' HIV care (including ART) is now scheduled to receive the majority of global HIV funding. WHO has resolved to treat 3 million people with ART by 2005. The US Congress has mandated that 55 per cent of all HIV international funding be devoted to HIV care, including ART. ART will undoubtedly be more widely available in the twenty-first century and will have profound effects on the HIV epidemic, whether or not we choose to measure such effects. The opportunity to merge HIV treatment and prevention into a single package so as to optimize public health benefit from ART has never been greater.

References

Angarano G, Monno L, Appice A *et al.* (1994) Transmission of zidovudine-resistant HIV-1 through heterosexual contacts. *AIDS* 8: 1013–14.

Bayer R (1991) Public health policy and the AIDS epidemic: an end to HIV exceptionalism. *N Engl J Med* 324: 1500–4.

Beckerman KP (2003) Long-term findings of HINET 012: the next steps. *Lancet* 362: 842–43.

Benais JP, Miara A, Brion S *et al.* (2000) Treatment of sexual assault: a multicentre study in emergency medico-legal units in the Paris region. *Program and Abstracts of the XIII International AIDS Conference*, 9–14 July 2000, Durban, South Africa, abstract TuOrC314.

Blower S, Farmer P (2003) Predicting the public health impact of antiretrovirals: preventing HIV in developing countries. *AIDScience* 3, no. 11.

Blower SM, Gershengorn HB, Grant RM (2000) A tale of two futures: HIV and antiretroviral therapy in San Francisco. *Science* 287: 650–4.

Blower S, Ma L, Farmer P, Koenig S (2003) Predicting the impact of antiretrovirals in resource-poor settings: preventing HIV infections whilst controlling drug resistance. *Curr Drug Targets Infect Disord* 3: 255–62.

Bollinger RC, Brookmeyer RS, Mehendale SM *et al.* (1997). Risk factors and clinical presentation of acute primary HIV infection in India. *JAMA* 278: 2085–9.

Bratistein P, Chan K, Beardsall A *et al.* (2001) How much is it worth? Actual versus expected costs of a population-based post-exposure prophylaxis program. Paper presented at the First IAS Conference on Pathogenesis and Treatment. Buenos Aires, Argentina, 9–11 July, abstract 153.

Brewer TH, Metsch L, Zenilman J (2001) Utilization of a public STD clinic by known HIV positive adults: decreased self reported risk behavior, increased disease incidence. *Sex Transm Infect* 12(suppl. 2): 158 Abstract.

Brown A, Frost S, Mathews W *et al.* (2003) Transmission fitness of drug resistant human immunodeficiency virus and the prevalence of resistance in the antiretroviral treated populations. *J Infect Dis* 187: 683–6.

Cardo DM, Culver DH, Ciesielski CA *et al.* (1997) A case–control study of HIV seroconversion in health care workers after percutaneous exposure. Centers for Disease Control and Prevention Needlestick Surveillance Group. *N Engl J Med* 337: 1485–90.

Cameron DW, Simonsen JN, D'Costa LJ *et al.* (1989) Female to male transmission of human immunodeficiency virus type 1: risk factors for seroconversion in men. *Lancet* 2: 403–7.

Cates W Jr, Chesney M, Cohen M (1997) Primary HIV infection – a public health opportunity. *Am J Public Health* 87: 1928–30.

CDC (Centers for Disease Control and Prevention) (1998) Management of possible sexual, injecting-drug-use, or other nonoccupational exposure to HIV, including consideration related to antiretroviral therapy. Public Health Service Statement. *MMWR Morb Mortal Wkly Rep* 47: 1–14.

CDC (2000) Serious adverse events attributed to nevirapine regimens for postexposure prophylaxis after HIV exposures – worldwide, 1997–2000. *MMWR Morb Mortal Wkly Rep* 49: 1153–6.

CDC (2001) Updated U.S. Public Health Service Guidelines for the management of occupational exposure to HBV, HCV, and HIV and recommendations for postexposure prophylaxis. *MMWR Morb Mortal Wkly Rep* 50: 1–42.

Chakraborty H, Sen PK, Helms RW *et al.* (2001) Viral burden in genital secretions determines male-to-female sexual transmission of HIV-1: a probabilistic empiric model. *AIDS* 15: 621–7.

Chakraborty H, Helms RW, Sen PK, Cohen MS (2003) Estimating correlation by using a general linear mixed model: evaluation of the relationship between the concentration of HIV-1 RNA in blood and semen. *Stat Med* 22: 1457–64.

Cohen J (2001) *A Shot in the Dark: The Search for an AIDS Vaccine.* New York: John Norton.

Cohen MS, Hoffman IF, Royce RA *et al.* (1997) Reduction of concentration of HIV-1 in semen after treatment of urethritis: implications for prevention of sexual transmission of HIV-1. *Lancet* 349: 1868–75.

Cohen MS, Dallabetta G, Holmes KK, Cates W (1999) Global prevention of HIV transmission. In: *The Medical Management of AIDS.* Philadelphia: WB Saunders, pp. 499–512.

Cohen MS, Hosseinipour MC, Kashuba ADM, Butera S (2001) Use of antiretroviral drugs to prevent transmission of HIV. In: Remington JS, Swartz M, eds. *Current Clinical Topics in Infectious Disease.* Oxford: Blackwell Science.

Coombs RW, Reichelderfer PS, Landay AL (2003) Recent observations on HIV type 1 infection in the genital tract of men and women. *AIDS* 17: 455–80.

Conlon CP, Klenerman P, Edwards A, Larder BA, Phillips RE (1994) Heterosexual transmission of human immunodeficiency virus type 1 variants associated with zidovudine resistance. *J Infect Dis* 169: 411–15.

Creese A, Floyd K, Alban A, Guiness L (2002) Cost-effectiveness of HIV/AIDS interventions in Africa: A systematic review of the evidence. *Lancet* 359: 1635–42.

Cu-Uvin S, Caliendo AM, Reinert S *et al.* (2000) Effect of highly active antiretroviral therapy on cervicovaginal HIV-1 RNA. *AIDS* 14: 415–21.

DeCock KM, Mbori-Ngacha D, Marum (2002) Shadow on the continent: public health and HIV/AIDS in Africa in the 21st century. *Lancet* 360: 67–73.

Delwart EL, Mullins JI, Gupta P *et al.* (1998) Human immunodeficiency virus type 1 populations in blood and semen. *J Virol* 72: 617–23.

Desquilbet L, Deveau C, Goujard C *et al.* (2002) Increase in at-risk behavior among HIV-1 infected patients followed in the French PRIMO cohort. *AIDS* 16: 2329–33.

Dukers NHTM, Goudsmit J, de Wit JBF *et al.* (2001) Sexual risk behavior relates to the virological and immunological improvements during highly active antiretroviral therapy in HIV-1 infection. *AIDS* 15: 369–78.

Dukers NHTM, Spaargaren J, Beijnen R *et al.* (2002) HIV incidence on the increase among homosexual men attending an Amsterdam sexually transmitted diseases clinic: Using a novel approach for detecting recent infections. *AIDS* 16: F19–F24.

Dyer JR, Kazembe P, Vernazza PL *et al.* (1998) High levels of human immunodeficiency virus type 1 in blood and semen of seropositive men in sub-Saharan Africa. *J Infect Dis* 177: 1742–6.

Eron JJ, Vernazza PL, Johnston DM *et al.* (1998) Resistance of HIV-1 to antiretroviral agents in blood and seminal plasma: implications for transmission. *AIDS* 12: F181–F189.

Fang C-T, Hsu H-M, Twu S-J *et al.* (2004) Decreased HIV transmission after policy of providing free access to highly active antiretroviral therapy in Taiwan. *J Infect Dis* 190: 879–85.

Farmer P (1999) *Infectious Diseases and Inequalities: The Modern Plagues.* Berkeley, CA: University of California Press.

Farmer P, Léandre F, Mukherjee JS *et al.* (2001) Community-based approaches to HIV treatment in resource-poor settings. *Lancet* 358: 404–9.

Farmer P, Leandre F, Koenig S *et al.* (2003) Preliminary outcomes of directly observed treatment of advanced HIV disease with ARVs (DOT-HAART) in rural Haiti. Paper presented at the 10th Conference on Retroviruses and Opportunistic Infections, Boston, Massachusetts, 2003, abstract 171.

Fideli US, Allen SA, Musonda R *et al.* (2001) Virologic and immunologic determinants of heterosexual transmission of human immunodeficiency virus type 1 in Africa. *AIDS Res Hum Retroviruses* 17: 901–10.

Fiore JR, Sugligoi B, Saracino A *et al.* (2003) Correlates of HIV-1 shedding in cervico-vaginal secretions and effects of antiretroviral therapy. *AIDS* 17: 2169–76.

Fleming DT, Wasserheit JN (1999) From epidemiological synergy to public health policy and practice: the contribution of other sexually transmitted diseases to sexual transmission of HIV infection. *Sex Trans Infect* 75: 3–17.

Galvin S, Cohen MS (2004) The spread of HIV: Sexual transmission, co-transmission and biological amplification. *Nat Microbiol*, January.

Garnett GP, Bartley L, Grassley, Anderson RM (2000) Antiviral therapy to treat and prevent HIV/AIDS in resource poor countries. *Nat Med* 8: 851–4.

Gerberdering, JL (2003) Occupational exposure to HIV in health care settings. *N Engl J Med* 348: 826–33.

Ghys PD, Fransen K, Diallo MO *et al.* (1997) The associations between cervicovaginal HIV shedding, sexually transmitted diseases and immunosuppression in female sex workers in Abidjan, Cote d'Ivoire. *AIDS* 11: F85–F93.

Gray RH, Wawer MJ, Brookmeyer R *et al.* and the Rakai Project Team (2001) Probability of HIV-1 transmission per coital act in monogamous, heterosexual, HIV-1-discordant couples in Rakai, Uganda. *Lancet* 357: 1149–53.

Gray RH, Li X, Wawer M, Gange S *et al.* for the Rakai Project Group (2003) Stochastic simulation of the impact of antiretroviral therapy and HIV vaccines on HIV transmission; Rakai, Uganda. *AIDS* 17: 1941–51.

Grohskpof LA, Smith DK, Kunches LK *et al.* (2002) Surveillance of post-exposure prophylaxis for non-occupational exposures through the US national registry. Paper presented at the XIV International Conference on AIDS, Barcelona Spain, 7–12 July 2002, abstract M0ORD1107.

Guay LA, Musoke P, Fleming T *et al.* (1999) Intrapartum and neonatal single-dose nevirapine compared with zidovudine for prevention of mother-to-child transmission of HIV-1 in Kampala, Uganda: HIVNET 012 randomised trial. *Lancet* 354: 795–802.

Harrison LH, Do Lago RF, Moreira RI *et al.* (2000) Demand for post sexual exposure chemoprophylaxis (PEP) for the prevention of HIV infection in Brazil. Paper presented at the 7th Conference on Retroviruses and Opportunistic Infections (CROI), San Francisco California, 30 January–2 February 2000, abstract 492.

Harrison LH, do Lago RF, Moreira RI, Mendelsohn AB, Schechter M (2001) Post-sexual-exposure chemoprophylaxis (PEP) for HIV: a prospective cohort study of behavioral impact. Paper presented at the 8th Conference on Retroviruses and Opportunistic Infections, Chicago, Illinois, 4–8 February 2001, abstract 225.

Hart CE, Lennox J, Pratt-Palmore *et al.* (1999) Correlation of human immunodeficiency virus type 1 in blood and the female genital tract. *J Infect Dis* 179: 871–82.

Hart GJ, Davis M, Imrie J, Davidson O, Williams I, Stephenson J (2001) 'If I'm not asked directly then I don't always tell people': disclosure of HIV status to sexual partners by gay men on HAART. *Int J STD AIDS* 12(Suppl 2): 185, abstract.

Henry K, Chinnock BJ, Quinn RP, Fletcher CV, de Miranda P, Balfour HH (1988) Concurrent zidovudine levels in semen and serum determined by radioimmunoassay in patients with AIDS or AIDS-related complex. *JAMA* 259: 3023–6.

Hightow LB, Leone PA, Macdonald P *et al.* (2003) Are colleges high transmission areas in the rural southeast? Insights from acute HIV surveillance. IDSA 2003, San Diego California, 9–12 October, abstract 609.

Hu J, Garner MB, Miller CJ (2000) Simian immunodeficiency virus rapidly penetrates the cervicovaginal mucosa after vaginal inoculation and infects intraepithelial dendritic cells. *J Virol* 74: 6087–95.

Imrie A, Beveridge A, Genn W, Vizzard J, Cooper DA (1997) Transmission of human immunodeficiency virus type 1 resistant to nevirapine and zidovudine. Sydney Primary HIV Infection Study Group. *J Infect Dis* 175: 1502–6.

Jackson JB, Barnett S, Piwowar-Manning E *et al.* (2003) A phase I/II study of Neviraphine for pre-exposure prophylaxis of HIV-1 transmission in uninfected subjects at high risk, *AIDS* 17: 547–53.

Jacquez J, Koopman J, Simon C, Longini I (1994) Role of the primary infection in epidemics of HIV infection in gay cohorts. *J Acquir Immune Defic Syndr* 7: 1169–84.

Janssen RS, Holtgrave DR, Valdisserri RO *et al.* (2001) The serostatus approach to fighting the HIV epidemic: prevention strategies for HIV infected individuals. *Am J Public Health* 91: 1019–24.

Kahn JO, Martin JN, Roland ME *et al.* (2001) Feasibility of postexposure prophylaxis (PEP) against human immunodeficiency virus infection after sexual or injection drug use exposure: The San Francisco PEP study. *J Infect Dis* 183: 707–14.

Kashuba ADM, Dyer JR, Kramer LM, Raasch RH, Eron JJ, Cohen MS (1999) Antiretroviral drug concentrations in semen: implications for sexual transmission of HIV-1. *Antimicrob Agents Chemother* 43: 1817–26.

Katz MH, Gerberdering JL (1998) The care of persons with recent sexual exposure to HIV. *Ann Intern Med* 128: 306–12.

Katz MH, Schwarcz SK, Kellogg TA *et al.* (2002) Impact of highly active antiretrovirial treatment on HIV seroincidence among men who have sex with men: San Francisco. *Am J Public Health* 92: 388–94.

Kiessling AA, Fitzgerald LM, Zhang D *et al.* (1998) Human immunodeficiency virus in semen arises from a genetically distinct virus reservoir. *AIDS Res Hum Retroviruses* 14 (Suppl 1): S33–41.

Koopman JS, Jacquez JA, Welch GW *et al.* (1997) The role of early HIV infection in the spread of HIV through populations. *J Acquir Immune Defic Syndr Hum Retrovirol* 14: 249–58.

Kravcik S, Victor G, Houston S *et al.* (1998) Effect of antiretroviral therapy and viral load on the perceived risk of HIV transmission and the need for safer sexual practices. *J Acquir Immune Defic Syndr* 19: 124–9.

Krieger JN, Coombs RW, Collier AC *et al.* (1995) Intermittent shedding of human immunodeficiency virus in semen: implications for sexual transmission. *J Urol* 154: 1035–40.

Lampinen TM, Critchlow CW, Kuypers JM *et al.* (2000) Association of antiretroviral therapy with detection of HIV-1 RNA and DNA in the anorectal mucosa of homosexual men. *AIDS* 14: F69–75.

Law MG, Prestage G, Grulich, Van de Ven P, Kippax S (2001) Modelling the effect of combination antiretroviral treatment on HIV incidence. *AIDS* 15: 1287–94.

Levine WC, Pope V, Boomkar A *et al.* (1998) Increase in endocervical CD4 lymphocytes among women with nonulcerative sexually transmitted diseases. *J Infect Dis* 177: 167–74.

Little SJ, Daar ES, D'Aquila RT *et al.* (1999) Reduced antiretroviral drug susceptibility among patients with primary HIV infection. *JAMA* 282: 1142–8.

Little SJ, Holte S, Routy J-P *et al.* (2002) Antiretroviral drug resistance among patients recently infected with HIV. *N Engl J Med* 347: 385–94.

Low-Beer S, Stoneburner RL (2003) Behaviour and communication change in reducing HIV: Is Uganda unique? *Afr J Aids Res* 2: 9–21.

Low-Beer S, Weber AE, Bartholomew K *et al.* (2000) A reality check: the cost of making post-exposure prophylaxis available to gay and bisexual men at high sexual risk. *AIDS* 14: 325–6.

Marks G, Richardson JL, Crepaz N *et al.* (2002) Are HIV care providers talking about safer sex and disclosure. A multi-clinic assessment. *AIDS* 16: 1953–7

Margolis A, Wolitski R, Parsons J, Gomez C (2001) Are healthcare providers talking to HIV-seropositive patients about safer sex? *AIDS* 15: 2335–7.

Marseilles E, Hoffman PB, Kahn J (2002) HIV prevention before HAART in sub-Saharan Africa. *Lancet* 359: 1851–6.

Martin JN, Roland ME, Bamberger JD *et al.* (2001) Post-exposure chemprophylaxis (PEP) for sexual exposure to HIV does not lead to increases in high risk behavior: The San Francisco Project. Paper presented at the 8th Clinical Conference on Retroviruses and Opportunistic Infections, Chicago, Illinois, 2–4 February 2001, abstract 224.

Mayer KH, Boswell S, Goldstein R *et al.* (1999) Persistence of human immunodeficiency virus in semen after adding indinavir to combination antiretroviral therapy. *Clin Infect Dis* 1999; 28: 1252–9.

Mbulaiteye SM, Mahe C, Whitworth JAG *et al.* (2002) Declining HIV-1 incidence and associated prevalence over 10 years in a rural population in south-west Uganda: a cohort study. *Lancet* 360: 41–6.

Miller M, Meyer L, Boufassa F *et al.* (2000) Sexual behavior changes and protease inhibitor therapy. *AIDS* 14: F33–F39.

Min SS, Corbett AH, Rezk N, Fiscus SA, Cohen MS, Kashuba ADM (2002) Differential penetration of protease inhibitors [PI] and non-nucleoside reverse transcriptase inhibitors [NNRTI] into the female genital tract [GT]. Paper presented at the World AIDS Conference, Barcelona, Spain, 2002.

Moatti JP, Prudhomme J, Coulibaly T *et al.* (2003) Access to antiretroviral treatment and sexual behaviours of HIV-infected patients aware of their serostatus in Cote d'Ivoire. *AIDS* 17: S69–S77.

Mocroft L, Ledergerber B, Katlama C *et al.* (2003) Decline in the AIDS and death rates in EuroSIDA: an observational study. *Lancet* 22–9.

Mofenson LM, McIntyre JA (2000) Advances and research direction in the prevention of mother-to-child HIV-1 transmission. *Lancet* 335: 2237–44.

Mofenson LM, Lambert JS, Stiehm ER *et al.* (1999) Risk factors for perinatal transmission of human immunodeficiency virus type 1 in women treated with zidovudine. Pediatric AIDS Clinical Trials Group Study 185 Team. *N Engl J Med* 341: 385–93.

Molla A, Vasavanonda S, Kumar G *et al.* (1998) Human serum attenuates the activity of protease inhibitors toward wild- type and mutant human immunodeficiency virus. *Virology* 250: 255–62.

Moodley D, Moodley J, Coovadia H *et al.* (2003) A multicenter randomized controlled trial of nevirapine versus a combination of zidovudine and lamivudine to reduce intra-partum and early postpartum mother-to-child transmission of human immunodeficiency virus type-1. *J Infect Dis* 187: 725–35.

Myles JE, Hirozawa A, Katz MH *et al.* (2000) Postexposure prophylaxis for HIV after sexual assault. *JAMA* 284: 1516–17.

Musicco M, Lazzarin A, Nicolosi A *et al.* (1994) Antiretroviral treatment of men infected with human immunodeficiency virus type 1 reduces the incidence of heterosexual transmission. *Arch Intern Med* 154: 1971–6.

159

Nagelkerke N, Jha P, Vlas S *et al.* (2002) Modeling HIV/AIDS epidemics in Botswana and India: impact of interventions to prevent transmission. *Bull WHO* 80: 89–96.

Nelson K, Celentano D, Eiumtrakol S (1996) Changes in the sexual behavior and a decline in HIV infection among young men in Thailand. *N Engl J Med* 395: 297–302.

Otten RA, Smith DK, Adams DR *et al.* (2000) Efficacy of postexposure prophylaxis after intravaginal exposure of pig-tailed macaques to a human-derived retrovirus (human immunodeficiency virus type 2). *J Virol* 74: 9771–5.

Pereira AS, Kashuba AD, Fiscus SA *et al.* (1999) Nucleoside analogues achieve high concentrations in seminal plasma: relationship between drug concentration and virus burden. *J Infect Dis* 180: 2039–43.

Pereira AS, Gerber JG, Smeaton L *et al.* (2001) The pharmacokinetics of amprenavir, lamivudine, and zidovudine in the male genital tract of HIV-1-infected men. Paper presented at the 8th Conference on Retroviruses and Opportunistic Infections, Chicago, 4–8 February, abstract 749.

Pilcher CD, Shugars DC, Fiscus SA *et al.* (2001) HIV in body fluids during primary HIV infection: implications for pathogenesis, treatment and public health. *AIDS* 15: 837–45.

Pilcher CD, McPherson JT, Leone PA *et al.* (2002) Real-time, universal screening for acute HIV infection in a routine HIV counseling and testing population. *JAMA* 288: 216–21.

Pilcher CD, Price MA, Hoffman IF *et al.* (2004a) Frequent detection of acute primary HIV infection in men in Malawi. *AIDS* 18: 517–524.

Pilcher CD, Tien HC, Eron JJ *et al.* (2004b) Brief but efficient: acute HIV infection and the sexual transmission of HIV. *J Infect Dis* 189: 1785–92.

Ping LH, Cohen MS, Hoffman IF *et al.* (2000) Effects of genital tract inflammation on HIV-1 V3 populations in blood and semen. *J Virol* 74: 8946–52.

Pinkerton SD, Holtgrave DR, Bloom FR (1998) Cost-effectiveness of post-exposure prophylaxis following sexual exposure to HIV. *AIDS* 12: 1067–78.

Porco T, Martin JN, Page-Shafer KA *et al.* (2003) Decline in HIV infectivity following the introduction of highly active antiretroviral therapy. *AIDS* 2003.

Quinn TC, Wawer MJ, Sewankambo N *et al.* (2000) Viral load and heterosexual transmission of human immunodeficiency virus type 1. *N Engl J Med* 342: 921–9.

Reddy S, Troiani L, Kim J *et al.* (2003) Differential phosphorylation of zidovudine and lamivudine (ZDV/3TC) between semen and blood mononuclear cells (MCs) in HIV-1 infected men. Paper presented at the 10th Conference on Retroviruses and Opportunistic Infections, Boston, MA, February.

Royce RA, Sena A, Cates WJ, Cohen MS (1997) Sexual transmission of HIV. *N Engl J Med* 336: 1072–8.

Rosenberg ES, Billingsley JM, Caliendo AM *et al.* (1997) Vigorous HIV-1-specific CD4+ T cell responses associated with control of viremia. *Science* 278: 1447–50.

Rosenberg E, Altfeld M, Poon SH *et al.* (2000) Immune control of human immunodeficiency virus type 1 after early treatment of acute infection. *Nature* 407: 523–6.

Ruiz MS, Gable AR, Kaplan EH, Stoto MA, Fineberg HV, Trussell, James, eds (2001) *No Time to Lose: Getting More from HIV Prevention*. Washington, DC: National Academy Press.

Schecter M, Do Lago RF, Ismerio R *et al.* (2002) Acceptability, behavioral impact and possible efficacy of post-exposure chemprophylaxis (PEP) for HIV. Paper presented at the 9th Conference on Retroviruses and Opportunistic Infections, Seattle, Washington, 24–28 February 2002, abstract 15.

Scheer S, Chu PL, Klausner JD, Katz MH, Schwarcz SK (2001) Effect of highly active antiretroviral therapy on the diagnoses of sexually transmitted diseases in people with AIDS. *Lancet* 357: 432–5.

Shelton J, Halperin DT, Nantulya V, Potts M, Gayle HD, Holmes KK (2004) Partner reduction is crucial for balanced 'ABC' approach to HIV prevention. *BMJ* 328: 891–3.

Si-Mohamed A, Kazatchkine M, Heard I *et al.* (2000) Selection of drug-resistant variants in the female genital tract of human immunodeficiency virus type-1-infected women receiving antiretroviral therapy. *J Infect Dis* 182: 112–22.

Speck CE, Coombs RW, Koutsky LA *et al.* (1999) Risk factors for HIV-1 shedding in semen. *Am J Epidemiol* 150: 622–31.

Stolte IG, Dukers NHTM, de Wit JBF, Fennema SA, Coutinho RA (2001) Increase in sexually transmitted infections among homosexual men in Amsterdam in relation to HAART. *Sex Transm Infect* 177: 184–6.

Stover J, Walker N, Garnett GP *et al.* (2002) Can we reverse the HIV/AIDS pandemic with expanded response? *Lancet* 360: 773–777.

Taylor S, van Heeswijk RP, Hoetelmans RM *et al.* (2000a) Concentrations of nevirapine, lamivudine and stavudine in semen of HIV-1-infected men. *AIDS* 14: 1979–84.

Taylor S, Back D, Drake S *et al.* (2000b) Antiretroviral drug concentrations in semen of HIV-infected men: differential penetration of indinavir, ritonavir, and saquinavir. Paper presented at the 7th Conference on Retroviruses and Opportunistic Infections, San Francisco, CA, abstract 318.

Tovanabutra S, Rovison V, Wongtrakul J *et al.* (2001) Male viral load and heterosexual transmission of HIV-1 subtype E in northern Thailand. *J Acquir Immune Defic Syndr* 29: 275–83.

Tsai CC, Follis KE, Sabo A *et al.* (1995) Prevention of SIV infection in macaques by (R)-9-(2 phosphonylmethoxypropyl)adenine. *Science* 270: 1197–9.

van der Straten A, Gomez CA, Saul J, Quan J, Padian N (2000) Sexual risk behaviors among heterosexual HIV serodiscordant couples in the era of post-exposure prevention and viral suppressive therapy. *AIDS* 14: F47–F54.

Vernazza PL, Troiani L, Flepp MJ *et al.* (2000) Potent antiretroviral treatment of HIV-infection results in suppression of the seminal shedding of HIV. *AIDS* 14: 117–21.

Wang SA Panlilo AL, Doi PA *et al.* (2000) Experience of healthcare workers taking post-exposure prophylaxis after occupational HIV exposure: findings of the HIV exposure Prophylaxis Registry. *Infect Control Hosp Epidemiol* 21: 780–5.

Wade NA, Birkhead GS, Warren BL *et al.* (1998) Abbreviated regimens of zidovudine prophylaxis and perinatal transmission of the human immunodeficiency virus. *N Engl J Med* 339: 1409–14.

Wainberg MA, Friedland G (1998) Public health implications of antiretroviral therapy and HIV drug resistance. *JAMA* 279: 1977–83.

Wawer MJ, Serwadda D, Li X *et al.* (2003) HIV-1 transmission per coital act, by stage of HIV infection in the HIV+ index partner, in discordant couples, Rakai, Uganda. Paper presented at the 10th Conference on Retroviruses and Opportunistic Infections, Boston, 2003, 40.

Wulfsohn A, Venter WDF, Schultze D, Levey M, Sanne IM (2003) Post exposure prophylaxis after sexual assault in South Africa. Paper presented at the 10th Conference on Retroviruses and Opportunistic Infections, Boston, Massachusetts, February 2003, abstract 42.

Zhang H, Dornadula G, Beaumont M *et al.* (1998) Human immunodeficiency virus type 1 in the semen of men receiving highly active antiretroviral therapy. *N Engl J Med* 339: 1803–9.

Zhang L, Ramratnam B, Tenner-Racz K *et al.* (1999) Quantifying residual HIV-1 replication in patients receiving combination antiretroviral therapy. *N Engl J Med* 340: 1605–13.

Challenges in Developing HIV Vaccines

7

Laurence Peiperl
Department of Medicine, University of California, San Francisco, USA

Susan Buchbinder
Director, HIV Research Section, San Francisco Department of Health, San Francisco, USA

Laurence Peiperl, MD is Assistant Clinical Professor of Medicine at the University of California San Francisco. He is an investigator in the HIV Vaccine Trials Network and serves on the leadership of several U.S. and international HIV vaccine trials. He directs the UCSF Center for HIV Information.

Susan Buchbinder, MD is the Director of the HIV Research Section and Associate Clinical Professor of Medicine & Epidemiology at the University of California San Francisco. She has published extensively in the area of HIV infection, risk factors and disease progression. She is a Principal Investigator for the San Francisco HIV Vaccine Trials Unit (HVTU), provides scientific direction and implementation of Phase I–III preventive HIV vaccine trials in San Francisco, leads the HVTN Phase III Committee, and directs site development in the Americas for HIV vaccine trials.

The principle behind vaccination is simple: exposing an individual to a harmless stimulus (the vaccine) that resembles some part of an infectious agent induces immunity that protects against disease if that infectious agent is later encountered. This approach has been extraordinarily successful over the past 200 years in ending or averting epidemics of such diseases as smallpox, polio, and influenza, and in protecting individuals against endemic illnesses such as rubella, measles, and hepatitis B.

On the other hand, no effective vaccines exist for a number of infections that cause millions of deaths each year, including malaria, tuberculosis, and AIDS. It is difficult to judge how long it will take to develop an HIV vaccine that is safe, efficacious, and practical for worldwide use. In 1984, shortly after HIV was identified as the virus that causes AIDS, US Secretary of Health and Human Services Margaret Heckler predicted that an HIV vaccine would be ready for testing 'in approximately two years'. Although small trials of HIV vaccines did begin in the late 1980s, two decades later no vaccine has been demonstrated to have even partial efficacy against HIV infection.

Pessimistic predictions may be no more accurate. In speaking of polio vaccine development in 1945, Australian scientist FM Burnet stated, 'While I was in America recently I had good opportunity to meet with most of the men actively engaged on research in poliomyelitis.... The part played by acquired immunity to poliomyelitis is still completely uncertain, and the practical problem of preventing infantile paralysis has not been solved. It is even doubtful whether it ever will be solved' (Robbins, 2004). This bleak assessment of the potential for developing an efficacious polio vaccine was made only 10 years before the licensure of the Salk polio vaccine, and 50 years later global eradication of polio appears within reach.

Insights gained during development of one vaccine have sparked the rapid development of others. For example, the realization that vaccines can be made from killed bacteria led to the development of vaccines against typhoid, plague, and cholera in the last part of the nineteenth century. Vaccines against diphtheria and tetanus, both based on toxoids (modifications of harmful proteins made by bacteria), were developed within several years of each other in the 1920s (Plotkin and Plotkin, 2004). Unfortunately, attempts to duplicate the recombinant protein approach that resulted in a successful hepatitis B vaccine in the 1980s have so far proved unsuccessful in protecting against HIV infection (Berman, 2003; Pitisutithum, 2004).

Vaccine development has also depended historically on empiric approaches and fortuitous events. Edward Jenner's vaccination of several people in the 1790s using material derived from cowpox set the course for the eventual eradication of smallpox. This breakthrough, perhaps the greatest in the history of medicine, emerged not from a detailed understanding of virology or immunology, but from an incremental advance over the ancient practice of variolation, in which fluid from active smallpox pustules was scratched into the skin or blown up the nostrils of healthy people (Crosby, 1993).

The appropriate balance between thorough understanding of mechanism and timely empiric evaluation constitutes a central debate in HIV vaccine development. To what extent should resources and time be devoted to basic virologic and immunologic studies aimed at optimizing potential HIV vaccines, as opposed to clinical trials of readily available vaccine candidates to evaluate efficacy without delay? Although it is not unusual for 20 or 30 years to elapse between identification of an infectious agent and development of an effective vaccine against it

Table 7.1 Length of time taken to develop selected vaccines.

Vaccine	Discovery of etiologic agent	Vaccine developed or licensed in US	Years elapsed
Typhoid	1884	1896	12 years
Pertussis	1906	1926	20 years
Polio	1908	1955	47 years
Measles	1953	1983	30 years
Hepatitis B	1965	1981	16 years
Rotavirus	1970	1998	28 years
Hepatitis A	1973	1995	22 years
Lyme disease	1982	1998	16 years
HIV	1983	???	>20 years

Source: AIDS Vaccine Advocacy Coalition. www.avac.org

(Table 7.1), the magnitude of the global AIDS epidemic makes developing an HIV vaccine a matter of the greatest urgency. This chapter provides an overview of the scientific, ethical, practical, and public health issues that pose challenges to current efforts to develop an HIV vaccine. Efforts to overcome these challenges have advanced not only HIV vaccine development, but also vaccinology, immunology, and international health in general.

The Process of Vaccine Testing

In earlier centuries, the most efficient way to test a vaccine was to give it to healthy individuals and then permit them to be exposed (or in some cases, actively expose them) to the microbe in question. If the individuals were protected, the vaccine was effective. If they became ill, or even died, they might be considered to have made a brave (if not entirely informed) sacrifice for their fellow human beings. Following World War II, the World Medical Association developed principles to guard against the kind of human experimentation that took place under Nazi governments. The resulting Declaration of Helsinki (available online at http://www.wma.net/e/ethicsunit/helsinki.htm), first adopted in 1964, states clearly that in medical research on human subjects, considerations related to the well-being of the individual study participant should take precedence over the interests of science and society. The principles of this Declaration have been incorporated into the guidelines of the International Conference on Harmonization and the United States Code of Federal Regulations, and provide an ethical standard to which US researchers must adhere when conducting research on human subjects anywhere in the world. (See 'Ethical Issues,' below.) To provide appropriate protections for human subjects and ultimately for consumers, the development of a new vaccine proceeds in stages.

Preclinical Testing

Before a product can enter human (clinical) trials, preclinical development must establish that it is not toxic in animals. In the United States, the Food and Drug Administration (FDA) Center for Biologics Evaluation and Research (CBER) provides advice to a vaccine developer regarding what animal safety studies are required to demonstrate safety of a given product. Immunogenicity (the ability of a vaccine to induce an immune response) is usually studied in preclinical experiments as well, although, as discussed below, the lack of a perfect animal model makes it difficult to extrapolate immunogenicity data to human beings. In practice, however, it is usually the demonstration of strong immune responses in animals, particularly non-human primates, and often the demonstration of vaccine-induced protection of animals against viral challenges with simian immunodeficiency virus (SIV) or SIV/HIV hybrids (SHIV) that motivate a vaccine developer to pursue human trials.

Clinical Safety and Immunogenicity Studies (Figure 7.1)

Provided that safety is demonstrated in animals, the first clinical trials of a new vaccine product are designed to assess safety in human beings. These Phase I trials usually enroll 10–20 participants at each dose being tested, and may proceed to higher doses if each successive dose is shown to be tolerated. Phase I trials contain a small number of placebo recipients to assure an unbiased assessment of side-effects. Subjects are randomly assigned to vaccine or placebo groups, and neither investigators nor subjects are aware of their group assignment until after the study is completed. Phase I trials also provide preliminary data on immunogenicity in humans, but are generally too small to permit accurate comparisons of different dose levels or dosing schedules. The FDA continues to review data and research protocols through all phases of clinical development.

If Phase I studies show a vaccine to be safe and well tolerated, Phase II studies may be undertaken to further assess safety, and also to study immunogenicity. Phase II studies, which generally involve between 100 and 1000 participants, may compare several doses, or dosing schedules, or combinations of different vaccines. Again, a double-blinded, placebo-controlled design is used to provide an assessment of 'background' symptoms and immune responses. In addition to providing an unbiased assessment of side-effects, this type of study design also ensures no given participant is guaranteed to have received the actual vaccine, and therefore the chance is minimized of increasing risk behavior under the optimistic assumption that one might be protected against HIV.

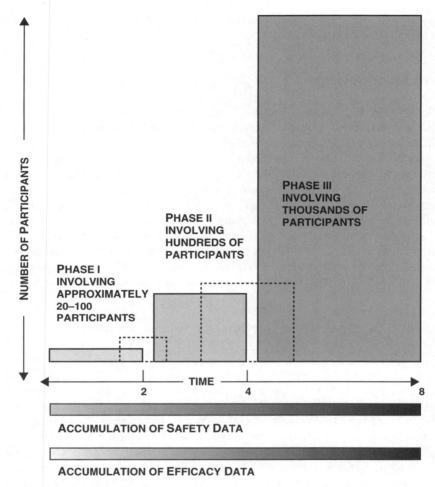

Fig. 7.1 Phases of clinical trials. Dotted lines suggest Phase I/II (also known as Phase IB or Phase IIB) or Phase II/III (also known as Phase IIB) trials, which have characteristics of both types of trial indicated. For example, a Phase I/II trial may have the scientific goals of a Phase I trial, but to permit global scope might have the number of participants usually associated with a Phase II trial. Approximate duration of trials is given in years. Pauses are often necessary between trials to review safety and immunogenicity data.

Clinical efficacy studies

If a vaccine regimen proves safe and immunogenic in Phase II, the next step is an efficacy (Phase III) trial to determine whether the vaccine actually protects against HIV. At the time of this writing, only two closely related HIV vaccine candidates have completed Phase III testing, and were not found to protect against HIV infection (Berman, 2003; Pitisutithum, 2004). To understand why so few efficacy trials have been undertaken despite some 20 years of HIV vaccine research requires consideration of the realities involved in testing an HIV vaccine.

First, the idea that a vaccine is immunogenic in Phase II testing suggests that researchers know what sort of immune responses are likely to protect against HIV, and can perform laboratory tests to determine whether the vaccine is eliciting such responses. In fact, as elaborated below, the laboratory correlates of protective immunity against HIV (if indeed such immunity exists in humans) are not known. One way to identify such correlates might be through a Phase III trial that compares the immune responses of subjects who become infected after receiving the candidate vaccine to those who have received the vaccine and remain uninfected. Of course, such an approach assumes that the vaccine being tested will protect some proportion of participants, and in any case cannot be used to select the first products to enter Phase III testing.

Second, the questions to be answered by an efficacy trial are debatable. Ideally, a vaccine would completely prevent subsequent infection by HIV. But if aborting infection is not possible, would it be useful to have a vaccine that slows HIV disease progression? What about a vaccine that might not prevent infection, but reduces the infectiousness of the vaccinee who subsequently becomes infected with HIV? Need an HIV vaccine be shown to be effective in specific subpopulations (women vs. men, heterosexuals vs. homosexuals, sexual vs. injection drug-use acquisition), or will summary estimates of protection across subpopulations suffice? Does efficacy need to be demonstrated in specific racial or ethnic groups, or against specific subtypes of HIV out of the many subtypes that are prevalent in different areas of the world? In the absence of data or philosophical consensus, each of these questions must be addressed, implicitly or explicitly, in designing a Phase III HIV vaccine trial.

Even if limited populations and specific viral subtypes are chosen for an efficacy trial, the fact that infection is a relatively infrequent event (generally less than 5 per cent per year even in high-risk populations) necessitates large study populations to assure that a trial has the statistical power to detect vaccine efficacy. Both government and industry have been understandably reluctant to undertake such trials without reasonably firm scientific evidence in favor of the vaccines being tested. The following section outlines some of the difficulties researchers face in obtaining this kind of evidence.

Scientific Challenges

Over the past two decades, research efforts directed at understanding the interactions between HIV and the immune system have led to advances in virology and immunology in general. Much of our knowledge of cellular immunology, and in particular the types, functions, and regulation of T lymphocytes, has developed in tandem with efforts to understand the immunopathogenesis of AIDS. HIV has also served as a paradigm case in the development of new laboratory methods to measure immune responses. Despite many advances, however, our understanding of how (and even whether) a vaccine might induce the immune system to protect against HIV infection remains limited. Our ignorance is the result of several factors discussed below.

Humoral and Cellular Immune Responses

We know that HIV infection elicits both antibody (humoral) and cellular immune responses. Antibodies, which are produced by B lymphocytes, are proteins that bind to three-dimensional structures such as the outer envelope protein of HIV, and may either inactivate the virus or facilitate its clearance from the body. Antibodies against specific microbes are responsible for immunity against many infectious diseases. An HIV vaccine that could elicit an effective antibody response would enable immunized individuals to clear the virus immediately following exposure, before it could enter cells and establish life-long infection. This ideal of 'sterilizing immunity' has been called the 'holy grail' of HIV vaccine research. We also know, however, that most naturally occurring antibodies that bind to HIV cannot effectively neutralize the virus.

In contrast to the humoral immune response, in which antibodies bind to foreign structures outside the body's cells, cellular immune responses, which are mediated by T lymphocytes, detect cells that contain infectious agents such as viruses, and prevent the further spread of infection by a series of interactions that result in killing of the infected cells. Cellular immunity seems unlikely to provide sterilizing immunity because an infected cell may harbor HIV in a latent form for many years without triggering a cellular immune response, and then begin producing active virus. Further, as discussed below, HIV can mutate to escape both humoral and cellular immune responses.

Models of Protection

There is no fully reliable model for immune protection against HIV. The vast majority of infected individuals develop disease if not treated, suggesting that the natural immune response is usually inadequate. A small minority of HIV-infected individuals remain healthy for years without treatment and show little evidence of HIV replication or immune damage. Studies of HIV-specific immune responses in these long-term non-progressors (LTNPs) suggest that both T helper (CD4) and T cytotoxic (CD8) immune responses directed against multiple components of the HIV virus are needed to maintain immunologic control of HIV in infected individuals (Rosenberg *et al.*, 1997; Kalams *et al.*, 1999). While specific genetic factors have been identified in a minority of LTNPs, these inherited factors are not directly applicable to HIV vaccine development (Cohen *et al.*, 1998; Flores-Villanueva *et al.*, 2001).

Another group that may provide insight into protection against HIV infection are people who are repeatedly exposed to HIV without developing evidence of infection. Unlike LTNPs, these individuals remain negative on repeated HIV antibody testing and have been called 'HIV exposed, persistently seronegative' (HEPS). HIV-specific CD8 T cell responses have been detected in a HEPS cohort of Kenyan sex workers, but whether these responses are actually responsible for protection is unknown (Kaul *et al.*, 2001).

A variety of animal models for HIV infection have been used, but none is ideal. In general, HIV does not cause disease in other species. Chimpanzees can be infected with HIV, but may control the infection without treatment, and as an endangered species are not generally available for research purposes. Macaques are more commonly used as research animals, and can be infected with the simian immunodeficiency virus (SIV). However, SIV differs from HIV significantly in the viral envelope protein, which is considered to be the prime target for an effective antibody immune response. Genetically engineered simian-human immunodeficiency (SHIV) virus strains containing SIV replication machinery and HIV envelope allow research into antibody responses against HIV (Letvin *et al.*, 2002). Nevertheless, human and simian immune responses are clearly not identical, and induction of (or failure to induce) protection in monkeys cannot be assumed to predict the effectiveness of a vaccine candidate in humans.

Immune Correlates of Protection

With neither a clinical nor a confirmed experimental model for immune protection against AIDS, we are left to speculate which immune responses (if any) will provide protection against HIV infection. For many infections that are preventable by existing vaccines, antibody immunity can be readily measured and serves as a reliable predictor of protection against future infection. For example, an individual with a positive blood test for antibody to the surface protein of hepatitis B virus is generally protected against infection with hepatitis B (regardless of whether that antibody is due to prior vaccination, response to natural infection, or passive immunization with gamma globulin).

In contrast, a positive HIV antibody test (outside of a vaccine trial) provides evidence that one is infected with HIV, but does not indicate protection from disease progression. Further, early human studies of HIV envelope protein vaccines showed that individuals developing an antibody response to the vaccine could subsequently become infected with HIV through risk activities (Kahn *et al.*, 1995). As noted above, two large efficacy trials of the VaxGen HIV envelope vaccines failed to show protection against infection, despite the development of appreciable antibody responses against the envelope protein (Berman, 2003; Pitisutithum, 2004). These studies were well conducted, with adequate recruitment, excellent retention of study subjects, and efficient study procedures.

These results do not necessarily mean that no future vaccine-induced antibodies will protect against HIV infection. At present, however, we do not know which (if any) antibodies provide protection, nor do we know how to create a vaccine that will elicit them. Studies of the three-dimensional structure of the HIV envelope protein and specific antibodies that bind to it and neutralize the virus suggest novel approaches, such as vaccinating with proteins that mimic three-dimensional envelope structures that take shape only after the virus binds to a cell. A study in newborn macaques suggests that a mixture of synthetically prepared neutralizing antibodies may protect against milk-borne transmission of a SHIV (Ruprecht *et al.*, 2003), but how to make a vaccine that elicits such antibodies, and whether they would prove effective against HIV in humans, is unknown.

Identifying correlates of cellular immunity is even more complex. Recognition and killing of an infected cell depends on the presence of viral components on the cell surface. We have learned that the particular components that appear on the cell surface, as well as the strength of the immune response that each component can elicit, vary from individual to individual and from one strain of virus to the next. It is therefore unknown which viral components are most important to include in a vaccine designed to elicit cellular immunity. Most likely, a variety of different components will need to be included in order for a vaccine to have any chance of inducing appreciable benefit through cellular immunity. Even if such a vaccine proves partially effective, determining which components or combination of components is providing the benefit, and whether the effect is limited to people of specific genetic makeup, may remain difficult.

Evasion of the Immune Response

As the epidemic has required us to expand our understanding of the virus and the immune response, researchers have identified an array of strategies that HIV has evolved to evade the human immune system. For example, the envelope structure tends to be highly disordered until the moment it attaches to the cell surface, leaving relatively little opportunity for the immune system to recognize, and mount an antibody response against, key viral surface structures (Myszka *et al.*, 2000; Kwong *et al.*, 2002). Antibody responses are further hindered by sugar molecules (glycosylations) covering the underlying protein structure and concealing it from antibodies.

Viral latency is another, very effective, strategy for avoiding the immune response. HIV integrates its genetic material into a cell's chromosomes shortly after infection, and before HIV proteins can be produced. The virus can therefore remain dormant in the cell for many years, undetected by the cellular response, until the cell begins producing new viruses (Chun *et al.*, 1997). Because T cell immunity can act only on virus within cells, and because cells infected with HIV can remain latently infected for many years without attracting killer T cells, cellular responses by themselves are not expected to eliminate HIV infection.

One of the most difficult challenges to vaccine development is posed by the ease with which HIV can change its structure without losing the ability to infect and cause disease. This ability to mutate results from a lack of precision in the molecular machinery that the virus uses to copy itself after it infects a new host cell. While a high error rate might appear to be a hindrance to viral reproduction, in fact this 'sloppiness' produces an enormous diversity of viral variants in each infected individual, thereby greatly increasing the chance that some variant will be able to escape from any given immune response. For example, the envelope protein contains variable loop structures that are able to undergo considerable mutation without impairing virus function. Because these loops are highly exposed and easily recognized as foreign, they act as decoys to the immune system, eliciting an antibody response that is ultimately ineffective as the loop structure mutates and escapes recognition. In fact, studies of infected individuals have shown that the virus can rapidly mutate to escape the natural antibody responses that occur following infection (Richman *et al.*, 2003; Wei *et al.*, 2003), and also to escape suppression by T cell immunity (Rosenberg *et al.*, 1997; Goulder *et al.*, 2001).

Viral Diversity

The diversity of HIV is not limited to the random multiplicity of strains existing in a given infected individual. Worldwide, the virus can be classified into at least 11 major subtypes (clades), which differ from one another substantially in their envelope proteins (Osmanov *et al.*, 2002). Further, two viruses of different subtypes can combine with one another if both infect the same individual, leading to circulating recombinant forms that are hybrids of the two parent subtypes. It is not known whether a vaccine that is protective against virus of one clade would also be effective against other clades or recombinant forms.

Viral diversity is matched by the diversity of the molecules (HLA) responsible for presenting peptide antigens to T cells in human beings. Some viral peptides are preferentially presented by HLA molecules associated with specific ethnic groups, raising the possibility that a given vaccine might be effective in some individuals but not others, according to their inherited HLA type.

Viral diversity also occurs in a non-random fashion over the course of infection in a given individual. To gain entry into cells in the early stages of infection, HIV preferentially uses a molecule (CCR5) found on immune cells close to the mucosal surface. Later in the course of infection the envelope protein in some viral subtypes switches its structure to gain entry via a molecule (CXCR4) found more exclusively on T helper cells. Whether this change in envelope structure is relevant to vaccine design, and whether the same immune response will protect both those exposed to HIV by mucosal routes and those exposed through non-mucosal routes (such as injection drug users) is unknown.

The laboratory conditions under which HIV is cultured can also lead to a form of diversity, with laboratory-adapted strains showing different properties than viral strains directly obtained from human beings (primary isolates). For example, the antibodies that neutralize laboratory-adapted viruses from which early envelope vaccine candidates were developed do not generally neutralize primary isolates (Wrin *et al.*, 1995). This form of diversity contributes to the difficulty of predicting vaccine efficacy from limited laboratory studies of vaccine-induced immune responses.

The Vaccine Pipeline

Many products have been considered as possible HIV vaccines, and approximately 80 have entered Phase I clinical trials. The HIV vaccine pipeline changes rapidly, and readers are referred to Internet sites such as the HVTN Pipeline Project (http://chi.ucsf.edu/vaccine) or the International AIDS Vaccine Initiative database (http://www.iavi.org) for updated summaries of HIV vaccine products in human trials.

No vaccines currently in clinical testing contain HIV itself. Live attenuated strains of HIV are not considered safe for human use, as retroviruses may mutate, recombine, and integrate into cellular DNA in ways that raise concerns over reversion to virulence or carcinogenesis. Similarly, the use of killed HIV raises concerns that failure of the inactivation process in even a tiny fraction of a vaccine lot could have disastrous consequences.

Products in the HIV vaccine development pipeline therefore contain only components of HIV, and can be divided into two general classes: those that are intended primarily to elicit a neutralizing antibody response, and those intended to elicit an effective cellular response. The antibody-inducing products are those that reflect the three-dimensional structure of the active virus, and typically remain outside the cell cytoplasm. These products, including proteins (generally the HIV envelope protein in one form or another) or component peptides of viral proteins, represent the first approaches taken in the early 1990s, with the rational expectation that neutralizing antibodies would provide the most effective means of clearing the virus before it could enter cells and cause damage to the immune system.

As evidence accumulated that available products were unlikely to elicit protective antibodies, attention turned to approaches that might elicit cellular immune responses that, even if they did not achieve sterilizing immunity, might keep the virus in check following infection. Such products, which must target viral antigens into the cytoplasm in order to stimulate a response by cytotoxic T cells, include non-pathogenic viral vectors (such as vaccinia, canary pox, replication-deficient adenovirus, and several others) engineered to carry genes encoding selected components of HIV; and a variety of DNA plasmid vectors encoding HIV peptides or proteins. These products include modified poxviruses (such as vaccinia and canary-pox), replication-defective adenoviruses, a variety of other viral vectors, and a variety of DNA plasmids. Because many of these products elicit limited antibody responses, current efforts seek to develop products or combinations that might induce both cellular and humoral immunity, and new peptide and protein products are also being developed.

However, even if a front-runner according to scientific criteria emerges among vaccine candidates, the race will not be over until efficacy is demonstrated and safety confirmed in well-conducted Phase III trials, and the product is then made available to those at risk worldwide. The subsequent sections of this chapter discuss the formidable challenges to HIV vaccine development that derive not from biology, but from ethical and practical issues.

Ethical challenges

While all clinical research involves ethical challenges, HIV vaccine development faces unique obstacles arising from the stigma associated with HIV infection or the behaviors that encourage its spread, the global nature of the epidemic, and the unique biological properties of the virus. The worldwide scope of the pandemic has focused public attention on the ethical issues involved in clinical research in general, and on HIV vaccine-related research in particular.

The ethical principles guiding HIV vaccine trial research are the same as those underlying all clinical research and are outlined in documents such as the US National Commission for the Protection of Human Subject's Belmont Report, the World Medical Association's Declaration of Helsinki, and the Council for International Organizations of Medical Science's International Ethical Guidelines for Biomedical Research Involving Human Subjects. Some additional issues specific to HIV vaccine research are discussed in the UNAIDS Guidance Document on Ethical Considerations in HIV Preventive Vaccine Research (UNAIDS, 2000), the result of a series of regional meetings with lawyers, activists, social scientists, ethicists, vaccine scientists, epidemiologists, representatives of non-governmental organizations, people living with HIV/AIDS, and health policy analysts to discuss ethical concerns in development of HIV vaccines. Here, we highlight five major ethical challenges to conducting HIV vaccine research that are making a major impact on the conduct of clinical research in general.

Research in Vulnerable Populations

To maximize the chance of detecting any benefit that a vaccine candidate might have, using the minimum number of study volunteers, and to ensure that the

173

resulting estimates of vaccine efficacy are broadly applicable to the population who will ultimately receive the vaccine, vaccine efficacy trials are conducted in populations at highest risk of acquiring the disease in question. For diseases that are vector-borne (e.g. malaria), or spread through casual contact (e.g. influenza), general populations can be enrolled in geographic areas where the diseases are endemic. Because HIV is spread most commonly through sexual contact or injection drug use, HIV vaccine efficacy trials can be conducted most efficiently in high-risk, HIV-uninfected individuals from populations in which sexual or injection transmission is occurring. Such populations are often involved in illegal or stigmatized activities, such as illegal drug use; exchange of sex for drugs, money, or services; or sexual activity between men. Such groups are considered 'vulnerable' because enrollment in trials may mark these volunteers as engaging in high-risk practices, and they may suffer additional discrimination or stigma as a result of participating in HIV vaccine research.

Even in regions of the world where HIV infection rates in the general adult population are high enough to justify enrolling vaccine trials without using specific behavioral eligibility criteria, discrimination and stigma may result from trial screening. Specifically, because such preventive HIV vaccine trials will exclude HIV-infected people, potential participants who are turned away from such trials may be perceived to be HIV infected, when in truth a number of other medical or operational criteria may have excluded the volunteer. Steps must be taken in conducting HIV vaccine trials to minimize the possibility of discrimination against trial participants or non-participants. Measures can be taken to protect the confidentiality of persons being screened or enrolled in trials. Staff can be trained to counsel volunteers about potential social harms that may arise out of participation, and to anticipate and prevent such occurrences. Community-wide activities can be undertaken to lessen the stigma associated with HIV risk and infection. Research units can conduct a variety of research activities that involve HIV-infected volunteers as well as those at low or high risk for HIV infection. This strategy benefits research efforts in the broader HIV-affected community, and may decrease the stigma associated with participating in HIV research in general.

Against this backdrop has emerged the suggestion that early safety studies of all vaccine candidates be conducted in study populations that are less vulnerable to harm or exploitation and that these studies be limited to volunteers in the country of the trial sponsor. This approach would require a sequential vaccine testing strategy in which vaccines would undergo safety testing in the sponsor's country, followed by safety studies in the eventual target population, followed finally by efficacy testing in those countries. Such an approach may lead to delays in testing without a clear benefit. A more beneficial approach might be parallel safety testing in the sponsor and host countries.

Social harms are not the only reason for concern in enrolling vulnerable populations in HIV vaccine trials. Concerns have been raised that study volunteers may harbor beliefs that the candidate vaccine is efficacious and may therefore increase their risk behavior during a trial. This issue is also relatively unique to HIV vaccine studies, in contrast to studies of vaccines against infectious diseases that are transmitted through casual contact or vectors. In HIV vaccine trials, study staff provide volunteers with ongoing counseling that includes warnings that the vaccine(s) being tested are of unproven efficacy, and that the participant may be getting a placebo rather than vaccine. Data from the first efficacy trial of an HIV vaccine candidate suggested that overall, participants reduced risk early in the trial, with a return to baseline levels over the three years of follow-up (Bartholow, 2003). However, comparison to a group of volunteers in a companion study that did not include a vaccine (or placebo), but otherwise provided similar risk-reduction counseling, suggested that these non-vaccine participants may have been more responsive to risk-reduction counseling than vaccine trial volunteers (Buchbinder *et al.*, 2003). These findings reinforce the need for ongoing, trial-specific counseling to minimize the risk of behavioral disinhibition resulting from vaccine trial participation.

Need to Support HIV Prevention in all Vaccine Trial Participants

An essential tension arises in conducting HIV vaccine efficacy trials. On the one hand, the only way to demonstrate HIV vaccine efficacy definitively is to enroll and follow high-risk volunteers, some of whom are randomly assigned to receive vaccine and others randomly assigned to receive placebo. If the HIV infection rate at the end of the trial is significantly lower in the group receiving vaccine compared with the placebo group, then the vaccine is demonstrated to be efficacious. On the other hand, we are ethically obligated to provide all study volunteers with the best prevention methods currently available, which may, in turn, drive down infection rates and limit our ability to answer the very question we set out to address. How can this tension be resolved?

Unfortunately, the resolution is relatively simple at the moment. All trial volunteers must receive the most effective prevention methods available (currently limited to counseling, condoms, and referrals), but unfortunately, despite the best prevention methods, HIV infection rates remain high in many populations. In the world's first vaccine efficacy trial, conducted in North America and Europe, HIV infection rates were 2.8 per cent per year over three years of follow-up in men who have sex with men enrolled in the trial, rates that are certainly high enough to assure that efficacy trials of reasonable size can reach a definitive assessment of vaccine efficacy. These infection rates occurred despite provision of state-of-the-art risk-reduction counseling and referrals to local prevention programs. In fact, if currently available counseling could drive down HIV infection rates to such low levels that vaccines could not be tested efficiently, we would not have such a pressing need for an HIV vaccine in the first place.

Several other ethical issues arise with regard to provision of prevention methods to vaccine trial volunteers. As more efficacious prevention methods are developed (e.g. behavioral interventions, STD treatment, vaginal and rectal microbicides), these too will need to be provided to HIV vaccine trial volunteers. The result may be that trials will need to be larger, have longer follow-up periods, or focus more on populations that maintain high infection rates despite these prevention methods. Questions arise as to whether provision of certain types of prevention methods (e.g. clean injection equipment for injection drug users) during trials will be possible if such methods are not available within the broader population or are illegal. Current vaccine trials use a placebo control, because there is no efficacious vaccine against which new vaccines can be compared. However, future vaccine candidates may prove to be partially efficacious. What level of efficacy must be demonstrated before that vaccine becomes the standard against which subsequent HIV vaccine candidates must be tested? These are issues currently being debated that will affect the design and implementation of future trials.

Vaccine-induced Positive Antibody Tests

HIV vaccines are designed to generate HIV-specific immune responses, including antibodies directed against HIV. Some vaccines are created to generate antibodies to multiple components of HIV, while others take a more targeted approach. Unfortunately, our current diagnostic methods for determining whether or not a person is HIV infected do so by detecting antibodies, even at low levels, against HIV. It is therefore imperative to be able to differentiate vaccine-induced antibody responses from true HIV infection. Volunteers who become HIV infected must be counseled about their HIV infection and referred for appropriate care and treatment (see discussion on access to treatment below). HIV antibody testing that is conducted as part of HIV vaccine trials is designed to be able to differentiate between vaccine-induced antibody and true HIV infection so that accurate information on HIV infection status can be given to participants throughout the trial. This has been a relatively straightforward process to date, because most vaccines include only a small number of HIV proteins, and often only parts of these proteins, allowing specialized antibody assays to discriminate between vaccine-induced antibody responses and true HIV infection. Newer vaccine products may require development of more specialized tests.

A different problem arises if trial volunteers receive HIV antibody testing outside of the vaccine trial site. In this situation, vaccine-induced antibodies may be incorrectly interpreted as representing true HIV infection, and volunteers may be given incorrect information. Trial volunteers may, in turn, incorrectly interpret this information by assuming they are infected (when the antibodies, in truth, were solely vaccine-induced) or by attributing the test results to the study vaccine (when they in fact result from actual HIV infection). Participants may also assume that receiving a positive antibody test result outside of the study means they received vaccine, rather than placebo; if they incorrectly assume that the vaccine will protect them, they may actually increase their risk of HIV infection. If the positive HIV antibody results are shared with others, the volunteer may be denied health or life insurance, employment, housing, or travel opportunities, as well as suffering other social harm or discrimination. For these reasons, trial volunteers are asked to go to the trial site for all HIV testing during the trial. In addition to routine HIV antibody testing during trials, volunteers should be encouraged to go to the trial site for interim testing, should it be required because of high-risk exposures or because of external requirements (e.g. insurance companies). Many trial sites will also offer ongoing testing after a vaccine trial is complete for the subset of participants who may have persistent HIV antibody, to ensure that future diagnostic tests for HIV infection reflect true HIV infection status rather than presence of vaccine-induced antibody.

Access to HIV Vaccines and Treatment for Vaccine Trial Volunteers

HIV advocacy groups have effected lasting changes in regulatory policy through their groundbreaking work in accelerating access to therapies proven effective in treating HIV infection. Their efforts have also established an essential role for community advisory boards in the development and implementation of ethical clinical trials. Although we do not yet have HIV vaccines proven to be efficacious in human beings, advocacy groups (AVAC) and international organizations (WHO-UNAIDS, 2000; Chang *et al.*, 2003) have led the dialogue regarding how to make such vaccines widely available once their efficacy is documented. Vaccine manufacturers recognize the need to provide their product to placebo recipients once the trial is over, if efficacy of their product is demonstrated. Providing vaccines to larger populations at risk of infection will mean addressing a number of operational and economic challenges, including manufacturing capabilities; infrastructure necessary to ship, store and administer vaccines; and payment for vaccines, particularly in developing countries or for uninsured persons in the developed world.

Infrastructure and availability are not new problems in vaccine development. The World Health Organization estimates that in 1998, one in four children worldwide failed to receive routine immunization with vaccines against common childhood infectious diseases. Even in the developed world, many efficacious vaccines have not reached their target population. For example, hepatitis B vaccines were first demonstrated to be efficacious in populations of men who have sex with men (MSM) in the US; however, a study of 3432 young MSM conducted in seven US metropolitan areas from 1994 to 1998 demonstrated that only 9 per cent had been immunized, while 96 per cent of the susceptible population had a regular source of health care or had recently accessed health care (Mackellar *et al.*, 2001).

Mechanisms must be developed for distribution of an efficacious vaccine even before testing of that product has begun, to speed its availability to the populations in greatest need.

A relatively small proportion of HIV vaccine trial volunteers will become HIV infected during the course of such trials. Much discussion has occurred about the ethical imperative to provide antiretroviral therapy to such volunteers. This is a particularly complex problem in HIV vaccine trials, where one of the primary objectives is assessment of vaccine effects on post-infection endpoints, such as HIV viral load and CD4 count. Many have argued that it would be unethical to follow volunteers for clinical or laboratory outcomes without providing them with therapy when they reach endpoints for which international organizations have recommended treatment. Some have argued that following vaccine trial volunteers without treating them would be tantamount to repeating the Tuskegee study experience, one of the most notorious examples of unethical research practices. In that study of the natural history of syphilis infection, a cohort of African American men in Tuskegee, Alabama, begun in 1932, continued to be observed without therapy despite the fact that a safe and effective treatment for syphilis (penicillin) was discovered during the course of the study.

After considerable discussion and debate, UNAIDS-sponsored regional meetings held in Geneva, Brazil, Thailand, Uganda, and Washington in 1997–1999 to discuss ethical issues in HIV vaccine trials reached the following conclusion: 'Care and treatment for HIV/AIDS and its associated complications should be provided to participants in HIV preventive vaccine trials, with the ideal being to provide the best proven therapy, and the minimum to provide the highest level of care attainable in the host country in light of the circumstances listed below' (UNAIDS, 2000). The 'circumstances' included the level of care and treatment available in both the sponsor (manufacturer) and host (clinical trial site) countries, including the availability of antiretroviral therapy outside of the research context, availability of infrastructure to provide treatment and care, and potential duration and sustainability of care and treatment for the trial volunteer. These circumstances may critically affect decisions about the level of care that may be provided in the host country. If adequate infrastructure were not available to provide sustainable care for volunteers, would it be ethical to provide care with inadequate infrastructure, or to stop treatment once the trial had stopped? On the other hand, would it be ethical to have different standards of care and access within a single trial that enrolls volunteers from multiple geographic locations?

While these discussions and debates continue, consensus is slowly growing that treatment must be provided to volunteers enrolled in HIV vaccine trials once they become infected and meet clinical and/or laboratory thresholds for initiation of therapy. These decisions are driven by the ethical imperatives stated above, but are also consistent with global efforts to improve health care infrastructure and provide antiretroviral therapy in regions of the world heavily affected by the HIV epidemic. Despite this consensus in principle, however, few countries or vaccine developers have determined how to cover the cost of such treatment in practice.

As treatment becomes more widely available, the scientific objectives underlying follow-up of HIV-infected volunteers take on a different emphasis. Rather than investigating the impact of the candidate HIV vaccine on HIV disease progression, studies should address the more complex question of the ability of the candidate vaccine to alter the natural history of HIV disease in the setting of treatment, including the potential for the vaccine to delay the need for treatment or alter the response to therapy. Addressing such questions will require that vaccine trial volunteers who become infected be enrolled in standardized research protocols and be provided fairly uniform access to antiretroviral therapy.

The prospect of developing and implementing such treatment protocols raises additional ethical and practical questions. How can uniform standards for a treatment trial be created if different trial sites have different standards for initiation of treatment or different regimens available to the populations? Need study volunteers enroll in a treatment trial to gain access to antiretroviral therapy? Will other therapy also be provided to participants (including prophylaxis against opportunistic infections)? Is it ethical to treat study volunteers without treating family members who have no other access to treatment? If family members are offered treatment only through the trial and only if the uninfected volunteer becomes infected, will volunteers increase their risk of infection during the trial in hopes of acquiring treatment for their family members? These issues will continue to be debated as approaches are pursued to permit ethical research that not only answers critical scientific questions but also maximizes benefit to study volunteers and limits the possibility of excessive inducements to volunteer. Because clinical research in HIV is both newsworthy and dependent on international collaborations, HIV vaccine research is bringing issues like these to the attention of communities, governments, multilateral organizations, and drug manufacturers worldwide. The resulting policies may determine the standards for conducting international clinical trials in many fields and for many years to come.

Developing and Testing Products for the Developing World

As discussed above, HIV can be classified into various subtypes (clades), each of which has a different global distribution (see IAVI report, August 2003: http://www.iavi.org/iavireport/0803/clades-vax.htm). While it seems unlikely that each viral subtype will define a protective immune response that does not overlap with other subtypes, there is at least a theoretical concern that candidate vaccines may have differential efficacy against different viral subtypes. Worldwide, subtype C infections account for the majority of HIV infections. Subtype B infection, most prevalent throughout the Americas, the Caribbean, Western Europe, and Australia, accounts for less than 15 per cent of infections worldwide. The vast majority of candidate HIV vaccines that have entered clinical trials have been developed using subtype B prototypes, although increasingly, the vaccine pipeline is including a variety of products directed against non-B subtypes. Developing countries have expressed considerably greater enthusiasm about testing vaccine products that are clade-matched for their local epidemics rather than those that are clade-mismatched. Investigators and government officials from some countries have even expressed a strong preference for testing products developed using country-specific viral strains, given viral diversity within clades in different geographic locations.

Issues of viral diversity may become considerably more complex as viral recombination becomes more widespread. Currently, many countries are experiencing mixed epidemics involving several subtypes, as well as an increasing number of infections with circulating recombinant forms, in which a single viral isolate comprises more than one viral subtype. Newer vaccine candidates are attempting to address the issue of viral diversity by using components representing multiple viral subtypes. This approach allows for development and testing of vaccines that could potentially be used in multiple regions of the world. While initial efficacy trials are likely to enroll volunteer populations in geographic regions matched by viral subtype to the candidate vaccine, future trials will be developed to assess the relationship of vaccine efficacy to viral diversity and will include subtype 'mismatched' populations.

Practical Challenges in Implementing Clinical Trials

Efficacy trials of HIV vaccines will require thousands of volunteers; the exact number required for each trial depends on background HIV infection rates in the study population, anticipated duration of follow-up, and the specific questions being addressed. Efficacy trials of vaccines against several other infectious agents (e.g. cholera, pneumococcus, hemophilus B, influenza) have required tens of thousands of volunteers, and the field trial of the Salk polio vaccine enrolled hundreds of thousands of volunteers, far larger than the sample sizes enrolled in the first HIV vaccine efficacy trials. Nonetheless, HIV vaccine efficacy trials face substantial challenges beyond size alone, including the geographic scope required of efficacy trials, the need for collaboration among the many groups conducting HIV vaccine and non-vaccine prevention research, and a tightly regulated research environment characterized by increasing monitoring and training requirements. We anticipate that a series of efficacy trials of multiple products will be necessary to arrive at an HIV vaccine that is highly efficacious against the myriad viral variants present worldwide. Such efforts will involve many geographic regions of the world; already, the HIV Vaccine Trials Network (HVTN), the leading HIV clinical trials network sponsored by the US National Institutes of Health, has clinical trial sites in 15 countries on four continents (http://www.hvtn.org). There are estimates that by the year 2010, more than 50 000 volunteers will be enrolled in currently planned HIV vaccine efficacy trials and an equal number of similar volunteers will be required for efficacy trials of non-vaccine HIV prevention strategies. These estimates reflect only those efficacy trials that are currently being planned and do not take into account the need for large numbers of study volunteers for Phase I and II trials nor the possibility of additional efficacy trials of products currently in earlier stages of clinical testing.

Building Clinical Trials Infrastructure

To conduct successful efficacy trials, investigators, staff, regulatory personnel, and community members at all participating sites must be fully engaged and acquire the requisite expertise to participate as full partners in research. Physical infrastructure – such as clinical trial sites, research pharmacies and laboratories, computer hardware and software and communication lines for exchange of data – must be established. Trials will also require local expertise in diverse technical fields, including epidemiology, biostatistics, clinical medicine, regulatory oversight, ethics, pharmacology, laboratory medicine, data management, counseling, community education, and techniques for recruitment and retention of volunteers. Countries participating in this research must often newly develop or expand existing ethical review boards and build specific expertise in the oversight of HIV vaccine trials. Additional staff training and staffing levels are being required to ensure adherence to an increasing list of regulatory requirements for conducting clinical trials.

Building clinical trials infrastructure requires resources and time, and uncertainties in the timing of future efficacy trials generates debate about when to begin new site development. There are no clear guidelines about the length of time that should be allotted to prepare new vaccine trial sites to participate in HIV vaccine trials. Sites with prior research experience, well-developed regulatory structures, and government approval to receive and test the candidate HIV vaccine can be ready to participate in efficacy trials several months after resources are dedicated to this purpose. More typically, several years are required after initial discussions with a potential new clinical trial site before requisite infrastructure and regulatory approvals are in place. Because many factors can affect the anticipated start date of efficacy trials – vaccine manufacturing or release problems, requirements imposed by local or national regulatory bodies, delays in enrollment or completion of Phase I/II trials, or disappointing safety, tolerability or immunogenicity results from such trials – it is difficult to anticipate with certainty when an efficacy trial will begin. A balance must be struck between early site development, which ensures adequate capacity to enroll vaccine efficacy trials rapidly, and delayed site development, which avoids wasting resources on fully staffed, idle vaccine trial sites. As mentioned above, involving vaccine trial sites in diverse research opportunities such as non-vaccine HIV prevention trials or HIV treatment trials may enable greater flexibility in site readiness.

In addition to infrastructure building, site development also requires assessment of HIV seroincidence in the local target population, and of the number of volunteers who can be expected to enroll at the site. Various methods exist to generate estimates of HIV incidence (Heyward *et al.*, 1994; Janssen *et al.*, 1998). Estimates must often be based on small longitudinal studies or extrapolated from cross-sectional studies; such estimates are generally imprecise, and conservative estimates should be used to avoid under-powering a study. Efficacy trials designed to measure indirect study effects (such as vaccine impact on HIV transmission) in addition to direct vaccine effects (on HIV infection rates or disease progression) will require additional planning to understand sexual or drug-using networks. One method for conducting such trials is the community randomized trial, in which pairs of similar communities are randomized to receive either vaccine or placebo. Such trials will require substantial efforts to develop collaborative relationships with multiple communities and characterize their HIV incidence and demographic and risk characteristics.

Building clinical trial capacity in developing countries requires long-term commitment of resources and ongoing training opportunities. Often, a limited pool of investigators is called upon to provide both research and clinical expertise in a variety of prevention and treatment areas. Investment must be made to provide training and support for new investigators to augment the existing pool of qualified individuals. Limited opportunities are available through US NIH-sponsored programs such as the Fogarty AIDS International Training and Research Programs (AITRP) and the Comprehensive International Program of Research on AIDS (CIPRA). Training opportunities are also needed for newly formed or expanded regulatory bodies and should ideally be provided by international organizations unrelated to the study sponsors, to avoid real or perceived conflicts of interest. The resources and training devoted to research infrastructure for HIV vaccine testing in developing countries can ultimately be leveraged to make these sites eligible for future participation in other types of medical research, so that they may remain as colleagues (and grow as healthy competitors) in the global research establishment.

Regulatory Issues

In contrast to the rapid policy changes enabling accelerated access to life-sustaining HIV treatments in the United States in the 1990s, HIV vaccine research remains largely 'business as usual' from a regulatory standpoint. Regulatory agencies worldwide remain understaffed and restricted by often inflexible processes by which they must review HIV vaccine trials. The emphasis on safety and liability in the US may be well adapted to protecting consumers from potentially dangerous products, but finds few opportunities for innovation to speed the development of new drugs in response to a global crisis. Under US regulation, a vaccine must undergo extensive animal testing and specified stages of human testing to address a standard set of concerns (which may or may not be strictly relevant to each type of vaccine being tested) and must be shown to be almost perfectly safe to merit licensing for widespread use. A country in which 30 per cent of the population is expected to die of AIDS might accept an accelerated development process or a different risk-benefit ratio, but regulations requiring that all US-sponsored research and US-based researchers comply with US standards preclude serious consideration of alternatives in international collaborations.

Moreover, review of multicenter protocols occurs not only at the federal regulatory and research network level, but at each individual research site, often by several committees, and also by each participating country, often at several in-country levels. To answer the same scientific question, however, the protocol must be consistent across all sites. The result is a labor-intensive effort to build an international consensus among researchers, community advisory boards, vaccine manufacturers, and other research program sponsors on the design of each protocol, with the knowledge that local review boards or national regulatory agencies may subsequently raise issues that will send all or part of the protocol back to the drawing board. Between regulatory and manufacturing issues, it is not at all unusual for initial human trials of an HIV vaccine to begin months or years later than originally planned. Given that approximately 14 000 new HIV infections occur each day worldwide (UNAIDS-WHO, 2003) the human cost of inconsistencies and inefficiencies in these systems is considerable.

Economic Considerations

Besides the scientific challenges outlined above, the vaccine developer must consider the economic incentives of vaccine development. Preclinical development and early clinical testing of a single product can be expected to require roughly US$100 000 000 in resources. If the product proves safe and immunogenic, an efficacy trial can be expected to entail further costs of at least that amount. If the vaccine then proves effective, the producer can expect to face the reality that the greatest need for the product is in hundreds of millions of people in areas where little or no resources exist to buy vaccines. Without major government incentives during the early years of the epidemic, is perhaps not surprising that the HIV vaccine development effort by major pharmaceutical companies was limited or non-existent. The recent movement toward public–private partnerships, for example the International AIDS Vaccine Initiative and the NIH-funded HIV Vaccine Trials Network, which can support international trials of privately developed vaccine candidates, appears to have 'jump-started' HIV vaccine development to some extent. The precedent of public–private partnerships against lethal diseases is not new. Before AIDS, private funding through organizations such as the March of Dimes, plus public funding, worked very effectively to foster the discovery and widespread implementation of an effective polio vaccine.

183

In societies that tend to define individual rights more clearly than concepts of common welfare, concerns over risk may discourage individuals and corporations alike from engaging in vaccine studies, as unforeseeable side-effects in healthy vaccine recipients could lead not only to personal injury, but also to professional or financial disaster. Motivation to develop HIV vaccines in particular may be further limited by the growing social and geographical gap between those threatened by the prospect of untreated HIV infection and those with the means to develop and test vaccines. Similar gaps did not exist for smallpox or polio, but are highly pertinent to tuberculosis and malaria.

Public Health Challenges

It is plausible that the first HIV vaccines to demonstrate efficacy against HIV infection or disease progression will have only low or moderate efficacy, rather than the high levels (>90 per cent) demonstrated by vaccines against hepatitis B, measles, and tetanus. 'Proof of concept' efficacy trials may be designed to detect very low levels of efficacy, too low to be considered for licensure but high enough to identify immune correlates of protection. Although the US FDA has not identified a specific efficacy criterion for licensure of candidate HIV vaccines, an FDA advisory committee reviewing plans for the first HIV vaccine efficacy trial suggested that the product being tested would be considered for licensure if the lower bound of the 95 per cent confidence interval for efficacy of that product exceeded 30 per cent (Hu *et al.*, 2003). It is not clear if that criterion will apply to future trials, nor how vaccine effects on surrogate markers of HIV disease progression (e.g. plasma viral load, CD4+ count) may be factored into future licensure decisions (Gilbert *et al.*, 2003). While the US FDA and European Agency for the Evaluation of Medicinal Products (EMEA) are likely to play an important role in the licensure of the majority of vaccine products, regulatory agencies in other countries will also play important roles in determining which vaccines receive regulatory approval and are ultimately used worldwide.

HIV differs from many other infectious diseases in being spread through behaviors that are often difficult to change for a variety of complex individual and societal reasons. If the prevalence of risk behaviors in a given community increases as a result of having a partially efficacious vaccine, the vaccine could paradoxically lead to increases in HIV transmission rates. A number of investigators have developed mathematical models to assess the impact of partially efficacious HIV vaccines on transmission rates, based on a number of assumptions about vaccine efficacy, vaccine coverage, transmission dynamics and rates of risk behavior change in the community (Longini *et al.*, 1995; Blower *et al.*, 2003; Gray *et al.*, 2003). Others have addressed the potential role of viral escape on vaccine efficacy (van Ballegooijen *et al.*, 2003). All of these models are limited by the veracity of the assumptions on which the models are based, but provide some insight into the possible outcome of vaccination programs based on these assumptions. Most such models suggest that modest to substantial increases in risk behavior could overcome the beneficial impact of a partially effective HIV vaccine. However, if administered in the context of prevention programs that maintain or reduce risk levels within a community, even vaccines of modest efficacy or those that do not prevent infection, but slow disease progression and limit infectiousness, could have a substantial impact on slowing the HIV epidemic.

The effect of HIV vaccine programs will also likely be influenced by choice of the target population, degree of coverage, and stage of the local epidemic. These factors and economic and logistical considerations will determine when and in what populations partially efficacious vaccines may best be used. The majority of vaccine programs target children or the elderly; few target high-risk subgroups or the general adult population. When an HIV vaccine is found to be efficacious, high-risk adults and adolescents would reasonably be part of the initial plan for immunization; some mathematical models suggest little additional benefit from expanding immunization programs to all adults in the setting of concentrated epidemics (Longini *et al.*, 1995). Given the high rates of HIV infection in adolescent populations (currently estimated to constitute 25 per cent of all infections worldwide) and the difficulty in targeting adolescent populations for immunization, highly efficacious HIV vaccines may reasonably be added to childhood immunization series in the future. However, licensure of vaccines for use in either children or adolescents will require inclusion of these populations in clinical trials. Such trials have traditionally been conducted after adult safety (and at times, after efficacy) trials for a variety of scientific, ethical, and logistical reasons, including differing pharmacokinetics of products in children compared to adults, issues of obtaining informed consent, difficulties in measuring and interpreting adverse events, and the belief that children should not be exposed to experimental products until these have been demonstrated to be safe in adults. Nonetheless, because drugs or vaccines may have different safety or efficacy profiles in children or adolescents, inclusion of children or adolescents in clinical trials is often required before products can be licensed for use in these subgroups. Adolescents, in particular, should be included in efficacy trials, as vaccine efficacy in this population could be affected by the difference in prevalence of cofactors for HIV infection (e.g. sexually transmitted infections, genital trauma during sexual intercourse, cervical ectopy) compared with adults. Sequential efficacy trials (testing first in adults, and then in adolescents) may lead to substantial delays in the availability of new drugs or vaccines for this population.

What the Future Holds

Because AIDS is a global epidemic, the HIV vaccine research effort must address global challenges to medical research, and can therefore lay the groundwork for benefiting human health in ways that extend even beyond the intended benefit of ending the HIV pandemic.

Already, HIV vaccine development efforts have had a beneficial effect on vaccine development in general. Because of safety concerns regarding standard strategies of whole-killed and live-attenuated vaccines, and skepticism about the efficacy of single-subunit recombinant proteins, substantial new development efforts have focused on DNA and viral vector vaccines. These techniques are already being brought to bear on other illnesses such as smallpox and Ebola. Additional research is focusing on cell-to-cell signaling molecules (such as cytokines) that may lead to improved vaccine adjuvants (substances given with a vaccine to increase the immune response). Advances in the field of T–cell immunology, including the development and standardization of laboratory methods to measure cellular immune responses, have similarly evolved in the context of HIV vaccine development.

The urgent need to develop a safe, broadly efficacious vaccine has also fostered the development of new non-governmental organizations, governmental initiatives, and public–private partnerships dedicated to moving the HIV vaccine field forward. The work of these organizations lays the groundwork for vaccines against other infectious agents as well. The International AIDS Vaccine Initiative is a public–private partnership established in 1996 with the mission to 'ensure that safe and effective preventive HIV vaccines are developed that are appropriate for use throughout the world, in particular in those regions most affected by HIV/AIDS' (http:// www.iavi.org). Among its accomplishments, this group has funded development and testing of several vaccine concepts directed against subtypes A and C, helped in developing a variety of innovative initiatives to address basic laboratory challenges, built clinical and laboratory infrastructure in a number of developing countries, published a newsletter to increase knowledge about HIV vaccines, and worked to raise general awareness of the need for an HIV vaccine. The AIDS Vaccine Advocacy Coalition (AVAC) is a community and consumer-based organization founded in 1995 'to accelerate the ethical development and global delivery of vaccines against HIV/AIDS' (http://www.avac.org). This advocacy group publishes an annual report focused on the major gaps in development of safe and efficacious vaccines, and through educational, analysis and policy work, identifies and attempts to address barriers to the development of a safe and efficacious HIV vaccine. The US NIH created the Dale and Betty Bumpers Vaccine Research Center (http://www.niaid.nih.gov/vrc) to conduct research on a variety of vaccines, with a particular emphasis on HIV vaccines. The infusion of resources and scientific expertise within a single institution holds much promise in advancing vaccine approaches to HIV and other infectious diseases. The South African AIDS Vaccine Initiative (SAAVI) was formed in 1999 to coordinate research, development and testing of HIV vaccines in South Africa (http://www.saavi.org.za). The European Vaccine Effort Against HIV/AIDS (EuroVac) includes investigators and laboratories from eight European countries to bring European preventive HIV vaccines into Phase I clinical trials (http://www.eurovac.net). The Canadian Network for

Vaccines and Immunotherapeutics (CANVAC) is a Canadian public–private partnership focused on vaccines against a number of infectious agents, including HIV (http://www.canvacc.org). Most recently, a global team of HIV vaccine researchers, public health officials, and policy makers have been discussing novel strategies to address pressing issues in vaccine discovery; product development; vaccine manufacture; laboratory standardization; regulatory, licensing and intellectual property; and clinical trials capacity (Klausner *et al.*, 2003). This group is developing short-, medium-, and long-range goals to attract and retain the best investigators to work on these issues, each of which could have a lasting impact on vaccine development in general, and may provide the resources and infrastructure for developing effective vaccines against the perpetual scourges of tuberculosis and malaria.

The implications of undertaking HIV vaccine development, and large efficacy trials in particular, are sobering. Multi-site trials will require international cooperation to ensure scientific validity, adequate enrollment and retention, and high standards for protecting the safety of volunteers. The costs range into the hundreds of millions of US dollars. Unresolved scientific questions, ethical controversies, and practical barriers each add uncertainty and delay. At any time in the process, a safety issue may arise that delays product development, or immunogenicity results for a vaccine candidate may prove disappointing, or reports may appear of new products that appear more promising, leading to difficult decisions on whether to continue development of existing products through a large and expensive efficacy trial, or to defer monopolizing available staff efforts and research volunteers until a 'better' candidate is ready to be tested.

Vaccine research must be done in collaboration with the communities who will test, and ultimately receive, the vaccines. Broad educational campaigns can bring about a greater appreciation for the potential of vaccines in general, and HIV vaccines in particular, to reduce the devastation of global epidemics. Responding to each of these challenges in the effort to develop an HIV vaccine will continue to transform and refine the way clinical research is conducted on a global level.

References

Bartholow B (2003) Risk behavior and HIV seroincidence in the US trial of AIDSVAX B/B. *AIDS Vaccine 2003*.

Berman PW (2003) HIV vaccine development. Paper presented at the Keystone Symposia Banff, Alberta, Canada.

Blower S, Schwartz E, Mills J (2003) Forecasting the future of HIV epidemics: the impact of antiretroviral therapies and imperfect vaccines. *AIDS* 5: 113–25.

Buchbinder S, Wheeler S, Vittinghoff E *et al.* (2003) Declines in risk behaviour are smaller in phase III vaccine trial participants that in non-vaccine trial control group. *AIDS Vaccine 2003*.

Chang M, Vitek C, Esparza J (2003) Public health considerations for the use of a first generation HIV vaccine. Report from a WHO–UNAIDS–CDC consultation, Geneva, 20–21 November 2002. *AIDS* 17: W1–W10.

Chun TW, Carruth L, Finzi D *et al.* (1997) Quantification of latent tissue reservoirs and total body viral load in HIV-1. *Nature* 387: 183–8.

Cohen OJ, Paolucci S, Bende SM *et al.* (1998) CXCR4 and CCR5 genetic polymorphisms in long-term nonprogressive human immunodeficiency virus infection: lack of association with mutations other than CCR5-Delta32. *J Virol* 72: 6215–17.

Crosby AW (1993) Smallpox. In: Kiple KF, ed. *The Cambridge World History of Human Disease*. Cambridge: Cambridge University Press, pp. 1008–13.

Flores-Villanueva PO, Yunis EJ, Delgado JC *et al.* (2001) Control of HIV-1 viremia and protection from AIDS are associated with HLA-Bw4 homozygosity. *Proc Natl Acad Sci USA* 98: 5140–5.

Gilbert P, DeGruttola V, Hudgens MG, Self S, Hammer S, Corey L (2003) What constitutes efficacy for a human immunodeficiency virus vaccine that ameliorates viremia: issues involving surrogate end points in phase 3 trials? *J Infect Dis* 188: 179–93.

Goulder PJ, Brander C, Tang Y *et al.* (2001) Evolution and transmission of stable CTL escape mutations in HIV infection. *Nature* 412: 334–8.

Gray R, Li X, Wawer M *et al.* (2003) Stochastic simulation of the impact of antiretroviral therapy and HIV vaccines on HIV transmission; Rakai, Uganda. *AIDS* 17: 1941–51.

Heyward WL, Osmanov S, Saba J *et al.* (1994) Preparations for phase III HIV vaccine efficacy trials: methods for the determinations of HIV incidence. *AIDS* 8: 1285–91.

Hu D, Vitek C, Bartholow B, Mastro T (2003) Key issues for the potential human immunodeficiency virus vaccine. *Clin Infect Dis* 36: 638–44.

Janssen RS, Satten GA, Stramer SL *et al.* (1998) New testing strategy to detect early HIV-1 infection for use in incidence estimates and for clinical and prevention purposes. *JAMA* 280: 42–8.

Kahn JO, Steimer KS, Baenziger J *et al.* (1995) Clinical, immunologic, and virologic observations related to human immunodeficiency virus (HIV) type 1 infection in a volunteer in an HIV-1 vaccine clinical trial. *J Infect Dis* 171: 1343–7.

Kalams SA, Buchbinder SP, Rosenberg ES *et al.* (1999) Association between virus-specific cytotoxic T-lymphocyte and helper responses in human immunodeficiency virus type 1 infection. *J Virol* 73: 6715–20.

Kaul R, Rowland-Jones SL, Kimani J *et al.* (2001) New insights into HIV-1 specific cytotoxic T-lymphocyte reponses in exposed, persistently seronegative Kenyan sex workers. *Immunol Lett* 79: 3–13.

Klausner RD, Fauci AS, Corey L *et al.* (2003) The need for a global HIV vaccine enterprise. *Science* 300: 2036–9.

Kwong PD, Doyle ML, Casper DJ *et al.* (2002) HIV-1 evades antibody-mediated neutralization through conformational masking of receptor-binding sites. *Nature* 420: 678–82.

Letvin NL, Barouch DH, Montefiori DC (2002) Prospects for vaccine protection against HIV-1 infection and AIDS. *Annu Rev Immunol* 20: 73–99.

Longini IM, Halloran ME, Rida W *et al.* (1995) AIDS: modeling epidemic control. *Science* 267: 1250–3.

Mackellar DA, Valleroy LA, Secura GM *et al.* (2001) Two decades after vaccine license: hepatitis B immunization and infection among young men who have sex with men. *Am J Public Health* 91: 965–71.

Myszka DG, Sweet RW, Hensley P *et al.* (2000) Energetics of the HIV gp120-CD4 binding reaction. *Proc Natl Acad Sci USA* 97: 9026–31.

Osmanov S, Pattou C, Walker N, Schwardlander B, Esparza J (2002) Estimated global distribution and regional spread of HIV-1 genetic subtypes in the year 2000. *J Acquir Immune Defic Syndr* 29: 184–90.

Pitisutithum P (2004) Efficacy of AIDSVAX B/E vaccines in injection drug use. Paper presented at the 11th Conference on Retroviruses and Opportunistic Infections, San Francisco.

Plotkin SL, Plotkin SA (2004) Short history of vaccination. In: Plotkin SA, Orenstein WA, eds. *Vaccines*. Philadelphia: Saunders/Elsevier, pp. 1–15.

Richman DD, Wrin T, Little SJ, Petropoulos CJ (2003) Rapid evolution of the neutralizing antibody response to HIV type 1 infection. *Proc Natl Acad Sci USA* 100: 4144–9.

Robbins FC (2004) The history of polio vaccine development. In: Plotkin SA, Orenstein WA, eds. *Vaccines*. Philadelphia: Saunders/Elsevier, pp. 17–30.

Rosenberg ES, Billingsley JM, Caliendo AM *et al.* (1997) Vigorous HIV-1 specific CD4+ T cell responses associated with control of viremia. *Science* 278: 1447–50.

Ruprecht RM, Ferrantelli F, Kitabwalla M, Xu W, McClure HM (2003) Antibody protection: passive immunization of neonates against oral AIDS virus challenge. *Vaccine* 21: 3370–3.

UNAIDS (2000) *Ethical Considerations in HIV Preventive Vaccine Research*. UNAIDS.

UNAIDS-WHO (2003) *AIDS Epidemic Update 2003*. Geneva: WHO.

van Ballegooijen M, Bogaards JA, Weverling GJ, Boerlijst MC, Goudsmit J (2003) AIDS vaccines that allow HIV-1 to infect and escape immunologic control. *J Acquir Immune Defic Syndr* 34: 214–20.

Wei X, Decker JM, Wang S *et al.* (2003) Antibody neutralization and escape by HIV-1. *Nature* 422: 307–12.

WHO-UNAIDS (2000) Future access to HIV vaccines. *AIDS* 15: W27–W44.

Wrin T, Loh TP, Vennari JC, Schuitemaker H, Nunberg JH (1995) Adaptation to persistent growth in the H9 cell line renders a primary isolate of human immunodeficiency virus type 1 sensitive to neutralization by vaccine sera. *J Virol* 69: 39–48.

189

Microbicides

8

Polly F Harrison
Director, Alliance for Microbicide Development, Silver Spring, Maryland, USA

Trisha L Lamphear
Research Associate, Alliance for Microbicide Development, Silver Spring, Maryland, USA

Polly F. Harrison, PhD, is Founder and Director of the Alliance for Microbicide Development, a nonprofit coalition of scientists, product developers, public health experts and advocates, whose goal is to accelerate the development of safe, effective and affordable topical microbicides. Dr. Harrison has been Senior Program Officer and Director of International Health at the Institute of Medicine of the U.S. National Academy of Sciences and has spent two decades living and working in the developing world as a medical anthropologist and policy analyst in a range of activities related to women's health and health development.

Trisha L. Lamphear, MPH, has been at the Alliance for four years, as an intern, research assistant, and currently as a Research Associate. For her Master's thesis, she conducted a pilot study on the knowledge and perceptions of college freshmen women around sexually transmitted diseases, HIV, and microbicides. At the Alliance, she does policy research and analysis, and works to inform policy-makers and educate constituencies about issues critical to microbicide research and development, which coincides with her own deep commitment to the health needs of women and children.

In preparing this article, the lead author, a medical anthropologist, was asked how a social scientist came to create a non-profit advocacy organization and, in that context, 'why microbicides?' The answer is a convergence of accumulated reasons and events that could not be ignored. Years of bringing up a family in the developing world and years of listening, clinically and ethnographically, to women's stories, made it clear that their search for health was not just about illness. It also served as a proxy for their often futile search for a better life, a strategy for achieving some control over harsh and intractable circumstances (Harrison, 1982). Access to what medicine could do to safeguard women's reproductive options and the health of their children seemed central to that search. And, as the HIV/AIDS epidemic extended its grip on ever-larger numbers of women, one had to recognize that their ability to protect against that lethal infection was fragile indeed (Stein, 1990; Epstein, 2004). A technology that could contribute to such protection appeared to be a 'no brainer'. Yet, unlike AIDS advocacy writ large, microbicide development was a cause without enough rebels, with insufficient and inconsistent funding, and with no industrial interest whatsoever. Thus, when even limited philanthropic support made it possible to assemble a coalition that would forge links among advocacy, research, and development in order to shape a visible, better integrated 'microbicide field', it was impossible to resist.

For well over a decade, there has been scientific and clinical interest in developing 'microbicides', topical applications that could provide protection against sexually transmitted infections. The basic idea is, however, considerably older. For over 50 years, vaginal applications containing such spermicidal surfactants as nonoxynol-9 had been used, alone and with barrier contraceptives, to reduce risk of unwanted pregnancy. While use of such preparations diminished as some women migrated to new contraceptive strategies, notably the pill, spermicides remained on the market, available over the counter at reasonable cost without the need for medical intervention or referral. By the 1970s, it had occurred to a few researchers that such products might also offer protection against sexually transmitted infections (STIs), an attribute expected to enhance their market appeal and spur greater use. Yet, even though some laboratory experiments indicated that 'N-9' (nonoxynol-9) and other similar compounds did, in fact, show activity against such common STIs as chlamydia, gonorrhea, and syphilis (Cutler *et al.*, 1973), research around this notion was scattered, scanty, poorly funded, and accompanied by little sense of urgency.

Impact of HIV on the Development of Microbicides

HIV would alter that scenario. HIV infections between men having sex dominated the early years of the epidemic, but as a heterosexual AIDS epidemic was revealed in Africa in 1983 (Baltimore, 2002), it became obvious that HIV/AIDS would inevitably impose an ever greater toll on women and, thereby, their newborn infants. Not until 1996, however, was there what UNAIDS considered a reliable tally of global HIV/AIDS incidence and prevalence. In 1996, UNAIDS estimated that women accounted for 42 per cent of new HIV infections globally (UNAIDS, 1996); by the end of 2002, that percentage had risen to 50 per cent, even higher in some parts of sub-Saharan Africa (UNAIDS, 2002). The same trend has prevailed in the United States, where women's share of annual new AIDS cases rose from 7 per cent to 26 per cent between 1986 and 2001 (CDC, 1986–2001). The great majority of these women – around 90 per cent in developing countries (UNAIDS, 2002) and 65 per cent in the United States (CDC, 2001) – contracted HIV through heterosexual contact, overwhelmingly from a husband or regular partner (UNAIDS, 2002). In sum, it can be fairly said that the global HIV-1 epidemic is essentially fueled by heterosexual transmission, which accounts for 80 per cent of the 40 million people now infected with the virus (UNAIDS, 2002).

It was not surprising, then, that the mid-1980s saw lively interest in revisiting the N-9-containing spermicides, now found to have rapid *in vitro* and, later, *ex vivo* efficacy against HIV (Malkovsky *et al.*, 1988). The fact that the US Food and Drug Administration (FDA) had categorized these products as 'GRAS' ('Generally Regarded as Safe') suggested that their testing in human subjects could be carried forward with greater speed and likelihood of safety. Thus, the 1990s brought a series of clinical trials of different N-9-containing formulations – a sponge, a film, gels – but the story had an unhappy ending. These products proved to have no efficacy against HIV and little efficacy against chlamydia or gonorrhea. Worse yet, they appeared to increase epithelial disruption and, correspondingly, the risk of HIV infection in frequent users (Kreiss *et al.*, 1992; Roddy *et al.*, 1998, 2002; Van Damme *et al.*, 2000, 2002; Wilkinson *et al.*, 2002; WHO/CONRAD, 2002). Evidence that N-9 also causes disruption of the rectal mucosa, thereby elevating risk of HIV infection during anal intercourse (Phillips and Zacharopoulos, 1998; Phillips *et al.*, 2000), generated additional and substantial concern. The result has been that both the Centers for Disease Control and Prevention (CDC) and the World Health Organization (WHO) have issued cautionary statements about the use of products containing nonoxynol-9, and some manufacturers of such products are reformulating them or, in a few cases, containing their distribution.

Parallel Tracks

But HIV was not the only epidemic. By the 1990s, the public health spotlight turned to capture another, 'hidden' epidemic of sexually transmitted diseases (STDs) in addition to HIV/AIDS (Leclerc *et al.*, 1988; Eng and Butler, 1996). In 1990, the WHO began a series of global estimates of the incidence and prevalence of just four curable STDs – chlamydia, gonorrhea, syphilis, and trichomoniasis – noting that adequate global data on other non-HIV STDs were fragmentary and elusive.

The findings were stunning, even in their incompleteness. In 1990, WHO reported 250 million new cases of those four STDs in women and men aged 15–49 worldwide; by 1995, the reported number was 333 million; and by 1999 the number was 340 million (WHO, 1990, 1990/1996). In 1996, a seminal study by the US National Academy of Sciences Institute of Medicine reported that more than 65 million persons in the United States were currently living with an incurable STI and that new cases were occurring at a rate of 15 million each year, two-thirds in persons under 25 and one-quarter in teenagers (Eng and Butler, 1996). Worse still, research was revealing a deeply destructive and persistent synergy between the two epidemics (Wasserheit, 1989, 1992). In themselves burdensome and often lethal, some non-HIV STIs were found to function as significant co-factors in HIV transmission and progression (Over and Piot, 1993; Cohen, 1998; Fleming and Wasserheit, 1999; Moriuchi *et al.*, 2000; Galvin and Cohen, 2004). In fact, some medical anthropologists and CDC researchers now refer to such co-occurrences as 'syndemics,' a term coined to label the biological and social synergies among two or more epidemics and the additional burdens of disease produced by such interactions (Milstein, 2001; Singer and Clair, 2003).

This synergy has particularly severe implications for women; by extension, their children; and by further extension, their families (Panos Institute, 1989; Temmerman *et al.*, 1992). In 1993, the World Bank estimated that in sub-Saharan Africa, women bore 80 per cent of the burden of disability caused by the non-HIV STIs (World Bank, 1993; Howson *et al.*, 1996). Further and more generally, a number of STIs are causally associated with preterm delivery, low birth weight, and subsequent morbidity and even mortality among the infants and children of infected mothers.

The reasons are a complex and potent interaction among gender physiology, culture, and economics. Biologically, women are more vulnerable to STIs in general than are men and less likely to exhibit the clear symptoms that might motivate timely and appropriate care. These basic vulnerabilities are compounded by women's lack of economic and social power in the many societies and situations where they cannot control sexual encounters; where they cannot insist on protective measures such as abstinence, mutual monogamy, or condom use; where attempts to do so may be met with punitive responses; and/or where economic pressures make sex work necessary to survival. For adolescent females, the picture is still bleaker. Anatomically more vulnerable to contracting these infections than are older women, girls have far more difficulty negotiating safer sex practices with partners, so that even early in the AIDS epidemic, women, on average, were becoming infected 5–10 years earlier than men (United Nations Development Program, 1993). More recent research finds only exacerbation of that trend.

A New Dynamic

The most dramatic change in the early history of microbicides was the way these coincident realizations sparked a new dynamic in the relationships among the work of science, the standard processes of bureaucracies, and the goals of

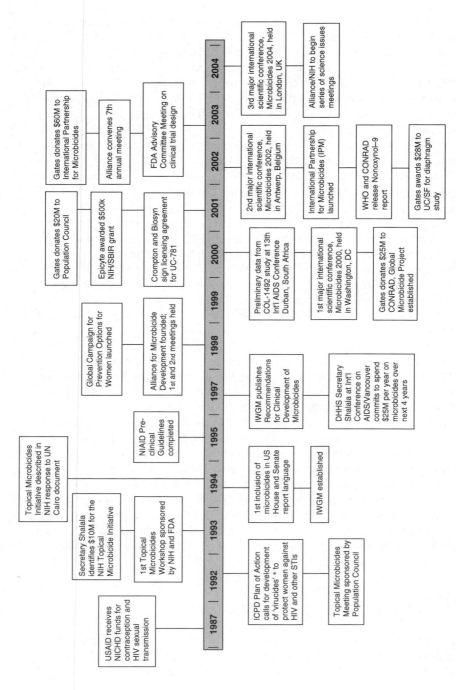

Fig. 8.1 Milestones in microbicide research and development. *NB: The term 'virucides' is still used in the British scientific community but is being largely overtaken by 'microbicides' as a term which anticipates that at least some of these candidates might also prevent sexually transmitted infections other than HIV.

women's health advocates. Learning from the activism of the 1980s which had pressed so hard and effectively on government, industry, and the scientific community to respond aggressively to the AIDS crisis, by the early 1990s public health researchers and activists were raising their voices to demand 'methods women could use' to protect themselves (Stein, 1990).

Figure 8.1 highlights key events in the evolution of the microbicide field. Some of the most noteworthy are the following. In 1992 the Population Council sponsored the first topical microbicide conference (Feldblum, 1992), in 1993 the National Institutes of Health made modest investment in a 'Topical Microbicide Initiative', and in 1994 the International Working Group on Microbicides (IWGM) was set up to facilitate interaction across the key public agencies (NIAID, 1997). In 1994, at the United Nations International Conference on Population and Development in Cairo, Egypt, 20 000 culturally, geographically, and organizationally diverse delegates negotiated a Program of Action that included a call for development of 'barrier methods, both male and female, for fertility control and the prevention of sexually transmitted diseases, including HIV/AIDS, as well as microbicides and virucides, which may or may not prevent pregnancy'. In Belgium, Canada, Great Britain, and the United States, researchers pursued the older question about other GRAS compounds that might make good microbicides, as well as new questions: Might compounds investigated as possible HIV therapies lend themselves to development as microbicides, and would that be especially true for compounds that seemed to be poorly absorbed, which might mean that they could make good topical applications?

Defining and Describing the Technology

The following definition unites the critical elements of this technology: 'A microbicide is a substance designed in various formulations to significantly reduce sexual transmission of HIV and/or other viral, bacterial, or protozoan pathogens when applied topically to genital mucosal surfaces prior to intercourse'. The key elements embedded in this definition are the intertwined concepts of topical application, variability in formulation, and timing. Microbicides, formulated as gels, creams, films, suppositories, or tablets, or designed as components of mechanical barrier methods – pre-loaded diaphragms or cervical caps, and sponges or rings slowly releasing active ingredients – are meant to be applied to the vagina or rectum to inhibit effective access by infectious pathogens. Timing of application is before sexual intercourse, with a span of compound activity responsive to behavioral preferences and efficacy during and after intercourse.

What is not immediately evident in this definition is the pivotal notion of 'control'. Microbicide research was propelled by the recognition that women's only defenses against HIV infection – abstinence, delayed initiation of sexual activity, mutual monogamy, the male condom – all require male cooperation to begin with and none are easily achieved in any event. Even in countries where the HIV epidemic rages, high levels of correct and consistent use of male condoms have proved hard to achieve and sustain (Foss *et al.*, 2003; Hearst and Chen, 2003). This is particularly (if somewhat paradoxically) true in stable relationships, since individuals willing or required to use condoms with 'outside' partners often resist using them with primary partners (Foss *et al.*, 2003), either because they do not perceive or are unwilling to acknowledge risk. Microbicides were, therefore, seen as a novel disease-prevention technology whose use women could determine and initiate, without the need for male acquiescence or even, perhaps, covertly. Furthermore, in circumstances where childbearing is tied to women's sense of self-worth, position in society, and often economic viability, microbicides with anti-infective potency but no negative effect on sperm would offer a clear comparative advantage over mechanical barriers, which are contraceptive by definition.

With HIV vaccines that could protect at-risk populations of both sexes a yet-distant option (McMichael and Hanke, 2003), and access to the newly developed female condom still limited by cost and acceptance (Meekers, 1999), it is not surprising that a multidisciplinary panel of eminent scientists recently ranked female-controlled methods of STI protection sixth in its list of the top 10 biotechnologies holding the most promise for improving health in developing countries in the next 5–10 years (University of Toronto, 2002).

How Microbicides Work

Chapter 2 of this book addresses the details of HIV transmission processes and relevant immune system functions. Still, to understand the ways microbicides might work, we need to revisit, if only briefly, the biological mechanisms by which HIV is transmitted sexually, even though our knowledge of these processes remains incomplete (Stevenson, 2003). For sexual transmission of HIV to occur, incoming virus must cross the multiple layers of genital mucosal epithelium and underlying connective tissue, the structure of which varies among vaginal, cervical, and rectal sites (Figure 8.2). The virus may achieve this in several ways: direct infection of epithelial cells; transcytosis through epithelial and specialized cells; transmigration of infected cells; uptake by intraepithelial cells; and/or, perhaps most importantly, circumvention of the epithelial barrier through physical breaches (Greenhead *et al.*, 2000; Stone, 2002; Shattock and Moore, 2003). Success in any of these transfers can result in virus–host cell interactions and local propagation of infection through infection of dendritic and CD4+ T cells and macrophages, dissemination to draining lymph nodes where extensive HIV replication and systemic infection are launched, and establishment of the lymphatic tissue reservoir that spreads infection to other organs and peripheral tissues (Pope and Haase, 2003).

Thus there are theoretically two potential target areas for microbicides: (1) the incoming pathogen and (2) the host mucosal cells that it infects through attachment or fusion (Stone, 2002; Turpin, 2002; Shattock and Moore, 2003). Each approach offers pluses and minuses, which suggests, as we will see later, that the best of all

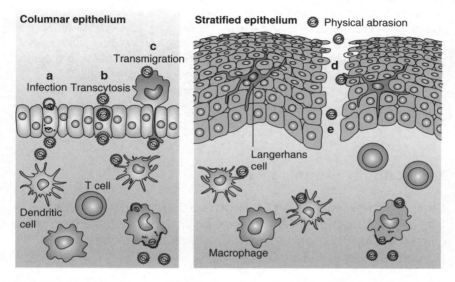

Fig. 8.2 Potential mechanisms of HIV transmission. Created by RJ Shattock, St George's Hospital Medical School.

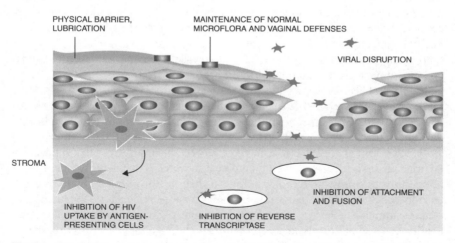

Fig. 8.3 Potential mechanisms of action for microbicide compounds. Created by RJ Shattock, St George's Hospital Medical School.

197

possible microbicide worlds may be some sort of combination. The greatest challenge in aiming at the incoming pathogen is, in the case of HIV-1, its enormous sequence variability, so that what needs to be targeted is its most conserved (least likely to change) features (Walker and Korber, 2001). Targeting the host mucosal cells will demand speed and efficiency of action, since the best chances of success are likely in the earliest stages of transmission in the relatively narrow window of opportunity when the initial interaction of virus with host cells and defenses occurs (Haase, 2001; Pope and Haase, 2003). Both target areas will require the active compound(s) to survive for enough time to provide protection even when diluted and distributed across the relevant mucosa (Shattock and Moore, 2003).

Figure 8.3 provides a biological 'map' to guide us through each target area and the relevant mechanisms of action. Its companion, Table 8.1, lists the candidate microbicides in each functional category.

Targeting the Incoming Pathogen

Blocking the Invader and Strengthening the Host – Physical Barriers, Lubrication, Maintenance or Enhancement of Normal Microflora, Mobilization of Natural Defense Mechanisms, Preventing Other STDs

There is consensus that susceptibility to sexually transmitted HIV infection is critically promoted by factors that, in various ways, compromise the integrity of the genital epithelium. These may include abrasion, trauma, hormonal status, micronutrient levels, use of certain intravaginal or rectal preparations, and ulceration or inflammation produced by other STIs or bacterial vaginosis. Therefore, one fundamental principle for microbicides is that they be formulated to provide lubrication, thereby coating the epithelial surface, reducing the risk of trauma, and providing at least a minimal physical barrier to infection.

The normal healthy vagina, in addition to the inherent toughness and protective multiplicity of its epithelial layers, further benefits from resident lactobacilli whose secretion of lactic acid and hydrogen peroxide provides a natural line of defense against invading pathogens, importantly including HIV (Kempf *et al.*, 1991; Klebanoff *et al.*, 1991; Martin *et al.*, 1999). This leads to another fundamental principle in the development of microbicides, which is that they absolutely must not perturb this protective ecology. Toward that objective, microbicide research has focused on strategies that would not only conserve but enhance the innate and adaptive immune defense systems by, for example, maintaining the natural vaginal acidity at virucidal levels in the presence of the alkalinizing effects of semen (Mayer *et al.*, 2001); supporting colonization by beneficial microflora (Vallor *et al.*, 2001) or engineering them to express a specific receptor for HIV to inhibit

Table 8.1 **Microbicides in development, by mechanism of action.**

Category	Products	Sponsor/Investigator
Acid buffers (3)	Acidform™ gel	Global Microbicide Project (GMP)
	Acidform™ tablet (AFT)	University of Auckland
	BufferGel™	ReProtect LLC
Adsorption inhibitors (11)	Carraguard™	Population Council
	Cellulose sulfate gel	Global Microbicide Project (GMP)
	Cellulose sulfate vaginal films (CS films)	University of Auckland
	Cellulose sulfate vaginal tablets (CS tablet)	University of Auckland
	Emmelle™ (dextrin-2-sulfate)	Medical Research Council (MRC)
	Polystyrene sulfonate gel (PSS gel)	Global Microbicide Project (GMP)
	Polystyrene sulfonate vaginal films (PSS films)	University of Auckland
	Polystyrene sulfonate vaginal tablets (PSS tablets)	University of Auckland
	Polyvinyl alcohol sulfate (PVAS)	University of Auckland
	Sulfonated hesperidin	University of Auckland
	Sulfuric acid reacted quercetin (SARQ)	University of Auckland
Devices (2)	FemCap device	FemCap, Inc.
	Foamer/cannula	Less-Cal Foods, Inc.
Entry and fusion inhibitors (21)	Anti-ICAM-1 antibody	Johns Hopkins University School of Medicine
	Betacyclodextrin	Johns Hopkins University School of Medicine
	C85FL	Weill Medical College of Cornell University
	Cellulose acetate phthalate (CAP)/Aquateric	New York Blood Center/Lindsley F. Kimball Research Institute
	Cyanovirin-N	Biosyn, Inc.
	DES10	AusAm Biotechnologies
	Doxovir™	Redox Pharmaceutical Corporation

(Continued)

199

Table 8.1 (Continued)

Category	Products	Sponsor/Investigator
	HIV antibody, HSV antibody	Mapp Biopharmaceutical, Inc.
	Human monoclonal antibodies (C2F5, C2G12, C4E10)	Polymun Scientific
	Hydrogels containing monocaprin	University of Iceland
	Invisible condom	Laval University
	K5-N, OS(H)	San Raffaele Scientific Institute/Glycores 2000 s r 1
	Mandelic acid condensation polymer (SAMMA)	Mount Sinai Medical School
	Novaflux proprietary product	Pennsylvania State University College of Medicine
	Phthalocyanines	Emory University
	Polymethylene hydroquinone sulfonate (PMHS)	Program for the Topical Prevention of Conception and Diseases (TOPCAD)
	Porphyrins	Emory University
	PRO2000/5 Gel	Indevus Pharmaceutical, Inc.
	Thrombospondin	Weill Medical College of Cornell University
	Transgenic plant extracts containing recombinant cyanovirin	Guy's Hospital
	VivaGel (SPL7013 gel)	Starpharma Ltd.
Replication inhibitors (5)	(+)-Calanolide A	Sarawak MediChem Pharmaceuticals, Inc.
	(−)-Calanolide B	Sarawak MediChem Pharmaceuticals, Inc.
	MC1220 (as a lead compound in dihydroxy alkyl benzyl oxopyrimidine series)	Idenix Pharmaceuticals
	Tenofovir (PMPA)	Gilead Sciences
	UC-781	Biosyn, Inc.
Surfactants (6)	Aldex antimicrobial cream	Medicine and Applied Sciences, Inc.
	Alkyl sulfates and related compounds (sodium dodecyl sulfate, ammonium dodecyl sulfate, etc.)	Pennsylvania State University College of Medicine

(Continued)

Table 8.1   (Continued)

Category	Products	Sponsor/Investigator
	C-31G (Savvy™)	Biosyn, Inc.
	GynaGel Vaginal Gel	Frontier Pharmaceutical, Inc.
	N-Halamine derivatives (polymeric biocides)	Auburn University
	Tutela	Telum Corporation
Uncharacterized mechanisms (6)	ASAP solution	American Biotech Labs
	PATH Proprietary 'BI'	Program for Appropriate Technology in Health (PATH)
	PATH Proprietary 'CO'	Program for Appropriate Technology in Health (PATH)
	Praneem Polyherbal	Talwar Research Foundation
	Spirulina platensis hot water extract	Earthrise Nutritionals
	Water-soluble organic salts of zinc	Patrick D'Kelly
Vaginal defense buffers (8)	Alpha-defensins	University of California Los Angeles, Mt. Sinai Medical Center
	Lactobacillus suppository	The Medicines Company
	Lactin-vaginal capsule	Osel, Inc.
	MucoCept HIV	Osel, Inc.
	Protected lactobacilli in combination with BZK	Biofem, Inc.
	Protegrins	University of California at Los Angeles
	Retrocyclin	University of California at Los Angeles
	VenaGel	Demegen

Total number of candidates in development: 62. This list will be reviewed by an expert panel in fall 2004 and may be modified subsequently.

infectivity (Chang *et al.*, 2003); somehow marshaling or synthesizing natural antimicrobial peptides (Cole and Lehrer, 2003) or proteins with innate antiviral activity (Moriyama *et al.*, 1999); or employing topical estrogens to thicken the vaginal epithelium (Marx *et al.* 1996; Smith *et al.*, 2004).

Finally, control of these infections can eliminate or limit their contribution to the epithelial inflammation and ulceration that may increase acquisition or transmission of HIV, even though much remains unknown about the precise mechanisms of these categories of pre-existing or coincident trauma, which are in any event often only observable microscopically (Keller *et al.*, 2003). Such remediation can be accomplished through discrete public health interventions to prevent or treat non-HIV STIs, or by microbicides offering efficacy against non-HIV pathogens, a possibility discussed later in this chapter.

Viral Disruption: Inactivation or Disruption of Membranes

The fact that HIV is prone to disruption and inactivation by many chemical agents (Shattock and Moore, 2003) was among the factors that spurred initial enthusiasm about the category of microbicides referred to as 'detergents,' 'surfactants,' or 'surface-active agents,' of which nonoxynol-9 is the best-known member. These agents act non-specifically to kill or inactivate invading viral or bacterial pathogens by disrupting their outer membranes. They produce comparable effects on sperm, and this spermicidal or spermiostatic potential continues to make them strategically important as components of a broadly effective preventive armamentarium. A related, although more recently developed, member of this category is the family of cyclodextrin derivatives that attack the specialized lipid domains or 'rafts' in viral and cell membranes (Khanna *et al.*, 2002), and naturally occurring cyclic peptides such as the defensins that punch holes in viral membrane (Cole and Lehrer, 2003).

However, because HIV, like any virus, must derive its membrane from the host cells, the risk is that a microbicidal compound that attacks the membrane of an invading pathogen non-specifically is likely to also disrupt host cell structure, to a greater or lesser degree depending on frequency of use and formulation. A persistent challenge in work with these agents – in fact, for microbicide development in general – is to find the right balance between efficacy against invaders and toxicity to normal host cells (Harrison *et al.*, 2003; Pope and Haase, 2003). Toward that objective, though to no avail as we noted earlier, new formulations of N-9 were developed that would release the compound in lower, longer-acting concentrations, either alone or in combination with other agents. Work on similar formulations continues for use with a few other surfactants, three of which are in clinical trials. Still, the advancement of surface-active agents in development has slowed dramatically in the wake of N-9's failure, and questions continue to be raised about the wisdom of further pursuing strategies targeting the viral membrane. Forthcoming clinical trials of the very few surface-active agents remaining in the development pipeline should help answer these questions in the next couple of years.

Inhibition of Viral Entry and Fusion – Targeting the Viral Envelope

The lack of specificity associated with compounds targeting the viral membrane is less of a problem with microbicide compounds that act more specifically by binding to the viral envelope (Env) surface glycoproteins gp120 and gp41. Stable binding to this Env complex is likely to impair its function and, in some cases, even cause permanent inactivation (Moore and Shattock, 2003), both potentially powerful effects. The challenges in targeting Env arise from the need for higher concentrations of compound in some cases and from the sequence variation that affects Env function directly, and is likely to require combinations of agents (Walker and Korber, 2001; Shattock and Moore, 2003). Nevertheless, the intervention opportunities offered by compounds inhibiting the earliest stages of viral infection – attachment, fusion, and absorption – are so compelling that they now dominate the length of the microbicide pipeline (Harrison, 2003).

Three different compound types fall into this category: (1) polyanionic molecules that recognize positively charged regions of gp120 in a non-sequence-specific manner, (2) monoclonal antibodies (mAbs), and (3) proteins and peptides that bind to specific sites on gp120 or gp41.

The first of these subcategories, the polyanionic molecules, alternatively referred to as anionic or sulfated polymers, or sulfated polysaccharides, are long-chain molecules made up of linked, negatively charged units whose precise mechanisms are various and not fully defined, although we know that they do not physically destroy HIV as do the surfactants. In some cases they seem to bind, specifically and sometimes irreversibly, to positively charged areas of gp120, thereby impairing Env function (Moulard *et al.*, 2000). Or they may behave non-specifically, when their large molecular size and high charge may make them behave as 'sticky' molecules that somehow interfere with the 'close encounter' required for infection to take place (Stone, 2002). Or they may interfere with more than one of the early events in the HIV-1 infection process (Mayer *et al.*, 2003). These compounds form the largest of the three subcategories of the attachment and entry inhibitors targeting the invading pathogen, and are sometimes spoken of as 'adsorption inhibitors.' They are also the oldest inhibitors to have been investigated as potential microbicides, with at least some published studies appearing at the very outset of the 1990s (Bugelski *et al.*, 1991). As a result, this subcategory contains several microbicide candidates that have had time to progress into the clinical stages of the development pipeline.

The advantages of these compounds are that, unlike surface-active agents, they seem not to damage host cells, and their large sizes mean that they are poorly absorbed through the epithelium, reducing the risk of systemic toxicity as well. They also seem to retain antiviral activity in the presence of semen without necessarily acting contraceptively, which suits them particularly well for developing country populations where conception and protection from HIV infection are both desired and necessary. Other positive characteristics of this category are that, in general, they are more easily formulated and inexpensive to manufacture, and all its members have displayed efficacy in animal models against other STI organisms, including chlamydia, gonorrhea, genital herpes, and trichomonas (Stone, 2002).

Major questions for this candidate group are whether its members are active against the most critical HIV clades, and whether the potency they display *in vitro*, particularly against HIV, will be similarly expressed in human subjects in the presence of cervicovaginal fluid and semen (Keller *et al.*, 2003). Answers to these questions may come from strategic combinations of comparative studies in animal models and subsequent effectiveness trials, but implementing such a strategy may be easier to discuss than to do. As is the case for HIV vaccines, there is as yet no animal model validated in clinical trials that can reliably predict efficacy in human subjects.

The monoclonal antibodies in our subcategory 2 are still in the earlier preclinical stages of exploration and act in various ways to inhibit pathogen activity. Recent research shows that vaginally applied mAbs can block infection by simian immunodeficiency virus (SIV) in a non-human primate model (Veazey *et al.*, 2003). Some mAbs may offer special promise due to their broad and potent neutralizing activity against the most commonly transmitted HIV-1 strains and the possibilities they offer for synergy in combination 'cocktails' (see discussion of 'Looking for Combinations', below) (Trkola *et al.*, 1995; Zwick *et al.*, 2001). It is also possible that mAbs could be expressed in transgenic plants. Prospects for such 'plantibodies' for a number of health applications are being actively pursued, and in one highly relevant case have shown to prevent vaginal HSV-2 transmission in a mouse model of the disease (Zeitlin *et al.*, 1998; Stoger *et al.*, 2002; Fischer *et al.*, 2003).

In subcategory 3, at present the most investigated compound is the bacterial protein cyanovirin-N (CV-N), which has low cytotoxicity yet displays broad activity *in vitro* and is so bulky that it may well impede more than one stage in attachment and fusion processes (Dey *et al.*, 2000). Identified and initially developed by the National Cancer Institute, CV-N is being advanced under a public–private partnership. First isolated from blue-green algae and subsequently reproduced through recombinant technology, the compound now raises the dilemma of how it and similar compounds can be manufactured plentifully and cheaply. One strategy being pursued is development of transgenic plant extracts containing recombinant cyanovirin.

Targeting the Host Mucosal Cells, Inhibition of Viral Entry and Fusion – Targeting Receptors and Co-receptors

It is also possible to interrupt the sequence of attachment, binding, and fusion on what we might call the 'host cell side of things'. Here the goal is not to aim at the invading virus but to specifically block the host cell surface receptors at which the virus binds. The prime targets in this view of the virus–cell fusion cascade are the dendritic cells in the host's immune system that carry a cell surface receptor called DC-SIGN, to which HIV-1 seems to attach initially (Nobile *et al.*, 2003); CD4, long known as the first receptor in the binding step of the fusion process, in which it plays a critical role as mediator (Sattentau and Weise, 1988); and the CCR5 and CXCR4 co-receptors, which are critical to completion of binding and ultimately virus–cell fusion (Dragic, 2001). The attack tools, so to speak, are again monoclonal antibodies, modified chemokines, and small molecule inhibitors. Monoclonal antibodies appear to offer promise in blocking all three types of cell surface receptors. Another line of inquiry is exploring the potential of such CCR5 receptor inhibitors as PSC-RANTES (Veazey *et al.*, 2004). The modified chemokines and small molecules do seem to lend themselves most appropriately to targeting the co-receptors CCR5 and CXCR4, although each approach will need to be assessed relative to the others for potency, cost, ease of delivery, and stability *in vivo* (Shattock and Moore, 2003).

Inhibiting Replication

The final category of microbicide compounds under investigation comprises those that interrupt the HIV life cycle after the virus has entered a target cell and proceeds to hijack it into making new viral copies. These compounds would do their work by acting to inhibit reverse transcription, an early step in this viral replication process, and/or to inhibit local spread or establishment of latent infection. Members of this class were originally developed as HIV therapeutics and only later considered for a possible preventive role. Potent antivirals that do not require cellular activation and may also be active against cell-free virus are now being pursued in topical formulations. These include several non-nucleoside reverse transcriptase inhibitors (NNRTIs), whose mechanism of action is to enter the host cell, lie in wait for any HIV genomes that have also somehow managed to enter, and in various ways disable their replication (Stone, 2002).

Three NNRTIs are about to enter Phase I clinical trials, and tenofovir, a nucleotide reverse transcriptase inhibitor (NRTI), recently entered a Phase I trial in the United States. Earlier in development are several entry inhibitors recently found to also offer potential as inhibitors of viral replication, which suggests several possibilities: that they are more broadly active than previously thought, that they might lend themselves to acting synergistically or additively when combined with other inhibitors (Ketas *et al.*, 2003), or that they are inherently 'combinations' since they intervene in more than one of the steps in the sequence of HIV infection. Whatever their precise mechanism or range of activity, the largest challenge for all replication inhibitors may be their potential for long-term toxicity should there be significant absorption into the systemic circulation, and the possible emergence of drug-resistant HIV strains (Stone, 2002) in a context of repeated or interrupted use. However, since viral escape from entry inhibitors is to be expected (Moore and Doms, 2003), compounds that function both as entry and replication inhibitors might well be strategically enticing as a double impediment to infection with some potential for synergy.

Looking for Combinations

Consensus is growing that it is unlikely that a microbicide product based on a single compound will provide full protection against mucosal HIV transmission, and that high levels of protection are likely to require a combination of compounds (Shattock, 2003). This should come as no surprise. Development and optimization of HIV therapies and prophylaxis have already confirmed the power of combination approaches, and HIV vaccine development is increasingly moving in a similar direction. The general principle is that combinations that can broaden coverage, diversify options, and thereby improve control over the various aspects of the HIV epidemic, make the most sense. We are, after all, just following a well-validated model of comprehensive prevention strategies that link multiple modalities and work synergistically to reduce risk (Gayle, 2003; Gross and Johnston, 2003a).

Applying this same framework to microbicides makes similar sense, and our growing understanding about infectious processes and the events and factors involved in viral–cell interactions makes it feasible to think early and well about strategies for developing combination microbicides. The tactics on which we can now focus would encompass combinations that might blockade multiple steps involved in HIV transmission, maximize activity through synergy among compounds, lower dosage requirements for each component, minimize potential development of resistance, and/or broaden the spectrum of diverse HIV strains or non-HIV STIs addressed by a given formulation (Shattock, 2003). For example, two or more inhibitors that are partially effective when used alone and that work by different or even the same mechanisms, could make a fully effective inhibitor when used in combination (Shattock and Moore, 2003). One could, for instance, imagine a single product that might simultaneously conserve or enhance the integrity of the vaginal environment or make it less hospitable to HIV, interrupt attachment to and entry of HIV into susceptible cells; and interfere with reverse transcription (Gross and Johnston, 2003a). Even closer to realization are combinations that may provide contraceptive efficacy (D'Cruz *et al.*, 2003). In fact, four of the six microbicides poised for effectiveness trials are expected to be contraceptive, and other microbicide candidates in preclinical development show effective inhibition of sperm function *in vitro* and contraceptive efficacy in the rabbit model (Table 8.2). Combination microbicides formulated to enhance pleasure, comfort, or cosmetic attractiveness might also enhance adherence to use (Gross and Johnston, 2003a), an utterly crucial factor in the ultimate public health effectiveness of these products.

The case for combination products with a broad spectrum of activity against non-HIV STIs is particularly compelling because of the potential contribution of such products to attenuating HIV transmission (Bowcut, 2003), and because of the increased utilization and, again, better adherence that might be motivated by products offering such multiplicity of protection. It is now habitual for developers of microbicide products to test them for efficacy against a range of STI pathogens to determine the potential scope of their activity. A pipeline profile derived from the Microbicide Research and Development Database (MRDD) designed and managed by the Alliance for Microbicide Development displays the breadth of potential efficacy offered by a number of microbicide candidates. Of roughly 50 microbicide candidates, almost half were found to have activity *in vitro* and in

Table 8.2 Microbicides in development: antisperm/contraceptive activity and activity against non-HIV sexually transmitted infections.

Compound name	Sperm	Hepatitis B	Herpes simplex virus	Human papilloma-virus	Chlamydia trachomatis	Haemophilus ducreyi	Neisseria gonorrheae	Treponema pallidum	Trichomonas vaginalis	Candida albicans
Acidform tablet (AFT)	I									I
Aldex antimicrobial cream	I	I	I				I			
Alkyl sulfates and related compounds	I		I,A	I,A	I		I			
ASAP solution									I	I
BufferGel™	I,A		I,A	A	I,A	I	I,A	I	I	
Cellulose acetate phthalate (CAP)	I		I,A		I	I	I,A		I	I
Cellulose sulfate			I		I					
Doxovir	I,A		I,A	I,A	I,A					
GynaGel vaginal gel		I	I,A	I,A	I	I	I	I	I	I,A
HX8 for HSV plantibody			I,A							
Invisible condom	I		I,A	I	I		I			

(Continued)

Table 8.2 (Continued)

Compound name	Sperm	Hepatitis B	Herpes simplex virus	Human papilloma-virus	Chlamydia trachomatis	Haemophilus ducreyi	Neisseria gonorrheae	Treponema pallidum	Trichomonas vaginalis	Candida albicans
Lactin vaginal capsule					I		I		I	I
Mandelic acid condensation polymer (SAMMA)	I, A	I	I	I	I		I			I
MC1220 (as a lead compound in dihydroxy alkyl benzyl oxopyrimidine series)			I			I	I			I
MucoCept HIV			I							
N-Halamine derivatives							I		I	I
Novaflux proprietary product	I									
PATH Proprietary 'BI'	I				I					I

(Continued)

Table 8.2 (Continued)

PATH Proprietary 'CO'	I		I		I		I	I
Polymethylene-hydroquinone sulfonate (PMHS)	I, A		I, A	I	I		I	I
Polystyrene sulfonate vaginal tablets (PSS)	I		I		I			
Polyvinyl alcohol sulfate (PVAS)					I	I		I
Porphyrins			I		I, A / I	I		
PRO 2000/5 gel	I, A		I, A		I / I	I / I		
Protected lactobacilli in combination with BZK			I					
Spirulina platensis hot water extract								
VivaGel (SPL7013)			I, A	A	I, A			
Water-soluble organic salts of zinc			I		I			I

I = *in vitro* activity; A = animal activity. Note: This list will be reviewed and updated by an expert panel in fall 2004.

209

animal models against herpes; one-third were found to have activity against chlamydia, gonorrhea, and human papillomavirus; and one-quarter had *in vitro* findings of activity against candida (Bowcut, 2003). How that will play out in human testing is impossible to predict; however, six of the candidates advancing to effectiveness trials include as secondary endpoints activity against non-HIV STIs and bacterial vaginosis (Bowcut, 2003) (see Table 8.2).

Devices and Desires

Another category of products comprises a range of physical barriers being explored for use in conjunction with different microbicide formulations to enhance the power of both prevention technologies. These include reusable or single-use cervical caps and diaphragms designed to either incorporate or deliver microbicidal formulations, as well as silicone intravaginal rings whose use would not necessarily be coitus-dependent but that could remain in place and slow-release microbicidal contents over longer periods of time to provide ongoing protection. For all of these, cost and ease of use in developing country settings will be the primary challenges, but their potential for higher effectiveness makes them a desirable research objective nonetheless, and recent and ongoing trials of diaphragms in Zimbabwe and South Africa indicate high levels of interest in this preventive technology among women at risk (Moench *et al.*, 2001; G Ramjee, personal communication).

Microbicides Growing Up

Whatever their spermicidal antecedents, microbicides are a brand-new technology, and drug development is typically punctuated with triage for various reasons, so it was expected that the structure and content of the microbicide R&D pipeline would change, by both attrition and growth. The most striking shift occurred in the number of surface-active agents, which fell by over half between 1996 and 2002 (Figure 8.4). That, too, was to be expected, given the N-9 disappointments, greater learning about what is needed to move from bench to clinic, more understanding of the exigencies of clinical trial design, and concerns about further advancing such agents despite the intrinsic appeal of their broad spectrum. Nevertheless, three of these agents are in clinical testing. The Invisible Condom™ based on sodium lauryl sulfate and being developed by Laval University, is entering Phase II expanded safety trials; Biofilm's benzalkonium-based product, is also in Phase II; and C-31G, known as 'Savvy'™, a combination of two amphoteric surface-active agents in a new formulation, is poised to enter Phase III effectiveness trials in 2004. Figure 8.5 provides an overview of new microbicide products currently in development that focus on prevention of HIV transmission.

More or less stable in their total number is the group of sulfated polysaccharides or anionic polymers. These naturally dominate the clinical portion of the

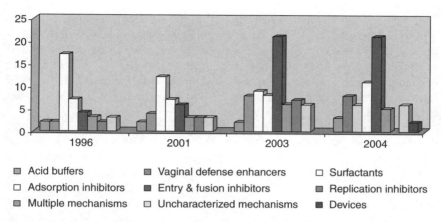

■ Acid buffers   ■ Vaginal defense enhancers   □ Surfactants
□ Adsorption inhibitors   ■ Entry & fusion inhibitors   ■ Replication inhibitors
■ Multiple mechanisms   □ Uncharacterized mechanisms   ■ Devices

Fig. 8.4 Structural changes in the microbicide development pipeline, 1994–2004. Source: Alliance for Microbicide Development.

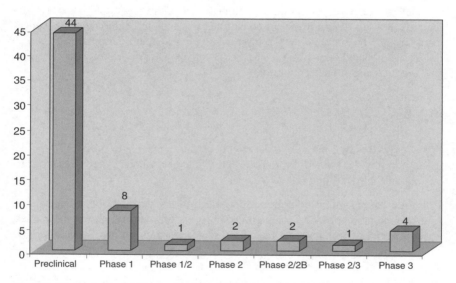

Fig. 8.5 Current microbicide pipeline with HIV as primary endpoint, 2004. Source: Alliance for Microbicide Development.

present pipeline since they have been the focus of research for over a decade. Two of these – the carrageenan-based Carraguard™ and dextrin-2-sulfate, trademarked as Emmelle™ – are about to enter Phase III effectiveness trials. PRO2000/5™, a naphthalene sulfonate, will be fielded shortly in two different concentrations: in a head-to-head Phase II/IIB screening trial with BufferGel™ and a Phase III trial with Emmelle™.

211

A different pattern characterizes the rest of the pipeline, reflecting its overall growth and the gradual engagement of scientists whose roots lie in different areas of basic HIV research. The total number of candidates that can be roughly classed as entry and fusion inhibitors is now three times what it was in 1996. The number of candidates with multiple and/or undefined mechanisms of action has also risen, reflecting the influx of new compounds still in early discovery and not yet fully characterized.

At the time of this writing, there were approximately 62 microbicide candidates in the microbicide pipeline (Figure 8.5). Of those, 18 are in some phase of clinical development; the rest require more preclinical research so that they can submit their application packages as Investigational New Drugs (IND) to the FDA in order to proceed to testing in human subjects. Estimates of the number of microbicide candidates in the development pipeline have ranged from 45 to 65 over the past three years, a variability that is largely a function of the arrival of new prospects and some sort of failure of older ones. It is also a function of the greater rigor that is being applied to the gathering of data about all candidates and associated research. An ongoing difficulty for evaluating this field has been, and remains, how to determine what constitutes a plausible candidate for advancement through the microbicide development pipeline so that funding support can be rationally allocated. This brings us to the players who are developing microbicides and how they are supported, or not.

The Players

Since early days in microbicide development, an increasing number of organizations and individuals have contributed to the field as a whole. Their roles are various but basically fall into three categories:

1. Entities doing microbicide research and, in a growing number of instances, also developing products. This group subsumes biopharmaceutical companies, non-profit research institutions, public-sector research groups, and individuals and groups doing 'supportive research,' for example, work on new animal model systems or development of non-invasive assays for clinical evaluation.
2. Public health and women's health groups advocating in various ways on behalf of the field and doing policy research and analysis to support those efforts.
3. Entities funding the work of both categories. The entities involved with microbicides and supportive research consist of a number of different sectors: biopharmaceutical companies, nonprofit research institutions, public-sector entities worldwide, and entities doing supportive research.

It would be impossible to list all of these entities, which are, in any case, largely represented in Table 8.1. Here, in alphabetical order, we introduce some of the key players whose work cuts across the microbicide field and its various needs.

Alliance for Microbicide Development (AMD)

The Alliance was established in early 1998 with a startup grant from the Rockefeller Foundation as an agent of change, at a time when progress in microbicide research and development was slow, fragmented, and severely under-funded. A coalition of over 200 representatives from small biopharmaceutical companies, non-profit research institutions, and health advocacy groups, the Alliance catalyzes support for its mission through advocacy; education; monitoring; research; trouble-shooting; convening and seeking consensus around critical issues; participating in a range of ad hoc partnerships; and networking across constituencies, disci-plines, and sectors. It is considered the principal and authoritative source of informa-tion about progress (or lack of progress) in microbicide research and development, as a neutral and objective convener and advocate around critical challenges in microbicide science and policy, and as a leader in interactions with the media.

Family Health International (FHI)

FHI is among the largest international public health non-governmental organiza-tions, managing research and field activities in over 70 countries to meet the pub-lic health needs of some of the world's most vulnerable populations. In addition to serving as the Coordinating and Operations Center for the HIV Prevention Trials Network (HPTN; see below), FHI is also conducting several non-HPTN micro-bicide trials. These include a Phase III trial of cellulose sulfate in collaboration with the Global Microbicide Project in Nigeria, two trials of C-31G (Savvy™) in Ghana and Nigeria, and a pre-exposure prophylaxis Phase I study of tenofovir (PMPA) in Cambodia, Cameroon, Ghana, and Nigeria.

Global Campaign for Microbicides (GCM)

Also established in 1998, as the Global Campaign for Prevention Options for Women, the GCM is a broad-based, international umbrella organization whose goal is to build support among policy-makers, opinion-leaders, and the general public for increased investment in microbicides and other user-controlled preven-tion methods. Its particular concern is the interests of end-users and assuring their protection. The Campaign is an equal partner with the Alliance in domestic legis-lative and media initiatives and with International Family Health in Great Britain in advocacy initiatives in Europe. It leads the field in its work with grassroots organizing in the United States, where it has 10 core sites, and has important advocacy initiatives in India and sub-Saharan Africa.

Global Microbicide Project (GMP)

The GMP was started with an award of US$25 million from the Bill and Melinda Gates Foundation as an independent project of CONRAD, the Contraceptive

Research and Development Program, an international collaborative organization. Its primary function is to develop and support cross-sectoral development of new microbicidal agents that specifically address the needs and perspectives of women across the length of the research and development pipeline, including authority to execute all phases of clinical trials of microbicides. It supports that function through a flexible and agile grants process that is unique in the microbicide field and critical to its continued advancement, and through development of clinical sites through implementation of clinical trials of key microbicide candidates.

International Family Health (IFH)

IFH is an international non-governmental organization in the United Kingdom dedicated to improving the sexual and reproductive health and rights of disadvantaged people in resource-poor settings. In a project funded by the European Community, the UK Department for International Development (DFID), and the International Partnership for Microbicides (IPM), IFH is collaborating with the Global Campaign for Microbicides, the Alliance, and other partners in efforts to raise awareness of microbicides among European donors, industry, regulatory bodies, and the scientific community; among developing-country policy-makers; and among HIV/AIDS, international development, women's health, and other activist organizations in Africa, Asia, and Europe.

International Partnership for Microbicides (IPM)

The IPM was launched in 2002 as the product of a two-year initiative by the Rockefeller Foundation and is presently funded by the Gates Foundation, Rockefeller, and grants from several European countries and the UK. Its goal is to improve the efficiency of efforts to deliver a safe and effective microbicide as soon as possible through implementation of a business model, strategic awards of contracts for specific candidate compounds or 'proto-products,' preparatory strengthening of key clinical sites, and preparation for product introduction.

Microbicides Development Programme (MDP)

The MDP is a five-year research collaboration sponsored by the UK's Department for International Development and administered by the Medical Research Council Clinical Trials Unit and Imperial College, London. In collaboration with institutions in Cameroon, South Africa, Tanzania, Uganda, and Zambia, the MDP is fielding trials of two candidate microbicides, dextrin-2-sulfate (Emmelle™) and PRO-2000/5™. Additionally, the MDP aims to develop new products to enter safety studies in the UK and Africa.

Population Council

The Population Council is an international non-governmental organization with staff in 18 developing countries, dedicated to improving the well-being and reproductive health of current and future generations around the world and achieving a humane, equitable, and sustainable balance between people and resources. Its Contraceptive Development Program has developed a candidate microbicide, Carraguard™, which is about to enter Phase III effectiveness trials in South Africa. The Council has also recently acquired an NNRTI (MIV-150), which may be more effective in attacking multiple strains of HIV in combination with Carraguard™. The Population Council also administers and participates in the Rockefeller-funded Microbicides Basic Science Network, which links five outstanding scientists charged with working on different, but complementary, aspects of research to facilitate the development of microbicides.

A frequently asked question is how each of these differs from the others, a question that seems to arise from the newness of the field and a historical paucity of financial resources, though it is not a question that seems to burden other comparable fields in any obvious way. Nevertheless, each organization does offer distinctive and critical comparative advantages; the challenge is to collaborate where there are overlapping interests, abilities, and needs, and to regard differences as a source of strength rather than some sort of intrinsic debility in the field as a whole.

Funding Development Efforts

Until recently, the paucity and discontinuity of resources flows have severely constrained microbicide research and development. Like vaccines in general and 'Third World' drugs for malaria, tuberculosis, and other tropical infectious diseases, microbicides are seen by industry as a 'public good' with little to offer in the form of appealing market share. Thus, except for provision of a few compounds for testing, applicators provided at cost, and some limited funding for conferences, there has been no investment to date by the large pharmaceutical industry in microbicide research and development.

Industry anticipation of poor returns in the early market life of microbicides is not irrational. A major study by the Boston Consulting Group of product evolution, likely market, product development costs and timing, and return on investment found that an initial investment in the first microbicide to reach the market would get a negative return between US$27 and $65 million, even if that first product were to have no competition and enjoyed a 100 per cent market share (Pharmaco-Economics Working Group, 2001). The analysis went on to conclude that significant positive returns would not be seen until the advent on the market of 'third-generation microbicides'; even then, returns would range from a negative US$49

Table 8.3   Funding for microbicide research and development: an overview (March 2004).

Source	FY 1997 *Actual*	FY 1998 *Actual*	FY 1999 *Actual*	FY 2000 *Actual*	FY 2001 *Actual*	FY 2002 *Actual*	FY 2003 *Actual*	Cum.
Philanthropic sector	1.4	2.1	5.5	27.2	8.0	5.1	17.8	67.1
International public sector	0	0	0.4	0.1	1.5	50.9	23.8	76.6
US public sector	26.8	25.3	32.3	34.6	61.3	75.2	78.8	334.3
Total	28.2	27.4	38.2	61.8	70.8	131.4	120.4	478.0

Source: Alliance for Microbicide Development.

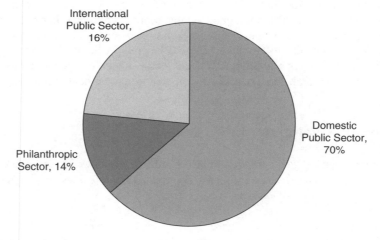

Fig. 8.6 Overview of sectors funding microbicides. Source: Alliance for Microbicide Development.

million to a positive US$428 million, depending on whether the microbicide in question became a niche product or a regular hygiene product.

Table 8.3 presents trends in funding for microbicide research and development beginning in 1997, the first year for which any significant amount of support of the field could be readily identified. Since that year, US$478.0 million has flowed into the microbicide field, of which 70 per cent, or over US$334.3 million, was provided by the US federal government (Figure 8.6), whose investment grew three-fold in that time frame.

The Public Sector: Government Agencies and Institutions

In the United States, three agencies play key roles in support of microbicide research and development: the Centers for Disease Control and Prevention (CDC), the National Institutes of Health (NIH), and the United States Agency for International Development (USAID). Of these, the NIH has provided approximately 77 per cent of all US government support for microbicide research and development, increasing its expenditures from US$21 million in FY1997 to US$58 million in FY2003, with US$63 million estimated for FY2004. Within the NIH, the dominant contributor has been the National Institute of Allergy and Infectious Diseases (NIAID). The main funding mechanisms employed by the NIH, as well as the CDC, are Requests for Applications and Proposals, some investigator-initiated grants, contracts for cross-cutting functions such as animal testing, and its Small Business Innovation Research (SBIR) grants program. CDC support for microbicide research fluctuated over this period, with an expenditure peak of US$4.7 million in FY2003. Support from USAID grew nine-fold, from US$2.1 million in 1997 to $17.9 million in FY2003, with a statutory provision of US$22 million for FY2004. It cannot be claimed that there would have been no US public-sector funding increases without advocacy efforts, but there is wide agreement that pressure from a range of advocacy groups and initiatives had undeniable and positive effects on the size of the increases.

As for the international public sector, no significant investments were made until FY2002, when the UK's Department for International Development provided almost US$24 million to the UK's Medical Research Council primarily for advancement of its dextrin-2-sulfate candidate, and the French Government provided US$41 million in support for its National Agency for Research into AIDS (ANRS) and implementation of clinical trials. Establishment of the IPM catalyzed additional funding from the governments of Denmark, Ireland, Norway, and the UK for the IPM's own program of product development and preparation for product access.

The Philanthropic Sector

Until FY2000, the philanthropic sector played a minor role in funding for microbicides, averaging a little under US$3 million in fiscal years 1997 through 1999. In 2000, the picture changed dramatically with major grants to the Population Council and the Global Microbicide Project. The total investment by the philanthropic sector from 1997 to the present amounted to US$67.1 million, of which the Bill and Melinda Gates Foundation contributed over 77 per cent. The Gates Foundation also provided the largest single contribution so far, US$60 million to the International Partnership for Microbicides, of which US$20 million was intended for targeted development of some key candidates. The Rockefeller Foundation has consistently supported the field at a more modest level, and was the first foundation to invest any funding in the field. The William and Flora Hewlett Foundation has been a modest but steady supporter, the Moriah Fund provided funding at a critical time for advocacy and policy work, and the American Foundation for AIDS Research (amfAR) has for the past four years given annual awards for AIDS research that always included support for some aspect of microbicide research.

Overall, however, microbicides have had to relive the earlier experience of HIV vaccines: skepticism, lack of industry interest, scanty and disjointed funding, competition from other technologies and diseases, substantial scientific and practical challenges, and a public sector uneasy about engaging in frank product development as a general matter. Like HIV vaccines, microbicides are pharmaceutical products that require levels of investment sufficient to support the entire pipeline process from early discovery to licensing, with costs escalating at each advance. Later stage clinical trials, whose costs have been rising steadily over the decade, are especially costly for both vaccines and microbicides because they are intended to prevent infection in presumably healthy populations. For both technologies, Phase III effectiveness trials require very large numbers of recruits who, furthermore, live in countries where HIV incidence must be high enough to provide a baseline comparator and where trial implementation may be quite challenging. Even though HIV vaccines benefit from surrogate markers that can provide at least minimal early evidence of efficacy, and even though microbicide trials must depend on user adherence that is far less easily measured than even repeated injections, both confront major difficulties in site capacity, trial implementation and, perhaps above all, costs.

Still, the microbicide field has learned from the experience of HIV vaccines that steady advocacy pressure and incremental scientific advances can together elicit capital inflows from the public and philanthropic sectors. The goal each technology seeks to achieve is getting something good enough medically and technologically far enough down the pipeline to evoke significant industry interest.

Microbicides Going Forward

Again like HIV vaccines, in fact like any new pharmaceutical product, large, basic, and complex questions must be answered all along the research and development pathway. The rampaging character of the HIV pandemic has, nonetheless, fueled a sense of urgency in afflicted populations that is not always obvious in the laboratories and hallways of science and bureaucracy. Still, there is an expectation that the new scientific tools that have emerged over the past few decades should have speeded things up more than has been the case. Thus, there is mounting impatience in a range of advocacy communities and a steady drumbeat pounding on scientists and bureaucrats to 'do it faster.' It is, of course, not fast enough.

This is surely true for microbicides. Since an HIV vaccine is years away and more challenging than once thought, since preventing HIV solely through behavior modification is hard to do and harder to sustain, and since the world's women really have nothing that assures their safety from a lethal disease, we must ask why progress in microbicide research and development has been so fragmented, fragile, and slow. We have already spoken of lack of interest on the part of the large pharmaceutical industry and the standard bureaucratic contortions that have affected everyone seeking adequate responses to the AIDS epidemic. In the case of microbicides, there are other explanations. Some reside in the scientific underpinnings of microbicide research and development; others are sociocultural and quite pragmatic.

Challenges in the Science

What scientific questions need to be answered in the field of microbicide research? Which of those are showstoppers, which fall into the 'nice to know' bin, and which must await answers from large-scale clinical trials? Some of the answers to the questions that follow are specific to microbicides; others are also needed by HIV vaccine developers, a realization that is drawing new researchers to the microbicide field. Mucosal immunology is the common ground for each field of inquiry, which may explain why we are starting to hear the terms 'mucosal barriers' and 'mucosal microbicides.'

Basic understandings

It has been repeatedly observed that the science of sexual transmission of HIV and non-HIV pathogens is poorly understood (Miller and Shattock, 2003). The fact that over 125 000 articles on HIV alone have been published in peer-reviewed scientific journals since 1983 (Fauci, 2003) should persuade us that our understandings about HIV in general are far broader and deeper than ever before, and surely sufficient for the pursuit of some quite sturdy hypotheses. Pivotal issues and questions remain unanswered, nonetheless, and while they need not be showstoppers, more certain responses could accelerate progress in the development of both HIV vaccines and microbicides. They are:

- We know much more about transmission of cell-free HIV than about transmission of cell-associated HIV (Miller and Shattock, 2003). What are the significant differences between those two routes of transmission and what do they mean for strategies for intervention? Or, must we assume that both viral sources will need to be targeted (Shattock and Moore, 2003) and invest more effort in evaluating candidates for their ability to block cell-associated HIV infection than has been the case so far?
- We also know much more about which co-receptors and other molecules are involved in virus–host cell interactions and how those interactions occur, though much remains to be known about the roles played by co-receptor expression

and usage in HIV-1 transmission and pathogenesis (Moore *et al.*, 2004). We also need to know much more about what types of cells, in what proportions, will be infected at each stage in transmission and infection, and about how, when, and with what speed infection is disseminated from the portal of entry and under what circumstances (Pope and Haase, 2003).

- We are increasingly secure in assuming that trauma, epithelial abrasions and breaks, inflammation, menstrual cycle, hormonal status, even micronutrient levels can play significant roles in viral entry and establishment and dissemination of HIV infection (Mostad *et al.*, 1997), but could benefit from a better grasp on the relative weight of each of those and how to account for them in microbicide development.

- We are seeing accumulating interest in interrupting the processes of HIV transmission at the earliest possible stage, since it seems that by the acute stage of HIV-1 infection, the immune system already faces an uphill struggle and its race with the virus may be effectively lost. This implies that the most critical focus for microbicides may well be at the beginning of transmission, that is, at the mucosal interface and initial virus interactions with host cells and defenses in different mucosal sites (Pope and Haase, 2003; Hu *et al.*, 2004).

Other models

Crucial to answering these questions is being able to take them from exploration *in vitro* to exploration in animal models. The best-established and most widely used such model for answering fundamental questions around HIV transmission and the potential efficacy of candidate microbicides is the rhesus macaque (Miller *et al.*, 1989). While this model is a good proxy for the anatomy, physiology, microflora, and natural acidity of the human vagina, it has been based on a single, high-dose inoculation of SIV or SHIV right after a single application of a microbicide. This does not really mimic either the pattern of repeated exposure of human subjects to potential infection or repeated use of a low-dose microbicide over time (Microbicide Initiative, 2002); recent efforts to develop such a model suggest that it is feasible (Otten *et al.*, 2004). Other non-human primate models are needed to assess product efficacy against non-HIV STIs, evaluate intra-rectal application, and grade microbicide candidates 'head to head.'

At the same time, the costs of such testing are high, and the microbicide field has been innovative in developing sophisticated *in vitro* models based on human tissue explants and small animal models for testing product efficacy and potential for toxicity. That said, while many microbicide candidate compounds show activity against HIV infection in *in vitro* assays and animal models, how do we know what that means for use in human beings? The answer is frustratingly circular: we cannot know the meaning of those assays and models until they are validated in clinical trials, but how can we predict enough from those assays to decide which clinical trials to do of what compounds and proto-products? The answer: We have to keep perfecting assays and design later-stage clinical trials so as to validate them, a task that should be commonly and strategically adopted by all implementing such trials.

Clinical evaluation

Because microbicides are intended for prolonged, repeated use, they must be indisputably safe (Mauck *et al.*, 2001; Lard-Whiteford *et al.*, 2004). The N-9 experience taught us that compounds designed to rapidly inactivate the incoming pathogen by disintegrating its lipid envelope can produce comparable damage in host cells lining the vagina, cervix, and rectum, permitting HIV ready access to primary target cells. The traditional clinical tools for assessing such local toxicity have been speculum-assisted naked eye and colposcopic examination. Yet, despite efforts by the CDC, CONRAD Program, and WHO to perfect and standardize these tools (WHO/CONRAD, 2000; Mauck *et al.*, 2000; Bollen *et al.*, 2002), there is agreement that they are not optimal and that other assessment and validation technologies are wanted (WHO/CONRAD, 2003). Basic questions have to do with defining 'normal' and 'healthy' (Priestley *et al.*, 1997); establishing baselines for product-related effects, particularly in settings where co-infections and hygienic limitations are rampant; and determining the significance of different epithelial disruptions and their causes. Another is whether these techniques can detect such crucial but subtle changes in the cervico-vaginal mucosa as the interference with host-defense mechanisms and induction of inflammation that may enhance HIV acquisition or transmission (Keller *et al.*, 2003). And, while there are ongoing efforts to craft new measures for assessing product safety such as quantitation of mediators of inflammation and immunity in genital tract secretions (Anderson *et al.*, 1998), the imminence of large effectiveness trials is ratcheting up pressure to expedite and validate this work. There is also mounting pressure to develop technologies for evaluating product safety in the rectal environment, presenting another, quite distinctive set of challenges (Roehr *et al.*, 2002).

Formulation

It may seem extreme to say that, in microbicide development, 'formulation is everything,' but in reality, that is not far off base when we recognize that, first of all, an unformulated active agent goes nowhere. Formulation, the vehicle in which the active ingredient is conveyed, stands at the junction of safety and efficacy where we wish to find lubrication and protection from surface trauma; conservation or restoration of the natural vaginal environment; lack of inherent systemic or local toxicity; mediation of any toxic effects deriving from the active agent itself; sufficient bioadhesiveness, dispersibility, and viscosity to be retained over the area at risk for a reasonable time in the presence of semen and bodily fluids and under the stress of intercourse; durability of efficacy, again over a length of time adequate to compete with an elusive virus; assurance that there is no undue systemic uptake;

possible enhancement of efficacy and, in the case of combinations, optimization of synergy and attenuation of any unanticipated antagonisms between active agents. Formulation science will also be essential to the newer microbicide concepts that are advancing pre-clinically, since some entry inhibitors and monoclonal antibodies will require manufacture at concentrations and volumes far beyond that needed for testing in non-human primates (Shattock and Moore, 2003). As is true for HIV vaccines (McMichael and Hanke, 2003), optimization of components and quantity manufacture will be major challenges for microbicides.

Formulation will also matter greatly to microbicide consumers. Even though research indicates that product safety and efficacy are the most important characteristics wanted in a microbicide, consumer behavior studies predict that cost, color, taste, physical consistency, ease of use, for some users unobtrusiveness and for others enhancement of sexual pleasure, all have potential for affecting the acceptability of and consistent and correct product use (Becker *et al.*, 2003).

Clinical trial design

Clinical trials of microbicides, especially large-scale multisite trials to assess effectiveness, are complex, resource-intensive, and costly; they also evoke tensions between ethical values and pragmatic needs (Stone, 2003). The central dilemmas in the design of these trials have been a focus of broad and intense discussion over the past year, culminating in a meeting of the FDA Anti-Viral Drugs Advisory Committee in August 2003 to address clinical trial design issues in the development of topical microbicides. The most contentious of those issues have to do with sample size, duration of follow-up, acceptable and desirable levels of effectiveness, statistical power, and number of control arms (Alliance for Microbicide Development *et al.*, 2003).

The greater problem is that, while there is consensus on some of these issues across the microbicide field, that consensus does not accord with current US regulatory positions, which are widely perceived as unduly exigent. At stake is the advancement to 'proof of concept' which is so critical for the microbicide field as a whole. Because there are yet no surrogate markers that could provide preliminary indicators of microbicide efficacy at earlier stages of the clinical trial sequence, as is the case for therapeutics and some vaccines, Phase III effectiveness trials are the only avenue to determining whether microbicides can actually 'work'. At this time, there is active discussion around the six microbicide candidates poised to advance through expanded Phase II safety trials and Phase III effectiveness trials in 2004. A current priority is to shape a collaborative strategy that will extract the maximum possible benefit from those trials. The goal is to assure that even if none of the candidate microbicides to be tested prove to have a level of effectiveness sufficient for licensing by regulatory authorities, the trials will still have strengthened capacities of sites for subsequent trials and generated crucial data, understandings, and procedures that can inform design and implementation of subsequent trials.

Clinical trial infrastructure

As work on microbicides and HIV vaccines accelerates, it is already apparent that the laboratory and clinical capacity of sites in countries where HIV incidence is, sadly, high enough to provide a baseline for evaluating the efficacy of a given preventive intervention, will soon be insufficient. The trials referred to above will need to recruit no fewer than 30 000 women in approximately 30 sites in. A number of entities are engaged in programs to build such infrastructure, as well as the ethical review and regulatory capacities that must underpin them. In the public sector, perhaps the most extensive efforts will be made under the European and Developing Countries Clinical Trials Partnership (EDCTP) and the Comprehensive International Program of Research on AIDS (CIPRA) supported by the US National Institutes of Health. The Wellcome Trust and Bill and Melinda Gates Foundation are also playing a role in bioethics and research and development capacity building in developing countries, and the WHO is about to embark on a program of regulatory strengthening and support. The NIH, the International AIDS Vaccine Initiative (IAVI), and the UK Medical Research Council also sponsor other sites and site networks. It has been suggested that vaccines and microbicides could be evaluated in combination and consideration is being given to setting up sites for both vaccine and microbicide trials, which could also incorporate treatment and care for local populations (Gross and Johnston, 2003a). A significant concern is how to address and negotiate competition for site capacity and strengthen capacity in a systematic, collaborative way (Godwin, 2003). At present, the general picture of the various efforts to create or strengthen clinical research capacity is somewhat disheveled. Notably, the NIH is rethinking the character and structure of the various HIV/AIDS-related networks it has been supporting, all of which will be recompeted over the coming year (NIAID, 2004).

The Future

The key questions here are how access and use can be assured once an effective microbicide becomes reality, and what impact this new technology might have on the AIDS epidemic and the lives of those for whom it could make a difference.

Assuring access and use

It is a truth, universally acknowledged, that a biomedical technology will have no effect on public or individual health if it is not used. In the case of microbicides, adherence to consistent and correct use is central not only to such effects, but to the optimal conduct and validity of the clinical trials of these technologies.

With this in mind, the microbicide field made a commitment to assurance of access from quite early days, despite skepticism about timing, given that there is neither a microbicide poised to enter the market nor proof of the principle that

223

such a technology could actually be effective. Historically, however, technological innovations have had mixed success in their introduction, some encountering significant obstacles and lengthy delays that might have been avoided with more thoughtful preparation (Becker *et al.*, 2003). This has been notably true in the case of some reproductive technologies and vaccines, particularly in developing countries. The nature of the AIDS epidemic makes it obvious that the delays of 10–15 years that have often characterized transfer of new technologies from the industrialized to the developing world would be intolerable and profoundly unethical. In addition, because much of microbicide research and development will continue to take place through a variety of public–private partnerships, matters of intellectual property and assurance of reasonable pricing tiers are best considered sooner rather than later (Godwin, 2003).

Introducing microbicides will be complex for a range of reasons. First, the earliest of these products will, like HIV vaccines, be only partially effective, with lower effectiveness than condoms in preventing HIV transmission. Second, they will also be 'user-controlled' vaginal products that will require recognition and discussion of sexuality and sexual practices that some providers, policy-makers, and potential users may find uncomfortable. Third, the fact that this new technology will offer women more power and control over their sexual lives may challenge present relationship structures and gender norms in ways that might be seen as threatening (Becker *et al.*, 2003).

Partial effectiveness, condom 'migration,' and the public health impact of microbicides

As with any new technology, it is almost instinctive to ask 'Is it necessary?' and 'What difference will it make?' Anticipating those questions, the London School of Hygiene and Tropical Medicine's (LSHTM) HIV Tools Project has worked for several years on model projections of the potential impact of microbicides on HIV and STD transmission. The LSHTM findings are that even employing conservative assumptions about microbicide anti-HIV efficacy (60 per cent) and coverage (20 per cent of groups in current contact with services), the three-year cumulative impact of use of a microbicide with 60 per cent anti-HIV efficacy could avert 2.5 million HIV infections among females, males, and children in lower-income countries. This, in turn, could produce direct cost savings to health systems in those countries of US$2.7 billion (US$ 2002) and another US$1 billion in productivity gains from preventing absenteeism and retraining and replacing workers. When a microbicide with anti-STD efficacy of 40 per cent is incorporated into these calculations, the HIV infections-averted figure rises to 2.7 million, direct cost savings to US$2.88 billion, and productivity benefits to US$1.13 billion (Watts *et al.*, 2002). These calculations are rather conservative since they do not take into account the costs of antiretroviral therapy, which would elevate the level of savings from microbicide use dramatically.

The HIV Tools Project then took on the question of 'condom migration', the term often used to describe the substitution of condoms for microbicides. A static mathematical model was employed to compare how different combinations of condom and microbicide use might affect individual risk of HIV and STD infection and identify the 'break-even' point at which any increased HIV risk associated with potential migration or substitution would be offset by the protection afforded by microbicides. The results were somewhat predictable but also reassuring in their detail. A 50 per cent HIV- and STD-efficacious microbicide could be used by groups using condoms with 25 per cent consistency or less without increasing their risk of HIV if they used microbicides in 50 per cent of sex acts. However, migration might increase risk where initial condom-use consistency (>70 per cent) and microbicide risk is high (<50 per cent of non-condom-protected acts). Given that condom use is erratic or low in much of the developing world (and not particularly consistent in the United States (Hearst and Chen, 2003), there are likely to be many situations in which the benefits of microbicide use would outweigh the negative impact of condom migration, and where microbicides could reduce HIV risk substantially (Foss *et al.*, 2003).

These are persuasive analyses and will be refined further. Nonetheless, they need to be translated into concepts that can be readily grasped by providers and consumers, concepts that will have to be framed differently in different settings. As just one example, a recent pilot study in South Africa (Becker *et al.*, 2003) found that the concept of 'partially effective' faded in priority in a context of high HIV risk and no preventive options. The opposite is true for college students in the US, for whom effectiveness equivalent to the male condom was paramount (Young-Holt *et al.*, 2004).

Access and the regulatory route

Most developing countries have limited regulatory infrastructure, so that approval of products for marketing are heavily influenced by the US FDA and European Medicines Evaluation Agency (EMEA). As indicated above, this is keenly felt in the microbicide field, where the imposition of standards appropriate to a US domestic market contends with quite different profiles of risks in countries with high and escalating rates of AIDS incidence and prevalence.

A variety of efforts are under way to address this. The World Health Organization has convened several meetings to take up these issues (WHO, 2002) and the European Commission is considering an amendment (Article 58 of EEC Council Regulation No. 2309/93) to new legislation that would provide for accelerated access to review for products whose primary user populations are in developing countries (European Parliament, 2003). Finally, an ad hoc working group of representatives from the HIV vaccines, microbicides, malaria, and tuberculosis communities is launching a legislative initiative in the US Congress to accelerate the development of prevention technologies against global disease which includes language directing the US FDA to enter into the global dialogue on these issues (Prevention Technologies Working Group, 2004).

A common theme across these efforts and communities is to shape a new regulatory framework to extend the mandate of Northern regulators so that they can make decisions based on the needs of developing countries rather than solely on Northern domestic markets. Another shared theme is to extend the mandate of those countries in the South with those which do have a regulatory infrastructure capable of implementing review and approval processes that would be recognized in similarly placed low- and middle-income countries (Godwin, 2003; Milstein and Belgharbi, 2004).

Common Cause and Shared Learning

Among the most heartening circumstances as we enter the twenty-first century is the shared view that there is synergy to be gained by strategic collaborations between AIDS prevention and treatment and between HIV vaccines and topical microbicides. Not so long ago, HIV vaccines and topical microbicides were seen as inherently competitive, for pragmatic reasons and because they were seen as intrinsically distinct. Topical microbicides are, after all, designed to act directly against HIV, while vaccines act indirectly by stimulating immune responses to combat HIV infection (Gross and Johnston, 2003a).

Now, however, one is more likely to hear that much can be learned by exploring the ways in which HIV vaccines and microbicides can complement each other as parallel prevention technologies. The first formal acknowledgment of such parallelism appeared at the Microbicides 2002 International Conference in Antwerp, Belgium (Johnston, 2002); since then it has been increasingly recognized, in advocacy contexts and most recently in a thoughtful series of articles and public presentations (Johnston, 2002; Gross and Johnston, 2003a,b,c; Nixon, 2003). Table 8.4 compares the two technologies in terms of their breadth, duration, and onset of protection, possible mechanisms of action, potential for combination to achieve other health outcomes, and fundamental biology.

At the most basic level, research into the molecular and cellular mechanisms of viral attachment and fusion, cell-to-cell transfer, and intracellular penetration are pivotal in the design of both vaccines and microbicides (Gross and Johnston, 2003a). Also highly relevant for both technologies are ideas about how HIV enters the body through different mucosal tissues, the relative contributions of vaginal and anal intercourse in HIV acquisition, the specific kind and quality of HIV that can be transmitted sexually, the varying vulnerabilities among different virus types, and potentials for neutralization of virus (Huff, 2003). Understanding being acquired about cervical-vaginal and rectal biology and HIV transmission and dissemination from those mucosal surfaces in the course of microbicide development could also provide insight into viral transmission through breast milk to infant oral

Table 8.4 Topical microbicides and HIV vaccines: a tabular comparison.

Protective characteristics	Topical microbicides	HIV vaccines
Breadth of protection	Mucosal transmission Sexual Vertical? Cross-clade, cross-subtype?	Mucosal transmission Sexual Vertical? Parenteral Clade or subtype specific?
Duration of protection	Time-limited Reversible Optimize long-acting delivery	Longer term Immune responses to vectors interfere with 2nd generation? Evaluate need to boost
Onset of protection Possible mechanisms of action	Rapid Block infection Mitigate disease? Reduce transmission	Delayed Block infection Mitigate disease Reduce transmission
Combinations to achieve other health outcomes	Anti-STD Contraceptive and non-contraceptive	Multiple childhood immunizations Other adult vaccines
Fundamental biology	Molecular processes of attachment Inter-cellular dissemination Early replication	Molecular processes of attachment Inter-cellular dissemination Post-latency activation, replication, assembly

From Gross and Johnston (2003a).

mucosa or gastrointestinal tract (Gross and Johnston, 2003a); it could also illuminate development of other systems for delivering drugs across mucosal barriers (Huff, 2003).

But the terrain shared by HIV vaccines and microbicides goes beyond overlaps in the basic science. A reality often ignored is that HIV vaccines and microbicides, once developed, will provide protection for both males and females. And, since both technologies are likely to be partially effective, certainly in the earliest product generations, utilizing them sequentially or simultaneously is likely to offer additive or synergistic benefits, particularly in populations at risk of other STDs or emergent HIV subtypes (Gross and Johnston, 2003a). Both technologies bear the enduring burden of stigma and discrimination around HIV and both confront challenges in preclinical evaluation of combination products. Both face big challenges in clinical trials: limited research and regulatory capacity; difficulties in recruitment, retention, and follow-up of large, high-risk, HIV-negative cohorts;

the transcendent need for true community engagement; assuring appropriate standards of care during and after trials; lags in regulatory approvals; manufacture of pilot and bulk lots; concerns about liability; and a daunting number of issues around access and distribution (Nixon, 2003). Correspondingly, both technologies would profit from application of their joint energies to improving strategies for assuring truly informed consent and other aspects of ethical trial conduct; clarifying and streamlining requirements to speed safe passage of candidates into and through the human trials sequence; expediting regulatory licensing decisions; harmonizing and maybe regionalizing approval criteria; planning for post-market monitoring; and integrating efforts to enhance local-level research and research capacity (Gross and Johnston, 2003b).

What the Future Holds

In 1996 the AIDS Vaccine Advocacy Coalition (AVAC) began a countdown from then-President Clinton's statement of commitment to finding a vaccine against AIDS; in 2003, AVAC published its most recent assessment, entitled *Five Years and Counting*. A similar countdown for microbicides in 2003 might have been entitled *Ten Years and Counting* if we were to start from the first named investment by the US government in microbicide research and development, US$10 million in 1993. Or, the title might be *Six Years and Counting*, starting from the commitment made by then-Secretary of Health Shalala to invest US$25 million federal dollars a year for the next four years in microbicide research.

As we move more deeply into the twenty-first century in 2004, the first wave of trials of the effectiveness of post-N-9 candidate microbicides will be fielded; how many of those there will be remains undetermined at the time of this writing. It must be observed, nevertheless, that the premier US government-funded trial – the head-to-head trial of BufferGel and PRO2000 – is not a full-fledged Phase III trial of effectiveness. Rather, it is an intermediate-size Phase II/IIb or 'screening' trial for which support in the advocacy community is at best mixed, and no US government effectiveness trial is planned as of the present. As a result, the first hopes of attaining the earliest proofs of microbicides as a preventive concept will rest on the funding and implementation of other trials of other candidates.

This could be viewed as a rather bleak picture, especially when we contemplate the daily tally of new HIV infections worldwide. In the case of microbicides, however, we believe it is more appropriate to see a half-full glass. The field is more evolved, better resourced, informed by newer lines of scientific inquiry, and enriched by learning from HIV/AIDS therapeutics and vaccines. After years of being the 'Cinderella' of HIV technologies, microbicides as a preventive technology have been integrated into the expanding dialogue on how to develop and provide medical products needed for global public health. Dismissal of microbicides as mere 'jams and jellies' has become truly inappropriate, and peer-reviewed articles reporting on microbicide research and research issues have risen dramatically from the total of 78 between 1992 and 1997 to a total of almost 350 such articles between 1997 and 2002. The pipeline has expanded substantially and its internal structure has shifted. The financial resource base for the field has grown correspondingly and become broader and more diverse. The field is now buttressed by a much expanded, more tightly integrated global and national advocacy base with better-honed public relations skills resulting in a rough tripling in media coverage of microbicides in each year beginning in 1998. All this has paid off in funding increases, significant legislative initiatives, and greater public awareness about microbicides as an important addition to the armamentarium against HIV/AIDS (Harrison, 2003; Norick, 2003). Very importantly, microbicides and the science surrounding their development are appearing with greater regularity at major scientific meetings.

Finally, as noted above, insights from the basic research underpinning the development of microbicides, HIV vaccines, and therapeutics are becoming shared and mutually productive terrain. Collaboration in the development of infrastructure for clinical trials and in their design and implementation should also serve both technologies and the populations they are intended to benefit. And, in conclusion, it is important to record that HIV therapeutics and vaccines, microbicides, and the technologies required with similar urgency to combat malaria and tuberculosis are increasingly linked. Each day, science discovers more about the biological and pragmatic interrelationships among these three great global killers and, each day, the advocacy for all the different strategies needed to address them is becoming correspondingly and more effectively co-mingled.

References

Alliance for Microbicide Development *et al.* (2003) FDA Antiviral Drugs Advisory Committee Meeting. *Microbicide Q* 1: 1–6.

Anderson DJ, Politch JA, Tucker LD *et al.* (1998) Quantitation of mediators of inflammation and immunity in genital tract secretions and their relevance to HIV type 1 transmission. *AIDS Res Hum Retroviruses* 14: S43–S49.

Baltimore D (2002) Steering a course to an AIDS vaccine. *Science* 296: 2297.

Becker J, Dabash R, McGrory E *et al.* (2003) *Paving the Path: Preparing for Microbicide Introduction: Executive Summary.* New York: EngenderHealth.

Bollen LJM, Kilmarx PH, Wiwawongwana P (2002) *Photo Atlas for Microbicide Evaluation.* Bangkok: Thailand MOPH–US CDC Collaboration.

Bowcut JC (2003) Microbicide activity against non-HIV pathogens. *Microbicide Q* 1: 5–7.

Bugelski PJ, Ellens H, Hart TK, Kirsch RL (1991) Soluble CD4 and dextran sulphate mediate release of gp120 from HIV-1: Implications for clinical trials. *J Acquir Immune Defic Syndr* 4: 923–4.

CDC (Centers for Disease Control) (2001) *HIV/AIDS Surveillance Report, Year-end Edition 2001*, Vol. 13, No. 2. Atlanta, GA: Centers for Disease Control.

CDC (2003) HIV/AIDS Surveillance Reports, 1986–2001. In: Kates J *et al.*, eds. *Women and HIV AIDS: Key Facts.* Menlo Park, CA: Kaiser Family Foundation.

Chang TL, Chang CH, Simpson DA *et al.* (2003) Inhibition of HIV infectivity by a natural human isolate of *Lactobacillus jensenii* engineered to express functional two-domain. *Proc Natl Acad Sci USA* 100: 11672–7.

Cohen MS (1998) Sexually transmitted disease enhance HIV transmission: no longer a hypothesis. *Lancet* 351: 5–7.

Cole A, Lehrer RI (2003) Minidefensins: antimicrobial peptides with activity against HIV-1. *Curr Pharm Des* 9: 1463–73.

Cutler JC, Singh B, Utidjan HM *et al.* (1973) Development of a vaginal preparation providing both prophylaxis against venereal diseases and contraception. *Br J Vener Dis* 49: 149–50.

D'Cruz OJ, Dong Y, Uckun FM (2003) Potent dual anti-HIV and spermicidal activities of novel oxovanadium (V) complex with thiourea non-nucleoside inhibitors of HIV-1 reverse transcriptase. *Biochem Biophys Res Commun* 302: 253–64.

Dey B, Lerner DL, Lusso P *et al.* (2000) Multiple antiviral activities of cyanovirin-N: blocking of human immunodeficiency virus type 1 gp120 interaction with CD4 and coreceptor and inhibition of diverse enveloped viruses. *J Virol* 74: 4562–9.

Dragic T (2001) An overview of the determinants of CCR5 and CXCR4 co-receptor function. *J Gen Virol* 82: 1807–14.

Eng T, Butler W, eds (1996) *The Hidden Epidemic: Confronting Sexually Transmitted Diseases.* Washington, DC: National Academy Press for the Institute of Medicine.

Epstein H (2004) Why is AIDS worse in Africa? *Discover* (February).

European Parliament (2003) Council of the European Union. Amended proposal for a regulation of the European Parliament and of the Council laying down Community procedures for the authorisation and supervision of medicinal product for human and veterinary use and establishing a European Agency for the Evaluation of Medicinal Products. Brussels, 12 June 2003.

Fauci A (2003) HIV and AIDS: 20 years of science. *Nat Med* 9: 839–43.

Feldblum P (1992) *Developing Virucidal Compounds for Intravaginal Use in Preventing the Sexual Transmission of HIV.* New York: Population Council.

Fischer R, Twyman, RM, Schillberg S (2003) Production of antibodies in plants and their use for global health. *Vaccine* 21: 820–5.

Fleming D, Wasserheit J (1999) From epidemiological synergy to public health policy and practice: the contribution of other sexually transmitted diseases to sexual transmission of HIV infection. *Sex Transm Infect* 75: 3–17.

Foss AM, Vickerman PT, Heise L, Watts CH (2003) Shifts in condom use following microbicides introduction: should we be concerned? *AIDS* 17: 1227–37.

Galvin SR, Cohen MS (2004) The role of sexually transmitted diseases in HIV transmission. *Nat Rev Microbiol* 2: 33–42.

Gayle HD (2003) Curbing the global AIDS epidemic. *N Engl J Med* 348: 1802–5.

Godwin J (2003) HIV vaccines, microbicides and treatments: Developing an agenda for action – a discussion paper. Canadian HIV/AIDS Legal Network, Montreal.

Greenhead P, Hayes P, Watts PS, Laing KG, Griffin GE, Shattock RJ (2000) Parameters of human immunodeficiency virus infection of human cervical tissue and inhibition by vaginal virucides. *J Virol* 74: 5577–86.

Gross M, Johnston PI (2003a) HIV vaccines and topical microbicides: a complementary combination. *Microbicide Q* 1: 5–9.

Gross M, Johnston PI (2003b) HIV vaccines and topical microbicides: a complementary combination – Part 2: Shared regulatory considerations. *Microbicide Q* 1: 8–12.

Gross M, Johnston PI (2003c) HIV vaccines and topical microbicides: distinctive regulatory considerations. *Microbicide Q* 1: 10–14.

Haase AT (2001) The pathogenesis of sexual mucosal transmission and early stages of infection: obstacles and a narrow window of opportunity for prevention. *AIDS* 15 (Suppl 1): S10–S15.

Harrison PF (1982) Mothers in distress. *CoEvolution Q* 36: 26–31.

Harrison PF (2003) By way of introduction. *Microbicide Q* 1: 1–4.

Harrison PF, Rosenberg Z, Bowcut JC (2003) Topical microbicides for disease prevention: status and challenges. *Clin Infect Dis* 36: 1290–4.

Hearst N, Chen S (2003) Condoms for AIDS prevention in the developing world: A review of the scientific literature. Unpublished paper, University of California, San Francisco.

Howson CP, Harrison PF, Hotra D, Law M, eds (1996) *In her Lifetime: Female Morbidity and Mortality in Sub-Saharan Africa*. Washington, DC: National Academy Press, for the Institute of Medicine.

Hu W, Watts P, Frank I *et al.* (2004) Blockade of attachment and fusion receptors inhibits HIV-1 infection of human cervical tissue. Paper presented at the 11th Retrovirus Conference, San Francisco, CA.

Huff B (2003) Women, men, and microbicides. *GMHC Treatment Issues* 17, September 2003.

Johnston PI (2002) Plenary presentation: mucosal vaccines and microbicides – similarities and differences: lessons (to be) learned. Microbicides 2002 Conference, Antwerp, Belgium, 13 May 2002.

Keller MJ, Klotman ME, Herold BC (2003) Rigorous pre-clinical evaluation of topical microbicides to prevent transmission of human immunodeficiency virus. *J Antimicrob Chemother* 51: 1009–102.

Kempf C, Jentsch P, Barré-Sinoussi F *et al.* (1991) Inactivation of human immunodeficiency virus (HIV) by low pH and pepsin. *J Acquir Immune Defic Syndr* 4: 828–9.

Ketas TJ, Klasse PJ, Spenlehauer C *et al.* (2003) Entry inhibitors SCH-C, RANTES, and T-20 block HIV type 1 replication in multiple cell types. *AIDS Res Hum Retroviruses* 19: 177–86.

Khanna K, Whaley KJ, Zeitlin L *et al.* (2002) Vaginal transmission of cell-associated HIV-1 in the mouse is blocked by a topical, membrane-modifying agent. *J Clin Invest* 109: 205–11.

Klebanoff S, Hillier S, Eschenbach D, Waltersdorph A (1991) Control of the microbial flora of the vagina by H_2O_2-generating lactobacilli. *J Infect Dis* 164: 94–100.

Kreiss J, Ngugi E, Holmes K *et al.* (1992) Efficacy of nonoxynol-9 contraceptive sponge use in preventing heterosexual acquisition of HIV in Nairobi prostitutes. *JAMA* 268: 477–82.

Lard-Whiteford SL, Litterst C, Matecka D, O'Rear JJ, Reichelderfer P, Yuen I (2004) Recommendations for the non-clinical development of topical microbicides for prevention of human immunodeficiency virus transmission. *J AIDS* 36: 541–52.

Leclerc A, Frost E, Collet M *et al.* (1988) Urogenital chlamydia trachomatis in Gabon: an unrecognized epidemic. *Genitour Med* 64: 308–11.

Malkovsky M, Newell Al, Dalgleish A (1988) Inactivation of HIV by nonoxynol-9. *Lancet* 1: 654.

Martin HL, Richardson BA, Nyange PM *et al.* (1999) Vaginal lactobacilli, microbial flora, and risk of human immunodeficiency virus type 1 and sexually transmitted disease acquisition. *J Infect Dis* 180: 1863–8.

Marx P, Spira AI, Gettie A *et al.* (1996) Progesterone implants enhance SIV vaginal transmission and early virus load. *Nat Med* 2: 1084–9.

Mauck C, Rosenberg Z, Van Damme L (2001) Recommendations for the clinical development of topical microbicides: an update. *AIDS* 15: 857–68.

Mauck C, Baker JM, Birnkrant DB *et al.* (2000) The use of colposcopy in assessing vaginal irritation in research. *AIDS* 14: 2221–7.

Mayer K, Peipert J, Fleming T *et al.* (2001) Safety and tolerability of BufferGel, a novel vaginal microbicide, in women in the United States. *Clin Infect Dis* 32: 476–82.

Mayer K, Karim SA, Kelly C, Maslankowski L *et al.* (2003) Safety and tolerability of vaginal PRO2000 gel in sexually active HIV-uninfected and abstinent HIV-infected women. *AIDS* 17: 321–9.

McMichael AJ, Hanke T (2003) HIV vaccines 1983–2003. *Nat Med* 9: 874–80.

Meekers D (1999) Patterns of use of the female condom in urban Zimbabwe (Research Division Working Paper No. 28). Population Services International, Washington, DC.

Microbicide Initiative, Science Working Group (2002) *The Science of Microbicides: Accelerating Development.* New York: Rockefeller Foundation.

Miller CJ, Shattock RJ (2003) Target cells in vaginal HIV transmission. *Microbes Infect* 5: 59–67.

Miller CJ, Alexander NJ, Sutjipto S *et al.* (1989) Genital mucosal transmission of simian immunodeficiency virus: animal model for heterosexual transmission of human immunodeficiency virus. *J Virol* 63: 4277–84.

Milstein B (2001) *Introduction to the Syndemics Prevention Network.* Atlanta: Centers for Disease Control and Prevention.

Milstein J, Belgharbi L (2004) Regulatory pathways for vaccines for developing countries. *Bull WHO* 82: 128–32.

Moench TR, Chipato T, Padian NS (2001) Preventing disease by protecting the cervix: the unexplored promise of internal vaginal barrier devices. *AIDS* 15: 1595–602.

Moore JP, Doms RW (2003) The entry of entry inhibitors: a fusion of science and medicine. *Proc Natl Acad Sci USA* 100: 10598–602.

Moore JP, Shattock RJ (2003) Preventing HIV-1 sexual transmission – not sexy enough science, or no benefit to the bottom line? *J Antimicrob Chemother* 52: 890–2.

Moore JP, Kitchen SG, Pugach P, Zack JA (2004) The CCR5 and CXCR4 coreceptors – central to understanding the transmission and pathogenesis of human immunodeficiency virus type 1 infection. *AIDS Res Hum Retroviruses* 20: 111–26.

Moriuchi M, Moriuchi H, Williams R, Straus SE (2000) Herpes simplex virus infection induces replication of human immunodeficiency virus type 1. *Virology* 278: 534–40.

Moriyama A, Shimoya K, Ogata I *et al.* (1999) Secretory leukocyte protease inhibitor (SLPI) concentrations in cervical mucus of women with normal menstrual cycle. *Mol Hum Reprod* 5, 656–61.

Mostad SB, Overbaugh J, DeVange DM *et al.* (1997) Hormonal contraception, vitamin A deficiency, and other risk factors for shedding of HIV-1 infected cells from the cervix and vagina. *Lancet* 350: 922–7.

Moulard M, Lortat-Jacob H, Mondor I *et al.* (2000) Selective interactions of polyanions with basic surfaces on human immunodeficiency virus type 1 gp120. *J Virol* 74: 1948–60.

NIAID (National Institute of Allergy and Infectious Diseases) (1997) *Topical Microbicides Program: Update 1997.* Bethesda, MD: National Institutes of Health.

NIAID (2004) AIDS Research Advisory Committee Meeting, 26 January 2004.

Nixon S (2003) Why invest in both microbicides and vaccines? Presentation at Canadian Microbicides Symposium, Ottawa, Canada, 30 October 2003.

Nobile C, Moris A, Porrot F *et al.* (2003) Inhibition of human immunodeficiency virus type 1 env-mediated fusion by DC-SIGN. *J Virol* 77: 5313–23.

Norick P (2003) The microbicide legislative and policy agenda: evolution and present status. *Microbicide Q* 1: 19–20.

Otten RA, Adams DR, Kim CN *et al.* (2004) Cellulose acetate phthalate protects macaques from multiple, low-dose vaginal exposures with an SHIV virus: new strategy to study HIV pre-clinical interventions in non-human primates. 11th Retrovirus Conference, San Francisco, CA.

Over M, Piot P (1993) HIV infection and sexually transmitted diseases. In: Jamison DT, Mosely WH, Measham A, Bobadilla J, eds. *Disease Control Priorities in Developing Countries*. New York: Oxford University Press, for the World Bank, pp. 555–28.

Panos Institute (1989) *AIDS and Children: a Family Disease*. London: Panos Institute.

Phillips DM, Zacharopoulos VR (1998) Nonoxynol-9 enhances rectal infection by herpes simplex virus in mice. *Contraception* 57: 341–8.

Phillips DM, Taylor CL, Zacharopoulos VR, Maguire RA (2000) Nonoxynol-9 causes rapid exfoliation of sheets of rectal epithelium. *Contraception* 62: 149–54.

Pope M, Haase AT (2003) Transmission, acute HIV-1 infection and the quest for strategies to prevent infection. *Nat Med* 9: 847–52.

Pharmaco-Economics Working Group of the Microbicide Initiative (2001) *The Economics of Microbicide Development: A Case for Investment*. New York: Rockefeller Foundation.

Prevention Technologies Working Group (2004) *The Project BioHealth Act of 2004*. Washington, DC: Prevention Technologies Working Group.

Priestley CJ, Jones BM, Dhar J, Goodwin L (1997) What is normal vaginal flora? *Gen Intern Med* 197: 23–8.

Roddy R, Zekeng L, Ryan KA, Tamoufe U, Tweedy KG (1998) A controlled trial of nonoxynol-9 film to reduce male-to-female transmission of sexually transmitted diseases. *N Engl J Med* 399: 504–10.

Roddy R, Zekeng L, Ryan K *et al.* (2002) Effect of nonoxynol-9 on urogenital gonorrhoea and chlamydial infection. *JAMA* 287: 1117–22.

Roehr B, Gross M, Mayer K (2002) Creating a research and development agenda for rectal microbicides that protect against HIV infection. Report from the Workshop, 7–8 June 2000 (Baltimore, MD) www.amfar.org/binary-data/AMFARPUBLICATION/download_file/28.pdf

Sattentau QJ, Weise RA (1988) The CD-4 antigen: physiological ligand and HIV receptor. *Cell* 52: 631–2.

Shattock R (2003) The rationale for combination microbicides: viral and cellular targets. *Microbicide Q* 1: 1–5.

Shattock R, Moore JP (2003) Inhibiting sexual transmission of HIV-1 transmission. *Nat Rev Micro* 1: 25–34.

Singer M, Clair S (2003) Syndemics and public health: reconceptualizing disease in bio-social context. *Med Anthropol Q* 17: 423–41.

Smith SM, Mefford M, Klase Z, Alexander N, Hess D, Marx PA (2004) Topical estrogen protects against SIV vaginal transmission without evidence of systemic effect. Paper presented at the 11th Retrovirus Conference, San Francisco, CA.

Stein Z (1990) Methods women can use. *Am J Public Health* 80: 460–2.

Stevenson M (2003) HIV-1 pathogenesis. *Nat Med* 9: 853–60.

Stoger E, Sack M, Fischer R *et al.* (2002) Plantibodies: applications, advantages and bottlenecks. *Curr Opin Biotechnol* 13: 161–6.

Stone A (2002) Microbicides: a new approach to preventing HIV and other sexually transmitted infections. *Nat Rev Drug Discovery* 1: 977–85.

Stone A (2003) Clinical trials of microbicides. *Microbicide Q* 1: 13–18.

Temmerman M, K'Oduol K, Plummer FA *et al.* (1992) Maternal HIV infection as a risk factor for adverse obstetrical outcome. *Int Conf AIDS* 8(2) pC283, abstract PoC 4232.

Trkola AB, Pomales H, Yuan B *et al.* (1995) Cross-clade neutralization of primary isolates of human immunodeficiency virus type 1 by human monoclonal antibodies and tetrameric CD4 IgG. *J Virol* 69: 6609–17.

Turpin JA (2002) Considerations and development of topical microbicides to inhibit the sexual transmission of HIV. *Expert Opin Investig Drugs* 11: 1077–97.

UNAIDS (1996) The status and trends of global HIV/AIDS pandemic. Official Satellite Symposium, 5–6 July 1996 Report. UNAIDS. 28 November 1996.

UNAIDS/WHO (2002) *AIDS Epidemic Update.* Geneva: UNAIDS, December.

United Nations Development Program (UNDP) (1993) *Young Women: Silence, Susceptibility and the HIV Epidemic.* New York: UNDP HIV and Development Program.

University of Toronto Joint Centre for Bioethics (2002) Top 10 biotechnologies for improving health in developing countries. Toronto, Program in Applied Ethics and Biotechnology, Canadian Program on Genomics and Global Health.

Vallor AC, Antonio MAD, Hawes SE *et al.* (2001) Factors associated with acquisition of, or persistent colonization by, vaginal lactobacilli: role of hydrogen peroxide production. *J Infect Dis* 184: 1431–6.

Van Damme L *et al.* (2000) Safety of multiple daily applications of COL-1492, a nonoxynol-9 vaginal gel, among female sex workers. *AIDS* 14, 85–88.

Van Damme L *et al.* (2002) Effectiveness of COL-1492, a nonoxynol-9 vaginal gel, on HIV-1 transmission in female sex workers: a randomized controlled trial. *Lancet* 360: 971–7.

Veazey RS, Shattock RJ, Pope M *et al.* (2003) Prevention of virus transmission to macaque monkeys by a vaginally applied monoclonal antibody to HIV-1 gp120. *Nat Med* 9: 343–6.

Veazey R, Offord R, Hartley O *et al.* (2004) Intravaginal PSC-RANTES protects against vaginal transmission of SHIV162P to macaques; implications for HIV microbicide strategies and pathogenesis. Paper presented at the 11th Retrovirus Conference, San Francisco, CA, February 2004.

Walker BD, Korber BT (2001) Immune control of HIV: the obstacles of HLA and viral diversity. *Nat Immun* 2: 473–5.

Wasserheit JN (1989) The significance and scope of reproductive tract infections among Third World women. *Int J Gynecol Obstet* (Suppl) 3: 145–68.

Wasserheit JN (1992) Epidemiological synergy: interrelationships between human immunodeficiency virus infection and other sexually transmitted diseases. *Sex Trans Dis* 19: 61–77.

Watts C, Kuraranayake L, Vickerman P, Terris-Prestholt F (2002) *The Public Health Benefits of Microbicides in Lower-income Countries: Model Projections.* New York: Rockefeller Foundation.

Wilkinson D, Ramjee G, Rutherford G (2002) Nonoxynol-9 spermicide for prevention of HIV and other sexually transmitted infections: systematic review and meta-analysis of randomised controlled trials. In: *Microbicides 2002*, Antwerp, Belgium. Abstract 5, Alliance for Microbicide Development, Silver Spring, MD, USA. http://www.itg.nbe/micro2002/Pages/Abstracts.html (accessed 20 March 2003).

WHO (World Health Organization) (1990/1996) *Global Prevalence and Incidence of Selected Curable Sexually Transmitted Infections.* Geneva: WHO, Department of HIV/AIDS.

WHO (1990) Sexually transmitted infections increasing by 250 million annually. Press release, 20 December 1990. WHO, Geneva.

WHO (2002) International regulatory issues in microbicide development: Preliminary Report from a WHO Consultation, Villars-sur-Ollon, Vaud, Switzerland, 4–6 March 2002. Unpublished document.

WHO/CONRAD (Contraceptive Research and Development) Program (2000) *Manual for the Standardization of Colposcopy for the Evaluation of Vaginal Products.* WHO/RHR/00.11–CONRAD/2000.1. Geneva: World Health Organization.

WHO/CONRAD (2002) *WHO/CONRAD Technical Consultation on Nonoxynol-9.* Geneva: World Health Organization.

World Bank (1993) *World Development Report 1993: Investing in Health.* New York: Oxford University Press.

Young Holt B *et al.* (2004) In press.

Zeitlin L, Olmsted SS, Moench TR *et al.* (1998) A humanized monoclonal antibody produced in transgenic plants for immunoprotection of the vagina against genital herpes. *Nat Biotech* 16: 1361–4.

Zwick MB, Wang M, Poignard P *et al.* (2001) Neutralization synergy of human immunodeficiency virus type 1 primary isolates by cocktails of broadly neutralizing antibodies. *J Virol* 75: 12198–208.

AIDS Behavioral Prevention: Unprecedented Progress and Emerging Challenges

9

Willo Pequegnat
Associate Director, Structural and International HIV/STD Prevention Programs of the Center for Mental Health Research on AIDS, National Institute of Mental Health, Bethesda, USA

Willo Pequegnat, PhD is Associate Director of the Center for Mental Health Research on AIDS at the National Institutes of Health (NIH). As the Senior Prevention Scientist, Dr. Pequegnat has primary responsibility for a wide range of national and international projects in behavioral preventive interventions, neuropsychological assessment, stress and coping, mental and physical functioning, and quality of life. She is a Principal Investigator (Staff Collaborator) on several NIMH studies including the Collaborative HIV/STD Prevention Trial in China, India, Peru, Russia, and Zimbabwe, the Multisite HIV Prevention Trial with African American Couples and the NIMH Healthy Living Project with HIV+ men and women. She plans and implements workshops, conferences, and national and international symposia, and represents NIMH on science policy-making committees and workgroups on a broad range of HIV/STD issues. She received her PhD in Clinical Psychology from the State University of New York.

In many areas of the world, the AIDS epidemic is out of control; unfortunately, developing countries with few economic resources are hardest hit with large increases in HIV incidence. People in the prime of life are most affected and as the epidemic matures, infection moves from the original high-risk groups to a broader cross-section of society and individuals become infected with HIV at younger ages (Gayle, 2000). The generation that should be parenting the next generation and participating actively in the workforce is experiencing the highest infection rates because AIDS has most severely affected people between the ages of 25 and 44 (CDC, 2004). In some African villages, there are primarily grandparents and children because the parent generation has died of AIDS. Tragically, all the gains made in the past 30 years in life span have been wiped out by HIV disease in many sub-Saharan countries where the life expectancy has again fallen to less than 40 years old. In countries with a long history of AIDS, a new phenomenon of child-headed households is emerging with unknown consequences for the children and for the social and economic well-being of those countries (Foster, 1998).

Prevention is still the only effective way to stem an even more devastating epidemic.

Progress in AIDS Prevention Science

In 1983 four US investigator-initiated HIV-related behavioral grants totaling US$200 000 were supported out of the US National Institute of Mental Health (NIMH) Director's discretionary fund (Miller *et al.*, 1990). The research in behavioral prevention rapidly accelerated and, by 1997, there was so much data from randomized controlled trials that the National Institutes of Health (NIH) held a Consensus Development Conference on Interventions to Prevent HIV Risk Behaviors. The Consensus Conference is a mechanism established by Congress to evaluate behavioral and biomedical research to determine whether the drug, technology, or intervention are ready to be implemented in public health agencies (NIH, 1997). The Consensus Conference is the closest mechanism that the US has to a Supreme Court for science. This was the first behavioral intervention selected for this format and it was based on a corpus of work that spanned only 12 years. The panel declared, 'Preventive interventions are effective for reducing behavioral risk for HIV/AIDS and must be widely disseminated' (NIH, 1997; NIH Consensus Development Conference Panel, 2000).

What accounts for this impressive advancement in behavioral prevention research? What are the challenges in mounting a scaled up behavioral prevention program internationally? What are emerging areas for future research? These questions will be addressed in this chapter.

Health Psychology Jumpstarted HIV/Sexually Transmitted Disease (STD) Prevention

In 1983, the US government held its first meeting of all agencies concerned about health to evaluate what should be done about the virus that was then known as HTLV-III. While the route of transmission was not yet understood, it was clear that there was a social and behavioral component. Therefore, Federal agencies

237

that had expertise in behavioral research were invited to participate. Investigators in behavioral medicine had been conducting research on the intersect between health and behavior since the late 1950s. Many of these strategies were based on social cognitive theories and they were quickly adapted by the first wave of researchers who moved into conducting HIV/STD prevention research.

While there were behavioral techniques that could be adapted to HIV prevention, investigators were initially hampered because there was a limited data base on sexual behaviors that put people at risk for HIV and understanding of the determinants of specific risky behaviors was poor. There was also minimal standardization in assessment instruments, especially for the subpopulations who were at greatest risk for HIV infection. Further, it was difficult to attract researchers into an AIDS research career because there was a perception of funding instability and stigma associated with the disease.

The initial period of HIV/AIDS research was characterized by overcoming these problems by conducting multiple KAB (knowledge, attitudes, behaviors) studies to identify the lifestyle of HIV symptomatic individuals and legitimizing AIDS as a research area. In 1985 when the ELISA test was developed so that asymptomatic individuals with HIV infection could be identified before they exhibited signs of the disease, investigators concentrated on adapting social cognitive approaches to prevent seronegative people from becoming infected.

Theoretical Framework for Prevention

The hallmark for HIV/STD behavioral prevention research has been its grounding in sound theory (Herek, 1995). All empirical research is based on assumptions – the challenge is to make those assumptions explicit so that interventions can be designed that permit those assumptions to be evaluated and modified.

In 1992, NIMH convened a meeting of the investigators whose theories of behavior change were used in the early years of AIDS prevention research: (1) health belief (Becker, 1988); (2) theory of reasoned action (Fishbein, 1980); (3) self-regulation and self-control (Kanfer, 1987); (4) social cognitive learning (Bandura, 1989, 1991); and (5) subjective culture and interpersonal relations (Triandis, 1980). They identified the following eight common factors that they believed can account for most of the variance in any given behavior: (1) intentions; (2) skills; (3) environmental constraints; (4) anticipated outcomes; (5) norms; (6) self-standards; (7) emotion, and (8) self-efficacy (Fishbein *et al.*, 1992; Fishbein, 1997).

Of the eight constructs, the first three were determined to be necessary and sufficient for bringing about behavior change. For example, a man who has decided to use a condom every time with casual partners (intentions), knows how to use the condom correctly (skills), and has a non-expired condom in his pocket when he decides to have sex (environmental constraint) will probably be successful.

The other five factors will influence how strongly and in what direction his intention for engaging in safer HIV/STD-related behaviors will be.

In addition to the theory-based approach, strengths of the HIV/STD prevention approach have been the utilization of a model of behavioral phases of research and a multiple level causal model. These phases and levels will be described and examples of research will be cited in the next two sections.

Phases of Behavioral Prevention Research

A model of phases of research that is methodologically similar to drug trials has been utilized: Phase I (discovery); Phase II (exploratory); Phase III (efficacy); and Phase IV (effectiveness) studies (Figure 9.1). This approach permitted better monitoring of the status of the research and advancement to clinical trials as rapidly as possible. This model also encouraged closing the gap between research and practice.

Phase I: Discovery Phase of Behavioral Prevention Research

Behavioral epidemiologic studies were conducted in Phase I to discover the knowledge, attitudes, and behaviors (KAB) of population-based samples. Surveys and

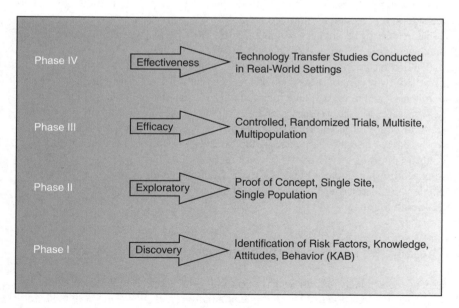

Fig. 9.1 Phases of behavioral prevention research.

qualitative methods were used to gain a more in-depth understanding of the determinants and antecedents of risk behaviors and the context in which they were occurring (Pequegnat *et al.*, 1995).

The data identified in this phase of research clarifies how different groups become infected with HIV and suggests intervention directions. For example, people living with HIV/AIDS due to male-to-male sexual contact rose by 20 per cent and heterosexual contact by 28 per cent between 1999 and 2002, while cases due to injection drug use in men only rose by 11 per cent. Among women living with HIV/AIDS heterosexual contact increased by 27 per cent but that attributed to injection drug use only grew by 12 per cent (CDC, 2004). Another example, is a study conducted by Choi and Catania (1996) at two different time points. Males were consistently more risky than women in three types of behavioral choices: (1) multiple partners; (2) more risky partners; and (3) not consistently using condoms. The gender and behavioral data in these two studies suggest the design of different prevention strategies even though each would target increased condom use (Szapocznik and Pequegnat, 1995).

Phase II: Exploratory Phase of Behavioral Prevention Research

When the initial HIV/STD risk factors are identified, the problem is explored in greater depth in Phase II studies and an intervention is designed to change the risk behaviors. These are usually single-site, single-population studies of moderate size to test the intervention concept.

There has been concern about effective HIV/STD prevention messages for adolescents. Jemmott and colleagues (1998) conducted a randomized trial with 659 African American 6th and 7th grade students in public schools to test the effects of two types of messages: abstinence and safer sex. The students were randomly assigned to one of three interventions: (1) the abstinence-based intervention; (2) the safer sex intervention; and (3) a general health promotion intervention (control condition). Adolescents in the abstinence intervention were less likely to report having sexual intercourse in the three months after intervention than were control condition participants, but not at 6- or 12-month follow-ups. Safer sex intervention participants reported more frequent condom use at all follow-ups and less unprotected sexual intercourse at three-month follow-up, but not at the 6- or 12-month follow-ups.

Phase III: Efficacy Phase of Behavioral Prevention Research

Having determined that an intervention will work, large randomized, controlled trials (RCTs) are conducted in multiple populations and sites using both behavioral and biological outcomes (Fishbein and Pequegnat, 2000; Pequegnat *et al.*, 2000).

The NIMH Multisite HIV Prevention Trial (Project Light) was a randomized, controlled, double-blind, study of a seven-session risk-reduction intervention based on the theory of behavior change versus a one-session state-of-the art counseling session (NIMH, 1998). A total of 3706 understudied and disadvantaged African American and Hispanic men and women were recruited from 37 STD clinics and primary health care clinics across the US. When the study was initiated, many people were skeptical that a social cognitive skills-based prevention program would work with low socio-economic status (SES) people.

People in the seven-session intervention reported significantly fewer unprotected sexual acts, had higher levels of condom use, and were more likely to use condoms consistently at the 12-month follow-up. The intervention also reduced in half the incidence of gonorrhea in men. If these behavioral changes were maintained for even one year, there would be a profound, cost-effective, public health impact in the communities that adopted this program (Holtgrave and Pinkerton, 2002).

Phase IV: Effectiveness Phase of Behavioral Prevention Research

Phase IV studies test how effective prevention programs are when delivered in public health clinics under real-life conditions. The tight controls of a randomized clinical trial are relaxed and the program is delivered by personnel committed to service not research. This is a critical and often overlooked step in putting an effective program into public health clinics where the interventions will stop the further spread of HIV/STDs (Kelly *et al.*, 2000a,b,c).

In a study by Kelly and colleagues (2000a,b,c), an intervention was conducted in collaboration with AIDS service organizations (ASOs) in 44 US cities to test which of different dissemination interventions effectively help organizations adopt the model and make it a part of their regular service program. The three different conditions were: (1) detailed procedural manuals and videos that could be used by the staff to learn how to offer the HIV prevention program; (2) the same manuals, videos, and procedural manuals; and in addition, their staff attended a two-day training workshop; and (3) the manuals, videos, procedure manuals, workshop and in a series of six-monthly consultation calls with the AIDS prevention researchers to problem-solve implementation of the intervention by the staff of the ASO. The results demonstrated that ASOs in the third condition were more likely to adopt the evidence-based intervention as a program.

This study has been replicated in 80 countries with non-governmental organizations (NGOs), who were randomized to either receive the intervention/manual and initial training or the intervention/manual, initial training, and on-going consultation on the internet during implementation. These results corroborate the original study (Kelly *et al.*, 2004).

241

Having described the phases of behavioral prevention research, the following section will describe some of the decisions in designing these successful prevention programs.

Levels of Prevention

In order to prevent an HIV/STD epidemic, individuals must change their risky behaviors. However, the intervention *per se* does not need to be delivered to the individual and interventions at multiple levels are necessary to mount an AIDS prevention social movement: individual, couple, family, community, and societal (Pequegnat and Stover, 2000; Waldo and Coates, 2000).

In addition to identifying the most effective level to introduce the prevention program, the developmental level and gender of the target population must be considered. If a pre-adolescent is not yet sexually active, a prevention program delivered to the parents that gives them the skills to help their children delay their sexual debut is appropriate. If the adolescent is sexually active, then an abstinence or sexual education program would be more appropriate. Prevention programs for a young adult couple would focus on condom skills and negotiating safer behaviors (Figure 9.2).

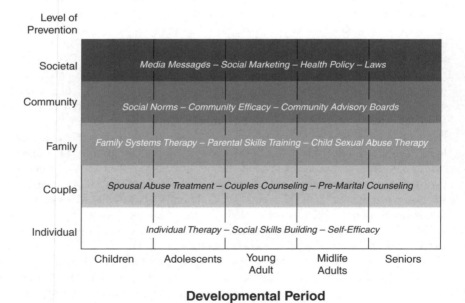

Fig. 9.2 Lifespan model for health promotion and disease prevention.

Individual-level Interventions

Multiple studies were conducted with individuals: adolescents (Rotheram-Borus *et al.*, 1991; Jemmott *et al.*, 1992; St. Lawrence *et al.*, 1995); young adults (Fisher *et al.*, 1996; O'Leary, 1999); women (Hobfoll *et al.*, 1994; Kelly *et al.*, 1994; DiClemente and Wingood, 1995; Kalichman *et al.*, 1996; Carey *et al.*, 1997; Belcher *et al.*, 1998); gay men (Valdiserri *et al.*, 1989; Peterson *et al.*, 1997; Roffman *et al.*, 1997); men (O'Donnell *et al.*, 1998; Celentano *et al.*, 2000; Bing, 2004); and the homeless and mentally ill (Nyamathi *et al.*, 1993; Carey *et al.*, 1995; Susser *et al.*, 1995; Kalichman *et al.*, 1995; Kelly, 1997; Kelly *et al.*, 1997b). For reviews of the individual-level interventions for these populations, see Kelly (2000) (gay or bisexual men and youth); Jemmott and Jemmott (2000) (heterosexual adolescents); Ehrhardt and Exner (2000) (women); and Rotheram-Borus *et al.* (2000) (heterosexuals).

Based on these studies, two significant Phase III studies were conducted that demonstrated efficacy with individuals: Project Light and Project Respect. (Project Light was discussed in the section on Phase III studies above.) Project Respect was a multisite randomized controlled trial that evaluated the relative efficacy of three interventions based on social cognitive theory with 5872 HIV-negative participants recruited from clinics (Kamb *et al.*, 1998). They were randomly assigned to receive one of the following: (1) two HIV education sessions; (2) two sessions aimed at increasing risk perception and condom use; or (3) four sessions of enhanced, skill-focused sessions. At three-month follow-up, 44 per cent of participants who received the brief two-session counseling and 46 per cent of those who received the enhanced four-session interventions were more likely to report no unprotected intercourse than those who received the risk education alone (38 per cent). These results were corroborated by the 30 per cent lower incidence of new STDs among brief and enhanced counseling participants as compared to controls.

Based on this corpus of HIV/STD prevention research, the essential components of an individual-level intervention are: perception of individual risk, opportunities to develop risk-reduction skills (condom use, negotiating safer sex), opportunities to practice role playing new behaviors *in vitro*, and weekly goals to practice new skills *in vivo*.

These components based on social cognitive approaches have been primarily used for individual behavior change. Couples and families, however, involve more complex relationships and require models that integrate communication and negotiation among multiple systems.

Couple-level Interventions

The predominant mode of HIV transmission worldwide is heterosexual intercourse and a mixed serostatus couple presents a major risk. A series of studies with couples provides compelling evidence of the utility of interventions at this level. In a study examining couples, Allen and colleagues (1992) offered a confidential HIV testing and condom program with 1458 childbearing women in Rwanda. While not originally designed as a couples study, 26 per cent of the male partners volunteered to view the educational video tape and receive an HIV test. Couples in whom both partners were tested were twice as likely to use condoms. The man's participation was also associated with significant reductions in HIV and gonorrhea rates among the women. Of concern was the finding that seropositive women with untested partners comprised the group least likely to use condoms, and the rate of HIV seroconversion in this group was more than twice that for women whose partners were tested and received counseling. The strongest predictors of condom use were a seropositive test result in the woman and HIV testing and counseling of the male partner.

Padian and her colleagues (1993) corroborated these results in a longitudinal intervention with mixed serostatus couples. Although the study did not use a control group design, these data suggest a positive impact of this kind of an intervention focused on skills building around condom use, development of better social skills and social support, and role plays of problem-solving on how to implement safer sexual behavior strategies. The proportion of couples reporting consistent condom use increased from 49 per cent at baseline to 88 per cent at follow-up. Among those couples at the 16-month follow-up no seronegative partner had become positive.

De Vincenzi and colleagues (1994) provide additional evidence for couple-level approaches in a study that delivered counseling and testing sessions every six months to mixed serostatus couples (196 women and 108 men). While it was a couple-level intervention, the outcome was focused on the 304 negative partners: 48.5 per cent of the couples used condoms consistently and despite a total of about 15 000 episodes of intercourse, no seronegative partners became infected; among those who did not consistently use condoms, 4.8 per cent seroconverted.

The final study is a randomized, controlled study of counseling and testing with both individuals and sexual partner dyads conducted in Kenya, Tanzania, and Trinidad with approximately 4000 participants (Voluntary HIV-1 Counseling and Testing Efficacy Study Group, 2000). They were randomly assigned to either counseling and testing intervention or to a health education control group. The proportion of HIV counseling and testing particpants who reported unprotected intercourse with non-primary partners declined by 35 per cent, relative to a reduction of 13 per cent among controls at the seven-month follow-up.

The results from these studies strongly support the efficacy of couples-level interventions, especially those combining counseling and testing in mixed serostatus couples. Many of the evidence-based individual prevention programs could be adapted for couples.

Family-level Interventions

In the first decade of AIDS research, most prevention efforts focused on the individual, but for every seropositive person, there is a constellation of family and friends who are also affected. Family members can play a role in preventing and adapting to HIV/AIDS by delaying initiation of sexual behaviors, engendering safer HIV/STD behaviors, and improving treatment adherence and quality of life (Pequegnat and Szapocznik, 2000).

Using Bronfenbrenner's (1979) ecological approach, Szapocznik and colleagues (2004) conducted a study to test the efficacy of Structural Ecosystems Therapy (SET), in decreasing HIV/STD risk in a sample of 209 HIV-seropositive, urban, low-income women by improving the psychosocial functioning of her family. SET is an intervention designed to restructure the patterns of relationships in a family to reduce stress and risky behaviors (e.g. using drugs and unprotected sex). The women were randomized into one of three conditions: SET, attention–comparison person-centered condition or a community control condition. Results of growth curve analyses over five time points revealed that SET was more efficacious than either of the control conditions in reducing psychological distress and family-related hassles. However, contrary to hypotheses, SET was not more efficacious in increasing family support. Latent growth mixture modeling analyses indicated that SET was most efficacious for women who, on average, were at or near the clinical threshold for psychological distress and for women with high levels of family hassles.

In a family study in two public housing complexes, 272 parents were randomly assigned to one of two conditions: (1) one group received the information packet covering all aspects of parental training and parent training sessions about how to talk to their children about HIV/AIDS and sex and (2) the other group received the information packet covering all aspects of the parent training (Krauss *et al.*, 2000). At baseline both groups of children reported similar levels of intentions to use condoms when they became sexually active. At the outcome assessment children whose parents received the training had significantly stronger intentions to use condoms and had fewer HIV-related worries (Krauss *et al.*, 1997a, b).

Family interventions can be effective because families exercise social control over their members and they can deliver HIV/AIDS prevention messages at teachable moments.

Community-level Behavioral Prevention Studies

In areas that currently have low HIV/STD prevalence but face an imminent increase, community-level HIV prevention approaches can be effective in stemming the further spread of HIV/STDs. These approaches target vulnerable at-risk segments of the community and attempt to reduce the prevalence and frequency of high-risk HIV/STD-related behaviors in these populations. Community-level behavior change interventions have the potential to reach large numbers of people, be cost-effective, and be feasible for implementation even in areas with limited economic and health care resources.

Rogers conducted research to explain how new behavioral trends became established within community populations (Rogers, 1983; Rogers and Shoemaker, 1971; Rogers and Kinkaid, 1981). Based on this work, he developed the Theory of Innovations (Rogers, 1983). He confirmed that there is a subset of people in a community who are opinion leaders – those individuals whose beliefs, practices, and behaviors are noticed and emulated by others.

In his editorial supporting the importance of community-level interventions, Kelly (1999) said, 'Ordinary people will, if asked and if properly assisted, do extraordinary things by taking on roles as AIDS prevention advocates to others in their own communities whether as volunteer peer advocates, popular opinion leaders, or as friends and neighbors'. Kelly and his colleagues (Kelly *et al.*, 1991, 1992a,b, 1997a) were the first to adapt the Theory of Innovations in multiple community-level behavior change interventions that engage popular opinion leaders (POLs) to redefine peer-group social norms. Their first study was conducted in three small southern cities with men patronizing gay bars. POLs were identified and trained in four sessions to deliver HIV/STD prevention messages to the patrons in the bars. Surveys were conducted in the bar at baseline and one year post-training of the POLs in a lagged baseline design. At baseline 33–42 per cent reported unprotected anal intercourse in the last two months. At follow-up those risk behaviors had been reduced 15–29 per cent below the baseline levels of risk behaviors.

Kelly (2004) has replicated these findings across multiple studies that incorporated elements of the POL model but added additional components to ensure that all the necessary intervention components were available in the community. For example, in gay bars, it is not necessary to introduce opportunities to engage in informal conversations because that is the *raison d'être* of going to a bar. However, when the POL was adapted for 18 low-income urban housing projects, opportunities to engage in informal conversations needed to be designed into the study because the women were not inclined to engage in social interactions in the housing project (Sikkema *et al.*, 2000). Risk-reduction workshops were first offered to all women living in the developments. In the control housing projects, this was followed by the distribution of AIDS education materials and condoms. In the intervention housing projects, social events and community activities were organized and carried out by health councils composed of women who were identified as popular among their female housing development neighbors. Risk behavior surveys were undertaken with all women living in all developments at baseline and at one-year follow-up. Women in the intervention housing developments reported any unprotected intercourse declined from 50 per cent to 38 per cent and the percentage of condom use increased from 30 per cent at baseline to 47 per cent one year later.

Another community-level HIV/STD prevention program was conducted by Kegeles and colleagues (1996) and used young MSM as POLs which was enhanced by an HIV/STD prevention publicity campaign and small-group risk reduction sessions in the community. Relative to a cohort in a comparison city, a cohort of young MSM in the intervention city showed reductions in sexual risk behaviors. Currently, the POL intervention is being adapted in an international Phase III two-arm randomized, community-level trial being conducted in five countries – China, India, Peru, Russia, and Zimbabwe. This is the first international test of this community-level prevention program based on the Theory of Innovations and these POLs are called community popular opinion leaders (C-POLs).

Communities with high HIV/STD incidence are often those where current social norms encourage high-risk behavior (e.g. social networks of intravenous drug users (IDUs)); therefore, using community-level interventions is critical to change those norms. Reductions of approximately 30 per cent from baseline levels in the prevalence of high-risk behavior among community population members have consistently been found and this is cost-effective and has public health significance.

Societal-level Interventions

There are differences in prevalence of HIV/STDs across and within countries. Structural, environmental, and social factors may indirectly affect these HIV transmission patterns, and examination at the societal level may provide some understanding of the determinants of individual risk.

Data from naturally occurring experiments provide tantalizing results and reinforce the value of a structural approach (Blankenship *et al.*, 2000; Parker *et al.*, 2000). The various types of societal-level interventions are model development, policy development, communications, mass media programs, and environmental interventions.

Although the causal role of social and physical factors has been studied in relation to violence and physical safety, it has received inadequate attention in relation to HIV risk behavior and its prevention (Werner *et al.*, 1992). The social and physical environment can support or constrain behaviors related to HIV/STD risks in high-risk communities. Increasingly, specific characteristics of the social environment (e.g. social norms held by peers) and the physical environment (e.g. number and types of places to congregate) have been identified as factors potentially associated with HIV risk behaviors (Cohen *et al.*, 2000). For example, collective efficacy (the extent to which adults in a neighborhood share and enforce a common but implicit standard of neighborhood conduct) is a powerful predictor of neighborhood violence as well as other behaviors that may be relevant to HIV risk (Sampson *et al.*, 1997). The code of the streets (where informal social norms are enforced in some contexts using subtle non-verbal and verbal cues) is another dimension that may be relevant to HIV-relevant risk behavior (Anderson, 1999).

Similarly, the existence of public spaces (such as parks, abandoned properties) where behavior can occur unobserved by others or where alcohol is available can encourage risky behaviors including those relevant to HIV transmission and prevention (Skjaeveland and Garling, 1997; Peirce *et al.*, 2000).

Model development

Poverty, power imbalances among classes of people, political strife, and lack of educational opportunities create the context in which infectious diseases can flourish. Many of these AIDS-relevant problems are beyond the purview of public health prevention research. However, investigators do use aggregate and demographic data (e.g. age of epidemic, GNP per capital, percentage foreign-born in population; religion; income equality; male–female literacy gap; male–female ratio; and percentage of male population in the military forces) to develop models that specify the causal pathways for infectious diseases (Over, 1998). Based on this guidance, legislators can develop effective policies that reduce the societal disease burden (Carael *et al.*, 1997; Hintzen and Lowe, 1995).

Policy development

Organizational regulations or State or Federal laws can have a huge impact on behavior. When it is illegal to purchase syringes, there is strong pressure to share needles in shooting galleries or other places because police will arrest anyone who is carrying a syringe. In 1992, a dramatic and well-publicized syringe law was passed in Connecticut which permitted the purchase of up to 10 non-prescription syringes in pharmacies (Groseclose *et al.*, 1995). Before the law was passed, only 19 per cent of IDUs were purchasing needles at a pharmacy, but after the law was enacted this proportion escalated to 78 per cent. Before law 52 per cent of IDUs shared needles, but after the law, this proportion dropped to 31 per cent (Watters *et al.*, 1994).

Another well-known example of a policy-change intervention is the 100 per cent condom program in Thailand. In 1990, the government enacted a policy of mandatory condom use in the brothels. The policy was implemented through a partnership of brothel owners, police, and public health clinics. Consistent condom use increased to over 90 per cent among sex workers, and diagnosable STDs declined by more than 75 per cent (Hanenberg *et al.*, 1994). These results were corroborated by the Thai military study, where the prevalence of HIV in new military recruits was 10.4–12.5 per cent before the policy change, but fell to 6.7 per cent after the policy was fully implemented (Celentano *et al.*, 2000).

Communications

A communications revolution is shaping the social dynamics and patterns of a new generation worldwide and reshaping those of the older generation

(DeGuzman and Ross, 1999). Computers give youth new types of control over their social communication, remove community and familial constraints, and permit the formation of new relationships beyond the local community. Sexuality is being dramatically affected by the Internet, and sex is the most frequently searched topic on the internet in the US (Cooper *et al.*, 1999).

Results from intervention studies being conducted using the Internet as a setting for HIV/STD prevention are not yet available. However, the report of a rapid increase in syphilis cases over a two-month period in San Francisco offers a glimpse of the Internet's potential impact. When investigated, all cases had originated in the same San Francisco gay male chat room on America Online. Seven men had 99 sexual contacts in the prior two months, and five of the seven were seropositive (Klausner *et al.*, 2000).

Mass media programs

Mass media programs based on social psychological principles and targeted to specific behaviors (condom buying, getting tested) can reach large numbers of people and result in widespread behavior change. Often these social marketing programs support other interventions at different levels.

In Switzerland, AIDS prevention advertising targeted to the general population and high-risk groups has been widespread and has been complemented by sex education and AIDS prevention efforts in schools (Dubois-Arber *et al.*, 1997). Annual telephone surveys of people aged 17–45 have been conducted to monitor behavior change. Despite concerns that this program might increase risky behaviors, no major changes in level of sexual activity (lifetime number of partners, frequency of sexual encounters in the past week) or potential exposure to risk of HIV transmission (acquisition of a new steady partner during the last year or of casual partners in the last six months). Systematic condom use with a new steady partner increased between 1988 and 1994, from 40 per cent to 64 per cent among 17- to 30-years olds and from 57 per cent to 72 per cent among those aged 31–45. Systematic condom use with casual partners increased from 8 per cent to 56 per cent between 1987 and 1994 among 17- to 30-year-olds and from 22 per cent to 42 per cent between 1989 and 1994 among those aged 31–45. Condom use was higher among those with multiple partners. Behavioral changes and stabilization of HIV prevalence have been observed in Switzerland. These results demonstrated the feasibility and utility of a mass media approach in a small country to deliver public health programs.

Environmental interventions

Environmental factors that may affect HIV risk behaviors have not been well studied. Some of these are social density, housing stability, number of alcohol beverage stores, design of bath houses, and access to purchasing condoms (e.g. dispensers in bars; 24-hour drugs stores). This is a promising avenue of research and may make a contribution to behavioral prevention research.

Contributions of Behavioral HIV/STD Prevention Research

Behavioral HIV/STD prevention research has improved the methodology and design of health prevention programs and has had a broad impact on health promotion/disease prevention research. Specific areas where there has been a contribution are: (1) utilization of the model of multiple level of causation; (2) early detection of disease; (3) theory-based prevention programs; (4) emphasis on Phase IV (technology transfer) studies; and (5) cost-effective studies of evidence-based interventions.

Because most health problems have multiple levels of causation, behavioral HIV/STD prevention research has promoted the multiple levels of causation model and encouraged the conduct of research at multiple levels. This is the only way to build a social health movement that will result in wide collective behavior change that will prevent the spread of epidemics.

HIV/AIDS has contributed to the development of prevention science by recognizing the importance of early detection of a disease so that behavior change can be implemented while the epidemic is nascent. If people who are infected are not diagnosed, the epidemic can spread rapidly and be undetected until there is a concentrated epidemic. In addition to early detection, HIV/STD prevention has focused on the role of social mixing of high-risk individuals across social networks as a factor that can fuel an epidemic.

While not originating the idea, HIV/STD prevention research has contributed to elevating the importance of theoretically based behavior change interventions and the public health necessity to move to behavioral randomized controlled trials as rapidly as possible. These strategies are diffusing to other areas where this has not been a strong tradition and work had languished at the descriptive level over multiple funding years.

Because of the urgency of averting the AIDS epidemic and the fact that many people in research in this area are either seropositive or have friends who are or have died from the disease, there has been an urgency to move efficacious programs into public health clinics as soon as possible. Technology transfer programs became a priority in the NIH AIDS Strategic Plan and multiple studies were conducted to examine different effective methods. The Centers for Disease Control and Prevention (CDC) developed a Prevention That Works Program where prevention programs that had been tested in a randomized controlled design were evaluated by a panel of experience to determine if they should be adopted by public health clinics and other places that provided health education. If they were approved, a team would develop a user-friendly prevention program that would be sold at a nominal price to public health agencies, clinics, and schools.

A related trend in HIV/STD prevention research that has contributed to prevention science broadly is the development of cost effective studies and the improvement of the methodology (Holtgrave *et al.*, 1996). Making the case for a tragedy that does not happen is difficult and AIDS researchers have conducted sophisticated studies on cost-effectiveness of evidence-based interventions that have provided persuasive data. Because of the scarcity of resources available for health promotion and treatment, evidence of cost-effectiveness will be extremely important in determining whether interventions are adopted by public health agencies in the US and in research in international settings.

Challenges for International Behavioral Research

While the plans to roll out treatment programs in the developing world are laudable, they will not be sufficient nor rapid enough to save this youthful generation from high rates of HIV and STDs. Even the WHO program called 'three in five' – that is, 3 million people treated in five years – rolls out on a time line that is too little, too late. Approximately 40 million people are estimated to be currently infected with HIV and other global plans to deliver HIV antiretroviral therapy (HART) in developing countries have not addressed developing the health care system needed to deliver treatment to the number of people that are in need. Behavioral prevention programs that are cost-effective, require few resources, and can be deployed quickly by non-governmental organizations are urgently needed.

The advances made in HIV/STD prevention research will be a tremendous advantage in scaling up a public health program in international sites. There are, however, some challenges to making progress internationally and it has raised some new issues: (1) cross-cultural adaptation, (2) trained behavioral prevention personnel, (3) research infrastructure, and (4) ethical conduct of research in developing countries.

Cross-cultural Adaptation

Many US studies have involved establishing cultural congruence of the study design, intervention, and assessment tools. In international sites, in addition to the cultural or linguistic differences, many of the at-risk populations are illiterate, which requires that the prevention programs are based on word of mouth and symbols that are easily understandable. Some of the concepts used in prevention programs in the US may not exist in another culture and so it is not a matter of translation but a significant adaptation to make that part of the program relevant. Another aspect of the culture that must be addressed in AIDS prevention is the institutionalized power imbalances between men and women, which means that women do not have the resources to support themselves and their children through legitimate employment. This can force them into a relationship with a man who may be non-monogamous or into commercial sex work. Because of gender roles, women often do not have the right to protect their own health from husbands. Consequently, extensive formative work needs to be conducted in order to adapt interventions that were developed in the US, Europe, or in other developing countries.

Trained Behavioral Prevention Personnel

In international settings, there is limited experience with behavioral prevention research and it may be difficult to identify appropriate in-country colleagues. There may only be a small cadre of investigators who have received excellent research training and have experience conducting behavioral research studies. Because there are so few of them in any developing country, people who are trained in different areas may fill behavioral research roles or the same trained individuals are frequently asked to participate in multiple studies in order to have host country visibility in the research application. This problem can be exacerbated when these investigators are recruited for positions at US universities. Because there has not been a strong behavioral prevention research program in these developing countries, in addition to investigators, there are not trained personnel who can immediately assume the staff roles (e.g. project director, assessors, facilitators) that are required to mount and conduct these behavioral prevention studies. While in the US it might be possible to advertise for and recruit personnel who only require training on the study protocol, this may not be realistic in an international site. The challenge internationally is to initiate a study while training the large staff that will be required to conduct all the demanding tasks required for a successful Phase III clinical trial. In addition, many of the interpersonal characteristics and required skills may be not be congruent with the country. For example, in many cultures, there is an authoritarian leadership style which may lead to facilitators who order group members to engage in certain behaviors rather than working with them to overcome their barriers to engaging in safer behaviors. In the early phases of research, it is often necessary to put in large teams of US staff to train the host country staff and to monitor the conduct of the study.

Research Infrastructure

The problems to be addressed in developing research infrastructure are similar to those for trained personnel. Laboratories, computer systems, library of user-friendly prevention studies, functional space for conducting behavioral prevention research must be developed at the same time that the study is being mounted. This can be stressful for both the US and host country investigators and staff at a time when multiple research activities should be in the field.

Ethical Conduct of Research

Prior to the HIV/AIDS epidemic, medical science had learned valuable lessons from high-profile ethical errors and misconduct in the Tuskegee syphilis study and the medical experiments on prisoners during the Third Reich. Over the last three decades there have been enormous strides made in awareness and sensitivity to the needs of vulnerable populations. The advent of international AIDS research in developing countries sponsored by developed countries has raised ethical dilemmas about studying stigmatized populations in cultures where randomized, controlled trials are not well understood.

While participants in developing countries will probably receive some benefits from participating in research, there are many ethical dilemmas which must be resolved at the beginning of the process of developing a joint research proposal. First, the research should be linked to the public health goals of the recipient country and not simply fulfill the scientific objectives of the donor country. A related concept is whether it is ethical to test an experimental or control intervention that is not and is unlikely to be the standard for care for people in that country. The dilemma is balancing the principle of beneficence for science and society at large versus the welfare of the research participants. Even investigators in developing countries can be coerced into approving a research study for the advancement of their scientific career rather than the public health priorities of their country.

In a resource-poor setting, what constitutes an undue incentive in a study rather than reimbursement for time and effort may not be clear. Participating in research may be the only way that the person has of gaining access to interventions – even those of unknown efficacy – and so participation may not be voluntary. Some of the reified concepts to protect against coercion, such as informed consent, may be a strange concept in that culture and not understood. Both the woman and her husband may assume that only he can give permission for her to participate in the research study but the Western investigator is not permitted to accept this consent. In order to gain the study benefits, the husband may demand that the wife participate and she may have not recourse.

The need for confidentiality highlights the importance of project staff selection and training from the project director, interviewer, facilitator, and even the driver. In small communities many people may know each other and activities that would jeopardize the research participant may be inadvertently observed or overheard by a project staff member who will gossip in the community.

253

Because the tradition of an Institutional Review Board (IRB) is a foreign concept, it may not be implemented in an impartial and appropriate way. People who have a vested interest in the research study may contribute to the decision-making. An application that is viewed as having limited benefit for the research participants may be approved because the funding will increase the budget of a local clinic and offer services that have not been available.

While many of these ethical dilemmas occur in conducting research in the US, they are magnified in international settings where the power imbalance may not lead to appropriate resolution or detection of ethical problems. However, to the extent that this heightened attention to ethical issues leads to greater consciousness of human rights and identifies moral principles that may be universal, the ethical conduct of all research may be improved.

What the Future Holds

Globalization of HIV/STD Prevention Research

Despite the challenges of conducting behavioral prevention research internationally, because 90 per cent of the world's HIV-infected populations live in areas of the world where only 10 per cent of the research is currently being conducted, globalization of HIV/STD prevention research will accelerate. Because of the prevalence of HIV/STDs in developing countries, there are many critical research questions that may only be answered in the international context. One of these is the effective delivery of both prevention and treatment interventions and the relationship between them on sero-incidence. Another is the impact of overcoming the stigma of HIV serostatus when large number of at-risk people in a community seek counseling and testing, and if necessary, treatment. There is also the impact of structural level interventions (policy change, media, environmental manipulation) on HIV/STD sero-incidence.

Modeling of Prevention Strategies

Because the resources to conduct specific studies are becoming more limited, mathematical modeling of the epidemic can be a powerful tool in assessing both where the treatment and prevention funds should be spent and what kind of prevention program designs will potentially avert the most cases of new infections. There are multiple mathematical models of the dynamics of the HIV epidemic that can be used as an HIV/STD behavioral prevention planning tool in designing HIV/STD prevention programs for emerging epidemics in developing countries. These models have wide applicability to AIDS prevention scientists, practitioners, and policy-makers (NIMH/ASIST, 2002).

Multiple-level Sustainable Interventions

Most research that is currently conducted occurs in the context of multiple prevention, treatment, and care programs being offered by multiple service providers. No research has evaluated the synergy of these multiple programs at multiple levels on the efficacy of the programs. They are tested as if they were only one intervention. An emerging area of research is examining the impact of individual, couples, family, community, and societal programs being offered in concert and the impact of this multiple-level approach on sustainability of the behavior changes.

Even if an AIDS vaccine is developed, HIV/STD behavioral prevention research will continue into the control of the transmission of HIV/STDs and into the development of prevention science. While the rapid advances in treatment and care have led to the impression that there is a cure for AIDS and therefore behavioral and biomedical resources can now be allocated to other health concerns, greater utilization of behavioral prevention programs can contribute to averting an impending epidemic in Asia and a worsening of public health in Africa. Developing countries are demanding treatment for HIV-positive people, but behavioral interventions are today's AIDS vaccine!

References

Allen S, Serufilira A, Bogaerts J *et al.* (1992) Confidential HIV testing and condom promotion in Africa: Impact on HIV and gonorrhea rates. *JAMA* 268: 3338–41.

Anderson E (1999) *The Code of the Street: Decency, Violence, and the Moral Life of the Inner City*. New York: W.W. Norton & Co.

Bandura A (1989) Perceived self-efficacy in the exercise of control over AIDS infection. In: Mays VM, Albee GW, Schneider SF, eds. *Primary Prevention of AIDS: Psychological Approaches*. Newbury Park, CA: Sage, pp. 128–41.

Bandura A (1991) A social cognitive approach to the exercise of control over AIDS infection. In: DiClemente R, ed. *Adolescents and AIDS: A Generation in Jeopardy*. Beverly Hills, CA: Sage, pp. 1–20.

Becker M (1988) AIDS and behavior change. *Public Health Rev* 16: 1–11.

Belcher L, Kalichman SC, Toppong M *et al.* (1998) A randomized trial of a brief HIV risks reduction counseling intervention for women. *J Consult Clin Psychol* 66: 856–61.

Bing E (2004) AIDS prevention with the Angolan military. Abstract, International AIDS Conference, Bangkok, Thailand, 11–16 July 2004.

Blankenship KM, Bray SJ, Merson MH (2000) Structural interventions in public health. *AIDS* 14 (Suppl 1): S11–S21.

Bronfenbrenner U (1979) *The Ecology of Human Development: Experiments by Nature and Design*. Cambridge, MA: Harvard University Press.

Carael M, Buve A, Awusabo-Asare K (1997) The making of HIV epidemics: What are the driving forces? *AIDS* 11 (Suppl B): S27.

Carey MP, Weinhart L, Carey KB (1995) Prevalence of infection with HIV among the seriously mentally ill: Review of research and implications for practice. *Prof Psychol Res Pract* 26: 262–8.

Carey MP, Maisto SA, Kalichman SC, Forsyth A, Wright I, Johnson BT (1997) Enhancing motivation to reduce risk for HIV infection for economically disadvantaged urban women. *J Consult Clin Psychol* 65: 531–41.

CDC (Centers for Disease Control and Prevention) (2004) Estimated numbers of persons living with HIV/AIDS by year and selected characteristics, 1999–2002 −30 areas with confidential name-based HIV infection reporting. *Surveillance Rep* 14: table 8.

Celentano DD, Bond KC, Lyles C *et al.* (2000) Prevention intervention to reduce sexually transmitted infections: A field trial in the Royal Thai Army. *Arch Intern Med* 160: 535–40.

Choi K-H, Catania JA (1996) Changes in multiple sexual partnerships, HIV testing, and condom use among U.S. Heterosexuals 18 to 49 years of age, 1990 and 1992. *Am J Public Health* 554–6.

Cohen DA, Scribner RA, Farley TA (2000) A structural model of health behavior: a pragmatic approach to explain and influence health behaviors at the population level. *Prevent Med* 30: 146–54.

Cooper A, Scherer CR, Boies SC, Gordon BL (1999) Sexuality on the internet: From sexual exploration to pathological expression. *Professional Psychol Res Pract* 30: 154–64.

DeGuzman MA, Ross MW (1999) Assessing the application of AIDS-related counseling and education on the Internet. *Patient Educ Counsel* 36: 209–28.

de Vincenzi I, for the European Study Group on Heterosexual Transmission of HIV (1994) A longitudinal study of human immunodeficiency virus transmission by heterosexual partners. *N Engl J Med* 331: 341–6.

DiClemente RJ, Wingood GM (1995) A randomized controlled trial of an HIV sexual risk reduction intervention for young African American women. *JAMA* 274: 1271–6.

Dubois-Arber F, Jeannin A, Konings E, Paccaud F (1997) Increased condom use without other major changes in sexual behavior among the general population in Switzerland. *Am J Public Health* 87: 558–66.

Ehrhardt AA, Exner TM (2000) Prevention of sexual risk behavior for HIV infection with women. *AIDS* 14 (Suppl 2): S53–S58.

Fishbein M (1980) A theory of reasoned action: Some applications and implications. In: Howe H, Page M, eds. *Nebraska Symposium on Motivation, 1979.* Lincoln, NE: University of Nebraska Press, pp. 65–116.

Fishbein M (1997) *Theoretical Models of HIV Prevention. Abstract Book: Consensus Development Conference on Interventions to Prevent HIV Risk Behaviors.* Bethesda, MD: National Institutes of Health.

Fishbein M, Pequegnat W (2000) Evaluating AIDS prevention interventions using behavioral and biological outcome measures. *Sex Transm Dis* 27: 101–10.

Fishbein M, Bandura A, Triandis HC *et al.* (1992) *Factors Influencing Behavior and Behavior Change: Final Report – Theorist's Workshop.* Rockville, MD: NIMH.

Fisher JD, Fisher WA, Misovich SJ, Kimble DL, Malloy TE (1996) Changing AIDS risk behavior: effects of an intervention emphasizing AIDS risk reduction information, motivation, and behavior skills in a college student population. *Health Psychol* 15: 114–23.

Foster G (1998) Child-headed households in the era of parental death from AIDS. Paper presented at the NIMH Annual research Conference on the Role of Families in Preventing and Adapting to HIV/AIDS, 29–31 July, Washington, DC.

Gayle H (2000) An overview of the global HIV/AIDS epidemic, with a focus on the United States. *AIDS* 14 (Suppl 2): S8–S17.

Groseclose SL, Weinstein B, Jones TS, Vallerooy LA, Fehrs LJ, Kassler WJ (1995) Impact of increased legal access to needles and syringes on practices of injecting drug users and police officers. Connecticut, 1992–1993. *J Acquir Immune Defic Syndr Hum Retrovirol* 10: 82–9.

Hanenberg RS, Rojanapithayakom W, Kunasol P, Sokal DC (1994) Impact of Thailand's HIV-control programme as indicated by the decline of sexually transmitted disease. *Lancet* 344: 243–5.

Herek G (1995) Developing a theoretical framework and rationale for a research proposal. In: Pequegnat W, Stover E, eds. *How to Write a Successful Research Grant Application: A Guide for Social and Behavioral Scientists.* New York: Plenum, 113–27.

Hintzen LP, Lowe R (1995) Socio-obstacles to HIV prevention and treatment in developing countries: the roles of the International Monetary Fund and the World Bank. *AIDS* 9: 539–45.

Hobfoll SE, Jackson AP, Lavin J, Britton PJ, Shepard JB (1994) Reducing inner-city women's AIDS activities. *Health Psychol* 13: 397–403.

Holtgrave DR, Pinkerton SD (2002) Consequences of HIV prevention interventions and programs: spectrum, selection, and quality of outcome measures. *AIDS* 14 (Suppl 2): S27–S33.

Holtgrave DR, Qualls NL, Graham JD (1996) Economic evaluation of HIV prevention programs. *Annu Rev Public Health* 17: 467–88.

Jemmott III JB, Jemmott LS (2000) HIV risk-reduction behavioral interventions with heterosexual adolescents. *AIDS* 14 (Suppl 2): S40–S52.

Jemmott III JB, Jemmott LS, Fong GT (1992) Reduction in HIV risk-associated sexual behavior among Black male adolescents: effects of an AIDS prevention intervention. *Am J Public Health* 82: 372–7.

Jemmott III JB, Jemmott LS, Fong GT (1998) Abstinence and safer sex HIV risk-reduciton interventions for African American adolescents: A randomized controlled trial. *JAMA* 279: 1529–36.

Kalichman SC, Sikkema KJ, Kelly JA, Bullto M (1995) Use of brief behavioral skills intervention to prevent HIV infection among chronic mentally ill adults. *Psychiatr Serv* 46: 275–80.

Kalichman SC, Rompa D, Coley B (1996) Experiment component analysis of a behavioral HIV/AIDS prevention intervention of inner-city women. *J Consult Clin Psychol* 64: 687–93.

Kamb ML, Douglas M, Rhodes JM *et al.* and the Project RESPECT Study Group. (1998) Efficacy of risk-reduction counseling to prevent human immunodeficiency virus and sexually transmitted disease. *JAMA* 280: 1161–7.

Kanfer F (1987) Self-regulation and behavior. In: Heckhausen H, Gollwitzer PM, Weinert FE, eds. Heidelberg, Germany: Springer-Verlag, pp. 286–99.

Kegeles SM, Hays R, Coates TJ (1996) The powerment project: A community-level HIV prevention intervention for young gay men. *Am J Public Health* 86: 1129–36.

Kelly JA (1997) HIV risk reduction intervention for person with severe mental illness. *Clin Psychol Rev* 17: 293–309.

Kelly JA (1999) Editorial: Community-level interventions are needed to prevent new HIV infections. *Am J Public Health* 89: 299–301.

Kelly JA (2000) HIV prevention interventions with gay or bisexual men and youth. *AIDS* 14 (Suppl 2): S34–S39.

Kelly JA (2004) Popular opinion leaders and HIV prevention peer education: Resolving discrepant findings and implications for the development of effective community programmes. *AIDS Care* 16: 139–50.

Kelly JA, St Lawrence JS, Diaz YE *et al.* (1991) HIV risk behavior reaction following intevention with key opinion leaders of population: An experimental analysis. *Am J Public Health* 81: 168–71.

Kelly JA, St Lawrence JS, Steven LY *et al.* (1992a) Community AIDS/HIV risk reduction: The effects of endorsement by popular people in three cities. *Am J Public Health* 82: 1483–9.

Kelly JA, Murphy DA *et al.* (1992b) AIDS/HIV risk behavior among gay men in small cities: Findings of a 6-city national sample. *Arch Intern Med* 152: 2293–7.

Kelly JA, Murphy DA, Washington CD *et al.* (1994) The effects of HIV/AIDS intervention groups for high-risk women in urban clinics. *Am J Public Health* 84: 1918–22.

Kelly JA, McAuliffe TL, Sikkema KJ *et al.* (1997a) Reduction in risk among adults with severe mental illness who learned to advocate for HIV prevention. *Psychiatr Serv* 48: 1283–8.

Kelly JA, Murphy DA, Sikkema KJ *et al.* (1997b) Randomized, controlled, community-level HIV prevention intervention for sexual risk behavior among homosexual men in U.S. cities. *Lancet* 350: 1500–5.

Kelly JA, Sogolow ED, Neuman MS (2000a) Future directions and emerging issues in technology transfer between HIV prevention researchers and community-based service providers. *AIDS Educ Prevent* 12 (Suppl A): 126–41.

Kelly JA, Heckman TG, Stevenson LY *et al.* (2000b) Transfer of research-based HIV prevention interventions to community services providers: Fidelity, adaption, and tailoring. *AIDS Educ Prevent* 12 (Suppl A): 87–9.

Kelly JA, Somlai AM, DiFranceisco WJ *et al.* (2000c) Bridging the gap between the science and services of HIV prevention: Transferring effective research-based HIV prevention interventions to communiuty AIDS service providers. *Am J Public Health* 90: 1082–8.

Kelly JA, Somlai AM, Benotsch, EG *et al.* (2004) Using distance communication technology to transfer HIV prevention interventions to service providers. *Science* 305: 1953–55.

Klausner JD, Wolf W, Fischer-Ponce L, Zolt I, Katz MH (2000) Tracing a syphilis outbreak through cyberspace. *JAMA* 284: 447–9.

Krauss B, Tiffany J, Goldsamt L (1997a) Parent and pre-adolescent training for HIV prevention in a high seroprevalence neighbourhood. *AIDS/STD Health Promotion Exchange* 1: 10–12.

Krauss B, Goldsamt L, Bula E (1997b) Parent-preadolescent communication about HIV in a high seroprevalence neighborhood. In: Sigman M, chair. Mother-adolescent communication about sexuality and AIDS. Symposium conducted at the Society for Research in Child Development Biennial Meeting, Washington, DC.

Krauss BJ, Godfrey C, Yee D *et al.* (2000) Saving our children from a silent epidemic: The PATH program for parents and pre-adolescents. In: Pequegnat W, Szapocznik J, eds. *Working with Families in the Era of HIV/AIDS*. Thousand Oaks, CA: Sage Publications.

Miller HG, Turner CF, Moses LE (eds) (1990) *AIDS: The Second Decade*. Washington, DC: National Academy Press.

NIMH (National Institute of Mental Health) Multisite HIV Prevention Trial Group (1998) The NIMH Multisite HIV Prevention Trial: Reducing HIV sexual risk behavior. *Science* 280: 1880–94.

NIMH (2002) *NIMH/ASIST*. CD-ROM.

NIH (National Institutes of Health) (1997) *NIH Consensus Statement: Intervention to Prevent HIV Risk Behaviors*. Bethesda, MD: US Public Health Service.

NIH Consensus Development Conference Panel (2000) National Institutes of Health Consensus Development Conference Statement. *AIDS* 14 (Suppl 2): S84–S96.

Nyamathi AM, Leake B, Flaskerud J, Lewis C, Bennett C (1993) Outcomes of specialized and traditional AIDS counseling programs for impoverished women of color. *Res Nurs Health* 16: 11–21.

O'Donnell C, O'Donnell L, San Doval A, Duran R (1998) Reductions in STD infection subsequent to an STD clinic visit: Using video-based patient education to supplement providers interactions. *Sex Transm Dis* 25: 161–8.

O'Leary A (1999) Preventing HIV infection in heterosexual women: What do we know? What do we need to learn? *Appl Prevent Psychol* 8: 257–63.

Over M (1998) The effects of societal variables on urban rates of HIV infection in developing countries: An exploratory analysis. In: *Confronting AIDS: Evidence from the Developing World.* Washington, DC: World Bank, pp.39–52.

Padian NS, O'Brien TR, Chang YC, Glass S, Francis DP (1993) Prevention of heterosexual transmission of human immunodefiency virus through couple counseling. *J Acquir Immune Defic Syndr* 6: 1043–8.

Parker RG, Easton D, Klein CH (2000) Structural barriers and facilitators in HIV prevention: A review of international research. *AIDS* 14 (Suppl 1): S22–S32.

Peirce RS, Frone MR, Russell M, Cooper ML, Mudar P (2000) A longitudinal model of social contact, social support, depression, and alcohol use. *Health Psychol* 19: 28–38.

Pequegnat W, Stover E (2000) Behavioral prevention is today's AIDS vaccine! *AIDS* 14 (Suppl 2): S1–S7.

Pequegnat W, Szapocznik J (2000) *Working with Families in the Era of HIV/AIDS.* Thousand Oaks: Sage Publications.

Pequegnat W, Page B, Strauss A *et al.* (1995) Qualitative inquiry: An underutilized strategy in AIDS research. In: Pequegnat W, Stover E, eds. *How to Write a Successful Research Grant Application: A Guide for Social and Behavioral Scientists.* New York: Plenum, pp. 113–27.

Pequegnat WM, Celentano D, Ehrhardt A *et al.* (2000) NIMH/APPC Workgroup on behavioral and biological outcomes in HIV/STD prevention studies: a position statement. *Sex Transm Dis* 27: 127–32.

Peterson JL, Coates TJ, Catanai JA *et al.* (1997) Evaluation of an HIV risk reduction intervention among African American homosexual and bisexual men. *AIDS* 10: 319–25.

Roffman RA, Picciano JF, Ryan R *et al.* (1997) HIV prevention group counseling delivered by telephone: An efficacy trial with gay and bisexual men. *AIDS Behav* 1: 137–54.

Rogers EM (1983) *Diffusion of Innovations,* 3rd edn. New York: Free Press.

Rogers EM, Kinkaid DL (1981) *Communication Networks: Toward a New Paradigm for Research.* New York: Free Press.

Rogers EM, Shoemaker FF (1971) *Communication of Innovations: A Cross-cultural Approach.* New York: Free Press.

Rotheram-Borus MJ, Koopman C, Haignere C, Davies M (1991) Reducing HIV sexual risk behaviors among runaway adolescents. *JAMA* 266: 1237–41.

Rotheram-Borus MJ, Cantwell S, Newman PA (2000) HIV prevention programs with heterosexuals. *AIDS* 14 (Suppl 2): S59–S67.

Sampson RJ, Raudenbush SW, Earls F (1997) Neighborhoods and violent crime: A multi-level study of collective efficacy. *Science* 277: 918–24.

Sikkema KJ, Kelly JA, Winett RA *et al.* (2000) Outcomes of a randomized community-level HIV prevention intervention for women living in 18 low-income housing developments. *Am J Public Health* 90: 57–63.

Skjaeveland O, Gäärling T (2002) Social-physical neighborhood attributes affecting social interaction among neighbors. In: Aragonéés J, Francescato G, Gäärling T, eds. *Residential Environments: Choice, Satisfaction, and Behavior.* Westport, CT: Greenwood, pp. 183–203.

St Lawrence JS, Brasfield TL, Jefferson KW, Alleyne E, Shirley A (1995) Cognitive-behavioral intervention to reduce African American adolescents' risk for HIV infection. *J Consult Clin Psychol* 63: 221–37.

Susser E, Valencia E, Miller M, Tsai WY, Meyer-Bahlburg H, Conover S (1995) Sexual behavior of homeless mentally ill men at risk for HIV. *Am J Psychiatry* 152: 583–7.

Szapocznik J, Pequegnat W (1995) Designing an intervention study. In: Pequegnat W, Stover E, eds. *How to Write a Successful Research Grant Application: A Guide for Social and Behavioral Scientists.* New York: Plenum, pp. 113–27.

Szapocznik J, Feaster DJ, Mitrani VB *et al.* (2004) Structural ecosystems therapy for HIV-seropositive African American women: Effects on psychological distress, family hassles, and family support. *J Consult Clin Psychol* 72: 288–303.

Triandis HC (1980) Values, attitudes and interpersonal behavior. In: Howe H, Page M, eds. *Nebraska Symposium on Motivation, 1979*. Lincoln, Nebraska: University of Nebraska Press, pp. 197–259.

Valdiserri RD, Leiter DW, Leviton LC, Callaban CM, Kingsley LA, Rialdo CR (1989) AIDS prevention among homosexual and bisexual men: Results of a randomized trial evaluating two risk reduction interventions. *AIDS* 3: 21–6.

Voluntary HIV-1 Counseling and Testing Efficacy Study Group (2000) Efficacy of voluntary HIV-1 counseling and testing in individuals and couples in Kenya, Tanzania, and Trinidad: A randomized trial. *Lancet* 356: 103–12.

Waldo CR, Coates TJ (2000) Multiple levels of analysis and intervention in HIV prevention science: Exemplars and directions for new research. *AIDS* 14 (Suppl 2): S18–S26.

Watters JK, Estilio JJ, Clark GL, Lorvick J (1994) Syringe and needle exchange as HIV/AIDS prevention for injection drug users. *JAMA* 271: 115–20.

Werner CM, Altman I, Brown BB (1992) A transactional approach to interpersonal relations: Physical environment, social context, and temporal qualities. *J Soc Personal Relationships* 9: 297–323.

The Evolution of Comprehensive AIDS Clinical Care

10

Kenneth H Mayer
Professor of Medicine and Community Health, Brown University Miriam Hospital, Providence, USA; Medical Research Director, Fenway Community Health, Boston, USA

Sreekanth K Chaguturu
Resident in Internal Medicine, Massachusetts General Hospital/Harvard Medical School, Boston, USA

Kenneth H. Mayer, MD is Professor of Medicine and Community Health, and Director of the Brown University AIDS Program, and the Brown-Tufts Fogarty (NIH) AIDS International Research and Training Program. He is Attending Physician in Infectious Diseases at Miriam Hospital, Providence, Rhode Island, Adjunct Professor at the Harvard School of Public Health and Medical Research Director at Boston's Fenway Community Health. He serves on the Board of Directors and on committees of amFAR, and was on the national board of the HIV Medicine Association, is a former board member of the Gay and Lesbian Medical Association, and serves on the editorial boards of several scientific publications including *Clinical Infectious Diseases*. He has co-authored more than 300 articles, chapters and publications and other publications on AIDS and related infectious disease topics, and is a frequent lecturer and presenter at national and international conferences. See section on The Editors for additional biographical information.

Sreekanth K. Chaguturu, MD received his undergraduate and medical degrees from Brown University and has worked as a clinical research fellow at the Y.R.G. Center for AIDS Research and Education in Chennai, India. He has coauthored multiple papers describing the natural history of HIV in southern India before and after the introduction of highly active generic antiretroviral therapy. He is currently training at Massachusetts General Hospital in Boston.

The impact of HIV/AIDS on the health care environment in the United States and throughout the world has been so profound and pervasive that it is almost impossible to remember what clinical care for patients with serious infections was like before the epidemic appeared. Many may not remember that during the first years of the epidemic, AIDS was often a rapidly fatal disease. Relatively soon after an individual came down with an opportunistic infection or other sign of severe immunodeficiency, the quality of life often declined quickly due to an increasing number of serious infections with multiple acute hospitalizations, until they died. This was the grim picture prior to the discovery of drugs capable of inhibiting the virus itself. Then, as now, effective prophylaxis for opportunistic infections in immunocompromised people was limited at best. Most of those who first suffered from the AIDS epidemic were relatively young and previously healthy. An AIDS diagnosis was tantamount to a death sentence, hence heartbreakingly difficult to deliver.

My work in AIDS started before the virus we now call HIV was discovered. Between 1980 and 1983, I (KHM) was in the middle of a three-year fellowship in Infectious Diseases at Brigham and Women's Hospital and Harvard Medical School in Boston, Massachusetts. At the time, my area of interest had little to do with the epidemic that would soon envelop the national consciousness and then the international scene. I was working in a molecular epidemiology lab at the hospital learning how to use DNA fingerprinting to track the spread of antibiotic resistance. I was also working one or two sessions a week at Boston's Fenway Community Health Center, as part of my desire to do community service and to gain wider clinical experience. Fenway was founded in 1971, as an outgrowth of Boston's era of progressive politics, and was known for being particularly responsive to the health care needs of gay men and lesbians. Several times a week, Fenway had special clinic sessions focused on diagnosing and treating the sexually transmitted infections of gay men, which were becoming increasingly common. In the early days of gay liberation, sex with multiple partners was considered culturally appropriate, and the most serious sequelae, sexually transmitted infections, were considered unpleasant, but manageable. Because of AIDS, this would soon change. An ever increasing number of patients at Fenway would become victims of AIDS, including some of our colleagues at the Center. The impact on how we cared for patients, interfaced with the community, and worked with each other would soon be profound.

So, in June of 1981, when the first reports of what came to be known as AIDS were published in *Morbidity and Mortality Weekly Reports*, I realized there was a significant congruence between my academic training program, and my 'moonlighting' job. (The aphorism was that one moonlighted at Harvard until becoming an assistant professor, and then one consulted.) However, although many of my mentors were intrigued by the immunological depradations of the emerging 'gay-related immunodeficiency disease' syndrome and were interested in trying to elucidate its etiology, there was little encouragement for me to try to understand the best ways to provide care for people living with AIDS.

By the spring of 1983, I had taken care of several dozen people severely compromised by the syndrome, whose etiology was still uncertain. I was able to collaborate with a public health graduate student and to collect blood specimens from gay men to assess the prevalence of asymptomatic immunosuppression and to create a repository, in hopes that a blood test would soon be available to identify people at risk for AIDS. We collected data on the men's sexual and recreational drug use patterns in order to better understand the specific practices associated with the spread of AIDS.

I had begun the interviewing process for faculty jobs at several medical schools, and most of the professors I spoke with were more interested in the laboratory skills I had developed to 'fingerprint' bacterial antibiotic resistance genes, rather than my clinical interests in understanding how AIDS was transmitted, or how to predict which gay men were most likely to sicken and die of the panoply of opportunistic diseases. One of my senior mentors at Harvard told me that since it was likely that AIDS was caused by an immunosuppressive lentivirus, it could take decades before effective therapy or a vaccine would be available. He questioned why I would want to dissipate my efforts as an antibiotic resistance researcher to focus on the clinical consequences of an incurable disease, limited to a small number of socially marginalized people.

I was fortunate to be able to take a faculty position at a Brown University teaching hospital that enabled me to continue my AIDS work at Fenway, while studying antibiotic resistance in Rhode Island. By the end of a decade the demands and complexities of HIV care and research continued to grow to become more than a full-time job. At this time more than 1000 people living with HIV receive their care at Fenway Community Health (its current name), and my colleagues at The Miriam Hospital Immunology Center care for almost 900 people living with HIV. The focus of this book is global, but even here in New England (not an epidemic epicenter) there are tens of thousands of people directly impacted by the spread of HIV, necessitating the development of new models of care for this complex, chronic viral-induced immunosuppressive syndrome.

Understanding Chronic Viral Immunosuppression

As the experience with the Infectious Disease Research faculty at Harvard Medical School indicated, at the outset of the AIDS epidemic there was no medical specialty that was devoted to the clinical care of patients with chronic viral diseases. Infectious disease programs trained researchers who tried to understand the pathogenesis of a wide array of microorganisms, public health researchers who tested vaccines and developed strategies to remove the vectors of infectious diseases (e.g. mosquito control for malaria) and a limited number of clinicians who diagnosed and treated infectious diseases. At the beginning of the AIDS epidemic less than 2000 physicians in the US had specialized training in infectious diseases and related disciplines. The therapeutic armamentarium to manage infectious diseases at the time consisted of antibacterial drugs, which tended to be used to treat acute infections for periods usually ranging from one to six weeks. There were no FDA-approved antiviral drugs that were designed for the long-term suppression of a serious systemic viral infection.

The principles of antibiotic therapy had evolved over more than five decades when the first patients who developed AIDS were diagnosed, and much of clinical infectious disease practice focused on the use of these drugs. The protocols for antibacterial treatment were relatively well established, but viral diseases usually were either self-limited and improved with time and were treated symptomatically, or were controlled with vaccinations (e.g. measles, mumps, rubella). The discovery of the human herpesviruses and their ability to remain latent in hosts for decades, established the ability of viruses to persist and evade immune surveillance. Rous had determined a virologic etiology for an avian tumor (Rous sarcoma virus) at the beginning of the twentieth century, so virologists for many years had perceived viral latency as an oncogenic facilitator, if not the primary cause of some tumors. However, at the time that the AIDS epidemic first surfaced, the links between immunosuppression, viral neoplasia, and opportunistic infections were not clearly delineated.

Starting in the late 1950s, oncologists determined that since cancer was due to wildly dividing cells, its manifestations could be arrested through the use of cytostatic agents. As patients lived longer after undergoing cancer chemotherapy, they became prey to opportunistic infections, since their normally dividing white blood cells were often as susceptible to the chemotherapy as the neoplastic cells, since the leukocytes normally divided to respond to new antigenic stimuli. Advances in transplant surgery in the 1970s were abetted by the use of immunosuppressive drugs to combat the normal host rejection of the foreign transplant. Patients who had undergone transplants were also susceptible to opportunistic infections, sometimes quite similar to those experienced by cancer chemotherapy patients. Immunologists, oncologists, and infectious disease specialists worked increasingly closely together in the diagnosis and management of these infectious complications, and were able to progressively understand why certain patients were susceptible to specific opportunistic infections, based on the loss of specific numbers and functions of white blood cell subpopulations. In most cases, the infectious disease specialist was a consultant to the oncologist, advising on specific drug regimens, but not becoming as involved in the complex social issues faced by people undergoing chemotherapy.

Advances in immunology in the 1970s created an understanding that certain cell surface markers could be used to classify the circulating leukocytes into subpopulations that had specific immunological roles. Polymorphonuclear leukocytes were associated with the control of many acute bacterial and fungal infections, while lymphocytes appeared to be more highly correlated with the regulation of cell-mediated immunity that prevented the reactivation of some of the latent herpesviruses, as well as curtailing the ability of ubiquitous environmental pathogens like *Pneumocystis carinii* to replicate in an immunocompetent host, and immune surveillance to prevent the development of certain tumors. Many of the observations that linked specific cell types to protection against certain infections and tumors were inductive, based on the increased incidence of these conditions if patients lost the cells because of chemotherapy, exogenous immunosuppression to prevent a transplant rejection, or an intrinsic immune deficiency disorder. Understanding of the role of specific lymphocyte subsets advanced greatly with the appearance of AIDS, since the hallmark lesion was the decline in the T helper lymphocyte subpopulation, associated with specific types of opportunistic infections and cancers.

The skills developed in diagnosing opportunistic infections in exogenously immunocompromised hosts were immediately transferable to the treatment of AIDS patients, and clinical care in the early years of the epidemic focused on the diagnosis of a wide array of life-threatening conditions in highly immunosuppressed patients, necessitating frequent hospitalization and palliative care. The time from an AIDS diagnosis to death was months to a few years in most cases, which expanded the duration of the clinical relationship between a classically trained infectious disease specialist and the patient, changing the earlier paradigm of the infectious disease specialist as a consultant. In many communities at the outset of the epidemic, patients infected with HIV were stigmatized because of the behaviors associated with the most efficient viral transmission (i.e. male homosexual behavior and injection drug use) and because of the fear of parenteral exposures and other professional contacts with bodily fluids posing a risk of transmission to health care workers. So, early in the epidemic primary care physicians who were gay or practiced in settings that cared for men who had sex with men or injection drug users became the other major group of 'HIV specialists.'

Thus, from the earliest days of the epidemic, several trends emerged regarding the human resource needs of the health care professionals providing care for the increasing numbers of people living with HIV:

1. The reorientation of infectious diseases as a medical specialty: Traditionally most infectious disease specialists tended to be disengaged consultants who focused on providing input to the primary physicians managing a case. With the advent of the AIDS epidemic, these specialists had to focus on long-term care for people living with HIV and needed to train the next generation of infectious disease doctors who could become primary care providers for people living with HIV.
2. The development of a subset of generalist physicians and other non-infectious disease subspecialists who focused on providing comprehensive HIV care. Many of these providers began their involvement with AIDS because of having medical practices that were oriented to providing care for men who had sex with men, or injection drug users, and subsequently kept abreast of new clinical information as it evolved through continuing medical education.

3. Subsequently, as the AIDS epidemic has matured, general training programs in internal medicine, family medicine, pediatrics and obstetrics and gynecology have been challenged to address what all residents and fellows – individuals who later will become independently practicing physicians – need to learn about HIV care, and whether to create specific tracks to train AIDS primary care physicians without subspecialty training (see below).
4. Since the epidemic shows no sign of diminishing, and no cure is in sight, and the medical management of HIV/AIDS has become more complex, the need to credential those who are competent to provide HIV care has grown, both to justify appropriate compensation from third party payers, and to address the expectations of people living with HIV and their advocates.

Adapting the Care Environment

For almost a full decade people with AIDS frequently required costly hospital care. Intensive care units swelled with critically ill patients, especially in hard-hit areas such as New York City and San Francisco. Initial estimates from the Centers for Disease Control (CDC) reported that the lifetime hospital costs of the first 10 000 patients identified with HIV totaled approximately US$1.473 billion or US$147 000 per patient (Hardy *et al.*, 1986). In the same article, lifetime indirect costs were estimated at US$4.8 billion, almost three and a half times more than direct inpatient costs. Several refinements of these figures have been published for the initial years of the epidemic and all have come to similar, overwhelming numbers for the cost of care. During much of the first decade of the HIV epidemic, state and local health departments, as well as hospitals were calling out alarms that AIDS could potentially bankrupt health budgets. These financial concerns did not abate when antiretroviral treatment (ART) started to become available, because the cost of only modestly effective medical regimens could readily exceed US$1000 per month per person (see below). And, since ART was much less effective than it is now, patients still suffered infectious episodes that required costly intensive care and went on to a downhill course when their infection became resistant to the limited supply of drugs available. As described in detail elsewhere in this book, one development of AIDS activism was to encourage community support through buddy programs. The rapid growth of such community support networks meant that medical professionals dealing with AIDS patients were also dealing with volunteer buddies who transported patients to appointments, helped with the activities of daily living (e.g. bathing, toileting, meals), and interacting with the patient's biological or chosen family. In all, the need to provide integrated, palliative care for many young people who often did not have traditional family supports, and/or were poor, socially marginalized, led to the development of a host of volunteer and community-based AIDS service organizations.

The early high mortality rate led to a sense of urgency for many health professionals and in some segments of the general population to find effective treatments for curbing the rising death toll from AIDS. As has been also covered elsewhere in this book, this 'race against time' resulted in the emergence of AIDS activism by groups hardest hit by the newly discovered epidemic – primarily from gay, white men. Early activism was based on an iterative process of building on lessons learned from the women's movement and gay liberation. The gay community stepped up with buddy organizations to help support the activities of daily living, such as shopping, caring for the home and transportation, with support services not yet funded publicly. Volunteers filled in gaps for people living in non-traditional environments, such as injection drug users and gay men, who often could not rely on immediate family. Medical professionals learned to interface with and sometimes rely on the assistance of the volunteers. Activist movements spread quickly from New York and San Francisco into other metropolitan areas throughout the United States, impacting various fronts in the AIDS epidemic: basic biomedical research, pharmaceutical industry practices, and local – eventually global – policy-making decisions. Our community-based AIDS research at Fenway Health Center, for example, worked with local activist organizations in the design of studies and recruitment of participants. Community-based prevention efforts became a two-way interactive process of non-medically trained activists and health centers, like Fenway.

Another way in which the care environment was affected was in the arena of drug approval. Activist organizations fought individually and collectively for changes to speed up the testing and approval of anti-AIDS drug treatments. After high-profile protests and lobbying, success came in 1992, when Vice President Dan Quayle and HHS Secretary Sullivan announced four FDA initiatives to accelerate access to new drugs and streamline the drug review process. The four initiatives included:

- Accelerated approval: Surrogate endpoints would replace death as an endpoint in evaluating drug efficacy. Additional testing would be done after approval to ensure product safety, but would allow drugs to reach markets one to three years earlier than under the previous system.
- Parallel track: HIV drugs would be available as early as possible in the drug development process to patients unable to participate in clinical trials.
- Safety testing harmonization: A cooperative agreement was established with the European Union, Japan, and the United States that would allow animal safety data in one country to be transferred to other countries, eliminating the need for duplicate testing.
- Outside expert reviews: Though the FDA would have final approval, they would seek external reviewers to sift through the backlog of new drug applications.

The National US Response

More so than in many developed nations, in the United States much of medical practice and health care delivery is planned and provided on the state, county or city level. For example, it is the states that license medical professionals, and award the necessary certificates to establish hospitals and clinics. The enormous costs of care, the stark death rates, and a mounting campaign from volunteer and community-based AIDS service organizations led to the recognition that a national government response was needed to increase access to care and treatment. Local and state health departments in the United States could not do it alone. Despite the introduction of zidovudine (AZT), the first antiretroviral medicine designed to fight HIV, its cost of approximately US$12 000 per patient per year was well out of the reach most people living with HIV (Arno and Feiden, 1992). In addition, since many individuals infected were between the ages of 20 and 40, they were unable to benefit from Medicare, the federally funded program in the United States that pays for and sets minimal standards for the care of the chronically ill. Seeing that state and local governments lacked all the resources needed to respond to the epidemic, Congress created state AIDS Drug Assistance Programs (ADAPs) to facilitate the purchase of AZT and in 1990 the ADAPs were incorporated into the newly enacted Ryan White Comprehensive AIDS Resources Emergency (CARE) Act. Thus, in a relatively short period of time in the US, AIDS altered the traditional ways America pays for and delivers health services. Ryan White brought together a number of individual programs that had come into existence between 1985 and 1990, and then added services, so that the US government was now funding a wide array of health care services for people living with HIV and AIDS (Table 10.1).

New Judicial Protections

AIDS also changed the health care environment through new judicial protections awarded to patients and families affected by the disease. In most instances, these new legal and ethical safeguards have been applied throughout the medical system. They are seen in a variety of areas from informed consent, medical record privacy, and health insurance coverage. This subject is discussed in greater detail in Chapter ??. As a practicing clinician and researcher in the field, a number of areas have been of particular importance to me. For example, in response to increasing concerns for people living with HIV/AIDS the Americans with Disabilities Act of 1990 prohibits discrimination against any qualified individual with a disability in employment, public services, telecommunications, and public accommodations. The Housing Opportunities for People with AIDS Act of 1991 provides housing assistance to low-income people living with AIDS. The National Institutes of Health Revitalization Act of 1993 provided authority for a permanent, independent Office of AIDS Research at NIH and requires the director of that office to 'act as the primary Federal official with responsibility for overseeing all AIDS research conducted or supported by NIH'. The Ticket to Work/Work Incentives Improvement Act of 1999 enabled states to create new Medicaid buy-in programs for working individuals with disabilities and authorizes state

Table 10.1   Programs under the Ryan White CARE Act.

Title I	Provides emergency relief grants to cities for health and support services for low-income and under- or uninsured people living with HIV and AIDS and their families. Services include health care and support services such as medical and dental care, prescription drugs, transportation, counseling, and home and hospice care
Title II	Provides formula grants to all 50 states, the District of Columbia, Puerto Rico, and US territories to improve the quality, accessibility, and organization of health care and support for those with HIV and AIDS. Services include direct health care and support, home and community-based care, assistance in continuing private health insurance coverage, and treatments and drugs that prolong life and/or prevent hospitalization through AIDS drug assistance programs
Title III	Provides grants for comprehensive primary health care services for people living with AIDS and at-risk populations, including women, the homeless, and substance abusers to slow transmission of the disease and provide early intervention through education, counseling, testing, and treatment. To qualify for funds, organizations must be public or gateway private entities
Title IV	Provides grants for coordinated HIV services and access to research for children, youth, women, and families. Applicants must demonstrate the ability to provide access to clinical trials or to establish links with providers offering clinical trials or other research
Part F	Added in 1996 to combine previously existing programs, this part includes: (1) 15 AIDS Education and Training Centers (AETCs) that provide training for health care professionals in early diagnosis and treatment of HIV infection; (2) the Dental Reimbursement Program, which assists dental schools and post-doctoral dental programs through grants for uncompensated costs incurred in providing oral health treatment to patients with HIV disease; and (3) the Special Projects of National Significance Program, which supports, through competitive grants, time-limited projects that demonstrate and evaluate innovative service delivery models for special populations with HIV disease

demonstration programs to provide Medicaid to workers with potentially severe disabilities, including HIV/AIDS, who are not yet disabled. Many of these legislative acts would not have been passed if it were not for the tireless campaigning of AIDS advocacy groups throughout the country.

However, these campaigns drew the ire of those working to improve the care and services provided to patients living with other diseases. A term arose in the early 1990s, arguing the special funding and programs for HIV was a form of 'exceptionalism'. 'Exceptionalism' is not a new concept – it first arose in 1972 when patients with end stage renal disease (ESRD) received Medicare benefits, even if they did not reach the age requirements. Though the ESRD program has faced a number of challenges, it has survived largely because eligibility is not dependent on income, but simply on the presence or absence of the disease (US Institute of Medicine, 1973). When AZT was introduced, many people living with the disease did not have insurance but had income levels above the limit for Medicare. ADAPs, as described above, were introduced to help expand coverage. However, with the introduction of protease inhibitors, ADAP programs, run by state governments, have experienced tremendous pressure. Across the United States, ADAPs saw costs increase by as much as 400 per cent in the first half of 1996 (National Alliance of State and Territorial AIDS Directors, 1996). At one point, nearly half of ADAP programs offered only limited access to protease inhibitors (Carton, 1996). On the one hand, a patchwork of programs has attempted to provide care for those who could not otherwise receive these costly treatments. There are those who argue that the 'absence of [benefits like those in the Ryan White Act] for persons with other stigmatizing diseases is troubling ... this discrepancy leaves AIDS exceptionalism vulnerable to the accusations of injustice' (Casarett and Lantos, 1998).

The success of AIDS activism in creating distinct and generous federal funding that targeted HIV/AIDS services, treatment and research has altered the way in which public health discourses are conducted around the allocation of resources for other serious and chronic illnesses. Specifically, organized coalitions for other diseases ranging from breast cancer to juvenile diabetes to Parkinson's disease have argued for their increased share of limited health care dollars. Though far from a widely accepted view in the HIV activist community, Martin Delaney, the founder of Project Inform, remarked, 'There are certainly other life threatening diseases out there. Some of them kill a lot more people than AIDS does. So in one sense, it is almost an advantage to be HIV positive. It makes no sense' (Stolberg, 1997).

To mobilize their constituents, celebrities have become increasingly involved as part of lobbying campaigns, in order to influence the public through the media. Earlier public health efforts such as the fight against polio through the March of Dimes and Jerry Lewis' Labor Day Telethons to raise funds for muscular dystrophy research have utilized celebrities and the media. However, the advent of AIDS and the publicity of the deaths of public figures such as Rock Hudson and Arthur Ashe, the infection of Magic Johnson, and the highly visible involvement of luminaries such as Elizabeth Taylor, brought about an unprecedented involvement of public figures advocating for health concerns. Activism surrounding HIV has created a new cultural norm for how diseases are discussed in public forums and how resources are mobilized in the public and private sector.

As new therapeutics continue to emerge, and as the epidemic continues to expand in America, the debate surrounding HIV exceptionalism will continue, and will have a significant impact on funding for other diseases. However, without a broadening of the constituencies that can benefit from programs such as Ryan

White CARE Act, funding for HIV programs will face an uncertain future during volatile economic times.

Transforming Infection Control

As epidemiological evidence grew in support of the theory that HIV was transmitted sexually and through blood and blood products, there was increasing fear throughout the medical establishment that high exposure to blood and blood products increased potential risk for contracting the virus. These fears were exposed to the public limelight in the late 1980s by Dr Lorraine Day, a prominent orthopedic surgeon who refused to operate on people with HIV (Goodman, 1988). In response, throughout the 1980s, various organizations set forth guidelines that transformed infection control practices. In 1982 the Centers for Disease Control published clinical and laboratory precautions that soon after were expanded to health care workers and allied health professionals (CDC, 1982, 1985, 1986). Subsequently the University of California at San Francisco AIDS Task Force, the College of American Pathologists and the American Hospital Association published similar recommendations to their respective constituents. (Conte *et al.*, 1983; College of American Pathologists, 1983; American Hospital Association, 1983). In the United States and most developed nations, health care systems quickly adopted similar guidelines in order to protect health care workers and patients, and to rebuild the trust of health care consumers.

In the late 1980s, the public developed a new fear as stories circulated regarding health care worker to patient transmission of HIV. The most compelling story was that of Dr David Acer, a Florida dentist who was diagnosed with HIV in 1987. He received his medical care some distance from his practice, while continuing to provide care for clients at his office. In 1989, Kimberly Bergalis, one of Dr Acer's patients, was diagnosed with AIDS. She denied a history of sexual intercourse, IV drug use, or a history of blood transfusion and reported treatment by a dentist whom she believed to have AIDS. Subsequently, six other patients in Acer's practice became infected with HIV. Genetic sequencing demonstrated that the viruses they carried were closely related, suggesting that Acer was the source of infection. The Bergalis family went on to wage a bitter and public battle for mandatory testing for all health care workers. Subsequent studies by the Centers for Disease Control revealed that because of the extremely low chance of transmission of HIV from provider to patient, mandatory screening of health care workers is unjustified. Nevertheless, the impact of the scare was significant. The health care environment had to adapt to legitimate concern that HIV could be spread either by negligence or deliberate intent from medical professionals to patients. Dentists started wearing surgical masks, emergency medical personnel donned protective gear when attending to people on the street, and health care facilities adopted a panoply of new safety measures.

Throughout the 1980s, as the number of cases of HIV rose among hemophiliacs, the public fear of blood products heightened. With increased public awareness of the risk for HIV transmission through blood transfusion, the public's fear of potential infection led to an increase in directed and autologous transfusions, resulting in an underutilization of blood bank services. In the United States they also faced numerous lawsuits from blood recipients who had contracted HIV from transfusions prior to the introduction of an HIV detection test. One highly celebrated tragic case was that of Arthur Ashe, a world-renowned tennis professional, who had acquired HIV infection from transfusion during coronary artery bypass surgery.

The American Association of Blood Banks (AABB), apprehensive that the alteration of universal donation policies would lead to fragmentation of the blood supply, and fearing an enormous financial burden they would face from lawsuits, established a number of reforms to regain the public trust. Over the course of the 50 years prior to the discovery of HIV, blood banks tested donations for syphilis and then hepatitis B surface markers. From 1985 onwards, seven additional tests were instituted in routine screening, including HIV, leading blood banks to perform over 95 million more tests on donations from 1985 to 1995 than in the prior 50 years (McCullough, 1993). Screening processes needed to change in order to determine at-risk individuals, and new surveys were designed to broach sensitive topics on sexuality. In addition, blood banks developed a donor deferral registry (DDR) to cross check donations with previously determined unsuitable donors (Grossman and Springer, 1992). In order to determine safety outcomes of the numerous reforms instated by the AABB, the National Blood Data Resource Center was founded in 1997 to collect, analyze, and distribute data on all aspects of blood banking and transfusion medicine (American Association of Blood Banks, 2003). The relatively small threat of transfusion-acquired HIV has led to tremendous improvements in quality and safety throughout the American blood banking system that would not have been initiated otherwise.

A New Care Model

Time went on and HIV/AIDS science improved. The tools for following a patient's disease and treating both symptoms and underlying viral infection advanced dramatically. Not only could we treat HIV, but we could also tailor and modify ART to an individual's need. Treatment decisions were an art, as well as a science, and remain so, but more effective medical therapy clearly led to a new care model. For example, as the natural history of HIV infection was mapped from numerous epidemiological and clinical studies, it became clear that CD4 T lymphocyte counts could be used to stage HIV disease. Results of CD4 T lymphocyte counts were used to determine when to initiate opportunistic infection prophylaxis and ART. However, CD4 counts had limited clinical utility in predictive progression of disease, and instead were used as an indirect or 'surrogate' marker of HIV disease progression (Mellors *et al.*, 1996, 1997).

In the 1990s, new technologies, including the polymerase chain reaction (PCR) assay, the branched DNA (bDNA) assay and the nucleic acid sequence-based amplification (NASBA) assay, made it possible to obtain accurate quantitative measurements of HIV RNA in plasma (Kievits *et al.*, 1991; Piatak *et al.*, 1993; Pachl *et al.*, 1995). These tests were used on samples from volunteers from the Multicenter AIDS Cohort Study (MACS), a project of the National Institute of Allergy and Infectious Diseases (NIAID). The MACS was one of the largest prospective HIV studies in the world. More than 5000 homosexual and bisexual men were enrolled into the MACS between 1983 and 1991 at MACS clinical sites in Baltimore, Los Angeles, Pittsburgh and Chicago. Each volunteer was seen every 3–6 months for an assessment of their virologic, immunologic, clinical, behavioral, and neurologic status.

Dr John W Mellors, of the University of Pittsburgh Medical Center, and his colleagues from MACS, found that the level of HIV RNA in a person's plasma was an excellent predictor of the risk of disease progression in conjunction with the CD4+ T cell count (Mellors *et al.*, 1996) (Figure 10.1). HIV RNA plasma levels proved to be a powerful predictor and were soon commonly employed not only to determine disease progression, but also to determine the relative effectiveness of antiretroviral drugs in clinical trials. Physicians found that if patients were failing antiretroviral regimens because the virus had developed drug resistance, the patient's viral loads would rise sooner than the CD4 counts would drop. However, just as CD4 counts were surrogate markers of disease progression, viral loads were surrogate markers of development of drug resistance. In order to have a more direct measure, physicians and scientists refined genotypic and phenotypic testing to determine development of resistance. These tests have allowed physicians to change drug regimens before significant morbidity or mortality can occur. This has arguably increased the quality of life for people living with HIV, while decreasing hospitalization and health care utilization costs.

This evolution in laboratory techniques to monitor HIV disease progression and response to treatment has had a profound impact on other viral chronic diseases – most significantly hepatitis C. Viral loads, in conjunction with liver function tests, are now routinely used to monitor patients living with hepatitis C. The number of laboratories capable of doing relatively complex laboratory procedures necessary to execute these tests has increased accordingly.

AIDS Specialty Practice

By the end of the first decade of the pandemic, HIV infection had been transformed from an acute to chronic disease process. This shift in perspective may be attributed to two trials sponsored by the National Institutes of Health, both of

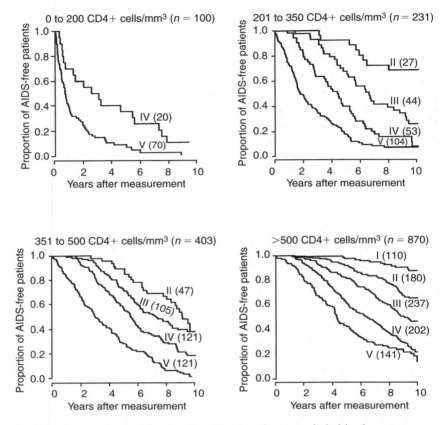

Fig. 10.1 Progression to AIDS based on CD4 lymphocyte and viral load measurements. From Mellors *et al.* (1996, 1997). Kaplan-Meier curves showing AIDS-free survival by HIV-1 RNA category among groups with different baseline CD4+ lymphocyte counts. The five categories of HIV-1 RNA were the following: I, 500 copies/ml or less; II, 501–3000 copies/ml; III, 3001–10 000 copies/ml; IV, 10 001–30 000 copies/ml; and V, more than 30 000 copies/ml. Numbers in parentheses are the sample sizes of the groups at baseline. Groups that were too small to provide estimates were omitted.

which terminated in 1989. The first demonstrated the efficacy of aerosolized pentamidine for prevention of the most common opportunistic infection at the time, *Pneumocystis carinii* pneumonia (Leoung *et al.*, 1990). The second trial demonstrated the effect of zidovudine in extending the natural history of HIV infection (Volberding *et al.*, 1990).

These new drug treatments created a new imperative – for the first time since the discovery of HIV, people who were at risk for infection had an incentive to be tested. From the perspective of health care financiers (government officials and insurance executives), AIDS could now be characterized by brief acute episodes requiring intensive hospitalization with longer periods of outpatient or nursing home care.

This model of care was further reinforced with the discovery of protease inhibitors, a new class of HIV drugs approved in 1996 (Collier *et al.*, 1996). Mass media outlets heralded the discovery as revolutionary, truly transforming HIV from an acute to chronic illness. *Newsweek* ran a cover story declaring 'The end of AIDS' where the authors reported '... though this is not the end of the plague ... this year's breakthrough does mark the end of our long-established way of thinking about the virus. Doctors are starting to consider HIV a chronic, manageable disease rather than a death sentence' (Leland, 1996). Another article in the same issue described triple drug therapy, also known as highly active antiretroviral therapy (HAART), as bringing people back from the brink of death. We were now seeing 'the Lazarus effect' (Leland, 1996).

As scientific advancements transformed the fundamental nature of HIV care, infectious disease specialists had to transform accordingly. Before the advent of ART, infectious disease specialists functioned as acute care managers. But with the introduction of HAART, care providers began to identify a number of complications of therapy, including the development of anemia, hepatitis, rash, metabolic and morphologic dysregulation. The evolution of HIV/AIDS as a chronic and complex disease has had several implications for patient care:

1. HIV care providers have become educated to monitor their patients for a wide array of clinical conditions, some related to the patients' risk behaviors (e.g. sexually transmitted disease screening), some related to HIV disease itself, and others related to anticipated complications of antiretroviral therapy (Table 10.2).
2. Clinicians have tended to delay the initiation of antiretroviral therapy until the patient is at increased risk for clinical progression from their immunodeficiency in order to avert medication-related complications (Table 10.3).
3. Generalists often needed to involve clinicians specialized in HIV care to assist in the management of HIV-infected patients' health maintenance issues (Dubé *et al.*, 2003). HIV care providers enjoy a close relationship with their patients, providing a major opportunity for primary and secondary prevention of non-HIV-related conditions.

However, a debate – which continues today – arose around the identification of an 'HIV specialist'. In order to determine Medicaid reimbursement rates for HIV care, various states or organizations have come up with similar, yet varied definitions of what constitutes an HIV specialist (HIV Medicine Association, 2003). However, most definitions have agreed that fellowship training in infectious diseases alone is not sufficient enough training to provide care for people living with HIV.

Two societies currently exist serving the needs of HIV care providers: the American Association of HIV Medicine (AAHIVM) and the HIV Medicine

Table 10.2   Comprehensive management of HIV-infected patients.

A: Relevant clinical history
Medical issues
Prior medical, surgical or psychiatric conditions
Current medications
Drug allergies
Prior or current infection with tuberculosis, sexually transmitted infections and/or
  viral hepatitis (A, B, or C)
Reproductive health history
Travel history
Immunizations
HIV-specific issues
    Duration of infection
    CD4 counts
    Plasma viral load measurements
    History of opportunistic infections or neoplasms
    Antiretroviral therapy history
    Prophylactic medications
    Nutritional history
Behavioral issues
Prior and current alcohol and other drug use
Cigarette and other nicotine use
Awareness of how HIV infection is transmitted, and current pattern of risk behaviors
Emotional status – presence of depression
Social issues
Family and other primary support systems
Employment/insurance status
Community involvement

B: Initial laboratory assessment
Complete blood count and differential
CD4 cell count
Plasma viral load (by branched DNA, PCR, or NASBA)
Serum chemistries: liver function tests, glucose, fasting lipid profile, BUN/creatinine
Syphilis serology (RPR or VDRL)
If status unknown, screen for hepatitis B and C
PPD and control
PAP smear for women
Toxoplasmosis serology
Chest X-ray, if (+) cough or constitutional symptoms
G6PD in appropriate populations

PCR, polymerase chain reaction; NASBA, nucleic acid sequence-based amplification; BUN,
blood urea nitrogen; RPR, rapid plasma reagin; PPD, purified protein derivative; G6PD,
glucose-6-phosphate dehydrogenase.

Table 10.3 Considerations regarding when to initiate antiretroviral therapy.

Clinical category	CD4 cell count and HIV RNA	Recommendation[a]
Acute HIV or <6 months after seroconversion	All	Treat
Symptomatic (AIDS, thrush, unexplained fever)	All	Treat
Asymptomatic	CD4 <200 cells/mm^3	Treat
Asymptomatic	CD4 200–359 cells/mm^3	Plasma HIV-1 RNA level (VL) of <20 000 in this CD4 strata is associated with low rates of progression; some experts would defer therapy
Asymptomatic	CD4 >350 cells/cubic mm	Defer. Some experts would offer treatment to patients with VL >55 000 since this defines a >15% risk of an AIDS-defining diagnosis in 3 years

[a] Recommendations are based on CD4 count and VL thresholds that define a 15% probability of an AIDS-defining diagnosis within three years. The strength of the recommendation depends on probability of adherence and prognosis for disease-free survival based on CD4 count and, to a lesser extent, on VL.

Association (HIVMA). The mission statement of HIVMA, which was founded by the Infectious Diseases Society of America is 'to provide an organizational home for medical professionals engaged in HIV medicine' (Infectious Diseases Society of America, 2003). AAHIVM, which was founded by several HIV primary care providers, describes itself as 'an independent organization of HIV specialists and others dedicated to promoting excellence in HIV/AIDS care ... advocacy and education' (American Academy of HIV Medicine, 2003).

The major difference between these organizations lies in their approach to credentialing care providers as HIV specialists. The AAHIVM has initiated an external credentialing service that is open to all practitioners, whereas HIVMA is seeking to grant a Certificate of Additional Qualification, which would be open primarily to generalists and infectious diseases specialists. One major debate about the process that each association has chosen for credentialing is that AAHIVM itself has taken on the responsibility for the certification process while HIVMA has worked with the American Board of Medical Specialties, the traditional agency responsible for medical specialists to develop a certification process analogous to that of other subspecialties.

Despite the various definitions of what constitutes an HIV specialist, or how these differences will play out, it is clear that the fundamental nature of HIV care has changed from acute to chronic care. Infectious disease training is heavily based on inpatient care, whereas with the advent of triple combination therapy, HIV medicine has become a largely outpatient-based disease. Many of the principles of the development of resistance are taught during an infectious diseases fellowship, which inform to a degree how antiretroviral therapy failure is managed. However, with HIV patients living longer, and the metabolic derangements encountered from antiretroviral therapy, chronic general medicine issues such as hypertension, diabetes, osteoporosis, and heart disease are becoming more relevant in the care of people living with HIV. The epidemic has matured in a way that needs these organization's complementary services. Credentialing will become increasingly formalized as the costs and complexity of care continue to increase.

Short-term Versus Long-term Care

Many comparisons have been made between the oncology and the HIV model of care. People living with cancer and HIV both receive drug regimens that have significant morbidity and toxicity. Both types of patients require frequent clinical visits to specialized physicians. One major difference between people living with cancer or HIV is that chemotherapy is generally a major short-term intervention, whereas antiretroviral regimens are currently a lifelong, continuous intervention. However, despite this difference, as chemotherapeutic and antiretroviral regimens improve HIV and many forms of cancer have been transformed into chronic diseases.

Both oncology and infectious diseases are inextricably tied to public health systems and public health approaches to disease prevention. As scientists learn more about environmental agents that can induce cancerous transformations in cells, public health officials have spent significant energy on reducing public exposure to teratogens. The most specific example is the fight against tobacco. HIV medicine has faced similar issues – for example, the inability to access clean needles has helped fuel the epidemic in certain areas. HIV however, unlike cancer, can be spread from one individual to another through direct contact. HIV care providers are increasingly forced to provide prevention messages at the individual level, while experiencing professional and personal pressure to engage at a community level.

As patients live longer with these chronic diseases, a host of services have arisen to meet the needs of these populations. Specialty ancillary services have been developed, including nurses, psychologists, psychopharmacologists, social workers, and field staff, to assist in the support and care of people living with HIV and cancer. This has proven to be critically important in helping people with living with HIV, since at the beginning of the epidemic, HIV spread predominately through disenfranchised groups – homosexual men, injection drug users, women and minorities. These groups had limited access to health care, and had few social support structures. Coping with a continuous, long-term treatment places great stress on intimate relationships, families and communities, and these support teams have become a critical part of retaining and providing top-quality care to traditionally disenfranchised groups. Many lessons have been shared between oncology and HIV patient support groups strengthening the services provided to both patient groups. Instead of splitting biological and psychosocial services, at the expense of the patient's quality of life, team structures and systems have developed to incorporate them into a relatively seamless continuum of care from home to hospital.

What the Future Holds

AIDS has been transforming the way health care is delivered in the United States and abroad. Specialists have had to adapt to the demands of providing broader primary care and primary care providers have had to learn aspects of technical specialty care. Both absorbed an enhanced appreciation for prevention. While many tests will still face us in the coming years, the lessons learned to date help inform our understanding of the future.

The Future of HIV Clinical Care in the US

A number of challenges will be faced as the United States faces its third decade of the HIV epidemic. Many of these challenges are not new: the government will need to continue to reduce the number of new HIV infections in the country, through targeting at-risk populations, tailoring interventions, reducing stigma, integrating prevention and treatments, and increasing prevention research. Also, there is a need to increase the number of people with HIV/AIDS who are in care by increasing the number of people who know about their HIV status, increasing access to care and coverage for people living with HIV/AIDS. These issues have come to prominence with the HIV Cost and Utilization Study. Although previous research has suggested that some segments of the HIV-infected population encounter serious difficulties in accessing care, the HIV Cost and Services Utilization Study (HCSUS) is the first study to demonstrate systemic, socioeconomic differences in access to HIV care across all regions of America (Bozzette *et al.*, 1998, 2001). Institutions will need to address the disproportionate impact of HIV on racial and ethnic minorities. Finally, the United States will need to maintain attention to the national epidemic while also responding to global crises.

The question that arises is whether the US public will be willing to help support and finance the numerous objectives in the country's continuing struggle against the epidemic. Recent polling suggests that the US public believes that

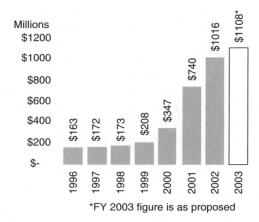

Fig. 10.2 Spending by the US on global HIV/AIDS; fiscal years 1996–2003. From Kaiser Family Foundation Global Spending on the HIV/AIDS Epidemic Report (October 2002) (Jennifer Kates).

federal government spending on HIV is necessary. Less than 10 per cent stated that the US government spends too much on HIV. Public opinion is also in favor of prevention (44 per cent) and vaccine research (41 per cent) over AIDS treatment programs (6 per cent) (Kaiser Family Foundation, 2003).

The Future of HIV Clinical Care Internationally

As the world confronts its third decade with HIV, ever increasing importance is being placed by the international community on combating the global spread of the virus. Though much is still necessary from public and private sectors in America and Europe, substantial progress has been made in curbing the spread of the epidemic, and bringing much needed access to treatment to people living with HIV in these areas. Much of this progress can be attributed to strong civil society movements that demand access and equity in care and treatment. Organizations have pushed governmental and corporate entities to streamline pharmaceutical approval systems, increase coverage for medication and treatment and provide ancillary services to people living with HIV.

The successes of these partnerships have provided the basis for the current generation of collaboration. As HIV continues to spread into resource-limited settings of Africa, Asia, and Latin America, the global community is recognizing the need to develop strategic partnerships that will allow transfer of resources – financial, intellectual or otherwise.

The United States began financing global HIV programs in the mid-1980s (Figures 10.2 and 10.3). Over the years, this amount has risen to US$1 billion in

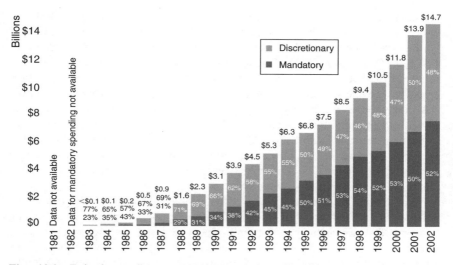

Fig. 10.3 Federal spending on HIV/AIDS by type (mandatory or discretionary), 1981–2002. From Kaiser Family Foundation Global Spending on the HIV/AIDS Epidemic Report (October 2002) (Jennifer Kates).

2002, accounting for 7 per cent of the US Government's total spending on HIV/AIDS. A majority of this increase has occurred in the last two years. Disbursement of funds occurs through five departments – State (through USAID), Health and Human Services (including the NIH, CDC, and HRSA), Agriculture, Defense, and Labor. This reflects the US Government's position that HIV is a potential destabilizing force on already critical situations around the globe. Thus, HIV is being increasingly viewed by public health and political leaders as a military, geo-political, and humanitarian issue. Whatever lens governments use to view the epidemic, one thing is clear – the commitment to fighting HIV globally is increasing. Yet, in a national survey by the Kaiser Family Foundation, only approximately 20 per cent believed that the US has a responsibility to fight HIV internationally, and almost 70 per cent stated that the US must first address domestic issues (Kaiser Family Foundation, 2003). The potential for the wider spread of HIV to destabilize many developing societies needs to be communicated to the public with greater clarity, as general opinion is more divided over the role of US funds internationally than domestically.

Access to care has increased in part from increased interventions from governments and civil society. Another major force increasing access to treatment has been the introduction of generic antiretroviral medications to the global market. Production of antiretroviral medications by generic manufacturers in developing countries has drastically reduced the price of combination HAART to around US$1 per day (Angerer *et al.*, 2001). Lower prices have allowed resource-limited centers to afford and administer HAART to HIV seropositive patients. However, widely accepted antiretroviral monitoring guidelines utilizing frequent CD4 T lymphocyte counts and HIV plasma viral load testing can cost upwards of US$1000 (Yeni *et al.*, 2002). The costs can be largely attributed to the patent-protected methods of nucleic acid amplification (PCR, bDNA, NASBA) and the complex machinery and reagents necessary for CD4 T lymphocyte quantification.

Fortunately, several important initiatives have arisen to address this problem. The World Health Organization in 2002 has released provisional guidelines for implementation and scaling up of ART in resource-limited settings (WHO, 2002). Research has emerged demonstrating that total lymphocyte count may serve as a surrogate marker for CD4 T lymphocytes, and p24 antigen may function as an alternative marker to plasma viral load.

Much of this research has occurred with bilateral North–South institutional collaborations. This model of research is providing a framework for multilateral networks that are helping to facilitate global research. In addition, increased global interactions have created a new generation of young health professionals who are comfortable working simultaneously in the developed and developing worlds.

Directly Observed Antiretroviral Therapy

Over the past few years, multiple antiretroviral medications have been developed that can be administered on a once-daily basis, including medicines in all three of the most commonly used therapeutic classes, including nucleosides like 3TC, FTC, ddI EC, abacavir; nucleotides like tenofovir; non-nucleoside reverse transcriptise inhibitors like nevirapine or efavirenz; and atazanavir and other protease inhibitors that are ritonavir-boosted.

A number of care providers have investigated the utility of integrating directly observed therapy (DOT) into HIV care after realizing the tremendous impact its implementation has had on tuberculosis (Mitty *et al.*, 2002). The initiation of DOT in the treatment of tuberculosis has improved cure rates in marginal populations. HIV and TB affect similar demographic groups globally, and DOT may serve as an important tool to deliver quality care while increasing adherence and decreasing the development of drug resistance. DOT for management of HIV infection has been effective among prisoners and in pilot programs in Haiti, Rhode Island, and Florida (Mitty *et al.*, 1999; Babudiere *et al.*, 2000; Farmer *et al.*, 2001; Fischl *et al.*, 2001).

Although DOT has successfully treated HIV infection in marginalized populations in the short term, a number of questions remain. HIV infection currently requires daily treament, sometimes up to three times a day, whereas there are substantially simpler regimens for TB. HIV infection must be treated lifelong, whereas TB is limited. Therefore, HIV DOT must not only deliver medicines, but additionally help develop the skills needed for independent medication administration. TB DOT programs do not have to confront these multitudes of challenges (Mitty *et al.*, 2002).

DOT programs to deliver HIV medications may be particularly efficacious if they are engrafted onto other systems that may rely upon institutionalized monitoring of daily adherence to medication regimens, such as methadone maintenance programs for opiate addiction (Clarke *et al.*, 2002). Moreover, for incarcerated populations once-daily antiretroviral regimens with observed adherence monitoring may optimize therapeutic responses and optimize patient care in such institutional settings (Wohl *et al.*, 2003). DOT is a promising strategy in improving the quality of care for many people with HIV, and is rightly considered 'a work in progress' (Mitty *et al.*, 2002).

References

American Academy of HIV Medicine (2003) http://www.aahivm.org/new/index.html (accessed 6 October 2003).

American Association of Blood Banks (2003) Highlights in Transfusion Medicine History. http://www.aabb.org/All_About_Blood/FAQs/aabb_faqs.htm#8 (accessed 17 October 2003).

American Hospital Association (1983) *A Hospital-Wide Approach to AIDS*. Advisory Committee on Infections within Hospitals, December 1983.

Angerer T, Wilson D, Ford N, Kasper T (2001) Access and activism: the ethics of providing antiretroviral therapy in developing countries. *AIDS* 15 (Suppl 5): S81–S90.

Arno PS, Feiden KL (1992) *Against the Odds: The story of AIDS Drug Development, Politics and Profit*. New York: Harper Collins.

Baudiere S, Aceti A, D'Offizi GP *et al.* (2000) Directly observed therapy to treat HIV infection in prisoners. *JAMA* 284: 179–80.

Bozzette SA, Berry SH, Duan N *et al.* (1998) The care of HIV-infected adults in the United States. HIV Cost and Services Utilization Study Consortium. *N Engl J Med* 339: 1897–904.

Bozzette SA, Joyce G, McCaffrey DF *et al.* (2001) Expenditures for the care of HIV-infected patients in the era of highly active antiretroviral therapy. *N Engl J Med* 344: 817–23.

Carton B (1996) New AIDS drug brings hope to Provincetown, but unexpected woes. *Wall Street Journal* 3 October 1996: A1.

Casarett DJ, Lantos JD (1998) Have we treated AIDS too well? Rationing and the future of AIDS exceptionalism. *Ann Intern Med* 128: 756–9.

CDC (1982) Acquired immune deficiency syndrome (AIDS): precautions for clinical and laboratory staffs. *MMWR Morbid Mortal Wkly Rep* 32: 577–80.

CDC (1985) Recommendations for preventing transmission of infection with HTLV-III/LAV in the workplace. *MMWR* 34: 681–95.

CDC (1986) Recommendations for preventing transmission of infection with HTLV-III/LAV during invasive procedures. *MMWR* 35: 221–23.

Clarke S, Keenan E, Ryan M, Barry M, Mulcahy F (2002) Directly observed antiretroviral therapy for injection drug users with HIV infection. *AIDS Read* 12: 305–7, 312–16.

College of American Pathologists (1983) *Proceedings of the Task Force on AIDS*. Fall.

Collier AC, Coombs RW, Schoenfeld DA *et al.* (1996) The AIDS Clinical Trials Group treatment of human immunodeficiency virus infection with saquinavir, zidovudine, and zalcitabine. *N Engl J Med* 334: 1011–18.

Conte JE *et al.* and the University of California San Francisco Task Force on the Acquired Immunodeficiency Syndrome (1983) Special report: infection control guidelines for patients with the acquired immunodeficiency syndrome (AIDS). *N Engl J Med* 309: 740–4.

Dubé MP, Stein JH, Aberg JA *et al.* for the Adult AIDS Clinical Trials Group (2003) Cardiovascular subcommittee guidelines for the evaluation and management of dyslipidemia in human immunodeficiency virus (hiv) infected adults receiving antiretroviral therapy: Recommendations of the HIV Medicine Association of the Infectious Disease Society of America and the Adult AIDS Clinical Trials Group. *Clin Infect Dis* 37: 613–27.

Farmer P, Leandre F, Mukherjee JS *et al.* (2001) Community-based approaches to HIV treatment in resource-poor settings. *Lancet* 358: 404–9.

Fischl M, Castro J, Mondoig R *et al.* (2001) Impact of directly observed therapy on long-term outcomes in HIV clinical trials (abstract 528). In: *Program and abstracts of the 8th Conference on Retroviruses and Opportunistic Infections (Chicago)*. Alexandria, VA: Foundation for Retrovirology and Human Health, p. 202.

Goodman E (1988) For doctors, an AIDS dilemma that's spreading with the disease. *Boston Globe*, 25 February.

Grossman BJ, Springer KM (1992) Blood donor deferral registries: highlights of a conference. *Transfusion* 32: 868–72.

Hardy AM *et al.* (1986) The economic impact of the first 10 000 cases of acquired immunodeficiency syndrome in the United States. *JAMA* 255: 209–15.

HIV Medicine Association (2003) HIV Quality Care network: HIV provider Definitions. http://www.hivma.org/HIV/HIVnet_ProDef.htm (accessed 6 October 2003).

Infectious Diseases Society of America (2003) HIV Medicine Association, http://www.idsociety.org/HIV/HIVMA/Announce_9-00.htm (accessed 6 October 2003).

Kaiser Family Foundation (2003) http://headlines.kff.org/healthpollreport/feature8/media/feature.pdf (accessed 17 January 2003).

Kievits T, van Gemen B, van Strijp D *et al.* (1991) NASBA isothermal enzymatic in vitro nucleic acid amplification optimized for the diagnosis of HIV-1 infection. *J Virol Methods* 35: 273–86.

Leland J (1996) The end of AIDS? *Newsweek* 2 December.

Leoung GS, Feigal DW Jr, Montgomery AB *et al.* (1990) Aerosolized pentamidine for prophylaxis against *Pneumocystis carinii* pneumonia. The San Francisco community prophylaxis trial. *N Engl J Med* 323: 769–75.

McCullough J (1993) The Nation's Changing Blood Supply System. *JAMA* 269.

Mellors JW, Rinaldo CR, Gupta P, White RM, Todd JA, Kingsley LA (1996) Prognosis in HIV-1 infection predicted by the quantity of virus in plasma. *Science* 272: 1167–70.

Mellors JW, Munoz A, Giorgi JV *et al.* (1997) Plasma viral load and CD4+ lymphocytes as prognostic markers of HIV-1 infection. *Ann Intern Med* 126: 946–54.

Mitty JS, McKenzie M, Stenzel M *et al.* (1999) Modified directly observed therapy for treatment of human immunodeficiency virus [research letter]. *JAMA* 282: 1334.

Mitty JA, Stone VE, Sands M, Macalino G, Flanigan T (2002) Directly observed therapy for the treatment of people with human immunodefiency virus infection: a work in progress. *Clin Infect Dis* 34: 984–90.

National Alliance of State and Territorial AIDS Directors (1996) Fiscal Status Update of State AIDS Drug Assistance Programs: Preliminary Findings from an August 1996 National Survey of State AIDS Programs. Washington, DC: National Alliance of State and Territorial AIDS Directors, 9 September: Table 1.

Pachl C, Todd JA, Kern DG *et al.* (1995) Rapid and precise quantification of HIV-1 RNA in plasma using a branched DNA signal amplification assay. *J Acquir Immune Defic Syndr Hum Retrovirol* 8: 446–54.

Piatak M, Saag MS, Yang LC *et al.* (1993) High levels of HIV-1 in plasma during all stages of infection determined by competitive PCR. *Science* 259: 1749–54.

Stolberg SG (1997) White House drops plan for Medicaid to cover cost of AIDS drugs for poor. *New York Times* 9 December: 14.

US Institute of Medicine (1973) Disease by disease toward national insurance: Report of a Panel on Implications of a Categorical Catastrophic Disease Approach to National Health Insurance. Washington, DC: National Academy of Sciences.

Volberding PA, Lagakos SW, Koch MA *et al.* (1990) Zidovudine in asymptomatic human immunodeficiency virus infection. A controlled trial in persons with fewer than 500 CD4-positive cells per cubic millimeter. The AIDS Clinical Trials Group of the National Institute of Allergy and Infectious Diseases. *N Engl J Med* 322: 941–9.

Wohl DA, Stephenson BL, Golin CE *et al.* (2003) Adherence to directly observed antiretroviral therapy among human immunodeficiency virus-infected prison inmates. *Clin Infect Dis* 36: 1572–6.

WHO (2002) Scaling up antiretroviral therapy in resource limited settings: guidelines for a public health approach. Available at www.who.int

Yeni PG, Hammer SM, Carpenter CC *et al.* (2002) Antiretroviral treatment for adult HIV infection in 2002: updated recommendations of the International AIDS Society-USA Panel. *JAMA* 288: 222–35.

The Ever-changing Face of AIDS: Implications for Patient Care

11

Jennifer Furin
Brigham and Women's Hospital, Division of Social Medicine & Health Inequalities, Boston, USA

David Walton
Partners In Health, Boston, USA

Paul Farmer
Brigham and Women's Hospital, Division of Social Medicine & Health Inequalities, Boston, USA

Jennifer Furin, MD, PhD is an Infectious Disease clinician and a medical anthropologist. Her areas of interest include the treatment of HIV and of multidrug-resistant tuberculosis in resource-poor settings. Dr. Furin divides her time between the Brigham and Women's Hospital in Boston, where she currently serves as Associate Director of the Howard Hiatt Residency in Global Health Equity and Internal Medicine, and clinical field sites in Peru, Haiti, Russia, and Boston.

David Walton, MD is a resident physician at Brigham and Women's Hospital in Boston, Massachusetts. He divides his clinical time between Boston and LasCahobas, Haiti, where he also serves as a resident physician at a rural health clinic treating primarily impoverished patients with HIV disease and tuberculosis. His scholarly work has been focused on the management of tuberculosis, HIV/TB co-infection, and the implementation of HIV treatment in resource-poor settings.

Paul Farmer, MD, PhD is a medical anthropologist and physician who has dedicated his life to treating some of the world's poorest populations and to the process of helping to raise the standard of health care in underdeveloped areas of the world. He is a founding director of Partners In Health, an international charity organization that provides direct health care services and undertakes research and advocacy activities on behalf of those who are sick and living in poverty. Dr. Farmer has worked in infectious-disease control in the Americas for nearly two decades and is a world-renowned authority on tuberculosis treatment and control. He is an attending physician in infectious diseases and Chief of the Division of Social Medicine and Health Inequalities at the Brigham and Women's Hospital in Boston, and medical director of a hospital, the Clinique Bon Sauveur, in rural Haiti.

After a mere two decades of existence, AIDS is now the primary infectious killer of adults in the world today. So far is its reach, in fact, that many health and education campaigns have been launched with the central message that 'nobody is safe from AIDS'. Indeed, biological risk for this pathogen is universal: but is it true that everyone is at equal risk from AIDS? Certainly, global rates of infection show that some populations are more at risk for infection than others, with a brunt of the pandemic being born by the poor of sub-Saharan Africa. And once infected with HIV, some populations are at increased risk of dying from the disease, due in large part to lack of access to medical care. Sadly, these two populations often intersect, with those most at risk for becoming infected with HIV – the poor, the marginalized, and the disenfranchised – also being those who have at their disposal the fewest resources to manage the disease.

This chapter will review the global distribution of HIV and AIDS and examine subepidemics that are illustrative of the unequal burden of HIV risk. It will also look at issues of treatment access and will examine several model and innovative programs that combine comprehensive HIV prevention and care with services aimed at addressing poverty and inequality. Experience from these programs shows that AIDS is more than simply a disease process that ravages the body: rather it is a biosocial phenomenon that has, as its root cause, poverty and gender inequality.

Understanding and managing AIDS in the world today means, fundamentally, understanding and managing it in a way that is cognizant of the social forces and factors that put people at risk of becoming infected with the disease and that make them sick once they have acquired it. It is only when a biosocial model is brought to bear upon this modern scourge that comprehensive care and hope for those who suffer can become a reality.

AIDS in the World: The Current Situation

Perhaps no other pathogen has affected modern man as profoundly as AIDS. It is currently the leading infectious killer of adults worldwide (WHO, 1999). In the

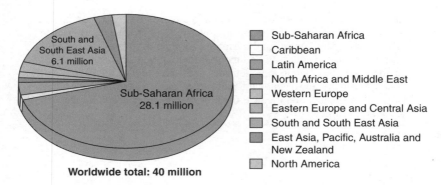

Fig. 11.1 Global distribution of adults and children living with HIV or AIDS at the end of 2001. From Lamptey (2002).

year 2002, it is estimated that 3 million people died of the disease and that the cumulative total of deaths was 28 million people (UNAIDS, 2002). In 2003, another 3 million deaths were registered along with 5 million new infections (UNAIDS, 2003). As of December 2003, it is estimated that more than 40 million people worldwide are infected with the human immunodeficiency virus (UNAIDS, 2003). No part of the world is untouched by AIDS, and the disease has been reported on every continent (UNAIDS, 2002). There is striking inequality, however, in its distribution. Not surprisingly, a majority of the world's AIDS cases are found in nations plagued by poverty, hunger, and underdevelopment. Figure 11.1 shows the global distribution of HIV infection at the end of 2001; similar trends have continued in 2002 and 2003.

Africa is home to more than 70 per cent of global AIDS cases, and in some populations, seroprevalence rates of over 35 per cent have been found (UNAIDS, 2003). It is estimated that between 25 and 28 million people with HIV and AIDS are currently living in sub-Saharan Africa and that between 3 and 4 million people are newly infected with HIV in this region each year (UNAIDS, 2003). Botswana is currently reported to have the highest prevalence of HIV with an infection rate estimated at 36 per cent; it is estimated that almost two-thirds of 15-year-old boys living in that country today will die of AIDS if infection rates continue at current pace (UNAIDS, 2002). In sub-Saharan Africa, women are especially susceptible to AIDS, with the percentage of women infected with HIV and sick with AIDS rising: an estimated 12.2 million women carry the virus compared with an estimated 10.1 million men (UNGASS, 2001). Women are 1.2 times more likely than men to be infected with HIV in sub-Saharan Africa. Among young women, this discrepancy is even more pronounced: a woman between the ages of 15 and 24 years is two and a half times as likely to be HIV infected as her male counterpart (UNAIDS, 2003).

AIDS has threatened the very development of sub-Saharan nations already mired in poverty. Because it strikes people in the prime of their lives, the workforce of

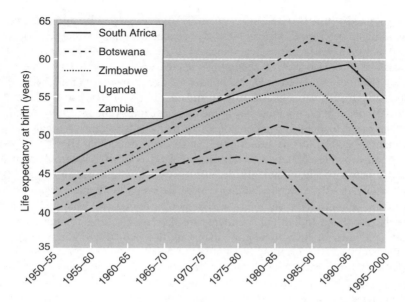

Fig. 11.2 Life expectancy in some countries in sub-Saharan Africa with a high prevalence of HIV. From Lamptey (2002).

many African nations has been decimated (WHO, 1999). What little gains have been made in terms of life expectancy are being reversed in many of the nations hardest hit by the disease (Figure 11.2). AIDS is also destroying the lives of families, as millions of children in Africa have been left orphaned by the disease (Unicef, 2000).

Although brisk debate about the nature of HIV transmission persists, most believe that HIV in sub-Saharan Africa is largely a sexually transmitted pathogen. This debate is important and should be buttressed by data gathered in the course of research that is as complex as the epidemic itself. However, poor-quality medical care – characterized by lack of access to basic primary health care and also by failure to follow universal precautions – lies at the root of many AIDS deaths in Africa. In order to fully integrate HIV prevention and care, it will of course be necessary to identify and differentially weight each important mode of transmission. But regardless of the route of infection, one conclusion is clear: the immensity and rapidity of HIV's spread has, as noted, reversed gains in life expectancy in many African countries. It is important to note that, for most of these countries, these curves are strikingly similar to projections advanced a decade ago by UNAIDS and by the WHO. Thus the worst-case scenarios for HIV have come to pass, as predicted, in the poorest parts of the world.

Even within the desperate situation in Africa, AIDS is strikingly patterned, with gender and income inequalities acting as major determinants of health. Some studies have shown that women are more than three times as likely as men to be infected with HIV (Boerma *et al.*, 2003). Although precise numbers may be impossible to determine, African victims of sexual and ethnic violence (Donovan, 2002) as well as war and physical upheaval (Eshete *et al.*, 1993; Mworozi, 1993) are also at increased risk of becoming infected and sick with HIV. One study among Sudanese refugees in Uganda under the age of five years found HIV to be responsible for 6.8 per cent of fatalities, and children with HIV had a case fatality rate of 30 per cent during their stay at the refugee camps (Orach, 1999). And HIV has been tied to debt and indebtedness in many sub-Saharan African nations (Odhiambo, 2003). As one author notes, 'there is no doubt that HIV/AIDS poses the greatest single challenge to the marginalized poor of Africa, where it has found a malnourished, vulnerable, defenseless host' (Odhiambo, 2003, p. 142).

Certainly, in Africa, we are facing a worst-case scenario. In many regions of the world, the worst may be yet to come. The poorer regions of Asia, including the densely populated Indian subcontinent, are the latest setting for the emerging AIDS epidemic. In 2003 alone more than 1 million people living in Asia and the Pacific acquired HIV, bringing the number of people living with the virus in this region to 7.4 million (UNAIDS, 2003). The spread of HIV in Asia appears to be largely fueled by injection drug use and the commercial sex trade. While many nations have national adult HIV prevalence of less than 1 per cent, given the densely populated countries found in the area, serious epidemics appear to be brewing. And certain populations – particularly injection drug users and commer-cial sex workers – are at elevated risk. In parts of China, HIV prevalence among injection drug users has been reported to be between 35 per cent and 80 per cent (UNAIDS, 2003). India is home to what is likely to be the continent's most disas-trous situation: an estimated 3.7 million people with HIV already live in this impoverished nation, and, as one author notes, 'India is also at war with poverty, illiteracy, and gender inequality, all of which make the fight against AIDS a more difficult battle' (Ratnathicam, 2001).

Three of Asia's most serious HIV pandemics are occurring in the countries of Thailand, Cambodia, and Myanmar, where HIV prevalence greater than 40 per cent has been documented among some groups of commercial sex workers (UNAIDS, 2003). Myanmar has one of the highest HIV rates in Asia, with one study estimating that 3.46 per cent of adults between the ages of 15 and 44 years are infected with HIV (Beyrer *et al.*, 2003). Not surprisingly, Myanmar is also plagued by a lack of public health infrastructure, with one author noting 'a World Health Organization report in 2000 concluded that of all its member states, only Sierra Leone had a health system that functioned worse than Myanmar's' (Cohen, 2003a, p. 1651). While government oppression may contribute to ongoing spread of the disease, lack of access to care no doubt contributes to the nation's death toll: although there are over 600 000 adults living with HIV in Myanmar, only a few hundred have access to antiretroviral treatment (Cohen, 2003a).

Nor are industrialized countries spared. Russia and the Ukraine, along with most other countries in Eastern Europe and Central Asia, claim the distinction of having the most rapidly expanding HIV epidemics. In 2003, some 230 000 people living in the region were infected with HIV (UNAIDS, 2003). As in Asia, the disease here is more closely tied to injection drug use, which itself is linked to a rapid rise in indices of social inequality (UNAIDS, 2002). Although the absolute number of AIDS cases in the former Soviet Union remains small, the epidemic is quickly spreading in Russia, with more than one-quarter of cumulative HIV cases being added in the year 2002 alone (UNAIDS, 2003). It is estimated that 1 million people between the ages of 15 and 49 are living with HIV in the Russian Federation, which is home to an estimated 3 million injection drug users (UNAIDS, 2003). HIV is closely linked with tuberculosis (TB) in the former Soviet Union (Schwalbe and Harrington, 2002). Prison-seated epidemics of TB, including drug-resistant strains, will be further fanned by the rapid rise in HIV incidence already documented among Russian prisoners (Farmer, 1999a; Coninx *et al.*, 1999). HIV is having a profound impact on the population dynamics in this region of the world, as it disproportionately affects young people; in Ukraine, for example, 25 per cent of people diagnosed with HIV are under the age of 20 years (UNAIDS, 2003).

Other Eastern European nations – such as the Czech Republic – are seeing rising rates of HIV, especially among commercial sex workers, a majority of whom are poor women who have migrated from Russia and the Ukraine (Resl *et al.*, 2003). Thus poverty and gender inequality are continuing to the fan the fires of HIV spread in this region of the world.

In Latin America and the Caribbean, several epidemiologic patterns of disease can be seen. Haiti – the region's poorest country – has also been the hardest hit by HIV. Haiti's national seroprevalence is estimated at 5–6 per cent and women are at increased risk compared with men in the region (UNAIDS, 2003). Other countries in Latin America and the Caribbean face smaller epidemics fueled by sexual transmission among men who have sex with men; in Peru, for example, seroprevalence among this group is estimated at 22 per cent; this number has risen from 18 per cent in 1998 (UNAIDS, 2003). In Brazil, HIV prevalence has remained relatively low, with rates among women attending antenatal clinics of less than 1 per cent in most regions, although in areas of high poverty, rates among such women as high as 3–6 per cent have been documented (UNAIDS, 2003). In some of the region's poorer countries, rates of HIV among women are rising. In Guatemala, for example, one study found that AIDS was responsible for 5 per cent of hospital admissions in one large regional hospital, even though general prevalence of HIV is estimated at less than 1 per cent. Among these hospital admissions, 30 per cent were women, a rising number compared to the early years of the pandemic in this region (Samayoa *et al.*, 2003). This study also demonstrated lack of access to basic HIV counseling and testing services for a majority of patients in the study, as 60 per cent were diagnosed with HIV when they presented with an illness requiring hospitalization. As in other regions of the world, even the relatively 'low burden' countries of Latin America show HIV is linked with inequality and poverty. In Mexican–US border towns, for example, high prevalence of HIV has been noted along with a dearth of public health services. The 'mobile populations' in these areas are also at increased risk of rape, other forms of violence, and poverty (Bronfman *et al.*, 2002).

Even within wealthy countries of the world, such as the United States, AIDS is a disease that is strikingly patterned along lines of social and gender inequality. The US currently shares less than 1 per cent of the global burden of HIV (CDC, 1996), although the number of people living with HIV in high-income countries is rising given improved life expectancy with antiretroviral treatment. Who are the individuals most at risk for becoming newly infected with HIV? More and more they are women and people of color (Zierler and Kreiger, 2000). Although it was first reported to be a disease primarily among men who have sex with men (CDC, 1981), HIV has taken root in the poor and marginalized communities of the United States where it remains entrenched. Although they make up only slightly more than 10 per cent of the US population, African-Americans accounted for approximately half of new HIV infections in 2003 (UNAIDS, 2003).

A study done in Atlanta found that lack of social capital, poverty, and income inequality were linked with higher rates of HIV, chlamydia, gonorrhea, and syphilis in the population studied (Holtgrave and Crosby, 2003). A study done on the neighborhood level in Boston found that the cumulative incidence of AIDS among people living in block groups where 40 per cent of the population was below the poverty line was seven times higher than among block groups where 2 per cent of the population was below the poverty line (Zierler *et al.*, 2000). Romero-Daza and colleagues found HIV infection to be strongly linked to violence and poverty among poor women living in America's inner cities (Romero-Daza *et al.*, 2003) and many studies have shown that women appear to be particularly vulnerable to the disease at the same time that they suffer from lack of access to care and treatment (Farmer *et al.*, 1996).

AIDS is now the leading cause of death among African-American women between the ages of 25 and 34 in the United States (UNAIDS, 2003). This may be due, in part, to lack of access to health care, even in a nation that boasts one of the world's leading health care systems. A study done in Los Angeles found that women and people of color were less likely to experience early HIV detection and be linked with appropriate treatment (Johnson *et al.*, 2003).

The figures presented above are dramatic: in slightly more than two decades, AIDS has become the number one infectious killer in the world. More than 40 million people are living with the disease worldwide. Of these 40 million, most are poor and suffer from a myriad other health and social concerns. In the areas of the world where HIV is expanding most rapidly, poor women are the people most likely to become infected. Thus, on a global level, when one takes a close look, the changing face of AIDS is more often that of a woman living in poverty.

Why is this the case? In order to understand the epidemiology of global HIV, it is important to take a biosocial approach to examining forces that place people at risk of the disease (Parker, 2002). Early in the course of the epidemic, it was largely felt that AIDS was a disease of men who have sex with men and of injection drug users (Farmer *et al.*, 2000). HIV 'risk groups' were highlighted, especially in the wealthy nations of the world. These risk groups included gay men, hemophiliacs, intravenous drug users, and, in the United States, a fourth risk group of being 'Haitian' was added to the list (Farmer, 1992). The categorization of these risk groups largely ignored the epidemic that was fast spreading across Africa, in which women were equally affected. Promiscuous sexual behavior was also often cited as a risk factor for acquiring the disease; in the poor countries of the world, however, such 'promiscuous' behavior was usually accounted for by at most 2 to 3 serially monogamous lifetime sexual relationships, and in a small study in Haiti, it was found that sexual relationships with soldiers or truck drivers were the riskiest of all (Farmer, 2002). A closer examination of risk for acquiring HIV reveals that it is often poverty and inequality that put people at risk for contracting HIV and for becoming sick from the virus once infection sets in (Farmer, 1996).

Stopping AIDS: How have We Done so Far?

What are the prospects for improvement in this grim scenario? Although the world's most advanced research institutions are turning their efforts towards the development of an HIV vaccine, progress has been slow (Nabel, 2001; Makgoba *et al.*, 2002; Esparza and Osmanov, 2003; WHO/UNAIDS, 2003). Thus the bulk of our interventions, in the short term, must consist of improved and integrated AIDS prevention and care. Physicians and social scientists should play a role not only in setting norms for such activities, but in assessing as honestly as possible the strengths and weaknesses of the tools currently at our disposal.

Despite two decades of experience in using information and education as the primary tools in HIV prevention, there have been, until very recently, no careful studies of the efficacy of these interventions. One meta-analysis of information and education campaigns concluded that, 'somewhat surprisingly, towards the end of the second decade of the AIDS pandemic, we still have no good evidence that primary prevention works' (Mayaud *et al.*, 1998). But there is increasing agreement that these tools, though of great importance, are of limited efficacy in precisely those settings in which they are most needed. Another study, conducted in urban Nicaraguan hotels, showed that aggressive information campaigns were actually associated with decreased condom usage (Egger *et al.*, 2000). A study done in India found that while more than 75 per cent of women surveyed understood how HIV is transmitted, only 8 per cent reported prevention methods. Of note in this study is that 30 per cent of the women surveyed reported being the victims of physical or mental abuse from their male partners (Shrotri *et al.*, 2003). It is important to draw sound conclusions from such studies, since there are obvious policy implications. 'Information and education campaigns' are necessary but inadequate; the outcomes of such campaigns are related to local social conditions (Farmer *et al.*, 1996). As one author of a study in Brazil notes: 'prevention campaigns aimed at certain groups often are not successful. One of the primary reasons for these failures is that the socioeconomic and cultural context of the target audience has been neglected by the campaigners' (McCalman, 2003, p. 565).

These sobering analyses, too long in coming, should not dampen our commitment to HIV education. Indeed, such efforts, especially among certain populations, might best be considered a global civic duty. Global health agencies should ensure, for example, that all who will come of age in the next few years have access to both accurate knowledge and effective preventive technologies. The WHO, for example, will consider 'AIDS prevention equity' – whereby correct and culturally appropriate information be imparted, along with existing prevention tools, to those most at risk of HIV infection – an important part of its AIDS portfolio. Countries such as Cambodia and Thailand have seen HIV infection rates fall at the same time that they have launched nationwide education and condom-use programs. Of note in these two countries is that education campaigns are tied to the provision of health and social services for recipients (Cohen, 2003b).

It is now clear that information and education campaigns will not in and of themselves inflect the incidence of HIV infections among the world's most vulnerable populations. Social conditions, rather than ignorance about HIV and its modes of transmission, are the primary determinants of risk in many of the poorest parts of the world. The dynamics of HIV risk for many people from quite different backgrounds can be evaluated. These people do not have a common language or culture; what they share is a position on the bottom rung of social structures.

Limitations to the Current Paradigm

The epidemiology of HIV, including the dynamics of risk, is instructive. But epidemiology tells only part of the story. The impact of HIV/AIDS on individuals, families, communities, and nations has been profound and touches hundreds of millions of people who are not themselves infected with HIV. Although no region has been spared, HIV has spread most rapidly in Africa, leaving an estimated 14 million children orphaned (UNAIDS, 2002; Wax, 2003). HIV has also fanned epidemics of tuberculosis, since the lifetime chances that quiescent infection with *Mycobacterium tuberculosis* will become active disease are increased 10-fold among HIV-infected people (Narain *et al.*, 1992). Moreover, people with HIV-associated tuberculosis transmit the air-borne disease to family members and other close contacts. Across southern Africa, rates of tuberculosis have more than trebled, and many conclude that the disease cannot be controlled without aggressive treatment of AIDS itself (Williams and Dye, 2003). Famine has been exacerbated by HIV, particularly in vulnerable regions of sub-Saharan Africa (de Waal and Whiteside, 2003).

There's much more to the story than can be readily measured by economists. Other social scientists are broadening the analysis to look at the impact of the disease on an array of events and processes. What are the myriad ways in which HIV arrests the development of poor communities? What is the cost, for example, of having millions of AIDS orphans? How does the disappearance of parents contribute to armed conflict, prostitution, and other social pathologies that accompany urban migration and attendant unemployment? What cost the 'burnout' registered among health professionals across Africa and in other settings where AIDS therapy is not available to those who need it most? In a study conducted in a Kenyan teaching hospital, for example, many young physicians were clinically depressed and announced their intention to abandon the practice of medicine. They listed AIDS and 'the poverty of the patients' as ranking reasons for their despair (Raviola *et al.*, 2002). In short, we are only now beginning to understand the social and economic toll of HIV/AIDS, which is heaviest in precisely those settings least prepared for a new threat to health and well-being.

When one examines the AIDS pandemic over the last two decades, the evidence is overwhelming that comprehensive programs linking HIV prevention and treatment are needed to turn to tide against this global killer. There is some reason to be optimistic that the future may hold these very things: at the turn of the century, a revolutionary idea was launched and the Global Fund to Fight AIDS, Tuberculosis, and Malaria (GFATM) was born (Poore, 2004). The goal of this initiative is for wealthy countries of the world to provide financial support to impoverished nations to deal with the three leading treatable infectious killers in the world today. Over a billion dollars has been pledged and GFATM has invigorated programs throughout the world to begin to tackle HIV in a holistic fashion. Much more is needed in terms of financial and human resources, however, if AIDS is to be dealt with in a truly comprehensive manner (Fleck, 2003).

AIDS: Access to Care

What is notable about the global pattern of HIV is not only its epidemiologic misalignment. It is shamefully ironic that the very populations most at risk for becoming infected with HIV and sick with the disease are also those populations least likely to have access to the advances in medical care that are making HIV a 'chronic, treatable disease' (Farmer, 1999b). No other pathogen in modern times has induced such brisk scientific enquiry. In 1996, a new class of drugs to treat HIV known as the protease inhibitors was developed and a cocktail of medications known as 'highly active antiretroviral therapy' – or HAART – was introduced, prolonging life and offering hope to those who were able to access these medications (Palella *et al.*, 1998). HAART is widely available in the United

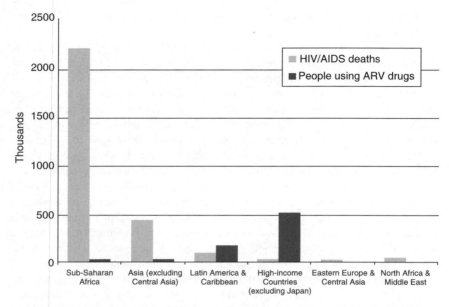

Fig. 11.3 HIV/AIDS deaths in 2001 and number of people using antiretroviral drugs by end of 2001: by region.

States and Europe, where people with advanced disease taking the drugs have been able to resume their activities of daily living, raising families, and continuing to work and enjoy fruitful lives. In the world's poor countries – and among the poor living in wealthy but inegalitarian societies – HIV remains a death sentence (Farmer, 2001). Figure 11.3 shows the proportion of AIDS deaths globally compared with the number of people receiving antiretroviral drugs and demonstrates that those most in need in the world are all too often those who go without.

Thus, even in the treatment of this disease, steep biosocial inequalities emerge. A young woman living in destitute poverty in rural Africa is more likely to become infected with HIV and at the same time is far less likely to access the medication that she needs to provide relief from this deadly disease. Even in countries such as the United States, where HAART is widely available, poor and marginalized populations are less likely to have access to treatment (Mukherjee *et al.*, 2003).

What is to be done to remedy this situation? How can care be brought to those most in need on a global level? The answers to these questions are not simple, and many in the field of global AIDS control have experienced professional burnout and fatigue in dealing with this crisis (Raviola *et al.*, 2002). If, however, HIV is understood as the biosocial phenomenon it is and efforts are made to treat it using comprehensive community-based approaches that are global in scope, the fruits of modern science may be brought to bear for those most in need.

Treating HIV Among the Poor: Integrating Prevention and Care

One of the chief lessons of recent years is the need for integrated AIDS prevention and care. Although there are studies reminding us of the need for constant and ongoing efforts to promote safe sex and good medical practice, there are no data to support the claim that increased access to AIDS care hampers prevention efforts. On the contrary, much emerging experience suggests that improving care will serve to directly strengthen prevention efforts. What accounts for the often stark division between AIDS prevention and care, which in the developing world has meant that, for most people living with HIV, there is simply no decent medical care available at all? The fact that it took 15 years to develop effective antiretroviral therapy for AIDS is regarded as a success by some; for the tens of millions who have died of AIDS, these victories come too late. But the fact that much was known about HIV and its modes of transmission well before effective therapy was available contributed, in both rich and poor countries, to a de-linking of HIV prevention and care (Farmer, 2000).

The results of this divorce have been extremely adverse. There are, to be sure, significant victories, but these have been tempered by failures that can be linked to a lack of integrated prevention and care. In the United States, for example, the introduction of antiretrovirals (ARVs) led to a striking decline in age-adjusted mortality among Americans living with AIDS (Fauci, 1999). And although AIDS remains the only ranking infectious cause of young adult mortality in the United States and Europe, there remain, in affluent countries, ongoing or growing sub-epidemics. As elsewhere, rates of HIV transmission vary by social standing. In the southern United States, for example, HIV continues to disproportionately affect ethnic minorities in urban conglomerations and is increasingly concentrated among people of color living in rural areas connected by major routes of commerce. Research conducted in rural North Carolina suggests that this epidemic is largely sexually transmitted and linked to racism and gender inequality (Rumley *et al.*, 1991). And even when local epidemiology differs, social inequalities of one sort or another remain part of the equation of both risk of infection and access to care. In urban Russia and the Ukraine, in contrast to the rural south of the United States, a rapidly emerging epidemic is, as already stated, attributable to injection drug use; among those most affected are the unemployed and, again, members of ethnic minorities. In other words, social inequalities remain linked to differential risk for HIV even in affluent or industrialized countries.

Prevention activities need to be designed with the local epidemiology of the disease in mind. In settings in which HIV is largely a sexually transmitted disease, information and education campaigns can save lives. In Thailand, for example, it is estimated that aggressive condom promotion targeting the military and commercial sex workers has resulted in significantly fewer new infections than had been predicted (Ainsworth *et al.*, 2003). In settings in which HIV transmission is linked more closely to injection drug use, harm-reduction strategies (e.g. the provision of clean needles as well as adequate therapy for addiction) have proven effective (Anon, 2003). But in each and every setting studied, the divorce of prevention and care – most marked in the poorest countries where a vanishing few of those in need of HIV care ever receive it – has crippled effective response to the disease and also heightened social stigma (UNAIDS, 2003).

The integration of HIV prevention and care will be a recurrent and unifying theme of global AIDS control efforts, in spite of a great diversity in subepidemics. In settings where HIV/AIDS is seen not as a private problem but as a public one, good public policy can prevent new infections and avert death among those already living with HIV. Of course there is far too much work at hand for there to be no division of labor regarding prevention and care: more human and financial resources are needed, and it is clear that some personnel, including activists, will be involved primarily in one sort of activity rather than another. At the same time, it is difficult to categorically class on-the-ground activities as contributing to 'prevention' versus 'care'. For example, most people would class the prevention of mother-to-child transmission of HIV (pMTCT) as a prevention activity. But implementing pMTCT programs has often called for improved prenatal care. Similarly, improving HIV care helps to destigmatize AIDS. Decreased stigma is associated with increased interest in voluntary counseling and testing (VCT), which is a cornerstone of effective HIV prevention and care (Farmer *et al.*, 2001). Improving HIV care, which necessarily means making ARVs available to those with advanced HIV disease, leads to a marked decrease in the number of opportunistic infections affecting people with advanced AIDS. Clinic time that had been dedicated to the management of thrush or diarrhea can instead be spent imparting important prevention information. In other words, ARVs can help to afford clinicians (whether doctors or nurses or community health workers) more time to reinforce prevention messages. Recently, some have attempted to move beyond sterile debates regarding prevention versus care and catalogued the mechanisms by which increased access to quality HIV care can strengthen prevention efforts, seeking to assess the likely impact of ARVs on the future of the epidemic in developing countries (Blower and Farmer, 2003). Ideally, the promise of treatment will increase the willingness of at-risk individuals to be tested, and the treatment itself may decrease infectiousness, but concerns have also been raised that wider use of ART may be associated with increased risk-taking behavior and transmission of drug resistant viral strains.

Certainly, more data are needed in order to craft sound policy and make clear recommendations to medical and public health specialists dealing with AIDS on a global level. But our database is scant in large part because so few patients in developing countries have access to quality AIDS care. Operational research is necessary to help us to define the role of ARVs in resource-poor settings, but to conduct operational research one must first have operations. Global health agencies should be committed to promoting integrated prevention and care of HIV/AIDS.

Brazil: Expanding Access to ARV

Far too few countries have introduced legislation to protect the rights of those liv-ing with HIV, including the right to effective therapy. Brazil is one country that has done so successfully. Although Brazil cannot be described as a socially egali-tarian country – indeed, indices of social inequality are high – it became one of the first nations in the world to mandate that access to HIV care be universal and free of charge to the patient. In a sense, then, AIDS was transformed from a pri-vate problem, one affecting individuals and their families, to a public one. By introducing innovative legislation, Brazil was able to build up Latin America's largest and best-functioning AIDS program. Indeed, many feel that widespread access to ARVs has helped destigmatize the disease in Brazil and thereby improved demand for voluntary counseling and testing. Although claims of causality are hard to prove, what is clear is that projections made over a decade ago, when it was predicted that Brazil would have a rapidly expanding epidemic, have not come to pass. Epidemiological surveillance data released in 2002 shows that HIV incidence has declined in recent years now that ARVs are widely avail-able: only 7361 new cases of HIV disease were registered in the first nine months of 2001, compared with the 17 504 cases registered in 2000 (Brazilian Ministry of Health, 2001). Furthermore, widespread ARV use has reduced hospitalizations and led to a substantial reduction in the incidence of tuberculosis and other oppor-tunistic infections. The Brazilian Ministry of Health estimates that cost savings for reduced hospital admissions and treatment of opportunistic infections between 1997 and 2001 have been close to US$1.1 billion. Projections based upon model-ing made in the early 1990s have been proven incorrect, as Brazil's HIV epidemic has contracted rather than expanded (Brazilian Ministry of Health, 2002).

In the summer of 2003 Mexico passed legislation similar to Brazil's and may reasonably hope for similar successes (Associated Press, 2003). Policy thus has an indisputable therapeutic effect on HIV/AIDS.

Treating HIV Among the Poor: Community-based Approaches

Countries far poorer than Brazil have been forced to focus their efforts elsewhere but can still claim positive results. In Haiti, a public–private partnership has intro-duced culturally appropriate HIV prevention and state-of-the-art HIV care to a population living in dire poverty. Haiti is the poorest nation in the Western hemi-sphere (UNDP, 2003). Not surprisingly, it is also the nation with the highest prevalence of HIV as well (UNAIDS, 2002). AIDS accounted for more than 5 per cent of deaths reported in Haiti in the year 2002 (PAHO, 2003) and it is believed the disease is grossly underreported due both to a lack of medical resources and stigma associated with the condition. There is poor public health infrastructure in the country and medical care is not available for a majority of the population. In spite of this, the population of Haiti is in desperate need of HIV treatment (UNAIDS, 2002). HIV has fueled the spread of other deadly diseases – especially tuberculosis (TB) – a disease with which it shares a noxious synergy (WHO, 2003).

In rural Haiti, where we work, an effort to manage HIV has been a routine part of medical care since the mid-1980s. Our group – known as Zanmi LaSante (Haitian Creole for Partners In Health) – first began to work in Haiti's rural central plateau region when the disease began to take off. Most of its victims were young men and women who were returning home from Port-au-Prince where they had gone to seek employment to support their families. When they became ill, they returned home to be cared for, adding to the burden of families barely able to make out a meager existence. Zanmi LaSante launched some of the first HIV prevention efforts in the region. In addition to providing culturally appropriate prevention and education campaigns, Zanmi LaSante introduced therapy to reduce maternal-to-child transmission in the early 1990s. Several physicians who work at our project in rural Haiti are also practicing medicine in the United States. Crossing between these two vastly different settings has allowed us to witness the miracles of modern HIV medicine and to attempt to bring them to our patients in rural Haiti. In 1998, we launched the HIV equity initiative whose goal is to bring state-of-the-art HIV treatment – including HAART – to our patients living in the heart of Haiti.

The project is community-based and relies on a cadre of community health care workers known as *accompagnateurs* to deliver care to patients. Once diagnosed with HIV, patients are evaluated clinically and assigned an accompagnateur to work with them throughout the course of their treatment. At the time we introduced HAART in Haiti, we had no access to sophisticated laboratory equipment to monitor CD4 counts – the foundation for guiding treatment in the wealthy nations of the world. Rather, we relied on what is termed a 'syndromic approach', with those patients demonstrating physical signs and symptoms of the disease being given priority for receiving antiretroviral treatment (Farmer *et al.*, 2001). All medications and services are provided to patients free of charge. The program has been widely successful: to date almost 1000 patients are receiving HAART and all have had a positive response to therapy, including weight gain, absence of opportunistic infection, and a return to activities of daily living.

We performed a small observational study of clinical outcomes in patients in our catchment area receiving community-based HAART. A group of 100 of these patients was compared with a group of 200 patients who were not receiving HAART and followed for a period of two years. Not surprisingly, the HAART-treated group did better across a range of clinical outcomes: they were more likely to be alive (not a single patient receiving HAART died), gain weight, and have improvements in their activities of daily living (ADL) scores. They were less likely to be hospitalized or to develop tuberculosis or other opportunistic infections.

Although small and observational in nature, these results show that even in the resource-poor setting of rural Haiti, effective AIDS treatment can be delivered effectively. Our excellent results, we feel, are due in large measure to the biosocial approach that is taken to treating the disease. Patients are not simply given antiretroviral therapy but rather are engaged in a system of care in which their accompagnateur monitors them on a daily basis. Adverse effects can be rapidly triaged and managed.

In addition to being given medication free of charge, each patient undergoes a detailed socioeconomic evaluation. Those with inadequate housing are offered rebuilding; those without access to work are enrolled in job programs. Nutritional support is provided for patients as a routine part of care, as weight and weight gain are key clinical indicators. Opportunistic infections are rapidly diagnosed and managed, again with the medications being given free of charge. Therapy is directly observed by accompagnateurs on a daily basis, allowing for close bonds to be formed between patients and provider and to guard against the development of antiviral resistance.

HIV prevention is closely tied to treatment. Prior to the introduction of HAART, people were reluctant to test and learn their serostatus, fearing there was little that could be done for them. With the introduction of HAART, however, interest in testing has risen sharply, and our clinics, which serve a catchment area of over 500 000 people, performed more than 25 000 HIV tests last year alone.

Finally, treatment of HIV has led to a reduction of stigma in our community. With the initiation of treatment, patients are seen to return take active roles in their community. Thus, HIV is no longer seen as the death sentence it once was. The broad social benefits of treating HIV in rural Haiti – including a return to work, ability to provide for families, and a continuation of education – contribute to the obvious medical ones of keeping patients alive and healthy. The program in Haiti is in the process of being replicated in five additional sites in the central plateau region and can serve as a model for management of HIV in other resource-poor settings, including Africa.

We have used a similar approach to providing HIV care to the poor living in urban Boston. In spite of geographic proximity to some of the leading health care institutions in the world, we have found that many patients living in the urban sectors of Boston have poor access to HAART. Many have lives that are characterized by disorder, and they struggle to make ends meet on a daily basis. Some are addicted to drugs; many are the victims of violence. They require comprehensive care to address their HIV, which is often only one problem on a long list of life-threatening conditions they face.

In order to provide such comprehensive care, our group founded the Prevention and Access to Care and Treatment (PACT) project in 1998. Patients are enrolled in PACT if they are found to be failing standard therapy for HIV. Each PACT patient is assigned a community health worker who visits them daily to observe them taking their HAART and to assist with any social or medical problems that the patient may be facing. PACT patients are given housing and food assistance, are helped in applying for medical insurance and other social benefits, and are given emotional and social support. To date more than 100 patients have been enrolled in the project and clinical outcomes among these patients are excellent, in spite of them being some of the 'most difficult to treat' HIV patients. HIV prevention is also a main focus of the PACT project, and efforts have been made to reach difficult to target populations – such as poor Latina women and men – through a variety of outreach efforts that also include community health workers. Thus, the model of community-based HIV care developed by our team in rural Haiti has been successfully transformed to benefit patients in inner-city Boston also suffering from inadequate access to care.

What the Future Holds

More than any other infectious pathogen, HIV challenges us to take a biosocial approach to understanding and treating disease. Those most at risk of acquiring HIV are at risk because they are poor and marginalized: their risk is a socially constructed phenomenon with biological consequences. It is no coincidence that the areas and populations of the world most afflicted with poverty, hunger, and civil unrest are the very same areas and populations most affected by HIV. Once infected with HIV, those most likely to become sick with and die from the disease are also victims of inequality. Life-saving treatment for HIV has been available for over half a decade, yet it reaches only a fraction of those who need it and virtually ignores the millions suffering with HIV who also happen to be poor. Innovative, community-based programs that take a biosocial approach to HIV management have been employed and are highly successful, even in the most resource-limited settings in the world. In rural Haiti and in urban Boston, we have found that community-based therapy administered by lay health workers that also takes into account the socioeconomic needs of patients can transform HIV into a disease that can be lived with, producing multiple social and medical benefits and decreasing stigma in the community as well. It is time to duplicate such efforts on a broader scale and change the course that HIV is taking in the world today.

More than a decade ago, the World Health Organization proposed a global strategy for preventing and treating HIV. At that time, the focus of efforts was on prevention of transmission through education; provision of health and social services to people living with HIV, including social and economic support; and mobilization of international efforts (WHO, 1992). Unfortunately, the proposed global strategy has proven to be inadequate in managing HIV in most settings. New infections continue, and the gap between those who have access to care and those who do not has only widened. In the year 2004, poverty and inequality now play an even bigger role than ever before in determining who lives and dies with HIV. Recognizing the limitations in its prior global plan, the WHO has since launched an aggressive campaign to strengthen ties between HIV prevention and treatment and to provide HAART to those who are in most desperate need. The initiative – known as the '3 by 5 strategy' – has as its goal the provision of comprehensive care, including antiretrovirals, to 3 million people with HIV by the end of 2005 (Gupta *et al.*, 2004). This is an ambitious and much-needed action plan for combating HIV disease and the global community is now poised to confront the AIDS pandemic on a new level.

What will be needed to meet the goals of the '3 by 5' initiative and to ensure that improved HIV-related prevention and care are provided to an increasing number of people worldwide? Examples from Haiti and Brazil show that in order to successfully treat poor people with HIV, comprehensive services that recognize the socioeconomic conditions in which HIV thrives must be put into place. Experience gives us reason to be optimistic that such services can be successful, even in the most resource-limited settings. Massive antiretroviral treatment scale-up and comprehensive treatment and prevention programs are needed in order to address HIV in Africa and in the other settings where it is exploding or poised to explode. This will require an influx of funding beyond that already promised by the GFATM. Furthermore, new public–private partnerships need to be formed and strengthened to provide care to the millions of people already infected in the world and to prevent infection in the hundreds of millions who are at risk. The AIDS pandemic is dynamic – both in terms of its epidemiology and its clinical treatment: where it has shown itself to be remarkably consistent is in its predilection for striking the poor and the weak. The power to change that face of AIDS is certainly within our reach. It will require us to break new scientific ground but perhaps more importantly, will also require innovation in the ways in which we seek to bring the fruits of modern science to those most in need. AIDS – like most of the world's infectious killers – is a disease of inequality. We must be cognizant of this and strive to overcome it in order to avert millions of needless deaths globally.

The authors of this chapter – who are all clinical AIDS care providers with experience in both the poor and wealthy countries of the world – are cautiously optimistic about what the future holds in terms of AIDS care globally. Certainly, when one looks at climbing rates of HIV infection worldwide, one can easily be overwhelmed by the magnitude of the problem. Indeed, it might appear that little has been successful in curbing the spread of HIV globally. And although much has been invested in AIDS science, most of the advances that have been made remain out of reach for the millions of AIDS sufferers in the world. Such pessimism, in our experience, often leads to inaction on the part of those who can, indeed, help turn the tide in the global war against AIDS. The WHO's '3 by 5' initiative is nothing short of inspiring, as it challenges us to meet global demand for AIDS care and treatment. With commitment of both human and financial resources – such as those of the GFATM – we feel that the goals of the '3 by 5' initiative can be met, although an unparalleled mobilization of public health capital will be required. We remain dedicated to this and to the mission of providing comprehensive AIDS services to all populations globally. It is both a medical and moral imperative and experience in even the world's most destitute settings has shown that such care is not only desperately needed but imminently possible. The future of AIDS care is ours to make. By using a biosocial approach to both understand and treat the disease, we greatly increase our chances of success for reining in this global scourge.

References

Ainsworth M, Beyrer C, Sourat A *et al.* (2003) AIDS and public policy: the lessons and challenges of 'success' in Thailand. *Health Policy* 64: 13–37.

Anon (2003) WHO declares failure to deliver AIDS medicines a global health emergency. *Bull WHO* 81: 776.

Associated Press (2003) Mexico to subsidize drugs for all AIDS patients. 5 August.

Beyrer C, Razak M, Labrique A *et al.* (2003) Assessing the magnitude of the HIV/AIDS epidemic in Burma. *J Acquir Immune Defic Syndr* 32: 311–17.

Blower S, Farmer P (2003) Predicting the public health impact of antiretrovirals: preventing HIV in developing countries. *AIDScience* 3: 11.

Boerma J, Gregson S, Nyamukapa C *et al.* (2003) Understanding the uneven spread of HIV within Africa: comparative study of biologic, behavioral and contextual factors in Tanzania and Zimbabwe. *Sex Transm Dis* 30: 779–87.

Brazilian Ministry of Health (2001) *Boletim Epidemiologico-AIDS*. Brasilia.

Brazilian Ministry of Health (2002) *National AIDS Drug Policy*. Brasilia.

Bronfman M, Leyva R, Negroni M *et al.* (2002) Mobile populations and HIV/AIDS in Central America and Mexico: research for action. *AIDS* 16 (Suppl 3): S42–S49.

CDC (Centers for Disease Control and Prevention) (1981) Kaposi's sarcoma and pneumocystis pneumonia among homosexual men – New York City and California. *MMWR Morb Mortal Wkly Rep* 30: 305–8.

CDC (1996) HIV/AIDS Surveillance Report. *MMWR Morb Mortal Wkly Rep* 45: 121–4.

Cohen J (2003a) Myanmar: the next frontier for HIV/AIDS. *Science* 301: 1650–5.

Cohen J (2003b) Thailand and Cambodia: two hard-hit countries offer rare success stories. *Science* 301: 1658–63.

Coninx R, Mathieu C, Debacker M *et al.* (1999) First-line tuberculosis therapy and drug resistant *Mycobacterium tuberculosis* in prisons. *Lancet* 353: 969–73.

De Waal A, Whiteside A (2003) New variant famine: AIDS and food crisis in southern Africa. *Lancet* 362: 1234–7.

Donovan P (2002) Rape and HIV/AIDS in Rwanda. *Lancet* 360: S17–S18.

Egger M, Pauw J, Lopatatzidis A *et al.* (2000) Promotion of condom use in a high-risk setting in Nicaragua: a randomized controlled trial. *Lancet* 355: 2101–5.

Eshete H, Heast N, Lindan K *et al.* (1993) Ethnic conflicts, poverty and AIDS in Ethiopia. *Lancet* 341: 1219.

Esparza J, Osmanov S (2003) HIV vaccines: a global perspective. *Curr Mol Med* 3: 183–93.

Farmer P (1992) *AIDS and Accusation: Haiti and the Geography of Blame*. Berkeley, CA: University of California Press.

Farmer P (1996) Social inequalities and emerging infectious diseases. *Emerg Infect Dis* 2: 259–69.

Farmer P (1999a) *Infections and Inequalities: The Modern Plagues*. Berkeley, CA: University of California Press.

Farmer P (1999b) Managerial successes: clinical failures. *Int J Tuberculosis Lung Dis* 3: 365–7.

Farmer P (2000) Prevention without treatment is not sustainable. *Natl AIDS Bull* 13: 6.

Farmer P (2001) The major infectious diseases of the world: to treat or not to treat. *N Engl J Med* 345: 208–10.

Farmer P (2002) *Pathologies of Power*. Berkeley, CA: University of California Press.

Farmer P, Connors M, Simmons J (1996) *Women, Poverty, and AIDS: Sex, Drugs, and Structural Violence*. Monore, ME: Common Courage Press, 1996.

Farmer P, Walton D, Furin J (2000) The changing face of AIDS: implications for policy and practice. In: Mayer K, Pizer H, eds. *The Emergence of AIDS: The Impact on Immunology, Microbiology and Public Health*. American Public Health Association.

Farmer P, Leandre F, Mukherjee J *et al.* (2001) Community-based approaches to HIV treatment in resource-poor settings. *Lancet* 358: 404–9.

Fauci A (1999) The AIDS epidemic: considerations for the 21st century. *N Engl J Med* 341: 1046–50.

Fleck F (2003) WHO issues global alert after grim report on HIV/AIDS. *British Medical Journal* 327: 693.

Gupta R, Irwin A, Raviglione M *et al.* (2004) Scaling-up treatment for HIV/AIDS: lessons learned from multidrug-resistant tuberculosis. *Lancet* 363: 320–4.

Holtgrave D, Crosby R (2003) Social capital, poverty, and income inequality as predictors of gonorrhea, syphilis, chlamydia and AIDS case rates in the United States. *Sex Transm Infect* 79: 62–4.

Johnson D, Sorvillo F, Wohl A *et al.* (2003) Frequent failed early HIV detection in a high prevalence area: implications for prevention. *AIDS Patient Care STDs* 17: 277–82.

Lamptey P (2002) Reducing heterosexual transmission of HIV in poor countries. *BMJ* 324: 207–11.

Makgoba M, Solomon N, Tucker T (2002) The search for an HIV vaccine. *BMJ* 324: 211–13.

Mayaud P, Hawkes S, Mabey D (1998) Advances in the control of sexually transmitted diseases in developing countries. *Lancet* 351 (Suppl III): S29–S32.

McCalman C (2003) Barriers and motivators for low-income Brazilian women in metropolitan Belo Horizonte: insights for AIDS prevention. *Health Care Women Int* 24: 565–85.

Mukherjee J, Farmer P, Niyizonkiza D *et al.* (2003) Tackling HIV in resource-poor countries. *BMJ* 327: 1104–6.

Mworozi E (1993) AIDS and civil war: a devil's alliance. *AIDS Analysis Africa* 3(6): 8–10.

Nabel G (2001) Challenges and opportunities for the development of an AIDS vaccine. *Nature* 410: 1002–7.

Narain J, Raviglione M, Kochi A (1992) HIV-associated tuberculosis in developing countries: epidemiology and strategies for prevention. *Tuberculosis Lung Dis* 73: 311–21.

Odhiambo W (2003) HIV/AIDS and debt crises: threat to human survival in sub-Saharan Africa. *Med Conflict Survival* 19: 142–7.

Orach C (1999) Morbidity and mortality amongst southern Sudanese in Koboko refugee camps, Arua District, Uganda. *East Afr Med J* 76: 195–9.

PAHO (2003) Country Profiles, Haiti, 2003. http://www.paho.org/English/DD/AIS/be_v24n1-haiti.htm

Palella F Jr, Delaney K, Moorman A *et al.* (1998) Declining morbidity and mortality among patients with advanced human immunodeficiency virus infection. *N Engl J Med* 338: 853–60.

Parker R (2002) The global HIV/AIDS pandemic, structural inequalities, and the politics of international health. *Am J Public Health* 92: 343–6.

Poore P (2004) The Global Fund to fight AIDS, Tuberculosis and Malaria (GFATM). *Health Policy Plan* 19: 52–3.

Ratnathicam A (2001) AIDS in India: incidence, prevalence and prevention. *AIDS Patient Care STDs* 15: 255–61.

Raviola G, Machoki M, Mwaikamboi E *et al.* (2002) HIV, disease plague, demoralization, and 'burnout': resident experience of the medical profession in Nairobi, Kenya. *Culture Med Psychiatry* 26: 55–86.

Resl V, Kumpova M, Cerna L *et al.* (2003) Prevalence of STDs among prostitutes in Czech border areas with Germany in 1997–2001 assessed in project 'Jana'. *Sex Transm Infect* 79: E3.

Romero-Daza N, Weeks M, Singer M (2003) 'Nobody gives a damn if I live or die': violence, drugs, and street level prostitution in inner-city Hartford, Connecticut. *Med Anthropol* 22: 233–59.

Rumley R, Shappley N, Waivers L *et al.* (1991) AIDS in rural eastern North Carolina – patient migration: a rural AIDS burden. *AIDS* 5: 1373–8.

Samayoa B, Arathoon E, Anderson M *et al.* (2003) The emergence of AIDS in Guatemala: inpatient experience at the Hospital General San Juan de Dios. *Int J STD AIDS* 14: 810–13.

Schwalbe N, Harrington P (2002) HIV and tuberculosis in the former Soviet Union. *Lancet* 360 (Suppl): S19–S20

Shrotri A, Shankar A, Sutar S *et al.* (2003) Awareness of HIV/AIDS and household environment of pregnant women in Pune, India. *Int J STD AIDS* 14: 835–9.

UNAIDS (United National Joint Programme on AIDS) (2002) *AIDS Epidemic Update.* Geneva: UNAIDS, December.

UNAIDS (2003) *AIDS Epidemic Update.* Geneva: UNAIDS, December.

UNDP (United Nations Development Programme) (2002) *Policy Paper on AIDS and Poverty Reduction Strategies.* Geneva: UNDP.

UNGASS (United Nations General Assembly Special Session) (2001) *UN Special Session Fact Sheets: Gender and HIV/AIDS.* Geneva: UNGASS, June.

Unicef (United Nations Children's Fund) (2000) *State of the World's Children 2000.* Geneva: Unicef.

Wax E (2003) A generation orphaned by AIDS. *Washington Post* 13 August, A01.

WHO (World Health Organization) (1999) *World Health Report 1999.* Geneva: World Health Organization.

WHO (2003) Harm reduction approaches to injecting drug use. http://www.who.int/hiv/topics/harm/reduction/en/

WHO/UNAIDS (2003) Global Report on HIV/AIDS 2003. WHO/UNAIDS, Geneva.

Williams B, Dye C (2003) Antiretroviral drugs for tuberculosis control in the era of HIV/AIDS. *Science Online* 14 August.

Zierler S, Krieger N (2000) Social inequality and HIV infection in women. In: Mayer K, Pizer H, eds. *The Emergence of AIDS: The Impact on Immunology, Microbiology and Public Health.* American Public Health Association.

Zierler N, Krieger N, Tang Y *et al.* (2000) Economic deprivation and AIDS incidence in Massachusetts. *Am J Public Health* 90: 1064–73.

Economics

12

Samuel A Bozzette
Department of Medicine, University of California San Diego, La Jolla, USA

Samuel A Bozzette, MD, PhD is a Health Services Researcher at the VA San Diego and The RAND Corporation, where he is Senior Natural Scientist. He is also Professor of Medicine at the University of California San Diego. He holds degrees from the University of Rochester (M.D), and the RAND Graduate School of Policy Studies (M.Phil; PhD; Policy Analysis), and is certified in Internal Medicine and Infectious Diseases. He is a Fellow of the American College of Physicians and the Infectious Diseases Society of America, and a member of the American Society for Clinical Investigation and the Association of American Physicians. His research involves treatment evaluation, clinical epidemiology, and health outcomes, policy and economics.

This chapter focuses on the economics of the HIV/AIDS epidemic in the United States. Prior to the HIV epidemic, study of the economics of infectious diseases was generally confined to acute conditions, the impact of chronic or endemic infection on the 'Third World', and a number of informal provider workforce studies predicting a great excess of infectious disease physicians. With the epidemic of chronic HIV infection came a large number of economic issues that had not been faced before by the infectious diseases community. How would the seemingly enormous costs of the growing epidemic be handled? The most affected groups included young people likely to be working in jobs without insurance or unemployed people. Those with private insurance often faced caps on expenditures. The ability to self-finance was rare. Local and state-based public insurance and the health care institutions lacked the resources. Federal (Medicare) coverage required a two-year waiting period for coverage after an often lengthy process to establish disability.

Where would the infrastructure for care come from? Surely the small number of infectious disease physicians, many of whom were consultants disinclined to provide ongoing care, could not be sufficient? Would hospitals in affected areas be overwhelmed? Would special AIDS wards be required, or even the restoration of the infectious diseases hospital system? How should outpatient care be organized? How could palliative and social services be incorporated? How could incentives in the public and private sectors be established to fund and conduct needed research?

All of these are economic issues, but all cannot be fully explored here. This chapter concentrates on the cost and financing of care, and on the implications of these factors for the organization of care. After a summary of current conditions, it will review key economic developments during three distinct phases of the epidemic. In this way, it will attempt to provide insights into the path that led here and a basis for forward extrapolation.

Summary of the Current Situation

The costs of the HIV epidemic in the US are indeterminate. On the front end, actual federal outlays are known but state data are less available. Capitation as well as stated reimbursement rates and billing levels are known for some private payers and providers, but actual payments and out-of-pocket costs are generally unknown. On the back end, utilization of health care resources and outcomes of HIV/AIDS patients in care are known reasonably well, allowing estimates of personal health costs. However, it should be remembered that the application of algebra to any of these available numbers would not yield the true cost or economic impact of HIV. For this, a large number of nearly imponderable resource effects would need to be resolved. Among these would be the effect of patients' and their caregivers' lost productivity, the direct cost of infrastructure for HIV care (including organizations, built structures, personnel, etc., to meet medical and non-medical needs), and the loss of benefits that are forgone when resources that could be put to other uses must be spent on HIV (opportunity costs).

The flux of health services and product utilization devoted to HIV engender costs in the realms of pharmaceuticals, outpatient care, hospitalization, and home care (acute, long-term, and palliative care). It shadows trends in the scope and nature of the epidemic in the United States but only imperfectly. This is in part because of changing clinical needs and trends in care, but also because many HIV-infected people receive no care at all, and because many appropriate HIV-related expenses are not attributable to individuals. However, it is mostly due to the fact that the largest proportion of the epidemic's real costs are something not discussed in any detail here: the indirect costs attributable to lost productivity.

According to Centers for Disease Control estimates, 500 000 Americans have already died with HIV infection, but the death rate is declining with the diffusion of increasingly sophisticated therapies into practice (CDC, 2003a, b). About 850 000–950 000 Americans are currently infected, with about 40 000 new infections per year (Fleming *et al.*, 2002). About three-quarters of the infected are aware of their infection, half are in care and somewhat fewer are receiving regular care (defined as one provider visit at least every six months) (Bozzette *et al.*, 1998; Fleming *et al.*, 2002).

The economic implications of this epidemiology include the following. Much of the future benefit of our response to HIV could come from investments directed to unmet need for prevention services and improved access to care. This could increase the proportion of individuals with known and unknown infection who are in care, so that prevention messages and medical therapies can be used to decrease transmission, the need for palliative care, and the burden on affected but uninfected people while maintaining the productivity of the infected. Under current systems, these expenditures cannot be attributed to any individual or even to any identifiable set of individuals; that is, they are public goods that must be supported by central allocations.

Direct personal expenditures are driven by the half of the infected population that is receiving regular and intermittent care. This spending can be expected to increase as increasing survival and unchanging incidence increase the number of people in care, and as initial and 'salvage' therapy becomes more complicated. These factors also imply a need for new investments in human and organizational capital as excellent HIV care moves further from the reach of non-expert practitioners and practices. Moreover, the trend to increased personal expenditures will be accelerated by success in improving access to care. This is especially true of people currently only receiving intermittent care as many of these individuals have relatively advanced disease and indications for expensive combination antiretroviral and other chemotherapy. More subtly, it will also be accelerated by success in improving access to high-quality care among the traditionally underserved groups – female, black and Latino, poor, unemployed, and uninsured. Studies have demonstrated that patients in these subgroups receive less care even when in regular care (Shapiro *et al.*, 1999); redressing this inequity will require additional expenditures in infrastructure and personal expenses (Steinbrook, 1998).

It is unclear how satisfying this new demand will be financed given the complex patchwork that is HIV coverage (Steinbrook, 2001). There are complicated overlaps and gaps in individuals' insurance coverage. Moreover, both individuals and provider institutions frequently depend on an array of safety-net and other programs that are generally not funded at the individual patient level.

Coverage by private insurance, at about 30 per cent of HIV patients in care, is much lower than the approximately 70 per cent coverage in the general population (Bozzette *et al.*, 1998). Further data from the same nationally representative sample of HIV/AIDS patients in care show that there are large regional variations in private coverage. For example, 45 per cent of patients in the West of the US have private coverage but less than 15 per cent of patients in the East.

Approximately 80 rather than 70 per cent of patients rely on public funds or are uninsured because of overlaps, dual coverage, and cross-financing (Goldman *et al.*, 2003). Some patients with private insurance have premiums paid by public funds. Some with private insurance lack or have limited pharmaceutical benefits, and receive drugs through public programs. Many who are uninsured chronically or at a point in time move intermittently on and off the Medicaid rolls, or they rely on county-level programs for the medically indigent, public hospitals, community-based health centers, and clinics supported by Title III funds of the federal Ryan White Comprehensive AIDS Resources Emergency (CARE) Act. The Ryan White CARE Act has been a vital source of federal funds for a variety of safety-net programs and facilities, including the AIDS Drug Assistance Program (ADAP), which is supplemented by local funds in many states.

Just less that 50 per cent of all HIV patients in care are enrolled in Medicaid. About 40 per cent of these patients (20 per cent of all patients in care) are also enrolled in Medicare. Conversely, as very few Medicare patients are not also enrolled in Medicaid, almost all Medicare patients are 'dual eligibles' (Goldman *et al.*, 2003). For most of the dual eligibles, services are provided by Medicare but drugs are provided by Medicaid. This is one of many situations in HIV financing that sets up perverse incentives. In this case, Medicaid programs spending more on better drug therapy do not obtain the benefits of the savings in hospital costs, which accrue to Medicare (Goldman *et al.*, 2001).

Total US federal spending on HIV/AIDS, which has been growing rapidly, is projected to exceed US$18.5 billion in 2004. The most rapidly growing and

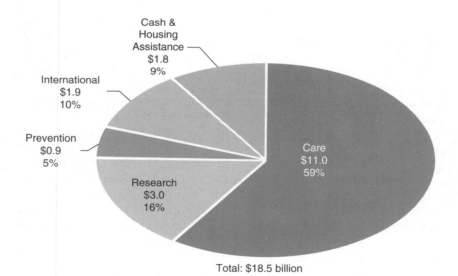

Total: $18.5 billion

Fig. 12.1 US funding for HIV/AIDS by category for Fiscal Year 2004 (in billions of dollars). Note that approximately 59 per cent of federal expenditures are for patient care, while 41 per cent are for prevention, research, assistance with living costs, and international HIV/AIDS efforts. From Summers and Kates (2004).

310

largest component of the total is, at approximately 60 per cent, direct expenditures for care. This growth has been such that, in a shift from the first 15 years of the epidemic, discretionary funding is not a majority of spending. Rather, entitlement funds, primarily through Medicare, Medicaid, and disability payments, account for the majority of expenditures. This increase is driven by two factors. The number of HIV-infected poor, unemployed, and disabled people who qualify for these programs is increasing, and the cost of providing services is growing (Kates and Sorian, 2000; Kaiser Family Foundation, 2003b). Prescriptions for highly active antiretroviral therapy (HAART) are now primary cost drivers in Medicaid as well as in ADAP, which operates under Title II of the Ryan White CARE Act. Nearly 90 per cent of ADAP drug expenditures are for HAART, and ADAP now comprises almost a third of the total CARE Act budget (Kaiser Family Foundation, 2003a).

As cost sharers in the Medicaid program and, in many places, in ADAP, states are also experiencing pressure on their health care budgets due to expanding caseloads and care intensity. The efficacy and expense of HAART has also increased

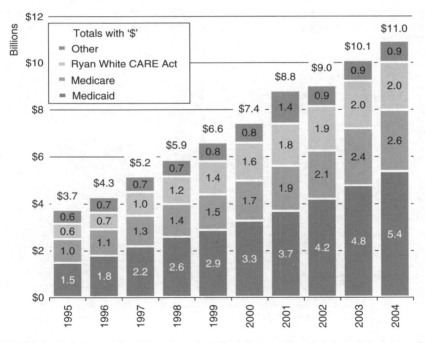

Fig. 12.2 US federal spending, 1995–2005, reflects substantial annual increases in spending for entitlement programs to care for the unemployed, disabled, and poor, as well as for covering the increasing cost of providing patient care services. From Summers and Kates (2004).

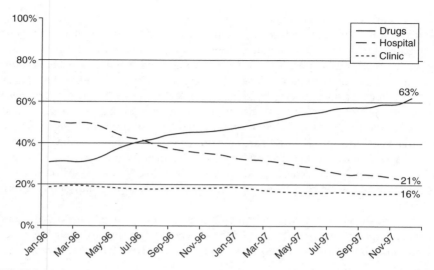

Fig. 12.3 Trends in components of costs, 1995–1997, in the United States demonstrate the increasing importance of outpatient drug spending as effective and expensive highly active antiretroviral therapy (HAART) came into widespread use. Adapted from Bozzette *et al.* (2001).

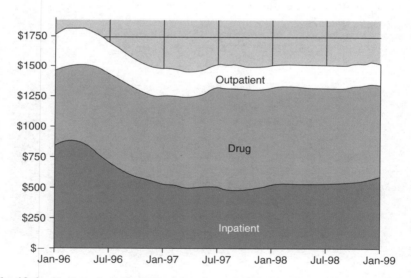

Fig. 12.4 The introduction of effective antiretroviral therapy reduced monthly per patient expenditures largely because the reduction in costs for treating opportunistic infections and inpatient hospital stays was greater than the increase in drug costs. From Bozzette *et al.* (2001).

pressure to expand Medicaid eligibility to greater numbers of HIV-infected people prior to disability status. However, the waiver process under Section 1115 of the Social Security Act requires states to demonstrate budget neutrality over the waiver period. Thus far, this process has been impeded by an inability to demonstrate the necessary budget neutrality. Doing so will require substantial discounts on drugs or the convincing evidence of offsetting savings, which may simply be unavailable in less ill, low utilizing patients.

Medicare does not cover drugs but can be expected to be an increasingly important source of financing for HIV services. Drives to improve access and improvements in therapy will lead to increases in Medicare rolls: more patients will survive to eligibility by aging or through the two-year waiting period for eligibility after receiving Social Security Disability Insurance. In addition, these programs tend to enroll sicker patients; the 50 per cent of patients covered by Medicare and Medicaid account for two-thirds of all direct spending on HIV care (Goldman *et al.*, 2003).

In summary, financing is problematic. Most HIV patients rely on a fragmented web of public funding and programs, or cling to private insurance. The result is wide disparities in quality of and access to care, with stunted growth and spread of care institutions (Shapiro *et al.*, 1999). However, the crisis in financing cannot fundamentally be due to total expense *per se*; the direct cost of HIV care has never accounted for more than 1 per cent of all annual direct personal health expenditures in the United States (Bozzette *et al.*, 2001).

Economic Evolution of the HIV Epidemic in the United States

Early Period: Chaos, Catastrophe, and Costly Hospitalizations

This economic phase started with the onset of the epidemic and ended approximately with the passage and implementation of the Ryan White CARE Act in 1990. Especially at the beginning of this phase, HIV was a catastrophic illness for patients and the health care system. Although earlier stages of the disease such as generalized lymphadenopathy and AIDS-related complex were recognized, patients usually presented with catastrophic AIDS-defining opportunistic infections requiring expensive and often prolonged hospital care. Survivors at one typical center had more than three hospitalizations per year (Seage *et al.*, 1986). Many patients developed severe neurological symptoms, contributing to a large need for palliative and home health care. The health care system was not prepared to meet these needs, which would have gone largely unmet were it not for hidden subsidies provided by countless volunteer hours. By the end of the period, antiretroviral monotherapy with zidovudine was widespread and providing periods of reconstitution or relief from progression. Effective prophylaxis against *Pneumocystis carinii* pneumonia, which was by far the most common presenting illness, was known. However, its use in practice, particularly among small providers, fell distressingly short of professional standards. Mortality from the disease declined throughout the period, but life expectancy was still very short at its end.

As care was dominated by the use of hospital services at the beginning of this period, early cost estimates were very high. Analyzing the first 10 000 cases of AIDS reported in the United States, Hardy *et al.* (1986) estimated an average life expectancy of 13 months and lifetime costs of a shocking US$147 000 per patient (in 1985 dollars). Most of this was due to hospital costs, but many AIDS patients required expensive care after discharge. In contrast, the cost of caring for the relatively few identified patients with early disease was quite low at less than US$500 per patient per year as only clinical follow-up in an outpatient setting was indicated. By the second half of the 1980s, Pascal (1987) estimated that hospital costs still dominated total costs, but that cost of personal care for a typical HIV patient over a 12-month lifetime had dropped to US$94 000. These lower costs were attributed both to a slow shift in the mix of patients toward early disease (as more of the iceberg's tip showed itself) and, more important, to increasingly better skills in caring for AIDS-related conditions.

Estimates of the total national direct or personal health care costs of treating HIV varied widely, but all increased sharply over time. For example, one of the best estimates put the cost of treatment between 1986 and 1991 at a total of US$37.6 billion (Pascal, 1987), while another forecast costs to rise from US$630 million in 1985 to US$8.5 billion in 1991 (Scitovksy and Rice, 1987).

The estimate of Arno *et al.* (1989) was in this range, but these authors also identified critical policy issues that vex to this day. These concerns relate to the need to deliver more and more expensive services, the price of pharmaceuticals already developed or developed partially at public expense; the lack of necessary financial commitments at the local, state, and federal government levels as well as in the private sector; and a critical lack of human and built infrastructure. Press coverage of the Arno *et al.* study summarized the concerns well: '[C]urrent services for testing, counseling, dispensing drugs and laboratory monitoring are "inadequate". San Francisco's health-care system is already overwhelmed with emergency rooms and outpatient clinics turning patients away because of too little money and too few care givers' (Herscher, 1989).

The cycle of undercompensation leading to an inadequate and soon overwhelmed system related to the 'Medicaidization' of HIV/AIDS care. This phenomenon was assured by the facts that infected individuals were often uninsured, that they tended to spend down to poverty levels, and that those with private insurance lost it is as they became more ill (Green and Arno, 1990). The loss of insurance secondary to the loss of work underscores the subtle nature of indirect costs: in this situation, the new out-of-pocket and public insurance costs are highly visible, but loss of that individual's contributions to society are not.

Middle Period: Transition to Integration Under Subsidy

The beginning of the middle economic period can be marked by the passage of the Ryan White CARE Act; the end came with the diffusion of highly active combination antiretroviral therapy (HAART) into practice. During this period, clinical management regularized and fears that hospitals would be overwhelmed receded. Stabilization for months to years and long-term remissions with maintenance therapy for opportunistic infections were common. At the same time, outpatient care of complications became much more complex. Both periodic hospital care and palliative care were still often required.

As standards and requirements for providing good care advanced, those cared for by experienced providers or practices experienced reduced progression, morbidity, and mortality (Bennett *et al.*, 1989; Kitahata *et al.*, 1996). This meant both that the course of disease ceased to be uniform, that the paradigm for excellent care began its shift from a hospital to an outpatient focus, and from generalist to HIV expert care.

Paradigmatic sites included the high-volume San Francisco General Hospital program, which emphasized a strong continuity between specialized inpatient wards and the clinics, and great deal of onsite research; the Owen Clinic of the University of California at San Diego, which evolved from a university-based gay men's clinic to an inpatient–outpatient program involving general medical wards; and the Fenway Community Health Center in Boston, which progressed from a small volunteer clinic for gay and transgender people to a comprehensive care environment conducting community-based research and administering complex treatments. These sites were quite different, yet all developed common elements including an intention to provide continuity of care, access to a comprehensive range of specialists, and use of non-physician providers, which over time came to prominently include case managers.

By the end of this period, most patients were cared for in larger practices that tended to use a model that included comprehensive care and inpatient–outpatient continuity. The clinical situation in HIV is well but not uniquely suited to this model, and clinical rationality has not been sufficient for it to dominate in other conditions amenable to centralized comprehensive care. In the case of HIV, the exotic and fear-inducing nature of the new disease and its concentration in specific areas led to natural concentrations of care in certain centers. In addition, the activism of the affected communities calling attention to gaps in services also contributed to the development of a comprehensive care model. Paradoxically, the development of the model was aided by its financial non-viability, a factor that simultaneously inhibited its diffusion; The former was because only those few institutions that saw it in their interest or mission to subsidize HIV care could adopt it and its attendant high level of organization. The latter was because diffusion of the organized comprehensive model was (and is) inhibited by the inadequacy of reimbursement.

The vast majority of patients had public insurance (particularly in the Midwest and East) or were self-pay, a misnomer for non-paying (particularly in the South). Financial incentives for providers to enter HIV care were non-existent, except in a few small areas such as part of Manhattan and West Los Angeles. Clinics such as the ones mentioned above were fueled by the fervor of volunteers and underpaid staff; donations and grants, often from community-based programs (e.g. AmFAR); and either direct subsidies from parent institutions, clinical research, or personal subsidies from research faculty and staff or trainees. Despite these successes, the system was severely constrained and new capacity was not being generated.

Many signs pointed to a critical lack of funds as a limiting factor despite infusions of federal resources in the form of grants, demonstration programs, and research infrastructure funds: the financial starvation of existing clinics, difficulty of starting new sites of care, increasing caseload, and increasing need for expensive pharmaceuticals (e.g. antiretrovirals, maintenance therapy for complications such as intravenous gancylovir). The Ryan White CARE Act was passed in 1990 to help alleviate the need for funding beyond that available from traditional sources.

The CARE Act remains a hugely important feature of the financing and economics of HIV in the United States, retaining a fundamentally similar structure as funding has increased from US$220 million in 1991 to US$2 billion in 2003 (Health Resources and Services Administration, 2003; Institute of Medicine, 2004). The purpose of the Act is

> to provide emergency assistance to localities disproportionately affected by the Human Immunodeficiency Virus epidemic and to make financial assistance to States and other public and private nonprofit entities to provide for the development, organization, coordination, and operations of more effective and cost-efficient systems for the delivery of essential services to individuals and families with HIV disease. (Ryan White CARE Act of 1990, P.L. 101–381, §2 Purpose)

The provisions of the CARE Act provided several overlapping types of grants. Title I grants are directed to highly affected centers (Eligible Metropolitan Areas or EMAs), which had to qualify based initially on the number of reported AIDS cases, then on the estimated number of living AIDS cases. There were originally 16 EMAs, a number that had grown to 51 by 2003. The size of a grant was determined both by a formula and by a supplemental grant process, but the results of the latter strongly correlate with the formula (base) award (Institute of Medicine, 2004). Local distribution of funds was determined by planning bodies and tended to emphasize support to infrastructure and direct provision of care to alleviate unmet medical and non-medical needs.

Title II grants go to states for various uses such as supporting provider networks, subsidizing the continuation of private insurance for individuals, and, very important, the purchase of pharmaceuticals. The latter, known as the AIDS Drug Assistance Program or ADAP, has come to be a major supplier of essential HIV chemotherapy. The amounts of the Title II grants are determined by a formula. Titles III and IV provide direct grants for various programs, the most important of which are the Title III-funded clinics and various early intervention programs and demonstration projects.

The crucial role of the CARE Act rests in the kind of support that it provides. Most notably, these include increases in funding at the margin to mitigate access difficulties through improved infrastructure and provision of HIV drugs and a range of subsidized services. At US$200 million in its first year and growing to US$600 million by 1995, CARE Act funding was not insubstantial, but by the end of this period, it was a small proportion of all federal spending on HIV. For example, in 1995, total federal spending was US$5.1 billion, US$2.5 billion of which was spent on Medicare and Medicaid and US$1.4 billion of which was spent on HIV-related research (Kaiser Family Foundation, 2003b; Summers and Kates, 2004). Of course, CARE Act allocations represent an even smaller percentage of all spending on the personal care of HIV patients, which was estimated to be US$6.7–7.8 billion in 1996, when CARE Act spending for all purposes was US$700 million (Hellinger and Fleishman, 2000).

Late Period: Pervasive Effects of Powerful Treatments

The first protease inhibiting antiretroviral therapy became available in December 1995, followed shortly by the first non-nucleoside reverse transcriptase inhibitor. These drugs had high acquisition costs, and were used only in combination with existing but only slightly less expensive drugs. However, combination antiretroviral regimens containing these drugs (highly active antiretroviral therapy or HAART) resulted in dramatic reductions in both HIV-related morbidity and mortality (Palella *et al.*, 1998). Such regimens rapidly diffused into the population under care, with about 60 per cent of all adults with less than 500 CD4+ cells receiving one of the newer drugs by the end of 1996. The changes in care that followed characterize the recent economic period of HIV care.

The introduction of these combination regimens and the attendant changes in the standards for monitoring care came with a fear of exploding expenditures because of the large incremental cost of providing these drug combinations. However, reports from various individual programs suggested that, over the short term, the introduction of protease inhibitors lowered or did not greatly increase overall costs. The explanation was that the increased drug costs were offset by lowered costs of managing opportunistic complications (Gebo *et al.*, 1999; Keiser *et al.*, 2001). Moreover, the costs of community-based support and palliative care were also decreasing.

Bozzette *et al.* (2001) used a nationally representative sample to estimate that the direct cost of care for HIV-infected adults in the United States declined from about US$1800 to less than US$1400 per patient per month in the first 36 months of care after the introduction of HAART. The drop in monthly costs was due to the fact that decreases in cost of treating opportunistic infections and all hospital costs were greater than the increases in drug costs. In that study, a sad confirmation of this effect was that hospital rather than pharmaceutical expenditures continued to be the largest component of cost only in groups with poor access to new drug therapies.

Although per patient per month costs declined, increases in lifetime costs of care are projected. This is because the reductions in monthly costs are not as great as the increases in life expectancy. However, models and data from some clinics all indicate that the increased costs represent a good value. That is, each yearly increase in life expectancy arising from treatment is purchased at a cost of US$13 000–23 000, values that are well within the range of those accepted as reasonably cost-effective in developed countries (Freedberg *et al.*, 2001).

Increased life expectancy among endstage patients with an unchanging incidence resulted in an increased prevalence of AIDS. At the clinic level, this meant a longer retention of patients without a decline in new entrants, and an increased caseload. In turn, the initial declines in total clinic budgets seen shortly after the introduction of HAART reversed as reductions in per patient per months costs were overwhelmed by the increased number of patients (Wallace *et al.*, 2003). Increasing federal expenditures for HIV care illustrate this point. Medicare and Medicaid spending increased dramatically from US$2.5 billion in 1995 to US$5 billion in 2000, to an estimated US$8 billion in 2004 (Kaiser Family Foundation, 2003b; Summers and Kates, 2004). Although considered discretionary, increases in Ryan White CARE Act spending from US$1 billion, to US$1.7 billion, to an estimated US$2.6 billion over the same intervals were driven in substantial part by the increasing cost of ADAP.

ADAP is the payer of last resort for increasing numbers of HIV patients who are either uninsured or whose drug regimens exceed the limits of private coverage. Federal ADAP spending tripled between fiscal year 1996, when it was US$52 million, to US$167 million in the following year. Since then, expenditures have grown annually to the FY 2004 level of US$749 million (Health Resources and Services Administration, 2003; Summers and Kates, 2004). ADAP is the sole repository of earmarked funding within Title II of the Ryan White CARE Act, and it is the most market-vulnerable link in the entire chain of escalating federal expenditures on HIV/AIDS care. As the fastest growing component of the CARE Act, it is a clear example not only of the policy dilemma that arises when a program does not appropriate the benefit that it generates (e.g. when savings from use of drugs paid by ADAP go to other programs), but also of the disconnect between the push to expand access and the pull to contain costs at both the state and federal levels.

As a federal–state partnerships ADAPs vary considerably across the states and US territories with respect to eligibility, range and organization of services covered, and amounts of annual voluntary allocation of Title I EMA and Title II base funds along with general revenue and other state-budgeted funds to the programs. For example, while all ADAPs require documentation of HIV status, the medical (CD4 count or viral load range) and financial means (Federal Poverty Level percentage-calibrated) criteria for eligibility differ across programs, as do the formularies and drug-purchasing systems. Most ADAPs serve a racially and ethnically diverse client base whose incomes average 200 per cent below FPL and a majority of whom are uninsured and in advanced stages of HIV disease. Most programs cover all FDA-approved antiretroviral drugs, but only 15 cover all recommended drugs for the prevention and treatment of opportunistic infections (Aldridge and Chou, 2003). Many states impose caps either on enrollments, expenditures, or both, in their ADAPs to reduce the rate of program growth.

The variations in accessibility and generosity across state programs translate to significant structural inequities in access to this essential element of HIV care. Where ADAP clients live affects their access to efficacious treatment regimens, and thereby their likelihood of a good outcome. Since the expensive drugs that ADAPs render accessible are cost-effective, ADAPs themselves should be cost-effective (Freedberg *et al.*, 2001; Johri *et al.*, 2002; Walensky *et al.*, 2002). This has been evaluated at the level of state policy. Models indicate that, were all states to increase the generosity of their ADAPs to the level of the most generous program, the total cost of HIV care (but not ADAP costs) would decrease over the short term (Goldman *et al.*, 2001). Moreover, employment of patients would increase, thereby generating new offsetting tax revenue (Goldman *et al.*, 2001). Related models based on the same data indicate that increasing eligibility for public insurance would reduce mortality, and easing the restrictive prescription drug policies associated with public insurance would reduce the gap in outcomes between those with public and private insurance (Bhattacharya *et al.*, 2003).

The increases in government outlays for HIV drugs and HIV care generally could accelerate due to a number of factors, including the number and complexity of patients. Numbers will continue to increase with increasing gains in longer term survival and, hopefully, with improved access for those lacking regular care. The need to manage treatment failure, resistance, increasingly complex combinations of increasing numbers of drugs, and a high prevalence of side-effects and co-morbidities in patients has again shifted the paradigm for patients in regular care. There is general agreement that primary care for HIV patients should be provided by physicians with specific expertise, whose care is characterized by better quality of processes and improved outcomes (Kitahata *et al.*, 2003). As such, the momentum for credentialing in HIV medicine is growing (Zuger and Sharp, 1997). Professional organizations, with the support of payors, are attempting to define an expert and to lobby for a certificate of added qualification in HIV medicine (HIV Medicine Association, 2003). States are considering whether to compel (as opposed to advise) health systems to make such providers available.

Samuel A Bozzette

What the Future Holds

It is certain that pressure on care financing will continue to build. It is also certain that one approach to cost containment will be attempts to reduce drug acquisition costs. One likely means of accomplishing this is to use the government's market (monopsony) power to force prices in the direction of the very low prices available in the developing world. While seemingly sensible in the short run, this is a dangerous strategy that must be approached with caution to avoid damage to future patients. Most patients who need ART will be in the developing world. Managing this market requires accepting either low returns that reveal feasibly low prices or conceding to use of generics that could compromise international intellectual property agreements. Removing the possibility of blockbuster returns by limiting pricing in the United States, the world's most lucrative market, could be a substantial disincentive to drug research and development. This could lead to curtailment of investment in this area, severely undermining innovation and emptying the pipeline of new HIV drugs to the detriment of future patients.

Access not only to chemotherapy but also to a full range of high-quality care will play an increasingly important role in the economics of HIV. Efforts to bring an increasing proportion of the infected into care will require central allocations of additional resources. Success will bring increased caseloads but not proportionate increases in personal expenditures: HIV-infected persons not in care are generally less ill than those in care. In the United States, we are in need of a comprehensive policy debate on how to create and structure incentives to enhance access to care and, especially difficult, to improve quality of care. The quality conundrum is whether to 'reward' good care, thereby withholding funds from sites with deficient care, or to provide additional resources to substandard sites in the hope of improving them. An additional issue is how to assess population-level quality, or quality across a region, and how to hold regional programs responsive and accountable to such measures.

Current regional and state allocations constructed under existing Ryan White CARE Act formulae seem unfair as the amount allocated per case varies by more than is reasonable across jurisdictions. According to a recent Institute of Medicine report, this inequity does not appear to be owing to the use of estimated living AIDS cases rather than reported HIV cases in the formula (Institute of Medicine, 2004). Rather, it is largely attributable to structural elements of the formula. For example, people residing in an EMA are double counted; once for local and again for state application. It is thus not surprising that all of the highly funded states have multiple EMAs and that all of the most poorly funded states have none (Institute of Medicine, 2004). Reform of the allocation mechanisms must be a priority for the next CARE Act reauthorization cycle.

CARE Act grantees and others require assistance in completing the shift of HIV care into a full chronic care model. The chronic disease model emphasizes continuity of comprehensive care. It identifies six elements for success: community resources, which traditionally have been a strong point in HIV care; health care organizations, which are evolving with the demand (and willingness to pay) for increased expertise; self-management support, which is well developed in HIV medicine, especially in relation to adherence; delivery system design, which must evolve with changing needs; decision support, which will likely become an essential element of managing antiretroviral therapy in the face of drug resistance; and clinical information systems, which are being increasingly used for clinical and for quality and outcomes tracking purposes (Bodenheimer *et al.*, 2002a,b). The challenge for the future is to establish incentives toward these activities.

With the transformation of HIV into a chronic disease, long-term issues will become increasingly important. Patients will need costly care for non-opportunistic conditions and diseases of aging. The notion of an AIDS diagnosis granting presumptive permanent disability must be carefully examined, as must the problem of benefits decreasing the likelihood of a return to employment. Finally, with continued progress, patients will face the happy burden imposed by the economics of retirement and old age.

References

Aldridge C, Chou L (2003) *Trends in Opportunistic Infection Drug Coverage and Spending.* National ADAP Monitoring Project Issue Brief No. 1584–04, National Alliance of State and Territiorial AIDS Directors, Kaiser Family Foundation, and AIDS Treatment Data Network. Menlo Park, CA: Henry J. Kaiser Family Foundation.

Arno PS, Shenson D, Siegel NF, Franks P, Lee PR (1989) Economic and policy implications of early intervention in HIV disease. *JAMA* 262: 1493–8.

Bennett CL, Garfinkle JB, Greenfield S *et al.* (1989) The relation between hospital experience and in-hospital mortality for patients with AIDS-related PCP. *JAMA* 261: 2975–9.

Bhattacharya J, Goldman D, Sood N (2003) The link between public and private insurance and HIV-related mortality. *J Health Econ* 22: 1105–22.

Bodenheimer T, Wagner EH, Grumbach K (2002a) Improving primary care for patients with chronic illness. *JAMA* 288: 1775–9.

Bodenheimer T, Wagner EH, Grumbach K (2002b) Improving primary care for patients with chronic illness: The chronic care model, Part 2. *JAMA* 288: 1909–14.

Bozzette SA, Berry SH, Duan N *et al.* (1998) The care of HIV-infected adults in the United States. *N Engl J Med* 339: 1897–904.

Bozzette SA, Joyce G, McCaffrey DF *et al.* (2001) Expenditures for the care of HIV-infected patients in the era of highly active antiretroviral therapy. *N Engl J Med* 344: 817–23.

CDC (Centers for Disease Control and Prevention) (2003a) *HIV/AIDS Surveillance Report: Cases of HIV Infection and AIDS in the United States, 2002.* Vol. 14. Bethesda, MD: National Center for HIV, STD, and TB Prevention, Centers for Disease Control, US Department of Health and Human Services. http://www/cdc.gov/hiv/ stats/hasr1402.htm

CDC (2003b) Increases in HIV diagnoses: 29 states, 1999–2002. *MMWR Morb Mortal Wkly Rep* 52: 1145–8.

Fleming PL, Byers RH, Sweeney PA, Daniels D, Karon JM, Janssen RS (2002) HIV prevalence in the United States, 2000. Paper presented at the 9th Conference on Retroviruses and Opportunistic Infections, Seattle, WA, abstract no. 11.

Freedberg KA, Losina E, Weinstein MC *et al.* (2001) The cost effectiveness of combination antiretroviral therapy for HIV disease. *N Engl J Med* 344: 824–31.

Gebo KA, Chaisson RE, Folkemer JG, Bartlett JG, Moore RD (1999) Costs of HIV medical care in the era of highly active antiretroviral therapy. *AIDS* 13: 963–9.

Goldman DP, Bhattacharya J, Leibowitz AA, Joyce GF, Shapiro MF, Bozzette SA (2001) The impact of state policy on the costs of HIV infection. *Med Care Res Rev* 58: 31–53.

Goldman DP, Leibowitz AA, Joyce GF *et al.* (2003) Insurance status of HIV-infected adults in the post-HAART era: Evidence from the United States. *Appl Health Econ Health Policy* 2: 85–90.

Green J, Arno PS (1990) The 'Medicaidization' of AIDS: Trends in the financing of HIV-related medical care. *JAMA* 264: 1261–6.

Hardy AM, Rauch K, Echenberg D, Morgan WM, Curran JW (1986) The economic impact of the first 10 000 cases of acquired immunodeficiency syndrome in the United States. *JAMA* 255: 209–11.

Health Resources and Services Administration (2003) *AIDS Drug Assistance Program (ADAP) Funding Overview.* Rockville, MD: Health Resources and Services Administration, US Department of Health and Human Services.

Hellinger FJ, Fleishman JA (2000) Estimating the national cost of treating people with HIV disease: Patient, payer, and provider data. *J Acquir Immune Defic Syndr* 24: 182–8.

Herscher E (1989) Huge cost calculated for early treatment of AIDS. *San Francisco Chronicle* 15 September. http://www.aegis.com/news/sc/1989/Sc890911.html

HIV Medicine Association (2003) *Qualifications for Physicians Who Care for Patients with HIV Infection.* Alexandria, VA: HIV Medicine Association.

Institute of Medicine, Committee on the Ryan White CARE Act: Data for Resource Allocation, Planning, and Evaluation (2004) *Measuring What Matters: Allocation, Planning, and Quality Assessment for the Ryan White CARE Act.* Washington, DC: National Academies Press.

Johri M, Paltiel AD, Goldie SJ, Freedberg KA (2002) State AIDS Drug Assistance Programs: Equity and efficiency in an era of rapidly changing treatment standards. *Med Care* 40: 429–41.

Kaiser Family Foundation (2003a) *AIDS Drug Assistance Programs.* HIV/AIDS Policy Fact Sheet. Menlo Park, CA: Henry J. Kaiser Family Foundation.

Kaiser Family Foundation (2003b) *Federal HIV/AIDS Spending: A Budget Chartbook, Fiscal Year 2002.* Menlo Park, CA: Henry J. Kaiser Family Foundation.

Kates J, Sorian R (2000) *Financing HIV/AIDS Care: A Quilt with Many Holes.* Capitol Hill Briefing Series on HIV/AIDS. Menlo Park, CA: Henry J. Kaiser Family Foundation.

Keiser P, Nassar N, Kvanli MB, Turner D, Smith JW, Skiest D (2001) Long-term impact of highly active antiretroviral therapy on HIV-related health care costs. *J Acquir Immune Defic Syndr* 27: 14–19.

Kitahata MM, Koepsell TD, Deyo RA, Maxwell CL, Dodge WT, Wagner EH (1996) Physicians' experience with the acquired immunodeficiency syndrome as a factor in patients' survival. *N Engl J Med* 334: 701–6.

Kitahata MM, Van Rompaey SE, Dillingham PW *et al.* (2003) Primary care delivery is associated with greater physician experience and improved survival among persons with AIDS. *J Gen Intern Med* 18: 95–103.

Palella FJ, Jr, Delaney KM, Moorman AC *et al.* (1998) Declining morbidity and mortality among patients with advanced human immunodeficiency virus infection. *N Engl J Med* 338: 853–80.

Pascal AH (1987) *The Costs of Treating AIDS under Medicaid: 1986–1991.* RAND Document No. N-2600-HCFA. Santa Monica, CA: RAND Corporation.

Scitovsky AA, Rice DP (1987) Estimates of the direct and indirect costs of acquired immunodeficiency syndrome in the United States, 1985, 1986, and 1991. *Public Health Rep* 102: 5–17.

Seage GR, III, Landers S, Barry A, Groopman J, Lamb GA, Epstein AM (1986) Medical care costs of AIDS in Massachusetts. *JAMA* 256: 3107–9.

Shapiro MF, Morton SC, McCaffrey *et al.* (1999) Variations in the care of HIV-infected adults in the United States: Results from the HIV Cost and Services Utilization Study. *JAMA* 281: 2305–15.

Steinbrook R (1998) Caring for people with human immunodeficiency virus infection. [Editorial]. *N Engl J Med* 339: 1926–8.

Steinbrook R (2001) Providing antiretroviral therapy for HIV infection. *N Engl J Med* 344: 844–6.

Summers T, Kates J (2004) *Trends in U.S. Government Funding for HIV/AIDS: Fiscal Years 1981 to 2004.* HIV/AIDS Policy Brief No. 7032. Menlo Park, CA: Henry J. Kaiser Family Foundation.

Walensky RP, Paltiel AD, Freedberg KA (2002) AIDS Drug Assistance Programs: Highlighting inequities in human immunodeficiency virus-infection health care in the United States. *Clin Infect Dis* 35: 606–10.

Wallace MR, Tasker SA, Shinohara YT, Hill HE, Chapman GD, Miller LK (2003) The changing economics of HIV care. *AIDS Patient Care and STDs* 15: 25–9.

Zuger A, Sharp VL (1997) 'HIV specialists': The time has come. *JAMA* 278: 1131–2.

Expanding Global Access to ARVs: The Challenges of Prices and Patents

13

Michael R Reich
Harvard University Center for Population and Development Studies, Cambridge, Massachusetts, USA

Priya Bery
Director of Policy & Research, Global Business Coalition on HIV/AIDS, New York, USA

Michael R Reich, PhD is Director of the Harvard Center for Population and Development Studies and Taro Takemi Professor of International Health Policy at the Harvard School of Public Health. He recently edited a book on public-private partnerships for public health (distributed by Harvard University Press, 2003) and is co-author of *Getting Health Reform Right: A Guide to Improving Performance and Equity* (Oxford University Press, 2004). He received his PhD in political science from Yale University and has been a faculty member at Harvard University since 1983.

Priya Bery, SM is Director of Policy & Research at the Global Business Coalition on HIV/AIDS, a New York-based alliance of international companies fighting the pandemic. She works to advance partnerships between business and government in Asia and other regions heavily affected by HIV/AIDS. Ms. Bery received her Master's of Science in Health Policy and Management from Harvard University in 2001, where she focused her research on HIV/AIDS and access to medicines. Prior to her study in public health, she worked on health and environmental legislation in the U.S. Senate as well as in development on maternal and child health issues in India.

In the first years of the twenty-first century, access to AIDS medicines reached the top of the global health policy agenda. In developed countries, expanded access to new medicines occurred in the mid-1990s and contributed to dramatic reductions in deaths due to AIDS (Mocroft *et al.*, 1998). In the United States, for example, AIDS mortality rates decreased by 75 per cent between early 1994 and mid-1997 – a decline attributable in large part to the intensive use of antiretrovirals (ARVs) (Palella *et al.*, 1998). Since 1997, the US Food and Drug Administration approved over 50 therapies that can slow or disrupt viral replication or treat opportunistic infections. These AIDS drugs included three types of ARVs (nucleoside reverse transcriptase inhibitors, non-nucleoside reverse transcriptase inhibitors, and protease inhibitors) used in various combinations. With these new medicines and falling prices, the treatment of people living with HIV/AIDS became increasingly cost-effective. AIDS interventions in developed countries, including the delivery of highly active antiretroviral therapy (HAART), produced dramatic survival benefits and averted many long-term costs related to opportunistic infections and hospitalization.

While AIDS medicines became available to most people living with HIV in the developed world (Rose, 1998; UNAIDS, 2000b, p. 86), they have remained difficult to obtain in most developing countries. Nevertheless, in the past decade a sea change occurred in global policy and thinking about access to AIDS medicines for the world's poorest countries. Previously, many people wondered if it was feasible or desirable to treat AIDS patients in poor countries. Today, many people expect and demand expanded access to AIDS medicines for patients throughout the developing world. This chapter provides an historical perspective on how progress was achieved in addressing the challenges posed by two key dimensions affecting access to ARVs in developing countries: prices and patents. The chapter also demonstrates how major obstacles were recognized and confronted through a contentious and iterative political process.

Expanding Access to Treatment

Of the world's estimated 34–46 million people living with HIV in 2003, over 95 per cent live in the developing world, with 25–28 million in sub-Saharan Africa (UNAIDS/WHO, 2003). Adult infection rates in sub-Saharan Africa are strikingly high – for example, 38.8 per cent of adults in Botswana are living with HIV/AIDS and 20 per cent of adults in South Africa – compared with 0.6 per cent in the US and 0.1 per cent in the UK (UNAIDS, 2000c). Of the total infected population globally, it is estimated that approximately 6 million people are in need of treatment is low and middle-income countries, since ARV therapy is initiated after a certain stage in disease progression. Yet only 400 000 individuals had access in late 2003 (WHO, 2003). The need is greatest in Africa, where the epidemic has advanced relentlessly. At the end of 2003, only 100 000 people had access to ARVs in sub-Saharan Africa (about 2 per cent of the 4.4 million people estimated in need), although this represented a substantial increase from only 30 000 people with access to treatment in 2001 (UNAIDS/WHO, 2003).

Why are these life-saving drugs not reaching those who need them? As explained throughout this book, various factors have combined to limit access to AIDS medicines in poor countries. The main obstacles include overwhelming national poverty, the epidemiology of the disease, the economics of the medicines, and the problems of health care systems in developing countries. Other factors have also shaped the limited access, including economic stagnation, political instability, and the devastating impact of stigma and discrimination, discouraging individuals from getting tested and seeking care, support, and treatment. The reluctance of political leaders and governments to respond publicly and aggressively to the HIV/AIDS pandemic has delayed the effective implementation of national policies (Caldwell, 2000). Even when some leaders have decided to fight the epidemic, the commitment of resources has often lagged behind. Tragically, the countries most affected by the AIDS epidemic have confronted the greatest problems in providing access to AIDS medicines.

In the past few years we have seen increasing leadership by governments, international institutions, private companies, and civil society to expand access to ARVs in the countries that need the medicines most. In September 2003, the World Health Organization announced a global program of '3 by 5' to provide 3 million people with ARV treatment by 2005. The United Nations' Millennium Development Goals give high priority to efforts that can halt and reverse the spread of HIV/AIDS by 2015. New partnerships, such as the Global Fund to Fight AIDS, Tuberculosis and Malaria, have emerged to help achieve these goals. And individual donor countries have made new financial aid commitments, such as the US$15 billion in the US President's Emergency Plan for AIDS Relief, known as PEPFAR, which announced its first grants in February 2004. Corporations have also made new investments to extend treatment to employees, families, and local communities. These efforts are designed to scale up access to ARVs, which otherwise, according to WHO estimates, could only reach less than one million people in the developing world by the end of 2005.

Affordability of medicines has been at the center of the debate over access to AIDS drugs in poor countries. This chapter explores the high cost of drugs to show how the debate evolved and how key issues have been addressed. We discuss how drug prices are set, and how patents affect the price of pharmaceuticals. We review five policy options for price and patent issues in expanding access to AIDS medicines in developing countries. We conclude with an assessment of other obstacles to access, in the context of the sharply reduced prices of AIDS medicines over the past decade. These other issues must be resolved to achieve sustained access to AIDS medicines in resource-limited environments.

Pricing Pharmaceuticals

In developing countries, most medicines are purchased by households with personal funds or less frequently by governments with public budgets (WHO, 1998). Both personal funds and government budgets are severely limited. For example, during the 1990s, average total health expenditure (public and private) per year was US$14 per person in Uganda and US$246 per person in South Africa, compared with US$4080 in the United States (World Bank, 2000). In sub-Saharan Africa, nearly 46 per cent of people live on less than US$1 a day (UNDP, 2001, p. 10). Poverty thus makes it impossible for individuals or governments to pay for the medicines that are needed.

For AIDS, the standard treatment in developed countries in the mid-1990s was HAART, which at that time cost up to US$21 000 per person per year (Freedberg *et al.*, 2001). Who paid for treatment critically affected access. In developed countries, most HIV patients received AIDS care and treatment through government programs or private insurance. In most developing countries, by contrast, only a small number of HIV patients received treatment through personal funds or through very limited programs run by governments or companies, while the vast majority of patients received no effective treatment at all. As a result, in the late 1990s, the call for expanded access to AIDS medicines in developing countries became a conflict over drug pricing.

In almost all countries around the world, there is public concern about the high price of pharmaceuticals because of financial strain on government health budgets and on household budgets for low-income patients. Most countries (other than the United States) regulate drug prices by implementing price controls, placing limits on company profits, or setting reimbursement rates under social insurance programs (Danzon, 2000). Governments struggle with a basic policy conflict between reducing drug prices to contain health expenditures and expand health services, and raising drug prices to create incentives for new drugs or provide subsidies for local manufacturers.

In general, producers set prices for drugs to capture some combination of the costs of research, development, production and marketing – plus profits – and compete with other companies that manufacture the same or similar products. The total cost of developing a new drug is hotly debated. According to the Pharmaceutical Research Manufacturers Association, member companies invested US$32 billion in research and development in 2002 (PhRMA, 2003). Joseph A DiMasi and colleagues estimate the full cost of developing a new drug at US$802 million (including the costs of unsuccessful projects and opportunity costs) (DiMasi *et al.*, 2003). One co-author, Henry Grabowski, explained in another article that 'new product approval incurred out-of-pocket costs of over $400 million. This includes money spent in the discovery, pre-clinical and clinical phases as well as an allocation for the cost of failures' (Grabowski, 2002, pp. 851–2).

Critics have countered that this figure overstates the costs of drug discovery and development (Young and Surrusco, 2001).

Prices for new drugs, however, do not always reflect full costs, as shown by the wide differences in prices for the same product. Prices for the same drug (produced by the same company) vary greatly both between and within countries, because of different corporate strategies, policy circumstances, tariffs, exchange rates, and negotiating conditions. For example, the list price of zidovudine (AZT), an ARV used in HIV combination therapy, was US$1.71 per 100 mg capsule in the UK and US$0.66 in Spain (in 2000) (UNICEF-UNAIDS *et al.*, 2001). According to Danzon and Kim (1998), comprehensive price comparisons of international drug prices incorporate a host of methodological issues involving measurement differences in average price levels. These problems can produce different results (depending on how they are addressed) and can undermine the validity of policy conclusions from price comparisons.

Multinational companies that develop new drugs seek to set high prices for their products in major markets (such as the United States) as a way to achieve high returns on the costs of drug development and marketing (Danzon, 2000). Markets with high prices thus pay a higher share of corporate research and development costs, leading to US charges of free-riding by European (and other) governments and consumers (Editorial, 2002). This situation has created an 'imbalance' in pharmaceutical innovation between the United States and Europe, with a recent report identifying possible negative consequences for Europeans due to delayed access to drugs, poorer health outcomes, and lower investments in research (Gilbert and Rosenberg, 2004).

Governments in poor countries typically have limited leverage in negotiations with pharmaceutical companies over prices, especially for single-source products (produced by a single company under a product patent). All developing nations account for only 16 per cent of sales in the global pharmaceutical market, with Africa representing only 1.3 per cent (IMS Health, 2002). Consequently, prices in poor countries often end up close to those in rich countries, and they can even exceed prices in rich countries when customs, tariffs, distribution, and pharmacy charges are included. For many poor countries, difficulties in negotiating lower prices for AIDS medicines (and other drugs) are also related to the nation's overall poverty, generally small market size, inefficient pharmaceutical purchasing system, and limited domestic pharmaceutical production capacity.

Responding to International Pressures to Lower Prices for AIDS Drugs

The past decade has witnessed a surge of international pressure to lower the prices for AIDS medicines in developing countries (Figure 13.1). Pressure came from AIDS activists, people living with HIV/AIDS, generic pharmaceutical companies, and non-governmental organizations (including Médecins Sans Frontières, Consumer Project on Technology, ACT-UP, and the Treatment Action Campaign). Activists and world leaders including Nelson Mandela drew global media attention to this issue in their opposition to the lawsuit brought (and eventually withdrawn) by 39 drug manufacturers against the South African government's Medicines and Related Substances Act of 1997, which sought to expand access to low-cost AIDS medicines through various measures (Park, 2002; Sidley, 2001). The activist pressure helped place the issue of access to AIDS medicines high on the international health agenda and onto the policy agenda of the United Nations and the G-7 countries in the last years of the twentieth century.

Facing these pressures, international agencies and pharmaceutical companies responded by setting up new mechanisms that promised to expand access in developing countries and by reducing some prices. The first effort to expand access was a UNAIDS project in Uganda and Côte d'Ivoire in 1997, called the Drug Access Initiative. In Uganda, for example, prices for a first-line regimen declined from about US$12 000 per year in 1997 to about US$7200 per year in 1999 (Okero *et al.*, 2003, p. 7). A more formalized process was established in May 2000 through the Accelerating Access Initiative (AAI). Through AAI, UNAIDS along with other co-sponsoring international agencies and six pharmaceutical companies set up a preferential pricing mechanism at the country level. As of June 2002, 19 countries had signed agreements on significantly reduced drug prices (WHO, 2002). These two efforts helped expand the delivery of AIDS medicines to HIV patients in participating countries, reaching about 76 000 people in Africa by June 2003 (IFPMA, 2003), still a small proportion of the people needing treatment. The two initiatives also marked major shifts in the global

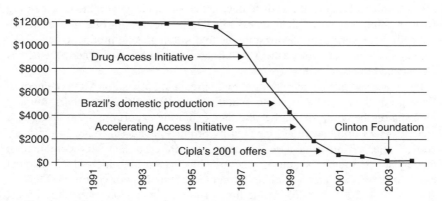

Fig. 13.1 Annual cost per person for triple-drug therapy in Africa (US$). Adapted from Quick (2001).

329

debate, making it legitimate to question the high prices of AIDS drugs for poor countries.

The first developing country to make a full-scale national commitment to provide universal and free access to ARVs for AIDS patients was Brazil. Brazil's 1988 constitution guarantees universal access to health care, and in 1996 Brazil passed a law that assures universal access to antiretrovirals (Lei no 9.313.996). This high-level political commitment was critically important for Brazil's efforts to expand access to treatment for people living with HIV/AIDS. The Brazilian government's policy of developing capacity for local production of generic products and its threats of compulsory licensing helped push down domestic prices for AIDS medicines (and raw materials) (Teixeira *et al.*, 2003). These strategies reduced the cost of ARVs in Brazil, although questions remain about how the country will sustain its national treatment program over the long term. Between 1996 and 2001, the average cost of treatment per patient decreased by more than 50 per cent in Brazil (Teixeira *et al.*, 2003, p. 82). Four years after the national treatment program was introduced, AIDS-related mortality had fallen by about 50 per cent, and each AIDS patient was only a quarter as likely to be hospitalized compared with the time before the national treatment program began (Rosenberg, 2001).

Brazil has been widely cited as a model of policy response for developing countries. But Brazil's response is not easily replicable in Africa, because of important differences: Brazil's relatively low prevalence of HIV (0.7 per cent in 2002 (UNAIDS, 2000c)), the country's relatively high income (US$2830 per capita in 2003), the strong national pharmaceutical industry, and its use of three World Bank loans to help finance the AIDS control program: US$160 million in 1993, followed by US$165 million in 1998, and an additional US$100 million in 2003 (World Bank, 2003)). Brazil also has a strong civil society movement that effectively put pressure on the government to adopt universal access to ARVs as official policy. Despite these differences, the Brazilian government is helping African countries expand their access to AIDS medicines, for example, by working with the government of Mozambique to develop generic production capabilities and in the interim provide them with Brazilian manufactured generic medicines (Associated Press, 2003).

India has also played an important role in reducing prices for AIDS medicines. Drug producers in India began to manufacture ARVs in the late 1990s, initially focusing on the domestic market and then exploring export opportunities. These generic AIDS drugs were not covered by product patents in India. In February 2001, Cipla, an Indian generic manufacturer, offered to sell ARV combination therapy at US$350 per person per year to Médecins Sans Frontières (MSF) and at US$600 per person per year directly to governments in poor countries (McNeil, 2001; UNDP, 2001, p. 106). At the time of the Cipla announcement, the lowest market price worldwide for triple combination therapy was just under US$10 500. Within one year, the lowest price for triple therapy had dropped to US$727 per person per year, a result of international pressure and competition by low-cost generics (Médecins Sans Frontières, 2003). WHO supported the role of generic manufacturers by including them in companies reviewed in the first international quality assessment of AIDS medicines in May 2001. In 2003, an updated version of this list included 74 products from 11 manufacturers (both branded and generic) for 11 ARVs and four combinations (WHO, 2003).

After the United Nations Special Session on HIV/AIDS in June 2001, a number of new partnerships and multisectoral coalitions emerged to help expand global access to ARVs, addressing both the cost of medicines and problems in delivery. The Global Fund to Fight AIDS, Tuberculosis and Malaria was established in January 2003 and allocated about US$2.1 billion in its first three rounds of grants, with about 59 per cent directed toward HIV/AIDS. The Global Fund estimates that an additional 500 000 people will receive ARVs over the next five years through Fund-supported programs. In May 2003, US President George Bush signed into law a five-year, US$15 billion commitment to fight HIV/AIDS in Africa and the Caribbean, which seeks to provide treatment to 2 million people. The business community is also working to increase the reach of treatment programs in partnership with the public sector, through such groups as the Global Business Coalition on HIV/AIDS (2003). For example, the mining company Anglo American is extending its employee treatment programs to the surrounding communities in South Africa through a new co-investment scheme with the Global Fund, the Henry J. Kaiser Foundation and the Nelson Mandela Foundation.

In the fall of 2003, prices for AIDS medicines dropped again, when the William J. Clinton Foundation announced a new partnership with Indian and South African generic producers and community organizations to provide triple-drug therapy at 38 cents per patient per day in Africa and the Caribbean. At these prices, the generic drug costs of AIDS treatment were cut by nearly 60 per cent (from the prevailing price of about US$1 a day). Until the Clinton effort, the lowest available price of the same three-drug regimen using brand-name ARVs was US$1.54 per patient per day (Schoofs, 2003). The new prices brokered by the Clinton Foundation will challenge the generic industry to deliver a continuous supply of high-quality drugs. But if sustainable, the prices could catalyze expanded access to treatment in a number of poor countries.

In May of 2004 the US government announced a major shift in AIDS policy to encourage the development of fixed dose combinations (FDCs) of ARVs. The government created a Fast Track Review System for AIDS Drugs designed to reduce approval time to six weeks. FDCs are single pills containing two or three drugs included in ARV triple combination therapy. At the same time, Bristol Myer-Squibb, Gilead, and Merck & Co., three manufacturers of branded ARVs, announced that they would work together to develop a combined, once-daily tablet. This is the first collaboration between patent-holders making single components of ARV triple therapy. People living with HIV/AIDS will benefit from simplified treatment regimens and potential cost savings by purchasing one pill instead of each drug separately. Fixed dose products have already been developed by Indian generic manufacturers and have been prequalified for first-line treatment in resource-limited settings by the WHO. Although these FDC products are currently used by people in developing countries, they are not permitted in the US President's Emergency Plan for AIDS Relief until they have been approved by the US government's new fast track program.

This review shows how prices for triple-drug AIDS therapy dropped dramatically in just four years, from 1999 to 2003, as prices fell up to 98 per cent – from US$12 000 a year to less than US$200 a year. Prices for a number of ARVs in many developing countries are now probably close to the marginal costs of production. These remarkable price declines have reduced price as a barrier to access for AIDS medicines for governments and many patients in developing countries. However, even at these lower prices, the cost of AIDS medicines remains far beyond the ability to pay for most people in developing countries except for the elite. Other obstacles also remain, including the lack of funding for AIDS medicines, debate among donors on the use of generic medicines and the lack of adequate facilities to treat and care for patients (as we discuss below). Moreover, pricing will persist as an important question for the next generation of ARVs, which are not covered by current agreements and policies. Prices for triple-drug therapy will also vary depending on the drug combination selected. Finally, if drug resistance increases, there would be a growing need for second-line (new) ARVs. A recent study in Europe reported a 10 per cent rate of HIV drug resistance for first-line drugs in newly infected individuals (van der Vijver *et al.*, 2003).

A critical factor that affects the pricing of new drugs is how the patent system operates at the national and international levels; we turn to this issue next.

How Patents Affect Drug Prices

The international patent system has been a major focus in the debate over access to AIDS medicines in developing countries. The past three decades have shown a global trend toward increased patent protection of pharmaceuticals, with a new international regime emerging since 1995, seeking to include more developing countries. This trend has been promoted by the international pharmaceutical industry, while critics (especially in the past decade) have argued that expanding patent protection has limited access to AIDS medicines by limiting competition from non-patented copies and thereby supporting high prices.

A patent is a set of legal rights, based on national law, providing the patent owner with the means to prevent others from making, using or selling a new invention for a limited period of time (for example, 20 years) (WTO, 2001b). These national laws operate within the rules of the international trade regime, which seeks to establish some consistency across national boundaries. Patents are intended to provide a balance between protecting economic incentives for innovators and promoting the public interests of society. Patents represent a form of intellectual property rights (IPR), which are designed to assure inventors that they (and not others) will receive economic returns on their innovative ideas, as a way of creating incentives to develop new products. (Other forms of intellectual property rights, such as trademarks and copyrights, are not considered in this chapter.) At the same time, the patent system allows public access to knowledge about innovations, as a way of promoting continued research and development by other parties.

National patent laws differ country by country. In general, rich countries tend to provide stricter protection of intellectual property rights, while poor countries tend to have limited protection and less effective mechanisms for enforcement. Not surprisingly, rich countries also tend to produce more intellectual property, and therefore have groups and individuals with strong incentives to seek effective protection. Countries at different levels of technological development thus have different needs and desires about a national patent system (Commission on Intellectual Property Rights, 2002).

For medicines, patents can be applied to new products, as a *product patent* for the chemical entity in a new drug, or to new processes, as a *process patent* for the method of producing the chemical ingredients for a medicine (WTO, 2001b). In general, poor countries seek to weaken the patent system, to promote cheap imports or allow the production and sale of cheap copies. They may then introduce a process patent system, as domestic companies are able to produce copies of existing products (which often are protected by product patents in other countries). Once a country's pharmaceutical industry can invent new products, the country typically changes its laws and moves to a product patent regime. Japan, for example, introduced product patents in 1976 (Reich, 1990), followed by Switzerland in 1977, Italy, Holland, and Sweden in 1978, and Canada and Denmark in 1983, with China in 1992–93, Brazil in 1996, and Argentina in 2000 (Lanjouw, 2003) (see Table 13.1).

Advocates for expanded access have argued that the international patent system, by supporting high prices and blocking the production and importation of generic medicines, has obstructed developing countries from obtaining cheaper AIDS medicines. According to these advocates, the obstructive role of patents has been enhanced by recent changes to strengthen the international patent system, which have been supported by the multinational pharmaceutical industry and by rich country governments (especially the United States). In short, advocates have argued that the patent system has protected the profits of drug companies in rich countries while ignoring the lives (and deaths) of HIV patients in poor countries.

Advocates for strengthening the international protection of patents, on the other hand, have argued that these intellectual property rights are essential as incentives to develop new medicines (including AIDS medicines). The research-based pharmaceutical industry has lobbied fiercely and effectively to enhance patent protection in international agreements and national laws around the world.

333

Table 13.1   Introduction of production patent protection and GDP per capita.

Country	Year of adoption	GDP per capita (1995 US$)
OECD countries		
Japan	1976	24 043
Switzerland	1977	36 965
Italy	1978	13 465
Holland	1978	20 881
Sweden	1978	21 896
Canada	1983	16 296
Denmark	1983	28 010
Austria	1987	25 099
Spain	1992	14 430
Portugal	1992	10 469
Greece	1992	10 897
Norway	1992	30 389
Recent Adopters		
China	1992–3	424
Brazil	1996	4482
Argentina	2000	8100
Uruguay	2001	6208
Guatemala	Future	1545
Egypt	Future	1191
Pakistan	Future	508
India	Future	450
Malawi	Future	156

Note: China GDP is for 1992; for countries adopting after 1992, the GDP per capita figure is for 1999. From Lanjouw (2003).

In short, the research-based pharmaceutical industry views the patent system as the essential cornerstone for their continuing drug development and commercial success (IFPMA, 2004). They argue more broadly that patent protection helps to promote economic development by providing incentives for innovation and investment (Rapp and Rozek, 1990). In brief, they argue that without product patents there would be few new drugs.

International Agreements Affecting Patents: The WTO and TRIPS

New institutions and mechanisms have been developed to address the differences in patent protection among nations and resolve conflicts that occur. The most important institution is the World Trade Organization (WTO), which was established as the global governing body of the international trade regime in 1994 as a result of the Uruguay Round of the trade negotiations in the General Agreement on Tariffs and Trade (GATT). The WTO sets the legal ground rules for international trade and promotes the objectives of non-discrimination, liberalization of trade barriers, competition, and transparency. As of April 2003, the WTO had 146 member countries.

Intellectual property standards for WTO members are established through the Agreement on Trade-Related Aspects of Intellectual Property Rights (TRIPS) of 1995. This mechanism sets a floor of IPR protection for countries and connects IPR to several international trade agreements. Prior to the TRIPS Agreement, over 40 countries (primarily poorer countries) did not provide any comprehensive product and process patent protection for pharmaceuticals (WHO, 2001). Under TRIPS, member nations are required to adhere to basic minimum standards for universal patent protection for any technological invention, including pharmaceuticals. Failure to comply with these rules brings the threat of trade sanctions and other adverse consequences. The expansion of patent protection through TRIPS drew broad support from the research-based pharmaceutical industry, which expected to benefit from increased protection of its patents around the world.

Countries that previously had no patent protection are now introducing it so that they can become members of the WTO. TRIPS provides some leeway for countries to bring their national legislation in compliance with agreement standards. The length of the period varies for developed and developing countries. Developed nations were required to apply all TRIPS provisions by 1 January 1996, one year after TRIPS was established; developing countries and transitional economies were given five years, until 1 January 2000; and least developed countries were given 11 years, until 1 January 2006 (WHO, 2001).

The 4th WTO Ministerial Conference, held in Doha, Qatar, in November 2001, extended this deadline until 2016 for the world's least developed countries. The meeting also produced the Doha Declaration on the TRIPS Agreement and Public Health, which asserted a priority to public health over intellectual property (WTO, 2001a). The Declaration stated, 'The TRIPS agreement does not and should not prevent Members from taking measures to protect public health', adding that TRIPS should be implemented in a manner 'supportive of WTO Members' right to protect public health and, in particular, to promote access to medicines for all'. The interpretation of the Doha Declaration in practical policy subsequently became a matter of vigorous debate. The Doha Declaration did not establish any new principles for TRIPS. Rather, it re-stated ideas contained in TRIPS and recognized that the poorest countries (without a well developed domestic pharmaceutical industry) 'could face difficulties in making effective use of compulsory licensing under the TRIPS Agreement' to gain access to medicines. In short, could a poor country use compulsory licensing under a public health emergency to import generic drugs that were protected by product patents (in the importing country), and if so, for which diseases and from which countries?

In August 2003, the WTO resolved some of these questions raised by the Doha Declaration. Without changing the TRIPS Agreement, the WTO General Council approved a statement supporting the importation of generic medicines into those developing countries that lacked pharmaceutical manufacturing capabilities, under certain conditions (WTO, 2003b). This represented an interim decision, intended to last until TRIPS is amended in the ongoing round of negotiations. The WTO declared that the decision removed the final 'patent obstacle' to cheap drug imports for poor countries. The WTO Director-General announced:

> The final piece of the jigsaw has fallen into place, allowing poorer countries to make full use of the flexibilities in the WTO's intellectual property rules in order to deal with the diseases that ravage their people.... It proves once and for all that the organization can handle humanitarian as well as trade concerns (WTO, 2003a).

How TRIPS Affects Access to ARVs

The debate over intellectual property rights and ARVs produced intense advocates on both sides. Supporters of IPR argued that strict enforcement of IPR is necessary for innovation and continued economic and social development, while critics of IPR countered that patent protection interferes with progress in human development in poor countries (UNDP, 2001, p. 103) by obstructing access to needed medicines and other products.

The TRIPS Agreement of 1995 is often interpreted as allowing for two mechanisms that could be used to expand access to cheaper versions of patented drugs:

- A *compulsory license* allows a government to grant a license to use a patent without permission of the patent holder, when the patent holder is either not using the patent within the country or not using it adequately (according to Article 31 of the TRIPS Agreement on 'other use without authorization of the right holder'). Under TRIPS, a compulsory license can be granted under certain circumstances, such as a national emergency or other circumstances of extreme urgency, and in the case of anti-competitive practice by the patent holder. This license would require that compensation be paid to the patent holder. The United States has used compulsory licenses for various technologies in the computer, recording, defense and other industries.
- *Parallel importation* provides access to lower-priced patented drugs by purchasing products marketed by the patent owner in one country (where they are sold at a lower price, such as Spain) and importing them into another country (where they are sold at a higher price, such as Britain) without the patent

owner's approval. Article 6 of TRIPS, by not settling or expressly prohibiting parallel imports, is interpreted as allowing for this kind of arbitrage.

The first case of a government's seeking to use compulsory licensing for ARVs occurred in August 2001, when Brazil's Ministry of Health announced steps to produce nelfinavir, a drug patented by Roche Laboratories, in a Brazilian government production facility in order to reduce the drug's price (Rich and Petersen, 2001). In 2000, Brazil had spent US$303 million on AIDS drugs, with about US$88 million (or 25 per cent of the total) on nelfinavir (Rich and Petersen, 2001). Roche responded to the government's announcement about compulsory licensing by offering to reduce the product's price in Brazil (more than the 13 per cent it previously offered, which the government had rejected as inadequate) – and an agreement was reached without a change in government policy. This case shows that countries like Brazil (with substantial resources, a domestic industry, political mobilization, and a large market) can use threats of compulsory licensing as leverage in price negotiations to achieve greater discounts. However, only a few developing countries resemble Brazil in these respects.

In March 2004, the government of Mozambique issued a compulsory license for manufacturing a triple combination of antiretroviral drugs to meet national needs. In doing so, Mozambique became the first African country to take this important step in implementing the Doha Declaration. Prior to this, no developing country had successfully used compulsory licensing or parallel importation to expand access to ARVs. However, the efforts by Brazil (and South Africa, as noted below) to implement national policies based on these two mechanisms advanced the international debate on access, even though the policies were not adopted. Later in 2004, several other developing countries issued a compulsory license for an AIDS medicine – and more are expected, especially if this mechanism proves to be effective in expanding access in practice.

Patents for AIDS Medicines

To what extent has the protection of patents affected access to ARVs in developing countries, especially since the start of TRIPS in 1995? A first step in answering this question is identifying where pharmaceutical companies have filed for patent protection for their products in developing countries. An analysis of 15 ARVs in 53 African countries found that eight products were patented in three or fewer countries, and four products were patented in 24–33 countries (Attaran and Gillespie-White, 2001). The authors suggested that these findings indicated a limited impact of patents on access. The study also found, however, that over half of the 53 African countries had patents on zidovudine and nevirapine, the two most commonly used drugs in combination treatments in developing countries, suggesting an important impact of patents for certain products in some countries (Boelaert *et al.*, 2002).

This study, designed to assess the impact of patents on the availability of AIDS drugs in Africa, generated significant controversy. On the one hand, the study supported the idea that pharmaceutical companies typically file for patents in countries where they expect significant sales. But the results also showed that some companies filed for patent protection in African countries where significant economic returns were unlikely (UNDP, 2001, p. 107). For example, one company (GlaxoSmithKline) filed for patents for two products in 33 and 37 African countries, including many that are unlikely to show significant sales volumes (such as Burundi, Comoros, Madagascar, and Rwanda). This finding suggests that other factors (in addition to expected markets and sales) can affect a company's decision to file for product patents in specific countries.

More generally, the impact of patents relates to the demand for medicines. In the developed world, strict patent protection does not affect demand or consumption because most consumers do not face the full cost of the drug (due to insurance coverage). In developing countries, most consumers must pay the cost of treatment out of pocket and therefore are not insulated from the costs of medicines. Inadequate health systems, lack of insurance and low wage rates exacerbate the impact of patents (through high prices) on access to treatment.

In developing countries where a significant national pharmaceutical industry exists (such as South Africa and Brazil, where local companies can produce some active ingredients) and a national patent system exists, patents can pose (and arguably did pose) an obstacle to access for ARVs through high prices. In those countries, the patent system prevents the production of patented ARVs as generic drugs. In such situations, countries have three options that comply with international trade law. First, they can manufacture AIDS drugs that were introduced *before* the start of product patent protection – as Brazil did for products before 1995 (when Brazil implemented product patents). Second, they can pressure companies to reduce their prices – again, as Brazil did through threats of compulsory licensing. Or third, countries can pass national legislation or declare a public health emergency in order to produce (or import) the drugs under a compulsory licensing system.

The application of trade strategies (like compulsory licensing and parallel imports) to expand access to ARVs generated a number of international conflicts. Developed countries (especially the United States) have threatened to cut foreign direct investment or retaliate in other ways if developing countries neglect or dilute patent protection (UNDP, 2001, p. 107). For example, the United States placed India, Thailand, and South Africa on the US Trade Representative's Special 301 Watch List in May 1998, because of the lack of adequate intellectual property protection. For South Africa, the United States objected to a 1997 amendment to the Medicines and Related Substances Act that appeared to allow the South African Minister of Health to revoke patent rights, in allowing for parallel imports, compulsory licensing, and registration of generic drugs (United States Trade Representative, 2000, p. 371).

Approaches for Expanding Access to Medicines for HIV/AIDS

Five broad approaches can be considered for expanding access to ARVs in developing countries: market-based approaches, differential pricing, trade policy-based approaches, bulk purchasing, and donations. The sustainability of each strategy depends not only on the affordability of the medicines but also on the ability to maintain incentives for future research and development by the pharmaceutical industry. Some of these approaches are being implemented, while others represent proposals that could be adopted. We briefly review each approach's advantages and disadvantages.

Market-based Approach

In a market-based approach, prices are set by companies, either through independent company decisions (as occurs mostly in the United States) or through negotiated agreements for each drug with governments and insurance providers. Governments can then purchase ARVs and other AIDS drugs according to their national priorities for AIDS and their health budgets. Brazil, for example, followed a market-based approach (by purchasing some products on international markets) but combined this with a trade policy-based approach (of threats to use compulsory licensing) along with external financing from World Bank loans and local production of certain AIDS medicines. A variation on a market-based approach is to support the creation of a global market for raw materials, which are then formulated into final products by local manufacturers. The WTO's 2003 interpretation of the Doha Declaration in effect allows the development of an international market of generics for the world's poorest countries through compulsory licensing mechanisms.

The primary disadvantage of this approach is that global inequities in drug access could continue for poor countries due to their limited capacity to negotiate with international companies and their limited budgets for AIDS care and treatment. The situation could change if companies continued to offer steep discounts in drug prices (for future as well as current products), if compulsory licensing through imports becomes feasible administratively, and if the Global Fund and donor governments offer adequate financing for AIDS-affected countries to procure ARVs . Though progress has been made, and the current price discounts have produced an expansion in access to AIDS medicines in developing countries, huge gaps remain.

Michael R Reich and Priya Bery

Differential Pricing

Differential pricing is a pricing system in which a significantly lower manufacturer's selling price is established according to a country's socioeconomic status (WHO and WTO, 2001). More generally, companies often charge different prices in different markets based on how much the market will bear. This method could also serve as a strategy for companies to maximize profits by increasing sales in each market and in previously inaccessible markets (Sherer and Watal, 2001). This method can also be used to set prices based on ability to pay in resource-poor settings, in order to expand access – and in those instances, it is sometimes called 'equitable pricing' (Grace, 2003).

For this pricing system to be sustainable, however, shipments between national markets would need to be prevented, so that products offered at lower prices in poor countries would not be resold in rich countries. This system can require a high level of cooperation among governments and patent holders, to assure that appropriate regulations and safeguards are effectively implemented. In countries with well-established drug regulatory systems, such as the OECD countries, this movement of products can be effectively controlled.

Price differentials can also have important political ramifications, as shown by US senior citizens who travel to Canada and Mexico to purchase cheaper drugs, and by the current policy debate over prescription drug prices in the United States (Ulik, 2003).

Differential pricing is often opposed by producers, but it can bring them some benefits by providing entry to new markets, expanding the volume of sales, and producing higher profits if priced above marginal cost. An important question is how prices would be set in a differential pricing system. Three options are:

1. *Internal company policy*: In this method, each company decides on its own criteria for price differentials. For example, Merck established a company policy to discount their ARV prices based on the UNDP's Human Development Index (HDI) and the level of AIDS incidence in each country (J Sturchio, personal communication, 2001). (The UNDP's HDI is a composite single-number ranking of countries based on life expectancy at birth, level of education and income per capita.)
2. *International-agency-facilitated price negotiations*: In this method, an international agency facilitates price negotiations for each country and each company. For example, UN agencies are working with six pharmaceutical companies on the Accelerating Access Initiative to secure reduced drug prices at the country level (UNAIDS, 2001). (Implementation of these agreements, however, has been slow and so far only a limited number of patients have received treatment.) Within such programs, companies have avoided joint discussions and decisions on price differentials, because such discussions can be illegal under anti-trust law (UNAIDS, 2000a).

3. *Distribution of price information*: Distributing information about prices of high-quality AIDS medicines available in the international market can help correct information asymmetries and assist buyers in their procurement negotiations. For example, the WHO, UNICEF, UNAIDS, and MSF have produced a price list to provide market information about drugs used in the treatment and care of HIV/AIDS (WHO *et al.*, 2003).

Increasingly, civil society groups, international non-governmental organizations (NGOs), and the business sector are engaging in independent negotiations with pharmaceutical companies as shown by the efforts of MSF, the Clinton Foundation, and Anglo American, among others. This experience can also help inform various parties (including governments, Global Fund country coordinating mechanisms, NGOs, and private companies) about the range of pricing options for specific AIDS medicines.

Trade Policy-based Approaches

A third strategy is to use international trade agreements plus national pharmaceutical policies to expand access to AIDS medicines – through the promotion of voluntary license agreements, the purchase of generic drugs, and the development of differential patent systems.

1. *Voluntary license agreements*: This method permits individual companies or patent holders to license their patented technologies (both products and processes) to firms in developing countries (Friedman *et al.*, 2003). These license agreements can allow local firms to produce the same drug at lower cost and thereby sell the product at a lower price. This option allows the patent holder to maintain property rights in certain markets and may require payment of royalties to the patent holder. GlaxoSmithKline, for example, decided to issue a voluntary license for Combivir to a South African generics manufacturer and then waived its rights to royalties (Reuters, 2001). In exchange, the South African company agreed to pay 30 per cent of net sales to a local NGO working on HIV/AIDS.
2. *Compulsory licensing*: Under the TRIPS Agreement, a country can administratively decide to use compulsory licensing and allow the importation or local production of drugs in a public health emergency, in order to obtain lower prices without permission of the patent holder. Such agreements, while legal, can result in legal disputes between the patent holder and user and can cause conflicts between the developing country government and patent holders or their governments. Under TRIPS, compensation must be paid to the patent holder, although the amount is set by the national courts. As noted above, several developing countries have recently issued a compulsory license for AIDS medicines, and other countries have threatened to do so.

3. *Differential patent system*: In this proposal, patent holders would be encouraged to patent drugs only in countries where they believed there was a substantial market. This approach could emerge through voluntary decisions by patent holders or regulated through international agreements and governing bodies. One proposal encourages patent holders to protect property rights in rich countries or in poor countries, but not both (Lanjouw, 2001). This would provide companies with patent protection in developed country markets (where they have the vast majority of sales and profits) and would cede developing country markets (where they have limited sales and profits) to low-cost producers.

Bulk Purchasing

Bulk purchasing allows for collaborative pharmaceutical procurement among countries with similar needs. Purchases are pooled at a national level, thereby expanding demand for the product and increasing the negotiating capacity of purchasers. This approach carries the potential for drug expenditure savings and improved procurement practices and could be applied on a regional or a global level. Pooled purchasing could simplify procurement for pharmaceutical manufacturers, but holds the risk of creating distortions due to monopsony (when there is only one buyer in a market). This mechanism also brings the added difficulty of coordinating an already complicated procurement process across countries. Pharmaceutical companies do not generally consider this approach an attractive option.

One example of global bulk purchasing is the Global Drug Facility for TB drugs, which was established in March 2001. This organization has achieved a reduction in drug prices of 30 per cent, pushing the cost of a six-month course of treatment to about US$10. The strategies have included a standardized set of drug products, a bulk-buying procurement system, and competitive bidding processes. In the first two rounds of applications, 12 countries were approved for support from the Global Drug Facility (Global Drug Facility, 2001).

A similar approach has been proposed for AIDS medicines through the Global Fund to Fight AIDS, Tuberculosis and Malaria. For example, a central procurement and distribution agency could help secure low prices for AIDS medicines through bulk purchasing agreements and could assure that recipients adopt integrated treatment and prevention regimens. Due to the challenges of bulk purchasing, the Global Fund currently supports procurement at the national level through bilateral agreements between governments and manufacturers.

Donations

Donations provide access to medicines through contributions from governments, NGOs, foundations, and corporations. A number of public–private partnerships have been established to expand access to AIDS medicines (IFPMA, 2001). These programs include Boehringer-Ingelheim's donation of Viramune (nevirapine) for prevention of mother-to-child transmission of HIV in developing countries (Viramune Donation Programme, 2002), and the donation by Pfizer Inc. (decided after repeated protests by AIDS activists) of the antifungal Diflucan (fluconazole) for treatment of opportunistic infections (cryptococcal meningitis and esophageal candidiasis) in 12 African countries and Haiti (and more countries over time). In Botswana, Merck & Co. is working with the Bill and Melinda Gates Foundation and Government of Botswana to support the African Comprehensive HIV/AIDS Partnerships (ACHAP). Merck decided to invest US$50 million over five years (along with US$50 million from the Gates Foundation) and is providing Crixivan (indinavir) and Stocrin (efevirnez) for the duration of the program.

Other pharmaceutical companies have made financial and product donations of various scales and in different geographic locations. Because donations are voluntary, these programs differ in their levels and duration of commitment. Whether significant donations of other AIDS medicines will occur in the future is uncertain. Some activists have opposed donation programs, because of questions about the continuity of supply for the long term and concerns that corporate donations are decided primarily for marketing reasons or tax benefits. They also argue that donations cannot provide a systemic solution to the great need for AIDS medicines in developing countries. Pharmaceutical company executives have disputed the charges about sustainability, marketing, and taxes; they have also responded that while donations cannot solve many of the problems of access, donations can make a positive contribution (Hardwick, 2001).

What the Future Holds

This chapter shows how the world made important progress in addressing the challenges that prices and patents posed to expanding global access to AIDS medicines. It demonstrates how major obstacles were recognized and removed through a contentious and iterative political process. The international regime of intellectual property rights was re-interpreted and re-negotiated to reduce its protection of high prices and its restrictions on generic production and exports. Research-based pharmaceutical companies and the international AIDS community altered standard business practices and pricing strategies in order to increase access to ARVs in the world's poorest countries. Prices for ARVs dropped precipitously in the developing world – in ways that few people expected. Pushed by activists, private companies and public agencies created a new potential for expanded global access to ARVs. Whether that potential will be achieved in practice remains to be seen; for millions around the world it is a case of too little too

Table 13.2   Seven key issues to be addressed in scaling-up access to ARVs.

1. Financing	Even at low prices, governments in developing countries lack sufficient funds
2. Procurement	Developing countries lack adequate procurement mechanisms for AIDS medicines
3. Infrastructure	Developing countries lack adequate health infrastructure in the public sector
4. Stigma and discrimination	Stigma and discrimination remain barriers to effective prevention, testing and treatment programs
5. Testing and diagnostics	There are a lack of testing facilities and low-cost diagnostics to support use of ARVs
6. Treatment protocols	The complexity of caring for AIDS patients remains a challenge
7. Operational experience	There is a lack of operational experience on the use of ARVs under field conditions

late. Cycles of price reduction will also be critical for new classes of ARVs, such as integrase inhibitors currently priced at US$20 000 per patient per year.

Political pressure from many sources helped achieve these changes. Activist pressure on drug pricing and corporate images had a major impact. Indeed, one could persuasively argue that activist pressures shaped and pushed the policy agenda in ways that multinational companies never anticipated (and did not desire). But other pressures also contributed, especially the emerging competition from generic producers in Brazil and India along with a growing recognition inside pharmaceutical companies of their global social responsibilities (Roberts *et al.*, 2002).

But even with greatly reduced drug prices and a stronger global generic market, AIDS medicines remain out of reach for the majority of people in most developing countries. The dramatic decline in prices has highlighted persistent problems in the purchasing, procurement and distribution systems. These difficult problems, not directly related to drug cost, must be addressed to achieve equitable and sustained access to AIDS treatment in the world's poorest countries. The WHO's '3 by 5' Initiative is currently developing comprehensive plans for the components related to scaling-up access to ARVs. We have identified seven key issues that require attention (Table 13.2).

1. Financing

Governments lack adequate funds to purchase and deliver ARVs, even at low prices. Current prices offered in developing countries to treat one patient for a year are still much higher than the annual per capita GDP of many of the hardest hit countries (UNAIDS/WHO, 2003). The development of long-term financing for AIDS treatment in developing countries remains a critical global priority. Developing country governments need to give higher priority to HIV/AIDS and mobilize existing and new resources to support national AIDS control strategies. Donor governments must also show more leadership to support responses to the epidemic through bilateral contributions and donations to international efforts such as the Global Fund to Fight AIDS, Tuberculosis and Malaria.

2. Procurement

Adequate mechanisms for ARV procurement do not currently exist. At present, each country is responsible for negotiating directly with individual companies on prices and conditions of procurement. This fragmented, market-based approach puts developing countries at disadvantage, because of limited information and market share. Initially, this approach was deliberately favored, as each national negotiation contributed to a further decline of prices. The situation is now different, because it is unlikely that prices will decline much further.

3. Infrastructure

The health infrastructure in many developing countries is inadequate to distribute and deliver ARVs safely and effectively to a significant portion of the infected population. In many poor countries, essential medicines do not reach people who need them, due to problems in financing, procurement, management, and delivery. Health centers and hospitals often lack adequate supplies of basic medicines, including antibiotics, antimalarials, and aspirin. Appropriate protocols for delivering ARVs will need to be designed and implemented in order to prevent the development of resistance. On the other hand, the business sector in developing countries often has private health facilities for employees and families and could play an important role in expanding access to treatment. To deliver ARVs in an effective and sustained way will require countries to improve the performance and equity of their health systems (Roberts *et al.*, 2004).

4. Stigma and Discrimination

Stigma and discrimination associated with HIV/AIDS are among the greatest barriers to the prevention of new infections and to expanded access to care, support, and treatment services that allow people living with HIV/AIDS to lead productive lives. Availability of treatment can help break down the stigma associated with people living with HIV/AIDS and encourage people to get tested and know their status. A number of existing ARV treatment programs report a low uptake of available services – commonly attributed to stigma associated with the epidemic, potential discrimination from lack of confidentiality, lack of support services, and high cost of diagnostics. Stigma and discrimination should be addressed as part of any comprehensive ARV treatment program.

5. Testing and Availability of Diagnostics

The fight for increased access to ARVs has highlighted the need for appropriate and cost-effective diagnostic support. Prior to the provision of antiretroviral therapy, individuals must be tested for HIV and have access to low-cost monitoring services to determine when they are ready for treatment. Over the years there has been an increase in the availability of a varied range of diagnostics to support voluntary counseling and testing, but over 90 per cent of individuals living with HIV do not know their serostatus. New diagnostics are easy to use and require minimal investment in infrastructure and training beyond mechanisms to ensure confidentiality and adequate counseling to support client needs. Improved diagnostic support is also essential to monitor the progression of the disease when on or off ARV therapy.

6. Treatment Protocols

Even if ARVs and other drugs were made available, major barriers remain to their effective use. Selecting which patients to treat and when in the disease progression will remain difficult decisions with important ethical implications (Daniels, 2004). Deciding on the optimum treatment regimens will be challenging, given the dearth of clinical trials and experience in developing countries. Ensuring compliance and monitoring the effects of treatment and drug resistance will be problematic, because of the general lack of sophisticated monitoring tests (CD4 counts and viral load). In addition, we cannot predict the effects on the health system of treating large numbers of AIDS patients for long periods of time. Treatment for HIV/AIDS also needs to be designed and implemented not as a stand-alone program but as part of a comprehensive prevention and care program. Treatment can serve as an entry point to assure these other components are in place to sustain broader care and support programs.

7. Operational Experience

An important obstacle to expanded access to AIDS medicines is the lack of operational experience on how to use ARVs under field conditions in poor countries.

Even if the medicines were made available for free (either through donations or external financing), we need guidelines on how to use them. Recent experiences in Botswana may help provide some answers about best practices in the African context. In particular, we need to understand how to deliver AIDS treatment in the private sector – including mission hospitals, employer facilities, and private practitioners – where quality of services tends to be higher than in public facilities. In order to assure that expanded access does more good than harm, there is a need for increased capacity and training of medical professionals and more systematic evidence about what works and what does not in providing AIDS treatment in the least developed countries.

These seven challenges continue to delay access to ARVs (and other AIDS drugs) for the majority of HIV-infected people in most developing countries. Proposals that seek to expand access to AIDS medicines will need to resolve these problems, and also address issues related to the allocation of resources for competing health and development problems. The international AIDS community grappled with the problems of pricing and patents, and produced several mechanisms that have greatly reduced the obstacles to access. Similar efforts will be needed for the remaining problems noted above, in order to assure expanded global access to effective AIDS medicines for the majority of affected people who live in the world's poorest countries.

Acknowledgments

The authors appreciate the helpful comments on earlier drafts from: Scott Gordon, Sofia Gruskin, Neeraj Mistry, Vinand Nantulya, Erica Seiguer, Jane Silver, Daniel Tarantola, and David Winickoff. An earlier version of this chapter was prepared as a policy brief with financial support from AmFAR (American Foundation for AIDS Research).

References

Associated Press (2003) Brazil to build AIDS drug factory in Mozambique. 5 November. http://www.aegis.com/news/ap/2003/AP031107.html

Attaran A, Gillespie-White L (2001) Do patents constrain access to AIDS treatment in poor countries? Antiretroviral drugs in Africa. *JAMA* 286: 1886–92.

Boelaert M, Lynen L, Van Damme W, Colebunders R (2002) Do patents prevent access to drugs for HIV in developing countries? Letter. *JAMA* 287: 840–1.

Caldwell JC (2000) Rethinking the African AIDS epidemic. *Population Dev Rev* 26: 117–35.

Commission on Intellectual Property Rights (2002) *Integrating Intellectual Property Rights and Development Policy*. London: Commission on Intellectual Property Rights, September.

Daniels N (2004) How to achieve fair distribution of ARTs in 3 × 5: Fair process and legitimacy in patient selection. Background paper for WHO/UNAIDS Consultation on Equitable Access to Care for HIV/AIDS, Geneva, 26–27 January.

Danzon P (2000) Making sense of drug prices. *Regulation* 23: 56–63.

Danzon PM, Kim JD (1998) International price comparisons for pharmaceuticals: Measurement and policy issues. *Pharmacoeconomics* 14 (Suppl): 115–28.

DiMasi JA, Hansen RW, Grabowski HG (2003) The price of innovation: New estimates of drug development costs. *J Health Econ* 22: 151–85.

Editorial (2002) Europe's addiction. *Wall Street Journal* 2 January.

Freedberg K, Losina E, Weinstein MC *et al.* (2001) The cost effectiveness of combination antiretroviral therapy for HIV disease. *N Engl J Med* 344: 824–31.

Friedman MA, den Bensten H, Attaran A (2003) Out-licensing: a practical approach for improvement of access to medicines in poor countries. *Lancet* 361: 341–4.

Gilbert J, Rosenberg P (2004) *Imbalanced Innovation.* Presented at the World Economic Forum at Davos. Boston, MA: Bain & Company. http://www.bain.com/bainweb/PDFs/cms/Marketing/addressing_innovation_divide.pdf (accessed 7 March 2004).

Global Business Coalition on HIV/AIDS (2003) Nine major companies commit to co-investment to expand community HIV/AIDS programs using corporate infrastructure. GBC, New York, 3 December. http://www.businessfightsaids.org/news_read.asp?sct=2&ID=9202&PR=1

Global Drug Facility (2001) GDF Factsheet. http://www.stoptb.org/GDF/whatis/docs (accessed 3 March 2002).

Grabowski G (2002) Patents, innovation and access to new pharmaceuticals. *Int Econ Law* 5: 849–60.

Grace C (2003) *Equitable Pricing of Newer Essential Medicines for Developing Countries: Evidence for the Potential of Different Medicines.* London: Department for International Development, and Geneva: World Health Organization. http://www.who.int/medicines/library/par/equitable_pricing.doc

Hardwick C (2001) Access to medicines in the developing world through partnerships. Background paper for the WHO/WTO Workshop on Differential Pricing and Financing of Essential Drugs. Høsbjør, Norway, 10 April.

IMS Health (2002) Projected global pharmaceutical market by year 2002. http://www.ims-global.com/insight/report/global/report.htm

IFPMA (International Federation of Pharmaceutical Manufacturers Associations) (2001) *Public/Private Partnerships: Industry Contributions to Improving Access to Medicines in the Developing World.* Geneva: IFPMA. http://www.ifpma.org/PPPs.htm (accessed 11 February 2002).

IFPMA (2003) *Expanded Access to AIDS Medicines: Initiatives of the R&D-Based Pharmaceutical Industry.* Geneva: IFPMA.

IFPMA (2004) Position statement on intellectual property and patents. http://www.ifpma.org/Issues/issues_intell.aspx (accessed 15 February 2004).

Lanjouw JO (2001) *A Patent Policy Proposal For Global Disease.* Policy Brief no. 84. Washington DC: The Brookings Institution.

Lanjouw JO (2003) *Intellectual Property and the Availability of Pharmaceuticals in Poor Countries. Innovation Policy and the Economy.* MIT Press 3: 91–130.

Lei no 9.313.996, Aceso Universal a Terapia Anti-Retroviral no Sistema Publica de Saude.

McNeil D (2001) Indian company offers to supply AIDS drugs at low cost in Africa. *New York Times,* 7 February.

Médecins Sans Frontières (2003) *Untangling the Web of Price Reductions.* www.accessmed-msf.org (accessed May 2003).

Mocroft A, Vella S, Benfield TL *et al.* (1998) Changing patterns of mortality across Europe in patients with HIV-1. *Lancet* 352: 1725–30.

Okero FA, Aceng E, Madraa E *et al.* (2003) *Scaling Up Antiretroviral Therapy: Experience in Uganda: Case Study*. Geneva: World Health Organization.

Palella FJ, Delaney KM, Moorman AC *et al.* (1998) Declining morbidity and mortality among patients with advanced human immunodeficiency virus infection. *N Engl J Med* 338: 853–60.

Park RS (2002) The international drug industry: What the future holds for South Africa's HIV/AIDS patients. *Minnesota J Global Trade* 11: 125–54.

PhRMA (Pharmaceutical Research Manufacturers Association) (2003) Industry Profile 2003. http://www.phrma.org/publications/publications/profile02/index.cfm

Quick J (2001) Ensuring access to essential drugs – framework for action. Presentation at the WHO/WTO Workshop on Differential Pricing and Financing of Essential Drugs. Høsbjør, Norway, 8–11 April.

Rapp T, Rozek R (1990) Benefits and costs of intellectual property protection in developing countries. *J World Trade* 24: 75–102.

Reich MR (1990) Why the Japanese don't export more pharmaceuticals: Health policy as industrial policy. *Calif Manage Rev* 32: 124–50.

Reuters (2001) GlaxoSmithKline Gives AIDS Drug Rights to Generic Maker. *New York Times* 9 October, p. C-4.

Rich JL, Petersen M (2001) Brazil will defy patent on AIDS drug made by Roche. *New York Times* 23 August.

Roberts MJ, Breitenstein AG, Roberts CS (2002) The ethics of public–private partnerships. In: Reich MR, ed. *Public–Private Partnerships for Public Health*. Cambridge, MA: Harvard Center for Population and Development Studies, distributed by Harvard University Press, pp. 67–85.

Roberts MJ, Hsiao W, Berman P, Reich MR (2004) *Getting Health Reform Right: A Guide to Improving Performance and Equity*. New York: Oxford University Press.

Rose DN (1998) AIDS drug regimens that are worth their costs. *JAMA* 279: 160–1.

Rosenberg T (2001) Look at Brazil. *New York Times Magazine* 28 January, p. 26.

Schoofs M (2003) Clinton program would help poor nations get AIDS drugs. *Wall Street Journal* 23 October.

Sherer FM, Watal J (2001) Post-TRIPS options for access to patented medicines in developing countries. *CMH Working Paper Series*, No. WG 4: 1, June.

Sidley P (2001) Drug companies withdraw law suit against South Africa. *BMJ* 322: 1011.

Teixeira PR, Vitória MA, Barcarolo J (2003) The Brazilian experience in providing universal access to antiretroviral therapy. In: *Economics of AIDS and Access to HIV/AIDS Care in Developing Countries: Issues and Challenges*. Paris: ANRS, Collection Sciences Sociales et Sida, pp. 69–88.

Ulik J (2003) Canada drug crackdown – buying cheap drugs north of the border may become more difficult. *CNN Money* 13 March. http://money.cnn.com/2003/03/13/news/drugs_canada

UNAIDS (2000a) *Accelerating Access to HIV/AIDS Care and Treatment in Developing Countries: A Joint Statement of Intent*. Final Draft. Geneva: UNAIDS, 8 May.

UNAIDS (2000b) *Report on the Global Epidemic: Care and Support for People Living with HIV/AIDS*. Geneva: UNAIDS, June.

UNAIDS (2000c) *Report on the Global Epidemic: Table of Country-specific HIV/AIDS Estimates*. Geneva: UNAIDS, June. http://www.unaids.org/epidemic_update/report/index

UNAIDS (2001) *Accelerating Access to HIV/AIDS Care, Treatment and Support*. Progress Report Updated November 2001. Geneva: UNAIDS. http://www.unaids.org/acc_access/Aaprogress1101.doc

UNAIDS/WHO (2003) *AIDS Epidemic Update: 2003.* Geneva: UNAIDS/WHO, December (UNAIDS/03.39E).

UNDP (United Nations Development Programme) (2001) *Human Development Report 2001: Making New Technologies Work for Human Development.* New York: UNDP.

UNICEF-UNAIDS Secretariat, WHO/HTP, and MSF (2001) *Sources and Prices of Selected Drugs and Diagnostics for People Living with HIV/AIDS.* Geneva, May.

United States Trade Representative (2000) *Foreign Barriers to Trade.* Washington, DC: USTR, March. www.ustr.gov/pdf/nte2000.pdf

van der Vijver DAMC *et al.* (2003) Analysis of more than 1600 newly diagnosed patients with HIV from 17 European countries shows that 10 per cent of the patients carry primary drug resistance: The CATCH study. Second International AIDS Society Conference, Paris, France, late breaker 1. Program and abstracts of the 2nd IAS Conference on HIV Pathogenesis and Treatment. Abstract LB1. 13–16 July.

Viramune Donation Programme (2002) http://www.viramune-donation-program.org (accessed 11 February 2002).

World Bank (2000) *World Development Indicators 2000.* Washington, DC: World Bank, figure 2.14.

World Bank (2003) Brazil: World Bank approves US$100 million for HIV/AIDS and STD control. News release no. 2003/406/LAC. Washington, DC: World Bank. 27 June.

WHO (World Health Organization) (1998) *Health Reform and Drug Financing: Selected Topics.* Geneva: WHO (WHO/DAP/98.3).

WHO (2001) *Globalisation, TRIPS and Access to Pharmaceuticals.* WHO Policy Perspectives on Medicines No. 3. Geneva: WHO.

WHO (2002) *Accelerating Access Initiative. Progress Report.* Geneva: WHO, June. http://www.who.int/hiv/pub/prev_care/isbn9241210125.pdf

WHO (2003) *Treating 3 Million by 2005: Making it Happen, The WHO Strategy.* Geneva: WHO and UNAIDS.

WHO, UNICEF, UNAIDS, and MSF (2003) *Sources and Prices of Selected Medicines and Diagnostics for People Living with HIV/AIDS.* Geneva: WHO, June. http://www.who.int/medicines/organization/par/ipc/sources-prices.pdf

WHO and WTO Secretariats (2001) *Report of the Workshop on Differential Pricing and Financing of Essential Drugs.* Oslo: Norwegian Foreign Affairs Ministry, Global Health Council, 8–11 April.

WTO (World Trade Organization) (2001a) *Doha Declaration on the TRIPS Agreement and Public Health.* WTO Doc. WT/MIN(01)/DEC/2, 20 November. Geneva: WTO. http://www.wto.org/english/thewto_e/minist_e/min01_e/mindecl_trips_e.htm

WTO (2001b) *TRIPS and Pharmaceutical Patents: Fact Sheet.* Geneva: WTO, April. http://www.wto.org/wto/english/tratop_e/trips/factsheet_pharm00_e.html

WTO (2003a) *Decision Removes Final Patent Obstacle to Cheap Drug Imports.* Press Release 350/Rev. 1. Geneva: WTO, 30 August.

WTO (2003b) *Implementation of Paragraph 6 of the Doha Declaration on the TRIPS Agreement and Public Health.* General Council Decision of 30 August 2003 (WT/L/540).

Young B, Surrusco M. (2001) *Rx R&D Myths: The Case Against the Drug Industry's R&D Scare Card.* Washington, DC: Public Citizen, July. http://www.citizen.org/documents/ACFDC.PDF

The African Experience 14

Salim S Abdool Karim

Deputy Vice Chancellor, University of Natal, South Africa.
Director, Centre for the AIDS Programme of Research in
South Africa (CAPRISA).

Salim S. Abdool Karim, MD, PhD is Deputy Vice-Chancellor for Research at the University of KwaZulu-Natal, Durban, South Africa, Professor of Clinical Epidemiology at Columbia University in New York, Adjunct Professor of Medicine at Cornell University, New York, and Director of CAPRISA (Centre for the AIDS Programme of Research in South Africa). Dr. Abdool Karim received his medical degree and PhD from the University of Natal, as well as degrees in Epidemiology from Columbia University, New York and in Public Health from the South Africa College of Medicine. In addition to his numerous awards and published papers, he serves on the Editorial Board of the Southern African Journal of HIV Medicine and Sexually Transmitted Disease, is Corresponding Editor of the International Journal of Infectious Diseases and is Associate Editor of AIDS Clinical Care.

Let us combine our efforts to ensure a future for our children. The challenge is no less.
Nelson Mandela – closing speech at the XIIIth international AIDS Conference, Durban, 14 July 2000

Soon after my arrival back from the United States in 1989 after being trained as an epidemiologist, I was inspired by the release of Mandela and the prospect of freedom and the need to address our country's greatest challenge – to build the new democratic South Africa. Having played an active role as an anti-apartheid activist, this was a dream come true. However, it was clear to me that this dream may be in jeopardy if AIDS was not dealt with adequately. This led to the first AIDS studies that I conducted in the early 1990s jointly with my wife, Quarraisha Abdool Karim, who was later to become the first National Director of the Government AIDS Control Programme in 1994 in the new democratic South Africa.

More than two decades later the AIDS epidemic has become a tragic reality and Africa is by far the worst AIDS affected region of the world, with eastern and

351

southern Africa in general more severely affected than western and northern Africa. The HIV/AIDS epidemic started tangibly in Africa in the late 1970s and early 1980s (Serwadda *et al.*, 1985), though some believe that HIV originated in Africa several decades before this. Heterosexual transmission is the predominant mode of spread of HIV infection throughout Africa, and with it, the concomitant HIV epidemic in newborns and young children through perinatal transmission. Homosexual transmission, intravenous drug use, unsafe injection practices and unsafe transfusions account for a small fraction of HIV infections in Africa.

By the end of 2001, the estimated total number of people infected with HIV in sub-Saharan Africa reached 29.4 million – over 70 per cent of the world's HIV infected population (UNAIDS/WHO, 2002). The average adult prevalence rate in Africa is 8.8 per cent, and 16 countries have infection rates exceeding 10 per cent (UNAIDS, 2001a). Approximately 3.5 million new infections occurred in Africa in 2002. An estimated 11.8 million young people (aged 15–24) and almost 3 million children under 15 are living with HIV (UNAIDS, 2002). Twenty per cent more African women than men are living with HIV.

So far, the AIDS epidemic in Africa has created 14 million orphans and it is predicted that the number will increase to 40 million by 2010 (UNAIDS, 2001b). Providing them with food, housing and education will test the resources and resolve of countries for many years to come.

The majority of deaths worldwide due to AIDS have been in sub-Saharan Africa, current statistics show that over 17 million Africans have died since the AIDS epidemic began in the late 1970s and more than 3.3 million of them were children (AIDS in Africa, 2003). An estimated 2.4 million Africans died due to AIDS in the past year and it is estimated that approximately 5500 funerals due to AIDS are held each day in Africa (Los Altos Rotary Club, 2003).

Sub-Saharan Africa is also home to roughly 90 per cent of the 800 000 infants who contract AIDS from their mothers before or during birth or as a result of breastfeeding, although this percentage is slowly declining as epidemics mature in other regions (UNAIDS, 2001a; UNAIDS/WHO, 2002). In some African countries, around 25 per cent of the pregnant women are infected with HIV.

The AIDS epidemic is devastating the most productive sector of the population by affecting young people in the prime of their lives, which is leading to dramatic changes in the projected age structure of the entire sub-Saharan region (UNAIDS/WHO, 2002). Life expectancy has been greatly diminished, dropping by 21 years from age 68 to 47, and in some parts of Africa life expectancy has halved to 34 years.

How Different Countries in Africa are Affected

Large variations in the presentation of the HIV/AIDS epidemic exist between individual countries in Africa (Figure 14.1, Table 14.1). In Somalia and Gambia the prevalence is under 2 per cent, whereas the national adult HIV prevalence rate in

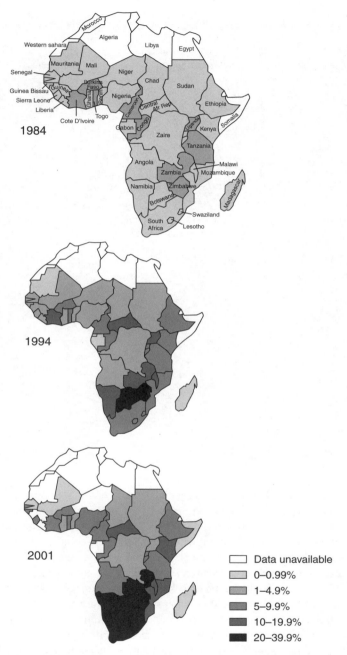

Fig. 14.1 The evolving AIDS epidemic in Africa. Source: UNAIDS/WHO (2002).

Table 14.1   Country-specific HIV/AIDS estimates for Adults 15–49 in Africa (2001).

Country	HIV prevalence (%)	HIV infections	Country	HIV prevalence (%)	HIV infections
Angola	5.5	317 185	Lesotho	31	305 040
Benin	3.6	105 444	Liberia	–	–
Botswana	38.8	295 656	Madagascar	0.3	22 614
Burkina Faso	6.5	327 990	Malawi	15	767 700
Burundi	8.3	239 621	Mali	1.7	86 632
Cameroon	11.8	833 670	Mauritania	–	–
Central African Rep.	12.9	222 138	Mauritius	0.1	667
			Mozambique	13	1 106 430
Chad	3.6	128 520	Namibia	22.5	184 500
Comoros	–	–	Niger	–	–
Congo	7.2	98 208	Nigeria	5.8	3 094 068
Côte d'Ivoire	9.7	761 838	Rwanda	8.9	334 284
Dem. Rep. of Congo	4.9	1 081 577	Senegal	0.5	22 605
			Sierra Leone	7	146 510
Djibouti	–	–	Somalia	1	40 150
Equatorial Guinea	3.4	7 174	South Africa	20.1	4 756 866
Eritrea	2.8	49 280	Swaziland	33.4	150 300
Ethiopia	6.4	1 852 928	Togo	6	129 120
Gabon	–	–	Uganda	5	514 500
Gambia	1.6	10 352	Tanzania	7.8	1 302 678
Ghana	3	291 000	Zambia	21.5	1 019 100
Guinea	–	–	Zimbabwe	33.7	2 013
Guinea-Bissau	2.8	15 596			
Kenya	15	2 299 950			

Source: UNAIDS/WHO (2002).

some other African countries has exceeded 30 per cent. For example, the rate in Botswana is 38.8 per cent, in Lesotho 31.5 per cent, in Swaziland 33.4 per cent, and in Zimbabwe 33.7 per cent (UNAIDS/WHO, 2002). Contrary to previous projections, HIV infection levels continue to mount, and some countries face a growing danger of rapidly growing uncontrollable epidemics. In Cameroon, HIV prevalence among pregnant women doubled to over 11 per cent among those aged 20–24 between 1998 and 2000, illustrating how the epidemic can surge suddenly (UNAIDS, 2001a). In West and Central Africa, where epidemics are less severe, the rate of new infections appears to be increasing. In eight countries in West and Central Africa, adult HIV prevalence has now surpassed 5 per cent (UNAIDS, 2001a).

South Africa has been hit especially hard and is the country estimated to have the largest number of people (5.3 million HIV-positive people as at December

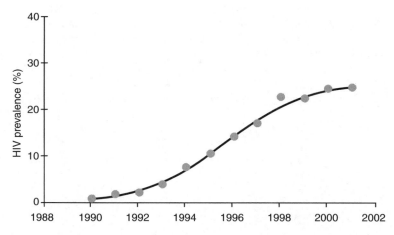

Fig. 14. 2   HIV prevalence from antenatal clinics in South Africa. Source: Gouws, 2005.

2002) living with HIV/AIDS (Figure 14.2). Every day in South Africa, an estimated 1700 people are newly infected with HIV (UNAIDS/WHO, 2002). Young
women are disproportionately affected and 60 per cent of all infected adults in
South Africa acquire their infection before age 25. It had been documented, as
early as 1992 (Abdool Karim and Abdool Karim, 1992), that adolescents (under
the age of 20 years) and young women in the early childbearing years (aged
20–24 years) had the highest rates of HIV infection, with HIV rates more than
four-fold higher among young girls than boys (Abdool Karim and Stein, 1999).
This pattern has continued. Throughout eastern and southern Africa, the prevalence of HIV in adolescent girls averages over five-fold higher than that in
teenage boys, and South Africa has been cited as the country with one of the
largest absolute ratios between girls and boys.

In South Africa, the rapid spread of HIV among adolescent girls and young
women has been described as explosive (Abdool Karim and Abdool Karim,
1999). In 1992, HIV prevalence in prenatal clinics in a rural sentinel district in
South Africa was estimated at 4.2 per cent. By 1995, HIV prevalence had increased
to 14.0 per cent and the highest prevalence was observed among young rural
women: 29.5 per cent within the 20–24 age group and 22.4 per cent within the
15–19 age group (Coleman and Wilkinson, 1997). In this same rural South
African district in 2001, HIV prevalence in prenatal clinics was 50.8 per cent in
the 20–24 year age group and 22.9 per cent in the 15–19 year age group. Temporal trends in age-specific prevalence and incidence rates of HIV infection in
prenatal clinics in this rural South African district are presented in Table 14.2 and
highlight the disturbingly high rates of new infection in young women under the
age of 25 years.

Table 14.2 Temporal trends in age-specific prevalence and incidence rates of HIV-1 infection in prenatal clinics in a rural South African district. Source: Gouws, 2005

Age group (years)	Prevalence (%)		Incidence (% pa)	
	1998	2001	1998	2001
15–19	21.1	22.9	10.0	8.9
20–24	39.3	50.8	14.6	12.1
25–29	36.4	47.2	11.5	10.2
30–34	23.4	38.4	7.4	7.4
35–39	23.0	36.4	4.5	5.1
40–44	12.3	26.7	2.6	3.5
Total	29.9	36.1	10.5	10.2

Finally, although both HIV-1 and HIV-2 occur in Africa, HIV-1 is by far the most common type yet in some parts of West Africa HIV-2 is more prevalent. HIV-2 is not transmitted as easily as HIV-1 and has contributed to a more regionalized distribution of the virus, which has become endemic in West Africa. HIV-2 is genetically more closely related to SIV than to HIV-1.

Risk Factors for HIV Infection in Africa

In sub-Saharan Africa the HIV-1 epidemic is now well established within the general population and virtually every segment of society is now affected by AIDS. The most important factors that have contributed and continue to contribute to severe HIV epidemics in sub-Saharan Africa include social and political instability, disruption of social support mechanisms and family structures, migrancy, high rates of other sexually transmitted infections (STIs), opportunistic infections, the subordinate position of women, and armed conflicts.

Population Migration

Truck drivers

Mobile populations have significantly influenced the spread of the HIV and this has been documented in several countries worldwide. Due to the migratory nature of their occupation, truck drivers often have multiple sexual partners. Towns located on main transportation routes throughout East Africa have high HIV prevalence rates relative to their surrounding rural areas and relative to national average HIV prevalence rates. Drivers often visit towns along the highway where there are restaurants, bars, lodges, and commercial sex workers (CSWs). CSWs, who are usually residents of the same towns, target the drivers as clients. These groups, besides transmitting HIV to each other, are also infecting regular partners, thereby significantly contributing to the spread of HIV and other STIs throughout sub-Saharan Africa as well as in other regions in the world (Marck, 1999).

In East Africa, the paving of the highway from Kinshasa in Zaire to Mombasa on the Indian Ocean may have helped to open the way for the HIV to spread. It is believed that up to 90 per cent of the CSWs working along the road who work in East Africa carry HIV. A study conducted at a weigh bridge 40 km east of Mombasa, Kenya in 1991–1992 showed that 26.1 per cent of 276 truck drivers were HIV-1 positive (Mbugua *et al.*, 1995).

In South Africa, a study done in 1998 to assess the HIV prevalence among truck drivers visiting sex workers along the national road linking the port city of Durban to the commercial heartland of Johannesburg, showed HIV prevalence among 320 truck drivers to be 56.3 per cent (95 per cent confidence interval (CI) 51–62 per cent) and very few (13 per cent) had used condoms during their last sexual encounter. Sixty per cent of the truck drivers reported having had an STI (discharge and ulcers) in the past six months and 83 per cent had received treatment. About 34 per cent always stopped for sex at the truck stops (Ramjee and Gouws, 2002).

All of the truck drivers from this study traveled to two or more provinces and 65 per cent traveled to neighboring countries such as Zimbabwe, Malawi, Mozambique, Zambia, Botswana, Namibia, Swaziland, and Angola.

Interviews with sex workers revealed that the men they had sex with came not only from South Africa but from other Southern African Development Community (SADC) countries such as Zimbabwe, Angola, Zambia, Mozambique, Botswana, Swaziland, and Namibia. Furthermore, the sex workers often travel with truck drivers to these countries, where they often have sex with other partners.

The high HIV prevalence and low condom use among truck drivers and sex workers, as well as the complex web of travel and sexual mixing, create a milieu that is conducive to the spread of HIV and other STIs (Ramjee and Gouws, 2002).

Migrant labor

Another large migrating population in South Africa is migrant laborers. Circular migration is fundamental to the way society is ordered in this part of sub-Saharan Africa and the migrant labor system in southern Africa that forces men to take jobs in distant cities to support their families, often keeping them away from their homes for extended periods, has been an important determinant of the spread of infectious diseases, and has contributed to the extraordinarily rapid spread of HIV (Lurie *et al.*, 1997; Lurie, 2000). Conjugal instability is a consequence of the migrant labor system and an urban/rural divide is created. Migrant populations create a market for commercial sex (Quinn, 1994) and high infection rates have been described in seasonal migrant workers (Lurie *et al.*, 2003). A survey in Carletonville, a gold mining area near Johannesburg, revealed that one-fifth of 88 000 miners were HIV positive, and 75 per cent of the almost 500 sex workers who serviced the miners were HIV positive. These circumstances place the partners of migrant workers in rural areas in a uniquely vulnerable situation for acquiring HIV.

Gender

In sub-Saharan Africa, women account for 58 per cent of all HIV infections, and infection rates among young women aged 15–24 are particularly important in influencing the epidemic curve for HIV in many countries. The growing disparity between male and female infection rates in Africa reflects the degree to which gender inequity is a major driving force in the epidemic in sub-Saharan Africa.

While young women and girls are probably more biologically prone to infection, this can only partially explain the large gender differences in HIV prevalence. Women and girls are commonly discriminated against in terms of access to education, employment, credit, health care, land, and inheritance. Many women, particularly those from impoverished backgrounds, see relationships with men (casual or formalized through marriage) as an opportunity for financial and social security.

Several studies have demonstrated that young women often form partnerships with older men who have some source of income and who are able to provide them with personal gifts and favors, as well as money for household necessities and school fees (Weiss and Gupta, 1998; Abdool Karim, 2001). Using a statistical simulation model that holds constant the ratio of male-to-female vs. female-to-male transmission probabilities, it has been shown (Garnett and Gregson, 2000) that the sex ratio of HIV prevalence increases as a function of women who have male partners 5–10 years older than themselves. These model predictions were confirmed using data from a population-based seroprevalence survey in rural Zimbabwe. Gregson *et al.* (2002) found that among sexually active respondents aged 17–24 years, older age of partner was a significant correlate of HIV infection.

Among young women who marry older men, their risk of infection increases if a husband is three or more years older than they are. The combination of dependence and subordination can make it very difficult for girls and women to demand safer sex (even from their husbands) or to end relationships that carry the threat of infection.

Youth

More than 40 per cent of people living with HIV/AIDS in sub-Saharan Africa are between the ages of 15 and 24, and young people account for more than half of all new infections in the region (UNAIDS, 2001b). Demographic and health surveys indicate that, on average, young people in the region begin having sex at an early age (average age of initiation is 13 years for boys, 14 for girls) and generally do not use condoms consistently. Early age of sexual initiation has been found to be associated with subsequent sexual behavior and risk of STIs, both in the USA (Greenberg *et al.*, 1992) and in Africa (Duncan *et al.*, 1990). In rural Zimbabwe, younger age of first sexual intercourse was associated with increased risk of HIV infection, while the mean age of first sexual intercourse was similar (18.5 years) for men and women (Gregson *et al.*, 2002). Moreover, very young girls are perceived as an 'HIV-free' group and are preferred as sexual partners by older men.

Sex Workers

Despite sex work being illegal in most African countries, desperate economic circumstances force many women to engage in commercial sex for survival in sub-Saharan Africa. This places them at risk of contracting HIV and transmitting the virus to their sex partners. Studies of sex workers at truck stops in South Africa between 1996 and 1999 found HIV prevalence was 50.3 per cent and an annual HIV incidence 20 per cent (Ramjee *et al.*, 1998), while in Harare, Zimbabwe, 86 per cent of sex workers were found to be living with HIV in 1994–1995.

Sexually Transmitted Infections

The transmission of AIDS by heterosexual intercourse is enhanced in the presence of STIs. Genital ulceration or inflammation caused by STIs increase the infectiousness of HIV-1-positive individuals and the susceptibility of HIV-1-negative individuals. The incidence of curable STIs is highest in sub-Saharan Africa, with 69 million new cases per year in a population of 269 million adults aged 15–49 (WHO, 2001). Table 14.3 shows the estimated incidence of the four most common curable STIs in people in sub-Saharan Africa. In South Africa, one survey in a rural prenatal clinic in KwaZulu Natal revealed that 70 per cent of the attendees had one or more STI (Sturm *et al.*, 1998).

Consequences of the AIDS Epidemic in Africa

HIV/AIDS has a widespread impact on many parts of African society, impacting on the individual, the family structure and society at large. HIV/AIDS dramatically affects economic activity and social progress and has become the biggest threat to the continent's development. UNAIDS estimates that AIDS is reducing the per capita growth in half of the countries in sub-Saharan Africa by 0.5–1.2

Table 14.3   Estimated incidence of curable STIs in people aged 15–49 in sub-Saharan Africa. Source: WHO, 2001

	Incident cases per year (millions)		
	Men	Women	Total
Syphilis	2.1	1.7	3.8
Chamydia trachomatis	7.6	8.2	15.9
Neisseria gonorrhoeae	8.2	8.8	17.0
Trichomonas vaginalis	16.2	15.9	32.1
Total	34.1	34.6	68.7

per cent annually. Life expectancy has halved in some countries and millions of adults are dying in their economically productive years. Many families are losing their income earners and the families of those who die have to find money to pay for their funerals.

As the epidemic progresses, the family unit is being eroded and the role of the household head is changing. Too many households are now headed by the elderly (such as grandparents – a situation referred to as a 'skipped generation'), a single parent whose partner has died, or the eldest child in a family which has been orphaned. In Kenya, Uganda, and Tanzania, the orphan rates have risen by 40–130 per cent since the onset of the AIDS epidemic. Children who are orphaned struggle to survive without a parent's care and frequently stop attending school in order to look after younger siblings (Johnson and Dorrington, 2001). Sub-Saharan Africa countries that are most severely affected by the AIDS epidemic have the lowest school enrolment rates in the world. In several African countries fewer than 50 per cent of 7–14 year olds are enrolled (Ainsworth and Filmer, 2002). Reasons for lower enrolment in school by orphans include a greater demand placed on children's time and grief. A decline in school enrolment is one of the most visible effects of the HIV/AIDS epidemic on education in Africa.

Companies of all types face higher costs of training, insurance, benefits, absenteeism, and illness. Skilled personnel in important areas of public management and core social services are being lost to AIDS. Essential services are being depleted and scarce resources are put under greater strain. As the epidemic matures, the health sector suffers the additional pressures of caring for those with AIDS.

In South Africa, the health system as it currently stands is still reeling from the history of inequity and apartheid that preceded democracy. The apartheid health care system was designed to provide private care to the 23 per cent of the population with insurance and an overburdened 'residual' state health care service for the poor. Thus, the majority of the country is served in a system that is over-crowded and with scarce resources.

The HIV/AIDS epidemic has exacerbated this problem. AIDS is now the leading cause of morbidity and death in sub-Saharan Africa including South Africa and the epidemic has therefore become an added burden on already strained health care systems. It is estimated that in 2002 there were between 4.5 million and 6.5 million people living with HIV and AIDS in South Africa and of this about 25 per cent (1.1–1.6 million people) were likely to be symptomatic, including 7 per cent (315 000–455 000 people) with clinical AIDS. Because HIV infection affects predominantly young adults, who are usually healthy, the epidemic is changing the demographic profile of hospital patients and placing an increased demand on health care services.

As a consequence, the South African health care system is being overwhelmed and the situation is unlikely to improve in the near future as the number AIDS cases is expected to climb sharply to an estimated 500 000 by 2005 and to 800 000, or double the current numbers, by 2010.

Furthermore, the full extent of the impact has not yet hit because of the length of the latency period between infection and the development of HIV-related illnesses. The individuals with AIDS who are now seeking health care are predominantly those infected more than seven years ago when prevalence of HIV was substantially below the current levels.

Not only has health utilization increased, but other illnesses that require attention (such as diabetes, infections, hypertension, etc.) are being crowded out by the increasing morbidity that AIDS brings.

Prior to the emergence of HIV in Africa, the continent was already experiencing a major tuberculosis epidemic. As the HIV epidemic has matured in sub-Saharan Africa, there has been a dramatic increase in the incidence of tuberculosis. Data on temporal trends in tuberculosis from one rural district in South Africa (Wilkinson and Davies, 1997) demonstrate trends that parallel the increase in HIV prevalence in the general population. Ongoing monitoring of tuberculosis in the 19 000 mineworkers employed by AngloGold demonstrated that tuberculosis cases have increased from 1174 per 100 000 in 1990 to 2476 per 100 000 in 1996, increasing primarily as a result of co-infection with HIV (Churchyard *et al.*, 1999). Tuberculosis is the most common first AIDS-defining condition in southern Africa (Churchyard *et al.*, 1999) and has become the leading cause of mortality among patients with HIV disease (Whalen *et al.*, 1996; Colvin *et al.*, 2001).

The worst of the epidemic clearly has not yet passed. In the absence of massively expanded prevention, treatment, and care efforts, the AIDS death toll on the continent is expected to continue rising before peaking around the end of this decade. Along with the increasing number of new cases and potential deaths due to AIDS, there is the specter of ever worsening adverse economic and social consequences.

HIV Prevention in Africa

A continuing rise in the number of HIV-infected people in Africa is not inevitable. Success is being achieved in some countries, and with greater governmental and societal awareness, plus the infusion of worldwide support for prevention strategies, there is hope that much can be accomplished.

Responses of African Governments

Some governments, such as Zimbabwe and Namibia, have aligned AIDS with homosexuality and have taken a strong anti-homosexuality stand. In these settings, government responses have tended to be slow, inadequate and generally ineffective. On the other hand, the positive and open approaches of countries like Botswana and Uganda have created vibrant programs of prevention and treatment which are hailed internationally and demonstrate that AIDS can be controlled.

South Africa has had a unique form of denialism in the epidemic in the highest echelons of political power. The first post-apartheid government of President Mandela was faced with the urgent need for reconciliation and nation building which took precedence over the need to accord AIDS the necessary priority and commitment. The current government, under the leadership of President Mbeki, is probably best characterized by its litany of errors in AIDS policy and for its failure to rise to the challenge that AIDS posed for South Africa. The creation of the Mbeki presidential panel, comprising denialists and orthodox scientists, marked the lowest point of the degeneration of the government's response into confusion and obtuseness. However, 2003 has seen a change of heart: in recognition of the extent of devastation caused by AIDS, the South African government made a far-reaching decision to provide free antiretroviral drugs in the government health care service.

Prevention Successes in Africa

Uganda was the first African country to show that prevention efforts can bring a widespread HIV/AIDS epidemic under control (Figure 14.3). HIV prevalence in pregnant women in urban areas has declined steadily for eight years in a row, from a high of 29.5 per cent in 1992 to 11.25 per cent in 2000. Uganda's prevention strategy focuses on a multi-pronged effort to provide information, education, and communication through decentralized community-orientated programs. These efforts have led to behavior changes; condom use by single women aged 15–24 almost doubled between 1995 and 2000/2001, and women in this age group are increasingly delaying sexual intercourse or abstaining entirely. In the capital, Kampala, almost 98 per cent of sex workers surveyed in 2000 reported that they had used a condom the last time they had sex.

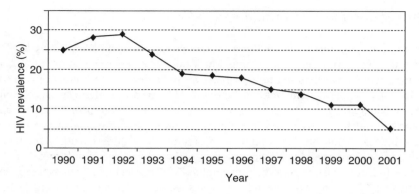

Fig. 14.3 HIV prevalence in Uganda over the last decade. Source: STD/AIDS Control Programme, Uganda (2001) HIV/AIDS surveillance report.

In South Africa, for pregnant women under 20, HIV prevalence rates fell from 21 per cent in 1998 to 14.8 per cent in 2002 (Department of Health, RSA, 2003). However, successful HIV prevention cannot be claimed until the number of new infections each year (incidence) starts to decline (Parkhurst, 2002). The good news is that there is evidence from some communities in South Africa that incidence rates are starting to decline. For example, in one rural South African community, the incidence rates in the 15–19 age group declined from 11.1 per cent (9.9–12.3) in 1999 to 8.9 per cent (7.0–11.0) in 2001 (Gouws, 2005). A major challenge now is to sustain and build on this success.

In Côte d'Ivoire the prevalence amongst female sex workers fell from 89 per cent to 32 per cent in the period 1991–1998. A partial explanation for this positive development was a higher frequency of condom usage, increasing from 20 per cent in 1992 to 78 per cent in 1998.

A decline in HIV prevalence has also been detected among young inner-city women in Addis Ababa, Ethiopia. Infection levels among women aged 15–24 attending antenatal clinics dropped from 24.2 per cent in 1995 to 15.1 per cent in 2001. However, this trend was localized and there was no evidence of HIV declines occurring elsewhere in the country.

HIV prevalence in Zambia also has declined significantly among 15- to 29-year-old urban women (down to 21.5 per cent in 2001 from 28.3 per cent in 1996). Behavior changes that have occurred in this region include urban men and women being less sexually active, having fewer partners, and using condoms more consistently (UNAIDS/WHO, 2002). Another positive example is Senegal, where prevention efforts initiated at the early stages of the epidemic managed to sustain a relatively low prevalence rate of 0.5 per cent. These are the some of the success stories that show us how prevention can succeed and what needs to be done to help to achieve this in the rest of the African continent.

Prevention in the Workplace

Increasingly, countries are focusing on the workplace as an essential venue for effective HIV prevention programs. In Zimbabwe, peer-education programs among factory workers led to a 34 per cent reduction in the incidence of HIV infections compared with factories randomized to the arm with no such programs (Katzenstein *et al.*, 1998). The government of Côte d'Ivoire, for example, has called on all businesses with more than 50 employees to establish HIV/AIDS committees, while the government of Cameroon envisions having agreements with 50 per cent of all businesses, requiring HIV/AIDS education for workers by 2005. In South Africa, periodic presumptive STI treatment for mineworkers has reduced STIs among workers and among sex workers from the community (Steen *et al.*, 2000).

Increasing Access to Condoms

In South Africa, as part of the government's efforts to scale up HIV prevention, public sector distribution of condoms increased from 6 million in 1994 to 358 million in 2002. Yet if more condoms were made available would they be used for the intended purpose? A study in South Africa to investigate what happens to the condoms which are distributed free of charge included 384 individuals who received more than 5500 condoms through public sector distribution. After five weeks, nearly 44 per cent of the condoms had been used during sex, roughly 22 per cent had been given away, and 26 per cent were still available for use. Fewer than 10 per cent of the condoms distributed by the government program had been lost or discarded, suggesting that individuals will use free condoms if they are made available (Myer *et al.*, 2001a).

Universal Education in Uganda

Since 1996, Uganda has provided free, compulsory education for all young people from 6 to 13 years. Uganda is using its schools to deliver HIV/AIDS education as part of a program that is well supported and seems to be successful (Rockefeller Foundation, 2002). Young women who are educated about HIV and AIDS tend to delay sexual debut or even abstain from sexual intercourse.

Community-based Programs in Response to HIV/AIDS

In an effort to integrate the governments' response to the HIV/AIDS epidemic, several countries in Africa have initiated community-based programs. An example of the community initiative is the provincial health department of KwaZulu-Natal in South Africa.

In response to the challenge and complexities of the impact of the epidemic in KwaZulu-Natal, the provincial government created the Provincial HIV/AIDS Action Unit (PAAU). The main task of this unit is to drive a coordinated government and non-government, including faith-based organizations, response to HIV/AIDS through coordinating preventative and support strategies against HIV/AIDS.

The Unit has embarked on a number of HIV/AIDS awareness and prevention campaigns in conjunction with communities. Some of its successful community initiatives include the training of a number of traditional leaders on HIV/AIDS, an aggressive HIV/AIDS awareness campaign targeting the taxi industry, and the integration of 484 HIV/AIDS communicators into a Community Health Worker program which consists of more than 2000 volunteers who run door to door campaigns. The establishment of these structures at the community level is necessary to facilitate effective community awareness programs and distribution of educational materials and information.

Furthermore, the PAAU is building capacity in communities for home-based care and is developing a database of all home-based care services in the province. A Community Capacity Enhancement Program has also recently been launched. This program seeks to enhance an integrated response to HIV/AIDS and poverty, through community conversations, an approach devised to get active community participation in intervention programs to combat HIV/AIDS. The Unit has succeeded in forming meaningful and lasting relationships and partnerships with various stakeholders including private sector, non-governmental organizations (NGOs), big business, churches, traditional structures, and government departments.

Prevention Gaps in Africa

Despite the successes described above, the positive trends do not yet offset the severity of the epidemic in Africa. Much of the progress is still occurring in localized settings. New infections continue to occur at a high rate in many countries and AIDS mortality is on the increase. Overall, a massive expansion in prevention efforts is needed, and although there is not one proven way to prevent new infections, the major components of a successful prevention program are well known. Youth-targeted behavioral interventions, scale-up of programs to prevent mother-to-child transmission, and supportive interventions to address gender inequities are required at scale in Africa.

Provision of Condoms

Condom accessibility will need to be drastically scaled up. In 2001 it was reported that the overall provision of condoms to sub-Saharan Africa is only 4.6 per man per year. An estimated 1.9 billion additional condoms would be needed to raise all countries to the average procurement level (about 17 condoms per man per year) of the six African countries that use the most condoms (Shelton and Johnson, 2001). It would cost an estimated $47.5 million a year to fill the 1.9 billion condom gap, excluding service delivery costs and production. However, based on data on condoms procured in public sector health facilities across South Africa, the estimated unmet need for condoms is probably closer to 13 billion (Myer *et al.*, 2001b).

Even if sufficient condoms could be supplied, they are not without their drawbacks, especially in the context of a stable partnership where pregnancy is desired, or where subordination of women prevents them from negotiating safer sex practices.

Provision of Voluntary Counseling and Testing

The provision of voluntary HIV counseling and testing (VCT) is an important part of any comprehensive national prevention and treatment program. The provision of VCT has become easier, cheaper, and more effective as a result of the availability of rapid HIV testing and therefore could be made much more widely available in many African countries. However, only an estimated 6 per cent of people who need HIV counseling and testing in Africa have access to it (Hauri *et al.*, 2005). The vast majority of those in Africa who are infected are unaware that they have HIV.

Targeted Behavioral Interventions

Although some countries have made enormous strides against the epidemic by supporting interventions targeting key populations, large numbers of people at highest risk for infection, such as youth and sex workers, do not have access to prevention programs. Only 8 per cent of out-of-school youth and more than one-third of in-school youth have access to prevention programs. In all, fewer than one-in-twelve sex workers and their clients is currently targeted by behavioral programs (UNAIDS, 2001a).

Prevention of Mother-to-Child Transmission

Currently the World Health Organization estimates that only 1 per cent of women who need programs for the prevention of mother-to-child transmission of HIV have access to these services. Yet sub-Saharan Africa accounts for roughly 90 per cent of the 800 000 infants who acquire HIV each year. Clearly the scaling up of such programs represents a central prevention priority in the region.

Broad-based HIV/AIDS Awareness

According to UNICEF, more than 70 per cent of adolescent girls (aged 15–19) in Somalia and more than 40 per cent in Guinea Bissau and Sierra Leone, have never heard of AIDS (UNAIDS, 2001a,b). Only 43 per cent of people at risk are reached by mass media awareness programs. Furthermore, even in areas where knowledge of AIDS is reasonable, women have serious misconceptions about how the virus is transmitted and underestimate their personal risk of acquiring HIV infection (Abdool Karim, 2001).

Diagnosis and Treatment of Sexually Transmitted Infections

The prevalence of STIs in many countries in Africa is high, accelerating the spread of HIV. In rural South Africa, nearly 9 per cent of adults have syphilis and almost one in 20 have gonorrhea (Colvin *et al.*, 1998). In Swaziland, more than half of the patients attending STI clinics tested in 2000 were HIV positive (UNAIDS/WHO, 2002), while seropositivity among STI clinic patients in Zimbabwe exceeded 70 per cent in 1995–1996 (WHO, 2001). It is estimated that only 14 per cent of people in Africa in need of STI services can obtain them at present.

Supportive Initiatives

Prevention strategies are more likely to be successful if they also address the social and economic conditions that accentuate vulnerability to HIV. Limited educational opportunity for girls, for example, is directly correlated with higher teen pregnancy rates and earlier initiation of sexual activity. In situations where a woman's economic security depends on a man, she may be less able to negotiate condom use. From a societal standpoint, countries that are too poor to support even a minimal health care infrastructure are unlikely to be able to provide VCT, STI diagnosis and treatment, or programs for the prevention of mother-to-child transmission.

HIV-related Treatment and Care in Africa

Treating and caring for the millions of Africans living with HIV/AIDS poses an enormous challenge to the continent and the world at large. Highly active anti-retroviral therapy (HAART) can transform the course of HIV infection into a manageable disease, as has been observed in many industrialized countries (van Praag and Perriens, 1996; Palella *et al.*, 1998; Bozzette *et al.*, 1998). However, in developing countries, where the disease burden is greatest, HAART has been largely unavailable. Even medication to treat opportunistic infections is not always available to those most in need. Until recently the routine use of antiretroviral treatment was thought to be technically and economically impossible in Africa.

The increasing availability of cheaper antiretroviral drugs and simpler drug regimens such as daily dosing drug combinations, and newer formulations such as triple drug combinations in a single tablet taken twice daily, increase the options and possibilities to enhance the quality of life for the millions living with HIV in Africa.

Access to antiretroviral therapy in Africa is slowly increasing and by the end of 2001, more than 10 African countries were providing antiretroviral therapy to people living with HIV/AIDS (UNAIDS, 2001a). The availability of resources from, among others, the Global Fund to Fight AIDS, Tuberculosis, and Malaria is a major step forward in the global effort against AIDS in Africa.

Botswana was the first country to begin a national AIDS treatment program providing antiretroviral drugs through its public health system. However, its ambitious antiretroviral drug program has been slow to get started. Of the 300 000 HIV-infected people, 110 000 were estimated to meet the criteria to qualify for treatment. The government aimed to enrol 19 000 people in the first year, but only 3500 were actually enrolled, highlighting a number of issues related to providing antiretroviral therapy. These include the education and training of health care workers and the capabilities of the health care infrastructure.

In South Africa, in addition to the handful of major companies (such as Anglo-Gold, De Beers, Debswana, and Heineken) and industries in the private sector, including the mines, utility companies, and clothing manufacturers that provide antiretrovirals to workers, the government has recently made a commitment to make antiretroviral therapy available in the public sector. The challenge now is to implement an approach that addresses both treatment and prevention in an integrated manner, in combination with building the capacity of health care professionals and an adequate infrastructure.

Among various models of HIV care provision, one proposed strategy that may be feasible for resource constrained settings is to integrate this care, including HAART provision, into the existing TB directly observed therapy (DOT) programs. This would allow for the opportunity to initiate HIV care and HAART for patients identified as HIV infected during TB treatment as well as to be able to continue such management for those who develop TB during HIV treatment.

However, stigma and discrimination are significant obstacles to the provision of AIDS treatment, since they form a major barrier to accessing HIV prevention, care, and support services. Despite the widespread availability of HIV voluntary counselling and testing services in many Africa countries, less than 10 per cent of HIV-infected people are estimated to be aware of their HIV status. One study has found that 50 per cent of adult Tanzanian women know where they could be tested for HIV, yet only 6 per cent have been tested (UNAIDS, 2001a). People living with

HIV and AIDS are afraid to disclose their HIV status, even to their primary sexual partner. More than half of all women who knew they had acquired HIV, and those who were surveyed by Kenya's Population Council, said they had not disclosed their HIV status to their partners because they feared it would expose them to violence or abandonment (UNAIDS, 2001a). Fear, in turn, perpetuates secrecy and denial of personal risk as well as the presence and scale of the HIV epidemic. Not only does denial affect prevention, it also presents a major challenge to the provision of antiretroviral therapy.

Transforming AIDS into a treatable disease has the potential to change community perceptions of people living with AIDS. For many individuals and couples in Africa, where HIV prevalence rates are high, finding out their infection status could expand their range of HIV prevention options.

What the Future Holds

The challenge of halting and ameliorating HIV/AIDS in Africa seems overwhelming but remains a possibility. To limit further devastation caused by AIDS in the African region several fundamental issues will need to be addressed.

First, the enormous barrier of stigma and denial needs to be resolved. Very few people are currently able to live openly with AIDS. Fear of discrimination often prevents people from getting tested, seeking treatment for AIDS, or from admitting their HIV status publicly. The denial and secrecy surrounding AIDS go hand in hand. The vicious cycle needs to be broken. There is a need for people who can withstand the stigma to openly live with AIDS. More HIV/AIDS-related education is needed in Africa since no policy or law alone can combat HIV/AIDS-related discrimination. The fear and prejudice that lies at the core of the HIV/AIDS discrimination needs to be tackled at both community and national levels.

The perception of AIDS needs to be transformed from a universally fatal disease, acquired through immoral sexual acts, to a disease like any other that can be treated and managed clinically.

Secondly, there is a need to tackle the gender-related violence and gender inequality. The inequality between men and women, as well as the economic deprivation that helps to drive the epidemic, must be addressed. The specific needs of women and girls need to be a key part of African HIV prevention programs. Although a long-term solution, it is still fundamental to work on these issues as part of the solution.

Thirdly, the high background rates of STIs need to be addressed and controlled.

Fourthly, additional resources are needed in Africa for HIV/AIDS. In 2000, it was estimated that $1.5 billion a year would make it possible to achieve implementation of successful prevention programs for the whole of sub-Saharan Africa at levels likely to impact on the further spread of HIV infection. This additional amount of $1.5 billion a year will enable the countries in sub-Saharan Africa to provide symptomatic and palliative care, prevent and treat opportunistic infections, and care for orphans. Providing antiretroviral therapy would add several billion dollars annually to this bill.

In the absence of adequate resources, lower cost innovative solutions need to be developed. Meanwhile, even small efforts could play a role before sufficient resources are in place for large programs. Donor funds, such as the Global Fund to Fight AIDS, Tuberculosis, and Malaria, are part of the solution addressing the resource shortage. This approach is not the complete solution – in many instances, African countries need more commitment from their own governments. In this regard, there are promising signs that some governments, such as Botswana, Rwanda, and Uganda, are responding in earnest.

Fifthly, there is a need for sufficient trained personnel to manage the implementation of large-scale programs and to provide the scale of health care needed. If successful antiretroviral treatment programs are to be implemented, the health infrastructure will also be challenged and stretched to support them.

Sixthly, the looming massive challenge is that of ensuring that the estimated 9 per cent of African adults who are HIV positive get the treatment and care they need. As antiretroviral drugs slowly become more widely available in Africa, efforts to improve the availability of voluntary counselling and testing are critical. Antiretroviral therapy together with prevention and treatment of opportunistic infections can result in significant gains in life expectancy and quality of life among people living with HIV; these benefits have been slow to come to Africa.

These are some of the serious challenges that African countries and their partners in the global community will have to face if they are to make a real difference to the epidemic.

For Africa, and South Africa in particular, there is a reality that needs to be acknowledged – a reality that thousands upon thousands are dying of AIDS, that prevention efforts for the most part have failed, and that there needs to be bold action. The turning point was the Durban AIDS conference where the silence surrounding AIDS was broken, due in part to the voices of activists, which were heard loudly and clearly. Indeed, South Africa is a good example of how advocacy and activism has shaped the response to the epidemic and where rationalism prevailed over denialism. The turning point is also, in part, the creation of the Global Fund and the US President's Emergency Plan for AIDS Relief (PEPFAR) as well as announcements of pharmacy price reductions. The price of drugs however, remains one small part of a larger challenge to identify, treat, and monitor the millions of AIDS patients in Africa and to care for the many orphans and broken families created by this devastating epidemic.

The tide has turned and there is no going back. Governments can no longer use the lack of donor funding as scapegoats. There is a clear voice of reason that is driven by the realization that AIDS is destroying the very fabric and economic driving force of society. Nothing less than energetic national commitment and political will are demanded to deal with this challenge and to reverse its ravishes.

> The challenge is to move from rhetoric to action, and action at an unprecedented intensity and scale. … For this there is a need for us to be focused, to be strategic, and to mobilise all of our resources and alliances, and to sustain the effort until the war is won.
>
> Nelson Mandela, June 2000

References

Abdool Karim Q (2001) Barriers to preventing human immunodeficiency virus in women: Experiences from KwaZulu-Natal, South Africa. *J Am Med Women's Assoc* 56: 193–6.

Abdool Karim Q, Abdool Karim SS (1999) South Africa: host to new and emerging epidemics. *Sex Transm Infect* 75: 139–47.

Abdool Karim Q, Stein Z (1999) Women and HIV/AIDS: A global perspective. In: *Women and Health.* Goldman M, Hatch M, eds. London: Academic Press.420–27.

Abdool Karim SS, Abdool Karim Q (1992) Changes in HIV seroprevalence in a rural black community in KwaZulu. *S Afr Med J* 82: 484.

AIDS in Africa (2003) http://www.aids-in-africa.net/aids-in-africa-history.htm (accessed October 2003).

Ainsworth M, Filmer D (2002) *Poverty, AIDS and Children's Schooling: A Targeting Dilemma.* World Bank Policy Research Working Paper 2885, September.

Bozzette SA, Berry SH, Duan N *et al.* (1998) The care of HIV infected adults in the United States. *N Engl J Med* 339: 1897–904.

Churchyard GJ, Kleinschmidt I, Corbett EL, Mulder D, De Cock KM (1999) Mycobacterial disease in South African gold miners in the era of HIV infection. *Int J Tuberc Lung Dis* 3: 791–8.

Coleman RL, Wilkinson D (1997) Increasing HIV prevalence in a rural district of South Africa. *J Acquir Immunodefic Syndr Retrovirol* 16: 50–3.

Colvin M, Abdool Karim SS, Connolly C, Hoosen AA, Ntuli N (1998) HIV infection and asymptomatic sexually transmitted infections in a rural South African community. *Int J STD AIDS* 9: 548–50.

Colvin M, Dawood S, Kleinschmidt I, Mullick S, Lalloo U (2001) Prevalence of HIV and HIV-related disease on the adult medical wards of a tertiary hospital in Durban, South Africa. *Int J STD AIDS* 12: 386–9.

Department of Health, RSA. (2003) *National HIV and syphilis antenatal sero-prevalence survey* in South Africa. Health Systems Research, Research Coordination and Epidemiology. Pretoria.

Duncan ME, Tibaux G, Pelzer A *et al.* (1990) First coitus before menarche and the risk of sexually transmitted disease. *Lancet* 335: 338–40.

Garnett GP, Gregson S (2000) Monitoring the course of the HIV-1 epidemic: the influence of patterns of fertility on HIV prevalence estimates. *Math Popul Studies* 8: 251–77.

Gouws E (2005). HIV incidence rates in South Africa. In: Abdool Karim SS, Abdool Karim Q, eds. *HIV/AIDS in South Africa.* Cambridge: Cambridge University Press (in press).

Greenberg J, Magder L, Aral S (1992) Age at first coitus: A marker for risky sexual behavior in women. *Sex Transm Dis* 19: 331–4.

Gregson S, Nyamukapa, CA, Garnett GP *et al.* (2002) Sexual mixing patterns and sex-differentials in teenage exposure to HIV infection in rural Zimbabwe. *Lancet* 359: 1896–903.

Hauri AM, Armstrong GL, Hutin YJF (2004) The global burden of disease attributable to contaminated injections given in health care settings. *Int J STD AIDS* 15(1): 7–16.

Hyde KAL, Ekatan A, Kiage P and Iarasa C (2002) *HIV/AIDS and Education in Uganda*: Window of opportunity. Rockefeller Foundation.

Johnson L, Dorrington R (2001) The impact of AIDS on orphanhood in South Africa: A quantitative analysis. Care Monograph No. 4. 2001. Centre for Actuarial Research, University of Cape Town, Rondebosch.

Katzenstein D, McFarland W, Mbizvo M *et al.* (1998) Peer education among factory workers in Zimbabwe: providing a sustainable HIV prevention intervention, XII International Conference on AIDS, Geneva. Abstract No. 33514.

Los Altos Rotary Club. Rotary AIDS Project (2003) The AIDS Pandemic: Current Worldwide Statistics. www.rotaryaidsproject.org/facts.html (accessed 27 October 2003).

Lurie M (2000). Migration and AIDS in southern Africa: a review. *South Afr J Sci* 96: 343–6.

Lurie M, Williams BG, Gouws E (1997) Circular migration and sexual networking in rural KwaZulu/Natal: Implications for the spread of HIV and other sexually transmitted diseases. *Health Transition Rev* 7: 15–24.

Lurie MN, Williams BG, Zuma K *et al.* (2003) The impact of migration on HIV-1 transmission in South Africa: A study of migrant and non-migrant men and their partners. *Sex Transm Dis* 30: 149–56.

Marck J (1999) Long-distance truck drivers' sexual cultures and attempts to reduce HIV risk behaviour amongst them: a review of the African and Asian literature. In: Cadwell JC *et al.*, eds. *Resistances to Behavioural Change to Reduce HIV/AIDS Infection.* Canberra: Australian National University, pp. 91–100.

Mbugua GG, Muthami LN, Mutura CW *et al.* (1995) Epidemiology of HIV infection among long distance truck drivers in Kenya. *East Afr Med J* 72: 515–18.

Myer L, Mathews C, Little F, Abdool Karim SS (2001a) The fate of male condoms distributed to the public in South Africa. *AIDS* 15: 789–93.

Myer L, Mathews C, Little F (2001b) Condom gap in Africa is wider than study suggests. *BMJ* 323: 937.

Palella FJ Jr, Delaney KM, Moorman AC *et al.* (1998) Declining morbidity and mortality among participants with advanced human immunodeficiency virus infection. HIV outpatient Study Investigators. *N Engl J Med* 338: 853–60.

Parkhurst JO (2002) The Ugandan success story? Evidence and claims of HIV-1 prevention. *Lancet* 360: 78–80.

Quinn T (1994) Population migration and the spread of types 1 and 2 human immunodeficiency virus. *Proc Natl Acad Sci* 91: 2407–14.

Ramjee G, Gouws E (2002) Prevalence of HIV among truck drivers visiting sex workers in KwaZulu-Natal, South Africa. *Sex Transm Dis* 29: 44–9.

Ramjee G, Abdool Karim SS, Sturm AW (1998) Sexually transmitted infections among sex workers in KwaZulu Natal, South Africa. *Sex Transm Dis* 25: 346–9.

Serwadda D, Sewankambo NK, Lwegaba A *et al.* (1985) Slim disease: a new disease in Uganda and its association with HTLV-III infection. *Lancet* 2: 849–52.

Shelton JD, Johnston B (2001) Condom gap in Africa: evidence from donor agencies and key informants. *BMJ* 323: 139.

Steen R, Vuylsteke B, DeCoito T *et al.* (2000) Evidence of declining STD prevalence following a core group intervention. Sex Transm Dis 27: 1–8.

Sturm AW, Wilkinson D, Ndovela N, Bowen S, Connolly S (1998) Pregnant women as a reservoir of undetected sexually transmitted diseases in rural South Africa: implications for disease control. *Am J Public Health* 88: 1243–5.

UNAIDS (2001a) *AIDS Epidemic Update – sub-Saharan Africa*. December. UNAIDS/01.74E-WHO/CDS/CSR/NCS/2001.2. Geneva: UNAIDS.

UNAIDS (2001b) *Children and Young People in a World of AIDS*. Geneva: UNAIDS.

UNAIDS (2002) *Paediatric HIV Infection and AIDS, UNAIDS Best Practice Collection*. Geneva: UNAIDS.

UNAIDS/WHO (2002) *Report on the HIV/AIDS Epidemic*. Geneva: UNAIDS/WHO.

Van Praag E, Perriens JH (1996) Caring for participants with HIV and AIDS in middle income countries. *BMJ* 313: 440.

Weiss E, Gupta RG (1998) Bridging the gap: addressing gender and sexuality in HIV prevention. Findings from the women and AIDS Research program. International Center for Research on Women, Washington, DC.

Whalen C, Okwera A, Johnson J *et al*. Predictors of survival in human immunodeficiency virus infected participants with pulmonary tuberculosis. The Makerere University-Case Western Reserve University Research Collaboration. *Am J Respir Crit Care Med*. 1996; 153: 1977–81.

WHO (World Health Organization) (2001) *Global Prevalence and Incidence of Selected Curable Sexually Transmitted Infections. Overview and Estimates*. Geneva: WHO.

Wilkinson D, Davies GR (1997). The increasing burden of tuberculosis in rural South Africa – impact of the HIV epidemic. *South Afr Med J* 87: 447–50.

Asia: Health Meets Human Rights

15

Chris Beyrer
Director, Fogarty AIDS International Training & Research Program, Johns Hopkins University, Bloomberg School of Public Health, Baltimore, USA

N Kumarasamy
Chief Medical Officer, YRG Centre for AIDS Research and Education, Principal Investigator-ACTU/HPTN052–Chennai site, Voluntary Health Services, Tharamani, India

H F Pizer
Health Care Strategies, Harvard Street, Cambridge, MA, USA

Chris Beyrer MD, MPH, is Associate Professor in the Departments of Epidemiology and International Health and founder of the Center for Public Health and Human Rights at the Johns Hopkins Bloomberg School of Public Health. He serves as Director of Johns Hopkins Fogarty AIDS International Training and Research Program and as Faculty for the JHU Fogarty Bioethics International Training Program. Dr. Beyrer is author of the 1998 book War in the Blood: Sex, Politics and AIDS in Southeast Asia (Zed Books, London, St. Martins Press, New York). He has worked extensively in developing nations including Thailand, China, India, Laos, Malawi, Uganda, Ethiopia, South Africa, Brazil, Russia, and Tajikistan. His numerous activities include HIV/AIDS professional training, HIV vaccine testing, and studying the health risks of sex workers opiate users. From 1992–1997 he was Field Director of the Thai PAVE and HIVNET studies based in northern Thailand.

N Kumarasamy, MD, PhD is Chief Medical Officer & Clinical Researcher at the Y.R.G. Centre for AIDS Research and Education Voluntary Health Services (VHS), Chennai, India. He has MD and PhD degrees from Madras Medical College, University of Madras with a specialty in Infectious Diseases. He also has completed postdoctoral training in HIV medicine at Johns Hopkins School of Medicine and Brown

University. He is the Chief Medical Officer at the VHS-YRG CARE Medical Centre in Chennai, India, Clinical Researcher for the YRGCARE/ Brown University, USA/NIH, USA collaborative research programs and Principal Investigator for the Chennai site for ACTG and HPTN trials of NIH's multi-site HIV study. His research focuses on the natural history of HIV in South India and the usage of antiretroviral drugs in developing country settings. Dr. Kumarasamy has published 55 original manuscripts.

H F Pizer, BA, PA is a medical writer, health care consultant and physician assistant. He is author, coauthor and editor of 13 books published worldwide in trade, mass market and professional editions, in English and in translation, about health and medicine. His books include the first for the general public on AIDS, organ transplants and stroke, and in women's health on coping with a miscarriage, natural family planning and artificial insemination. He is cofounder and Principal of Health Care Strategies, Inc a health care consulting firm in Cambridge, Massachusetts that provides program evaluation and management consulting services. He was founder and President of New England Medical Claims Analysts, a health care cost containment consultancy. He has written about the rising cost for health care in the United States and is former President of the Massachusetts Association of Physician Assistants. See section on The Editors for additional biographical information.

There is a growing awareness that HIV/AIDS epidemics, as well as many other important public health threats, are significantly worsened by government negligence, communal strife, social vulnerability, and societal denial. We have enough evidence of success in HIV prevention in states as diverse as Australia and Senegal to know that major epidemics of HIV are preventable. Yet they continue to occur. In at least some cases, unnecessary HIV epidemics are the consequence of chronic human rights violations and failures of public policy. This is the case in a number of Asian states, where at the beginning of the third decade of the AIDS epidemic we are at last seeing widespread awareness at the highest levels of government and the media that strong measures are needed. Asia is the world's second most HIV/AIDS-affected region after sub-Saharan Africa, with an estimated 7.6 million cumulative HIV infections by the end of 2003 (UNAIDS, 2003). To date Asia has been fortunate compared with Africa. Given the enormous populations of the region, so far the AIDS burden does not come close to the devastation in sub-Saharan Africa. But India alone, at just over a billion people, has more than twice the entire population of sub-Saharan Africa, so even small increases in HIV infection rates could lead to enormous numbers of people with AIDS (Figure 15.1).

Caution and diligence must prevail. Asia's epidemics are newer than in Africa and the West. More than half of the infections in Asia are in people under age 25. The Asian epidemics in India, Cambodia, Burma, Thailand, the Russian Far East,

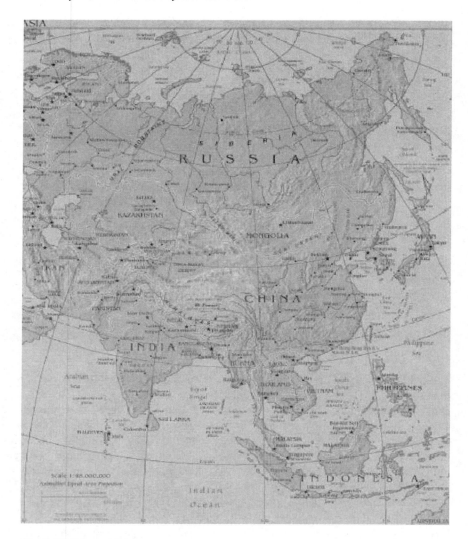

Fig. 15.1 Map of Asia.

and southern, south-western, and north-western China, have been explosive, not well predicted, and generally have been poorly managed. With the exception of Thailand, and some heartening trends in Vietnam and Cambodia, Asian governments have been slow to respond to the threat of AIDS.

Asia is arguably the most culturally, linguistically, geographically, economically, and politically diverse area on the planet. The enormous disparities across the region foster an equally uneven distribution of HIV risk and prevalence. The

376

Japanese enjoy one of the world's highest life expectancies, the people of Laos one of the lowest. In 2000, Burma's health care system was ranked the second worst in the world by the World Health Organization (WHO), while Singapore, South Korea, and Taiwan have health standards rivaling or surpassing those of much of Europe.

The national responses to AIDS in Asia have been as diverse as the states themselves. Democracy and civil society are growing in strength in South Korea and Indonesia, while Nepal, most of Central Asia, and Pakistan face deepening social turmoil and dictatorship. Burma and North Korea are two of the most repressive governments anywhere in the world and fail to meet the needs of their peoples on virtually every social indicator. Non-governmental organizations (NGOs), proven partners in AIDS prevention and care, vary widely in their presence, independence and efficacy across Asia. They are and have been prominent in Thailand, but virtually non-existent in North Korea (Nelson *et al.*, 1996).

North-East Asia, particularly Japan and South Korea, have seen cases of HIV among gay men and blood product recipients since the 1980s, but have not had generalized outbreaks and appear very unlikely to do so. South-East Asia, in contrast, is currently among the most affected subregions. Three states are most severely affected. Cambodia has the highest population prevalence in Asia at over 3 per cent of adults. It is followed by Burma and Thailand. Like Cambodia, Burma is poorly equipped to battle HIV while Thailand has become a model for how to respond to heterosexual spread, if not that related to injection drug use (Nelson *et al.*, 1996).

Of great concern are more recent outbreaks in three major Asian states: India, with its enormous population across a vast and diverse area, has the largest number of cases, and epidemics are brewing in China and the Russian Far East. Rates of infection in Central Asia so far have been low or are unknown, but recent trends suggest a concentrated epidemic is underway among drug users in Kazakhstan, Iran, and Russian Siberia (Beyrer, 2002). As we will discuss in more detail, so far the incidence and risk of HIV infection has been largely confined to intravenous heroin abusers. The problem is that in other areas of Asia, the pattern has been for HIV to move from intravenous drug users to the more general population. Within nations the incidence and risk of HIV varies widely based on local or regional political, economic and cultural conditions. For example, in India six states – Andra Pradesh, Karnataka, Maharashtra, Manipur, Nagaland, and Tamil Nadu – have by far the majority of cases. Table 15.1 illustrates the uneven burden of HIV/AIDS across Asia.

India may now have the largest number of HIV-infected citizens of any single country worldwide, with an estimated number of at least 4 million (UNAIDS, 2003). While the majority of these appear to be among heterosexuals of childbearing age, India also has experienced significant spread among drug users, blood products recipients, and among men who have sex with men. Indeed, given the diversity of the subcontinent, virtually every major route of HIV spread has been identified, with striking variations across those states for which reasonable data exist. The highest rate by state is Manipur, in India's isolated and troubled north-east, where the epidemic resembles that seen in Yunnan China (see below).

Table 15.1   Estimated HIV/AIDS cases, population rate, and 1999 AIDS deaths for selected Asian countries (based on UNAIDS data).

Country	People living with HIV/AIDS	HIV rate (per cent)	AIDS deaths in 1999
South-East Asia			
Cambodia	220 000	4.04	14 000
Burma	750 000–1 million[a]	2–5	Unknown
Thailand	755 000	2.15	66 000[b]
Malaysia	49 000	0.42	1900
Philippines	28 000	0.07	1200
Laos	1400	0.05	130
Indonesia	52 000	0.05	3100
South Asia			
India	3 700 000	0.70	310 000
Nepal	34 000	0.29	2500
Pakistan	74 000	0.10	6500
Bangladesh	13 000	0.02	1000
East Asia and the Pacific			
China	500 000	0.07	17 000
Japan	10 000	0.02	150
Korea	3800	0.01	180
Papua NG	5400	0.22	450
Central Asia and Russia			
Russia	170 000	0.18	850
Kazakhstan	3500	0.04	<100
Afghanistan[c]	–	–	–
Iran[c]	–	–	–

[a] Burma (Myanmar) estimates are higher than UNAIDS figures, estimated at 530 000 infections in 2000, but based on incomplete reporting since 1995.
[b] Thailand has lost an estimated 300 000–350 000 citizens to AIDS since the start of the Thai epidemic in 1988–1989.
[c] Data not reported to UN for Afghanistan and Iran.

For now it is largely related to the trafficking in heroin from Burma, Manipur's problematic neighbor to the east (Manipur State Department of Health Services, 1997). Tamil Nadu in the traditional Hindu south, and Maharashtra, with its capital Mumbai, are the second and third most affected areas, and in these regions sexual spread predominates, driven significantly by large, and largely denied, sex industries, and by chronic high rates of sexually transmitted infections.

India's heterosexual epidemic most closely resembles that of Thailand's, where a significant proportion of young men use commercial sex services before and often after marriage, while the majority of young women are sexually inexperienced and uneducated until marriage. These young women are exposed to HIV through the processes most highly valued in their cultures: monogamous marriage, child-bearing, and young motherhood. Indeed, in both India and Thailand the single most important risk factor for HIV infection among women is marriage (Gangakhedkar *et al.*, 1997). Those women who are found to be HIV infected are almost universally identified in pregnancy. As we shall discuss later in the chapter, this mode of transmission is due to traditional gender roles that victimize women. For the women it is too late to protect themselves and they face the risk of transmission to their infants.

The patterns of HIV spread across Asia have differed in some important ways from those seen in Africa and the West. With the exception of Cambodia, where HIV spread began in the sex trade, the initial spread of HIV was a critical factor among injecting drug users in the period 1988–1990. This was at least a decade later than in the West and probably more than a decade later than in Africa (Beyrer, 1998). As described in greater detail below, it was common for drug users to form an initial and important 'high-risk' group in the epidemics in Thailand, India, Burma, Malaysia, China, Pakistan, and Vietnam (Crofts *et al.*, 1998). Since then the virus has become widespread among sex workers and their clients. The scale of the region's sex trade and the large number of young men using commercial sex services was a public shock and embarrassment. From the communities of intravenous drug users and at-risk sex groups, the Asian epidemic spread to wider populations of sexually active adults and their infants.

One big question is China, where, by 2003, there were perhaps less than 2 million people out of a total population of well over one billion living with HIV (UNAIDS, 2003). China is one of the world's most rapidly developing economies and societies in the world, and along with rising incomes it is seeing increasing social dislocation. Millions of mostly poor people are moving from the rural countryside to the cities. There is no certain answer as to what this will mean for the spread of HIV, but it is known that societal dislocation and flux are known risk factors for this epidemic. The extent of spread due to the poorly understood, but certainly large outbreaks of HIV associated with blood donors in China's huge blood products industry could increase estimates of HIV prevalence by 1- to 3-fold.

Sri Lanka, Pakistan, and Bangladesh appear to be at an earlier stage of an HIV epidemic than India. They are vulnerable, as all are poor and have weak public health systems. HIV is present in all three countries. In addition, Sri Lanka remains embroiled in a longstanding civil war, and Pakistan and Bangladesh have extensive social and religious barriers to HIV prevention. Bangladesh, in particular, is poised for a serious outbreak of HIV. It has an extensive and highly stigmatized sex industry with some of Asia's largest brothels, high rates of other sexually transmitted diseases (STDs), and a dense and very young population. Pakistan faces the additional challenges of an extensive narcotics industry with large numbers of young addicts, active heroin trafficking from Afghanistan, and a recent suspension of civilian rule. The UN Drug Control Program estimated that Pakistan had

3 million injecting drug users in 2000, a huge population at risk (UNDCP, 2000). Nepal is also at risk for a major HIV epidemic in the coming years. A major issue is the extensive trafficking of Nepali women and girls into the Indian sex industry, where they are among the most vulnerable and disenfranchised of workers.

Another big question will be the availability of treatment. At this point relatively few people in Asia, and almost none in the poorest nations, receive antiretroviral medicines. It does not matter whether they are symptom-free, have full-blown AIDS, are pregnant, or have been exposed to the virus. Even in India where a new generic drug industry producing antiretrovirals for world export is flourishing, most people do not have access to HIV screening and sophisticated medical therapy.

It is perhaps fair to write that the Asian experience of HIV/AIDS may not be so much about what has happened, but what could happen in the world's most populous and diverse region. The underlying problems that contribute to the virulence of the epidemic are enormous. Arguably they may be considered human rights issues that demand regional and world attention. The final section of this chapter speaks to the interface of public health and political measures needed to prevent disaster.

AIDS Enters South-East Asia

AIDS in South-East Asia is a valuable lens for analyzing the epidemic throughout the region. The population of mainland South-East Asia is estimated to be about 344 million. After sub-Saharan Africa, it is the locale most impacted by AIDS (UNAIDS, 2002). All the conditions that promote the spread of HIV are present. The area is densely populated, ethnically varied, and economically and politically diverse. It includes relatively affluent Singapore and Brunei, where the epidemic remains limited, and very poor nations like Cambodia, Burma, and Laos, where HIV has taken hold. The risk of a broad AIDS epidemic in the emerging economies of south-eastern China, Thailand, and Vietnam probably falls in between these two extremes. As in the rest of the world, AIDS in South-East Asia is largely associated with poverty and a low level of general economic development. South-East Asia has large areas of extreme economic deprivation in both remote rural and urban areas. Primitive conditions in housing, education, transportation and communication, sanitation, water supply, and access to health care are serious problems wherever poverty exists. In many Asian states, disparities in health are wide and ethnic minorities and tribal peoples receive inferior medical treatment or have virtually no access to modern health care services.

South-East Asia has a diverse political and cultural spectrum that affects the HIV/AIDS problem. There are emerging democracies, military dictatorships, Islamic Republics, and three of the last five nominally communist states (China, Laos, and Vietnam). As we shall discuss, a critical factor is that South-East Asia has two of the world's leading heroin exporters – Burma and Laos. It is recognized that HIV/AIDS is present and spreading along the major heroin trade routes. Along with the drug trade, trafficking in young women and girls for sexual exploitation occurs in these areas, creating conditions ideal for the spread of HIV (Beyrer, 2001).

The Thai Experience

HIV-1 became a significant health risk in South-East Asia between 1988 and 1990, later than in other parts of the world. Thailand was the first Asian country to suffer a widespread epidemic of HIV-1 and the Thai experience with HIV is still by far the best described, documented, and understood (Weniger *et al.*, 1991). The Thai response offers a model for successful intervention at the national level in a developing country.

The first case of AIDS in Thailand was documented in 1984 in a homosexual man who was probably infected through sexual contact with a Western lover. A second documented case was found in a man who had been employed in a gay bar. He was a sex worker who had not been abroad, but had had multiple male and female, Thai and European, sex partners. The virus was now circulating within a subsection of Thai society and the country was in its 'first wave' of the epidemic.

In 1988 Thailand had approximately 50 000 injection drug users (IDUs). Between 1985 and 1987 the prevalence of HIV among Thai IDUs was probably negligible, perhaps 0–1 per cent, but in 1988 the number acquiring HIV seems to have taken off. In one study the prevalence of HIV infection in 1988 went from about 1 per cent in August to about 40 per cent in October, a staggering rate of sero-conversion of about 5 per cent per month (Weniger *et al.*, 1991). The epidemic was in now in what might called a 'second wave' that would quickly eclipse the first. HIV was still largely isolated within a community of young urban men living atypical lifestyles, but the foundation was being set for greater dissemination of the virus.

At first the Thai government and Thai society were reluctant to admit openly they had a problem. This was not unique. Throughout Asia this attitude was the norm. HIV/AIDS was thought of as an aberrant problem in permissive Western nations. Some believed that Asian 'family values' would keep the virus confined to social outcast groups like IDUs, sex workers, and gay men. The feeling was that 'Asian' or 'Confucian' ways were different from the West and would protect the general society. Some even suggested that Asians were genetically resistant to HIV.

Attitudes began to change as data came in on the HIV infection rate among women in the sex industry. Until 1989 only about 1 per cent of female sex workers in Thailand were HIV positive. A year after the explosion of HIV was noted among IDUs, a similar rapid increase in seroconversion was noted among female sex workers in Chiang Mai. The infection rate went from 1 per cent to 44 per cent in a mere six months. By 1991, the national rate of HIV infection among female sex workers was thought to be about 15 per cent. Northern Thailand, where Chiang Mai is a gateway, was particularly hard hit. Northern women make up less than

10 per cent of the overall population, but more than one-third of the country's sex workers come from this relatively poor and more rural part of the country. Thailand was now in what might be called a 'third wave' of its epidemic. These women generally were from a different social network from IDUs and the people who frequented gay bars. HIV was now spreading within a much larger group of the women themselves, their clients, and their clients' other sexual partners. As this wave grew it threatened the much larger population of sexually active adults in Thailand (Siraprapasiri *et al.*, 1994).

By 1991, HIV was about five times as common among young men in northern Thailand as in the rest of the country. Now the country was in a 'fourth wave' of the epidemic. Its most affected provinces were rural and in the north, places that typically lagged behind Bangkok in economic and social development. In 1991 tracking studies showed that about 10 per cent of men drafted into the Thai army from the upper northern part of the country were HIV positive, while only about 2 per cent of draftees from Bangkok were HIV positive. In the north, traditionally it was common for a man to start his sexual life in a brothel. On payday, during festivals and holidays, and after drinking, men go in groups to brothels. Epidemiological tracking demonstrated that the more a man went to a brothel the more likely he was to be HIV positive upon entering the army. It became increasingly clear that there was a link between the increasing incidence of HIV among army inductees and the occurrence of brothels, cafes, and massage parlors offering sex services.

The growing mass of epidemiological data caused both the Thai government and Thai society generally to take notice of what was happening. To its credit the government responded. In 1989 the Ministry of Public Health established a surveillance system to study sentinel groups, principally sex workers, soldiers, and IDUs. In 14 towns and cities around the country, teams of health workers screened high-risk individuals every six months. The information they amassed was critical to understanding what was going on (Phoolcharoen *et al.*, 1998).

Confronting Traditional Sex Roles

As time progressed it became clear that what was seen in Thailand would be applicable to the rest of Asia. Throughout Asia it has been common for men of privilege and high economic standing to have multiple wives and other sex partners. This was true in Thailand and persisted to modern times, especially in the north and other traditional communities. This time-honored pattern for the upper class was converted to a trade in young women more generally. It is not that traditional Thai, or Asian, society openly accepted sex outside marriage, but sex outside of marriage was quietly accepted. The social code permitted one type of behavior for public consumption, while it offered quiet tolerance for different behavior in private life. As long as it was not openly spoken of, men could have sex outside of marriage. This was disastrous for the spread of HIV.

Economic circumstances and traditional values combined to force some women into the sex trade. Dutiful children are supposed to be responsible for the family, including the debts of profligate and irresponsible fathers. For a young woman from a poor background this might mean having to go into the sex trade to pay off a father's gambling, drug using, and drinking debts. Again, this might be quietly accepted. A young woman would leave the village to work in the city in the sex trade and send money back home. Upon returning she would be accepted back in the village and home, but perhaps 40 per cent of returning sex workers also brought back HIV (Siraprapasiri *et al.*, 1994).

For Thais, as throughout Asia, one of the most difficult aspects of the epidemic was to openly confront the commonality of sex outside of marriage and prostitution. It is one thing to quietly allow it, but quite another to acknowledge that it could be so widespread as to spread a lethal virus that threatened the entire society. Unfortunately, conservative sexual culture plus silence offers an ideal context for transmitting HIV. The epidemiology is simple. The number of female sex workers is relatively small, but the number of their male partners is huge. Lacking education, money, freedom, and power, the female sex worker can do little to protect herself and her clients. Soon after starting to work in the sex trade, the young woman becomes infected with HIV and passes it on to many male clients. These men bring HIV home to girlfriends and wives. Women become pregnant, and fetuses and infants are exposed. This might be called the 'final wave' of the epidemic. It progressed more slowly than the prior waves, but its impact was far wider.

This scenario in Thailand was repeated elsewhere in Asia, especially in South-East Asia. In the final wave the new cases of women with HIV were usually women who had had only one sex partner in their entire life. This is being seen now in India. In addition to the pain of contracting a potentially fatal disease, the social realities are extremely painful for individuals, families, and societies overall. The years of societal and governmental denial serve to delay taking the steps needed to protect citizens. Widespread government programs were required to educate men on the need to use condoms and to establish a culture where women working in the sex trade are able to insist on condom use. Massive public education, in addition to the provision of free and low-cost condoms, is an essential preventive measure, but to do this requires the taboo to be openly acknowledged.

The Thai Government Responds

After the first in-depth risk factor studies were published in 1991 and 1992, the Thai government openly accepted that unprotected sex in brothels was the driving force behind the HIV/AIDS epidemic. The Ministry of Health did not decide to try to close brothels or arrest sex workers, but to promote safer sex through a national campaign. They called it, the '100 per cent Condom Campaign.' The Ministry distributed tens of millions of condoms to brothels, massage parlors, bars, and nightclubs. The existing national network of STD clinics started educating sex workers in condom use. Every time a sex worker came to clinic, she was given 100 free condoms, plus training. Signs were put up in even the lowest cost sex venues: 'No condom, no refund, no service.'

Outreach was performed through the efforts of public health nurses who went to sex venues. Gender-specific counseling was established. Night-shift teams visited sex venues during working hours. One team in Chiang Mai focused on gay bars; another worked with female sex workers, offering prevention services, STD care, counseling, a safe place to talk, and later anonymous HIV testing and counseling. Effort was made to deal with people on a one-to-one basis. The Ministry of Health set up research projects to monitor and clarify how the epidemic was spreading. Public health efforts were directed to reducing HIV transmission among IDUs. Needle exchange and harm reduction programs were established. One study determined that a decline in needle sharing from 20 per cent to 10 per cent would avert 21 774 new HIV infections by 2006 and 81 761 new infections by 2020 (Thai Working Group on HIV/AIDS Projections, 2001).

There was active collaboration between the Thai Army, Thai agencies and numerous NGOs from abroad, such as the Centers for Disease Control and the National Institutes of Health (NIH) in the United States, the World Health Organization, Unicef, the Thai and International Red Cross, the European Union, and university-based projects from institutions in North America and Europe. Collaborations between Chiang Mai University (CMU) in northern Thailand and Johns Hopkins University (JHU) in the United States began in 1991 and have continued. In 1992 the JHU-CMU was awarded the first of the PAVE grants (Preparation for AIDS Vaccine Evaluations) from the NIH, which supported cohort development, laboratory capacity building, and intensive behavioral research. In 1993 Thailand became the first developing country to have a national plan for HIV vaccine research. It has now done the world's first HIV vaccine efficacy trial in developing countries, and is participating in the second – clear evidence of the extraordinary commitment of Thai scientists and officials to participating in the search for solutions to the pandemic. History will show this was a remarkable effort on the part of the Thai people and its government.

Empowering Women, Protecting Society

It is a violation of human rights when Asian women acquire HIV because of mistreatment, abuse, and government negligence. The subordination of women that traditionally has been a hallmark of Asian society is one of the ugly factors that put women at risk and serves to spread the epidemic. If there is one potentially positive impact of this terrible epidemic, it is to bring to the forefront that traditional gender roles are fueling this public health tragedy and that there is an immediate need for greater social equality between women and men. This is an area in which HIV, public health, and human rights inexorably come together. Empowering women through modernizing gender roles holds promise for both combating AIDS and bettering society generally.

In traditional Asia boys are pampered and celebrated while girls are treated with disappointment and indifference. A boy is given few responsibilities in the home and offered extensive educational and career opportunities. A girl is raised to become a wife and mother. Her family saves for her dowry not her education. As a girl matures she is supposed to be silent about sex. To speak openly about it implies she is promiscuous and hence unfit for marriage (Solomon, 2003; Solomon *et al.*, 2003). She must be a virgin when she marries. Some women engage in anal intercourse, a documented risk factor for HIV transmission, in order to be virgins on their wedding night (Weiss *et al.*, 2000). Once married, a woman is judged by the number of children she has. Using a barrier contraceptive that might protect her against HIV transmission can be seen as an affront to her primary role as a mother. Research conducted in south India found that only 23 per cent of women felt comfortable encouraging condom use with their primary partner and only 5 per cent would refuse sex without a condom (Srikrishnan *et al.*, 2001). Young men also are not supposed to inquire about or discuss sex. For a man to admit lack of knowledge about sex or HIV transmission is a sign of diminished masculinity. In this covert environment dangerous myths abound, for example that having sexual intercourse with a virgin will cure a man's STD (Solomon, 2003; Solomon *et al.*, 2003).

For the most part, a young married woman has had only one sex partner, her husband, and his HIV risk becomes her risk. Before marriage she may not know his sexual history and is unlikely to bring up the subject. Once married reducing the number of sex partners for her is not an option. She cannot refuse sex, regardless of what he does. That would mean giving up children, an option few women can accept or that society would condone. She cannot insist on using a condom. Using a condom would admit he has engaged in risky behavior like having a mistress, frequenting a brothel, having sex with men or injecting drugs. And, he would have to put the condom on. Anal intercourse aside, in terms of HIV there is no higher risk sexual activity for a woman than the regular unprotected intercourse required for conceiving. Women are probably biologically more susceptible to HIV infection than men, because during vaginal intercourse the female genital tract is more vulnerable than the male genital tract to HIV. Women also more readily acquire many other STDs and this further increases their susceptibility to HIV. The female condom may prove to be an improvement, but it requires male approval. As discussed in Chapter 8, microbicides may some day prove to be an effective method of protection.

Over 40 per cent of new HIV infections occur among women globally, most through sexual transmission (UNAIDS/WHO, 2001). As in Africa (see Chapter 14), by far the most common HIV risk factor for an Asian woman is to be married. In India it is estimated that as many as 46 per cent of people with HIV are women and the majority of them acquired HIV during sexual relations with their husbands (National AIDS Control Organization, 2001). In one study, nearly 90 per cent of the women in south India reported being monogamous and marriage was their only risk factor for HIV (Newman *et al.*, 2000). It is the behavior of their husbands – typically having sex outside of marriage – that puts them at risk. These women are usually asymptomatic when they test HIV-positive; they learn they are infected with HIV in the process of going for routine prenatal care or because their husbands test positive (Kumarasamy *et al.*, 2003).

In the rapid modernization throughout much of Asia there is both promise and risk. Gender relationships are changing as Asian economies and societies move forward. Women's attitudes and their ability to assert themselves in the choice of prospective marriage partners are changing. In a study among female factory workers in northern Thailand, young women said they strongly favored men who did not visit sex workers and the sexual history of their future partners was an important criterion for marriage (Natpratan *et al.*, 1996). This is a marked contrast to their mothers' generation, where visits to sex workers were often preferred over husbands having mistresses. Young Thai women, especially in the urban middle class, are increasingly like their cohort in the West. One consequence is a greater frequency of voluntarily engaging in premarital sex, called 'serial monogamy'. This is a process of trial and error in which women and men try out their relationship. Usually it entails contraception and a greater sense of equality between the sexes than previously seen in Asian society. The recent societal acceptance of premarital sex is a risk factor in spreading HIV, while the empowering of women to be more equal partners in sexual relationships serves to reduce risk.

Perhaps the greatest threat and promise in the arena of changing sexual mores is in China and India, where there are enormous populations of young adults who are increasingly educated, mobile, and independent of traditional social patterns (Beyrer, 2003b). China is undergoing several major social transformations that interact with HIV. Social mobility, long restricted by national policy, is now possible in the new China. Since Deng Xiao-Ping's Open Door Policy, an estimated 100–110 million rural residents have left the land. This is called the 'floating population.' For the most part it is poor and poorly educated, with limited access to health care, health information, and social services. Should HIV spread in this group, and it may already have, it is uncertain whether China can and will respond effectively. Prostitution, once successfully suppressed by the Communist Party, has also made a dramatic return to China. While precise estimates are lacking, sex workers are found, sometimes in astonishing numbers, in virtually every Chinese city and town. STDs, almost eradicated from China by the 1960s, have also made a dramatic return. Syphilis rates, in particular, have more than doubled in each of the last several years (Chen *et al.*, 2000). The rapid rise in these infections is occurring in cities like Shanghai and Guangzhou, home to burgeoning sex industries and increasingly affluent young people. It is fair to say that the control of STDs, including HIV/AIDS, will be something of a test case for the new China as it will be in other parts of rapidly developing parts of Asia. China's old communist policies of tight social control that extended deep into the life of family and community were effective while brutal. They seem unlikely to return and clearly no longer are workable in this changing society and economy (Cohen *et al.*, 2000).

One of the most extreme and disturbing manifestations of the subordination of females in Asia is the trafficking in young girls and women for sexual exploitation, indentured servitude and prostitution. This practice is a modern version of slavery. It is a throwback to times when women were chattels and spoils of war. That such harsh violations of human rights exist in the twenty-first century is an outrage that demands immediate and effective international condemnation and transnational action. This is an area in which the public health community with its research tools for documenting violations and their downstream effects can have a profound impact. The trafficking of women and girls and their subsequent sexual exploitation, largely – but not exclusively – for work in prostitution, is the underpinning for a host of health problems including HIV/AIDS. Recent research work proposed a five-stage model for analysis and intervention: pre-departure travel and transit; destination; detention, deportation, and criminal evidence; and integration and reintegration. Exploited individuals face specific health-related problems at each stage; different interventions are required based on the phase the person is in. These girls and women are usually selling sex. They need screening and treatment for STDs, including HIV infection. They need professional attention to other medical conditions and to mental health. They suffer isolation, shame and fear. They feel and are trapped. Programs can assist individuals in becoming free from bondage and to advocate for change in economic, cultural, and political realities (Gushulak *et al.*, 2000; Zimmerman *et al.*, 2003).

Drug Use and Trafficking

It is estimated that 80–90 per cent of the world's heroin comes from Asia. Drug abuse and drug trafficking, particularly in injected heroin, along with the exploitation of individuals in the drug trade, are human rights problems with serious public health sequelae. The border areas between China and Burma are routes for trafficking in women for sex work. For example, sex and drug trafficking worked to spread HIV to the economic zone of Pingxiang on the highway and train crossing from Vietnam to China (Beyrer, 2001). Early in the Thai epidemic epidemiologists recognized the link between AIDS and injecting drugs. HIV in Asia spreads along known heroin trafficking routes, particularly from the Golden Triangle of South-East Asia and the Golden Crescent of Central Asia. Intravenous drug use continues to be the predominant risk factor for HIV in Malaysia and Vietnam, accounting for about 60–70 per cent of HIV infection (UNAIDS, 2000). The principal heroin producers in the Golden Triangle are the Lao People's Democratic Republic and Burma. The primary heroin producers in the Golden Crescent are Afghanistan and Pakistan (Yu *et al.*, 1999; Beyrer *et al.*, 2000a,b; Quan *et al.*, 2000). In both regions government policing is inadequate. Ethnic minorities grow the opium poppy as a much needed cash crop (US Department of State, 2002). For example, trafficking within Burma emanates from the Shan and Wa hills in the far north-eastern corner of the country, an area populated primarily by relatively independent ethnic minorities. This region is poorly controlled by the Burmese central government. Heroin moves within the country and from Mandalay, the largest city in northern Burma to India. This is a region where the association between HIV and drug trafficking is clear and striking. The prevalence of HIV among IDUs in Burma is estimated to be among the highest in the world at between 60 and 95 per cent (Myanmar Ministry of Health, 2000). Here, as in other parts of Asia, HIV eventually spread from IDUs to sex workers, IDUs' sex partners, and then to the more general population of wives and children (Beyrer, 2002).

For some time the HIV epidemic among ethnic minority drug users in China was largely restricted to an area running east along the Burma border in Yunnan Province. For many years this has been a first destination point for heroin export from Burma to China. Nearby Vietnam also has been affected. However, the problem then spread to other provinces with a significant rise in the prevalence of HIV among IDUs (Yu *et al.*, 1996). The current UNAIDS estimate is that there are perhaps 500 000 cumulative infections in this population, but there is concern that the virus may be spreading rapidly. It must be emphasized that the estimates are highly imprecise. Dramatic increases in both drug use and HIV have also been noted in Xinjiang Province in the north-west, which now has the highest population rate of HIV after Yunnan (Shao *et al.*, 1999). Guangxi Province, on the border with Vietnam, is the third most affected area, again largely among drug users of ethnic minority origin. Large in geography and population, and poor in socio-economic status, Sichuan Province in the south-west has the fourth highest number of AIDS cases. In addition to poverty, isolation, and the misfortune of being on known heroin trafficking routes, these provinces all have a high proportion of ethnic minorities in their populations. The extent to which these people are neglected by the central government is a health and human rights issue.

DNA fingerprinting technology has been used effectively to trace HIV variants and track the epidemic. The work documents a tight connection between heroin trafficking, uptake of injection drug use, and HIV spread (Beyrer *et al.*, 2000b). It also supports the connection between civil strife, drug trafficking, and HIV. Tracking studies from Burma, Laos, and Afghanistan verify the connection between the narcotics economy and insurgencies (Momoura *et al.*, 2000). Civil strife and inadequate policing are present in these areas, along with a paucity of health services in areas where there is civil strife.

Asia has lagged behind Europe and North America in establishing harm reduction and drug treatment programs (Gray, 1995; Des Jarlais and Friedman, 1998). Pilot projects have been set up in India, Nepal, and Vietnam, but their scope is limited. Except perhaps in Thailand, there has not been sufficient acknowledgment that these services are needed. With support from Médecins Sans Frontières and the Soros Foundation, the Russian Far East and Vietnam are virtually the only Asian states with active harm reduction programs for drug users. China, Malaysia, and Burma have very limited treatment programs, or focus, as in Malaysia, almost exclusively on incarceration. This is a human rights and health issue. Needle exchange programs are, of course, feasible in Asia; the question is one of political will and societal acceptance. The obstacles to setting up these programs appear to fall into three categories. First, they are seen as condoning or facilitating injecting drug use. Second, they face legal, security, and policy challenges. 'Safe' domains have to be set up where IDUs can get treatment, education, and referral without risking arrest. A third issue is to insure adequate funding and coverage. Unsafe injection practices promote epidemics of other blood-borne pathogens, like hepatitis C. The underlying need is clear. The problem is societal acceptance and governmental implementation.

At this point, far less is known about the interaction of the heroin trade and HIV in the Golden Crescent than is known about the epidemics in South and South-East Asia. It is generally assumed that the incidence of HIV is much lower in Afghanistan and Pakistan than it is along the trafficking routes of the Golden Triangle. Data are limited. Time will tell how these parts of Asia will be affected.

Blood Transfusion

China has seen an HIV threat arise via its blood supply and the problem exists in other developing areas of Asia. It is not well documented, but may emerge in coming years as a more significant challenge than heroin trafficking. There is mounting evidence of HIV transmission among paid professional blood *donors*, as well as recipients. Chinese culture has strong traditional restrictions on blood donation. Blood is seen as a vital essence. Removing it from the body is viewed as a threat to health. This led to chronic shortages of blood for transfusion and the development of a lucrative industry in procuring and selling blood and blood products. Private, often unlicensed firms, buy blood from young adults in impoverished rural zones for sale in urban centers. Blood collection techniques in this shadow industry have been inadequate. Equipment is reused, with inadequate attention to sterilization and with insufficient screening of donors. The result has been rural areas with very high rates of HIV and other blood-borne diseases, including hepatitis B, hepatitis C, and syphilis. Beijing hurriedly passed new legislation to outlaw these practices, but enforcement has been sporadic and ineffective (Beyrer, 2003a). Past experiences with government failures to control unsafe blood supplies in Japan and France suggest that this situation is potentially explosive from a political, as well as a public health perspective. The Chinese authorities sought to suppress information from the scientific community that highlighted the negligence. Both the repression of the medical professionals who brought this situation

389

to light and the lack of government oversight of the transfusion system are public health and human rights issues.

India also has serious and unresolved issues related to the safety of blood supplies and medical procedures. WHO estimated in 1998 that perhaps a fifth of all of India's infections, up to 1 million cases, were due to improperly screened blood and blood products. And again, young mothers, with high rates of anemia in pregnancy and frequent needs for transfusions after delivery, have been disproportionately affected. After years of denial and inaction about the safety of the blood system the Indian government is responding. India is a democracy and its political culture differs from that of other states in Asia. Its leaders are more accountable. The problems facing India are daunting, particularly given her huge population of young, poor, illiterate and socially marginalized citizens.

Widening Access to Modern Care

There is an immediate need to make modern antiretroviral therapy (ART) and medical services available to all individuals, regardless of socio-economic status and nationality. This is a human rights issue, as well as a medical necessity. Without medical therapy HIV infection is still largely a death sentence. At the time of this writing, there are probably at least 7–8 million people in Asia living with HIV/AIDS. Even if the most effective and robust preventive measures are implemented quickly, there almost certainly will be additional individuals infected with the virus. Should these individuals not get modern ART, the death toll will be enormous.

Time is of the essence to do what is needed. To date relatively few Asians with HIV/AIDS have access to state-of-the-art ART and the medical follow-up required for treatment to be effective. Thailand is arguably the furthest along among the mid-lower income states. Access to highly active antiretroviral therapy (HAART) is close to universal in the wealthy states, such as Japan and Singapore, but these countries have relatively small numbers of patients requiring care. Asian nations generally have limited nationally funded public health systems, as they exist in Western Europe and Canada. While the United States does not have a national health system, people with HIV have access to testing and treatment through private insurance and public programs. In Asia it is a wholly different matter. For example Thai citizens have some access to antiretroviral medications, but Burmese and Laotians, particularly in the mountain zones, cannot access HIV testing, much less AIDS care (Cohen, 2003).

India is a prime example of the problems that must be addressed in Asia and the hurdles to overcome in doing so. After South Africa, India has the second highest number of AIDS cases. Even at US$1 a day, the cost of ART is far beyond what the poor can pay (India's average per capita income is about US$500 a year). Nehru's India started on a socialist model, but she was far too poor to provide universal health care. While India is fortunate to have a generic drug industry that manufactures most of the known antiretroviral medications, the government has yet to develop a comprehensive agreement with the industry on pricing and supplying the drugs.

But India is taking note of the immediate need. In November 2003 the government announced its intention to provide free ART to HIV-positive new parents and children under 15 in the six states with the highest prevalence of infection. To that point, ART had been available to prevent mother–child transmission, but otherwise not to any significant extent compared to the reality on the ground. The stated goal of the Indian government is to eventually provide ART to all individuals with AIDS. This will take some time and in order to succeed, the government will have to work out agreements with the nation's pharmaceutical industry, expand health delivery systems for testing and treatment follow-up, and effectively integrate a huge influx of international assistance.

Until now HIV/AIDS programs in India have been funded primarily by international donors. The Global Fund to Fight AIDS, TB, and Malaria has promised US$100 million in support over the upcoming five years. Other international donors, such as the World Bank, the World Health Organization, and the Bill and Melinda Gates Foundation have been prominent in helping India with its HIV/AIDS epidemic. Much more needs to be done to make treatment for the poor a reality. The effort is going to be extremely complicated and challenging. One positive downstream effect may be to modernize and extend the primary health care system: out of a negative may come a positive (Waldman, 2003).

The good news is there are emerging examples of programs that demonstrate a comprehensive approach to prevention and care. YRG CARE (Y.R. Gaitonde Centre for AIDS Research and Education) is one example. It is a non-profit organization that offers voluntary counseling and testing (VCT), prevention, and care services in Chennai, India. In the last 10 years, over 7900 clients have accessed VCT services. The center is unique in two regards: it provides referral care to its 6000 registered patients to its own hospital of 21 beds and an intensive care unit, and it was among the first in India to prescribe generic HAART. On an ongoing basis, the center evaluates the financial ability of patients to procure HAART and to maintain adherence to treatment regimens. Currently the center is one of the largest private purchasers of generic HAART in the country (Figure 15.2).

In 1998, the annual per patient cost of a protease inhibitor-based HAART regimen reached upwards of Rs. 31 000 (current exchange rate, US$1 = Rs. 45). Since that time prices have steadily declined, and the introduction of generic nevirapine in 1999 to the India market has allowed prices to reach Rs. 1400 by the end of 2002 for a non-nucleoside-based HAART regimen. Currently nevirapine-based HAART is available in India as a one-pill, twice-daily combination. Improved availability and affordability of generic HAART appears to encourage patients to come for VCT, perhaps because HIV is no longer perceived to be a fatal disease. Nevertheless, social stigma remains a profound hurdle (YRG Base Care Model Report, 2004).

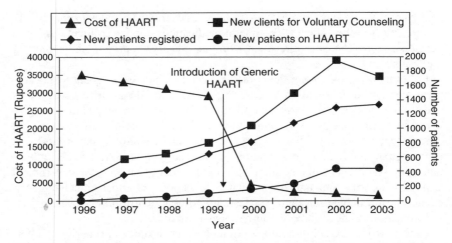

Fig. 15.2 Cost of antiretrovirals provided by YRG Care, Chennai, India, 1996–2003.

What the Future Holds

Asia does not currently face the same crushing AIDS burden as much of Africa. Yet, there is clear and compelling evidence that many nations already have severe epidemics and others are currently undergoing early phases that may presage future wide spread. The window of opportunity to respond to HIV in Asia may be narrow and closing. The time for immediate action is now. To date the experience of Asian nations in recognizing and confronting the challenges is diverse. A consequence of this uneven experience is that while the risks are known, the future is difficult to calculate. Truth is, the epidemic must be engaged on a variety of the battlefields discussed earlier: injection drug use and drug trafficking, the sex trade and trafficking in young girls and women, the empowerment of women generally, sex education and the provision of condoms, insuring the safety of the blood supply, improving access to primary health care for the poor, and access to antiretroviral medications for individuals already infected with HIV. In every aspect, much more needs to be done to provide up-to-date medical treatment for people living with HIV and AIDS. The extent of East–West cooperation will be an indication of the willingness of Asian states to admit and deal with the problem.

There is an immediate need to deal with injecting drug use. Opium, heroin, and amphetamine production in Burma, Afghanistan, and Laos, as well as the ready availability of drugs throughout the region are challenges for the foreseeable future. Heroin from Central Asia, including Tajikistan, and potentially Turkmenistan, may further complicate control efforts. States that already have a significant number of IDUs with or at-risk for AIDS include the Central Asian Republics of the former Soviet Union, especially Kazakhstan; and China, India, Thailand, Burma, Malaysia, and Vietnam. The potential for epidemic spread among drug users in Pakistan and Iran is there. Throughout Asia there is a general lack of attention to drug treatment and harm reduction measures that might mitigate the spread of HIV. Thailand has voluntary drug detoxification services, but does not currently allow methadone maintenance. Vietnam and the Russian Far East (with support from Médecins Sans Frontières and the Soros Foundation) are virtually the only Asian states with active harm reduction programs for drug users. China, Malaysia, and Burma have very limited treatment programs or focus, as in Malaysia, almost exclusively on incarceration.

Immediate transnational attention must be directed against the trafficking of women and girls for sex work and in what amounts to modern day slavery. Trafficking in women occurs across Asia. It is a despicable practice that makes HIV prevention a complex and politically sensitive issue. Source countries from which significant numbers of women are trafficked include Burma, Thailand, Vietnam, Russia, Uzbekistan, Nepal, Laos, China, and the Philippines. Destination countries include Thailand, China, Cambodia, India, Russia, Sweden, the United States, and the European Union. Countries in which trafficking of women occurs within the state for the domestic sex industry include China, Russia, India, Thailand, Cambodia, and Burma. Trafficking and sexual slavery are human rights abuses and crimes against the individual. All of the countries listed above, say the United States, are signatories to the United Nations Convention on the Rights of the Child, which explicitly bars both trafficking and child sex work. Yet in 2000, the trafficking industry appears, if anything, to be increasing. A social and personal harm in its own right, this is a major source of HIV epidemic potential, and one that will require regional and international cooperation to resolve.

Beyond the sex trade, Asia has large populations of internal migrants, migrant laborers, internally displaced persons, refugees, and workers in industries requiring mobility such as fisheries, shipping, trucking, and trade. As is Africa, social mobility has played important roles in HIV spread and is likely to be a growing source of social vulnerability. Crucial populations at risk include the 1–1.2 million Burmese refugees and migrants in Thailand, China, India, Bangladesh, and Malaysia; a large number, probably more than 3 million of Afghans in Pakistan; and migrant and/or overseas workers from Thailand, the Philippines, Indonesia, Laos, and other states. Asia's labor and migration laws lag strikingly behind what is needed to protect these individuals. Policies for workers and migrants with HIV are contradictory, often punitive, and often beset by barriers to providing preventive services and care that might limit the spread of HIV.

Frank and effective sexual health education and programs are woefully inadequate across Asia, and have been limited by a wide range of social, cultural, religious, and, in the case of the several communist states, political barriers to practical and evidence-based policies. While some states, including Thailand and South Korea, have been successful in implementing effective sexual health programs through Family Planning services, many lag sharply. Where political or social barriers are easing, the lack of local expertise will remain a barrier.

The social status of women and girls, and with it their educational and economic opportunities, must modernize. The everyday subordination of women that is the result of traditional Asian gender roles is perhaps the most important risk factor to be tackled. The majority of Asian women currently infected with HIV, plus the number who may in the future become infected, are young, married, and monogamous. They are the victims of their husbands' behavior. Subordinate social status, long-established sexual mores, a lack of education and poverty are known underpinnings of the powerlessness that women face in the traditional family setting. These women are unable to insist on spousal monogamy, deny sexual relations to their husbands or require their husbands to use condoms. Their future infants and children also are at risk. If not confronted openly on a societal level, these issues pose an enormous challenge to Asian mores. Yet, the subordination of women is an undeniable underpinning for a widespread heterosexual epidemic. India, Nepal, Pakistan, and Bangladesh are especially vulnerable, but no Asian nation is immune.

Attention must be directed to improving the safety of blood and blood products, and the safe delivery of these products through the health care pipeline. The World Health Organization estimated that in 2000 only one-third of the world's blood supply could be considered safely screened for HIV and other blood-borne infections (UNAIDS, 2002). In Japan, South Korea, Thailand, Taiwan, Singapore, and Malaysia this issue was resolved in the late 1980s. However, major problems with blood safety will continue to be a serious problem in many nations. Donor aid and enhanced political will are required in many countries, especially India, China, Russia, Nepal, Bangladesh, Burma, Cambodia, Laos, and Papua New Guinea. This process could be politically contentious in China and India, where official inaction, corruption, and profiteering in the blood products industry remain significant barriers to reform.

The Armed Forces also have a major role to play in HIV prevention and face important security issues if they fail to prevent HIV among their troops. HIV is an STD. Prevention programs directed at STDs have been a regular part of military health services since at least World War I. The UNTAC experience, where HIV spread rapidly among troops of the Indian, Pakistani, Indonesia, US, and Uruguayan armies, should stand as a warning to all concerned. The Thai prevention program directed at military recruits through condom promotion and sexual health education is the best example for how to do this effectively. Young men in the military are a high-risk group that must be targeted with strong prevention measures.

Based on what has been discussed, it is perhaps helpful to suggest a practical Asian Action Plan.

1. End official denial. It will take political will to make necessary policy changes. Resource-constrained governments must partner openly with international organizations.

2. Start seeing HIV/AIDS as a public health and human rights problem.
3. Reform and expand drug treatment and harm reduction for injecting drug users.
4. Develop national programs to disseminate frank sexual health messages. Target all at-risk groups with appropriate programs for adolescents, young adults, and women and men of childbearing age.
5. Institute effective regulation and monitoring of blood safety and supplies and implement universal precautions in health care settings.
6. Establish intensive prevention programs for military and police, particularly troops involved in international peacekeeping.
7. Recognize the rights of sex workers. Provide sex workers with condoms, along with testing and education. The Thai experience teaches that sex workers can be empowered to require condom use.
8. Establish cooperative regional and transnational programs against the trafficking of women and girls into the sex industry.
9. Establish antidiscrimination laws to protect people living with HIV and their families.
10. Develop government support for orphaned children to attend school.
11. Build funding for HIV/AIDS impact assessments and prevention programs into development projects that are planned throughout Asia over the next decade, such as highways, bridges, and other infrastructure.
12. Make a commitment to honest scientific inquiry regarding the epidemiology of the HIV transmission and to impartial evaluation of prevention and treatment efforts.
13. Make a commitment to developing the health care infrastructure necessary to provide everyone with HIV access to effective antiretroviral treatments.

References

Beyrer C (1998) *War in the Blood: Sex, Politics, and AIDS in Southeast Asia*. London: Zed Books/New York: St. Martins Press.
Beyrer C (2001) Shan women and girls and the sex industry in South-east Asia; political causes and human rights implications. *Soc Sci Med* 53: 543–50.
Beyrer C (2002) Human immunodeficiency virus (HIV) infection rates and heroin trafficking: fearful symmetries. *Bull Narcotics* LIV: 103–16.
Beyrer C (2003a) An epidemic of denial: stalled responses to HIV/AIDS in China. *Harvard Int Rev* 25.
Beyrer C (2003b) Hidden epidemic of sexually transmitted diseases in China: crisis and opportunity. *JAMA* 289: 1303–5.
Beyrer C, Razak MH, Lisam K, Wei L, Chen J, Yu XF (2000a) Overland heroin trafficking routes and HIV-1 spread in South and Southeast Asia. *AIDS* 14: 75–83.
Beyrer C, Razak MH, Chen J, Yu XF (2000b) Patterns of HIV spread associated with drug trafficking. *Proceedings of the Global Research Network Third Annual Meeting*, Durban.

Chen XS, Gong XD, Liang GJ, Zhang GC (2000) Epidemiologic trends of sexually transmitted diseases in China. *Sex Transm Dis* 27: 138–42.

Cohen J (2003) AIDS in Asia. *Science* 301(5640): 1613–1796.

Cohen MS, Ping G, Fox K, Henderson GE (2000) Sexually transmitted diseases in the People's Republic of China in Y2K: back to the future. *Sex Transm Dis* 27: 143–5.

Crofts N, Reid G, Deany P (1998) Injecting drug use and HIV infection in Asia: The Asian Harm Reduction Network. *AIDS* 12 (Suppl B): S69–78.

Des Jarlais DC, Friedman SR (1998) Fifteen years of research on preventing HIV infection among injecting drug users: what we have learned, what we have not learned, what we have done, what we have not done. *Public Health Rep* 113 (Suppl 1): 182–8.

Gangakhedkar R, Bentley ME, Divekar AD *et al.* (1997) Spread of HIV infection in married monogamous women in India. *JAMA* 278: 2090–2.

Gray J (1995) Operating needle exchange programmes in the hills of Thailand. *AIDS Care* 7: 489–99.

Gushulak BD, MacPherson DW (2000) Health issues associated with the smuggling and trafficking of migrants. *J Immigrant Health* 2: 67–78.

Kumarasamy N, Solomon S, Flanigan T, Hemalatha R, Thyagarajan SP, Mayer K (2003) Natural History of HIV disease in Southern India. *Clin Infect Dis* 36: 79–85.

Manipur State Department of Health Services (1997) Status paper on implementation of national AIDS control programme (Manipur) Imphal, November.

Motomura K, Kusagawa S, Kato K *et al.* (2000) Emergence of new forms of human immunodeficiency virus type 1 intersubtype recombinants in central Myanmar. *AIDS Res Hum Retroviruses* 16: 1831–43.

Myanmar Ministry of Health (2000) *National HIV/AIDS Sentinel Surveillance Reports, 1998, 1999,* Yangon.

National AIDS Control Organization (2001) *Surveillance for HIV Infection/AIDS Cases in India.* Ministry of Health and Family Welfare, Government of India.

Natpratan C, Nantakwan D, Beyrer C *et al.* (1996) Feasibility of Northern Thai factory workers for HIV vaccine trials. *Southeast Asian J Trop Med Public Health* 27: 457–62.

Nelson KE, Celentano DD, Eiumtrakul S *et al.* (1996) Changes in sexual behavior and a decline in HIV infection among young men in Thailand. *N Engl J Med* 335: 297–303.

Newman S, Sarin P, Kumarasamy N *et al.* (2000) Marriage, monogamy, and HIV: a profile of HIV-infected women in South India. *Int J STD AIDS* 11: 250–3.

Quan VM, Chung A, Long HT, Dondero TJ (2000) HIV in Vietnam: the evolving epidemic and the prevention response. *J Acquir Immune Defic Syndr* 25: 360–9.

Phoolcharoen W, Ungchusak K, Sittitrai W, Brown T (1998) Thailand: lessons from a strong national response to HIV/AIDS. *AIDS* 12 (Suppl B): S123–35.

Shao Y, Su L, Sun XH *et al.* (1999) Molecular epidemiology of HIV infections in China. Paper presented at the Fifth International Congress in AIDS in Asia and the Pacific, Kuala Lumpur.

Siraprapasiri T, Ungchusak K, Thanprasertsuk S, Akarasewi P (1994) HIV seroconversion rates among female sex workers in Chiang Mai, Thailand: a multi cross-sectional study. *AIDS* 8: 825–9.

Solomon S (2003) Stopping HIV infection before it begins in women. Paper presented at the 10th Conference on Retroviruses and Opportunistic Infections, Boston, MA, oral abstract 114.

Solomon S, Buck J, Chaguturu SK, Ganesh AK, Kumarasamy N (2003) Stopping HIV before it begins: issues faced by women in India. *Nat Immunol* 4: 719–21.

Srikrishnan AK, Morrow K, Ganesh AK *et al.* (2001) Same risks, disparate perceptions: challenges to microbicide acceptability in the Chennai Community. Paper presented at the 6th International Conference on HIV/AIDS in Asia and the Pacific, Melbourne, abstract #O777.

Thai Working Group on HIV/AIDS Projections (2001) *Projections of HIV/AIDS in Thailand, 2000–2020*. Bangkok: Thailand, Ministry of Public Health, AIDS Division.

UNAIDS (United Nations Joint Programme on HIV/AIDS) (2000) *Report on the Global AIDS Epidemic*. Geneva: UNAIDS.

UNAIDS (2002) *Report on the Global HIV/AIDS Epidemic*. Geneva: UNAIDS.

UNAIDS (2003) *Report on the Global HIV/AIDS Epidemic*. Geneva: UNAIDS.

UNAIDS/WHO (Joint United Nations Programme on HIV/AIDS and World Health Organization) (2001) *AIDS Epidemic Update: 2001*. Geneva: UNAIDS/WHO.

UNDCP (United Nations Drug Control Program) (2000) *Annual Report 2000*. Vienna: UNDCP.

US Department of State, Bureau of International Narcotics and Law Enforcement Affairs (2002) *International Narcotics Control Strategy Report*. Washington, DC: US Department of State.

Waldman A (2003) India plans free AIDS therapy. *New York Times* 1 December.

Weiss E, Whelan D, Rao GG (2000) Gender, sexuality and HIV: making a difference in the lives of young women in developing countries. *Sex Relationship Ther* 15: 233–45.

Weniger BG, Limpakarnjanarat K, Ungchusak K *et al.* (1991) The epidemiology of HIV infection and AIDS in Thailand. *AIDS* 5 (Suppl 2): S71–S85.

Yu EHS, Xie Q, Zhang K, Lu P, Chan LL (1996) HIV infection and AIDS in China, 1985 through 1994. *Am J Public Health* 86: 1116–22.

Yu XF, Chen J, Shao Y, Beyrer C *et al.* (1999) Emerging HIV infections with distinct sub-types of HIV-12 infection among injections drug users from geographically separate locations in Gunagxi Province, China. *J Acquir Immune Defic Syndr* 22: 180–8.

YRG Base Care Model Report (2004) Integrated prevention, care, and support services. http://www.popcouncil.org/pdfs/horizons/yrgcrbsmdl.pdf (accessed 21 April 2004).

Zimmerman C, Yun K, Watts C *et al.* (2003) The health risks and consequences of trafficking in women and adolescents: findings from a European study. London. *Lancet* 363: 565.

How HIV/AIDS Changed Gay Life in America – And What Others Can Learn from Our Experience

16

John-Manuel Andriote
Washington, DC, USA

John-Manuel Andriote has reported on HIV/AIDS since finishing a
master's degree at Northwestern University's Medill School of Journalism
in 1986. His award-winning 1999 book *Victory Deferred: How AIDS
Changed Gay Life in America* (University of Chicago Press) was hailed
by *Kirkus Reviews* as, "The most important AIDS chronicle since Randy
Shilts' *And the Band Played On.*" After three years as senior editor for
Family Health International's Institute for HIV/AIDS, Andriste in 2004
formed Health & Science Reporting (www.hsreporting.com), a Washington
DC-based consulting practice providing documentation services to HIV/
AIDS and other health projects working in the developing world.

We have made great strides in the United States toward managing HIV infection as
a chronic condition rather than the always-fatal illness it was in the 1980s. Today
stories abound of people with AIDS brought back from the brink of death – what
has been called a 'Lazarus experience', thanks to the combination therapies of
antiretroviral medications that emerged in the mid-1990s. By the time the AIDS
epidemic reached its two-decade mark, American AIDS service organizations
had added return-to-the-workforce programs to their service menus as living with
HIV became more common than dying from AIDS, at least in the United States.

But those fortunate enough to have access to antiretroviral drugs comprise only a
small fraction of the estimated 40 million people worldwide living with HIV/AIDS,

398

the vast majority of them in developing countries with marginal health care services and limited resources. An astonishing 23 million men, women, and children already have died from AIDS, most of them in sub-Saharan Africa. Political leaders, such as the current president of the United States, who refused to address the pandemic on public health and humanitarian grounds alone, seem finally to be realizing that HIV/AIDS – exactly like terrorism – is a threat to national security.

The premature deaths of extraordinary numbers of young, working-age citizens threaten to undermine already-fragile economies in countries south of the equator. Not only that but, much like the anger that fuels terrorism, HIV/AIDS festers and spreads amidst poverty and hopelessness. People without hope and a healthy self-respect do not typically make healthy choices, for themselves or their sexual partners. This is why caring for the infected and preventing the spread of HIV are as much about instilling hope and nurturing prospects for a productive future as they are about delivering antiretroviral medications and instructing on safer sex.

Today the world is realizing that gay people were not crying wolf in the 1980s when we shouted and demanded attention and resources for a deadly epidemic that was killing people we knew and loved – and would not go away, no matter how assiduously it was ignored, denied, and blamed on gay men. At last, larger, more realistic amounts of money are beginning to be channeled to the world's hardest-hit countries, already staggering beneath the weight of poverty, inadequate health care services and cultural attitudes that stigmatize the infected and prevent those who most need it from receiving HIV testing and treatment.

But even in the United States, particularly among its gay male residents, we are still far from where we need to be. By the end of 2002, some 886 575 AIDS cases had been reported in the US since 1981. Of them, nearly 500 000 were men who had been at risk of infection through sex with other men (CDC, 2002). It is stating the obvious to say that HIV/AIDS still disproportionately threatens American men of all races who have sex with other men (the CDC calls them MSM regardless of how they choose to label their sexual behavior). A resurgence of new sexually transmitted diseases (STDs) and HIV infection related to drug abuse among certain segments of the gay community beginning in the late 1990s shows us that HIV prevention must both continue and be continually updated to be relevant for each new generation. Even the not-so-young need to be reminded that sex still carries the same risks today as it did when we first heard of AIDS.

This chapter looks at the variety of ways in which gay Americans organized responses to HIV/AIDS in the 1980s and 1990s. It aims to show the many ways AIDS changed gay life in America, as well as how gay people shaped and influenced America's response to the epidemic. It explores some of the lessons gay Americans learned that can benefit individuals, communities, and even countries facing their own growing epidemics. It recalls the earliest efforts to organize care and support services for the ill, prevent the spread of HIV using targeted and explicit education, and transform the culture of medicine by empowering patients to be informed consumers of health care services. It looks at what gay people learned about doing politics in Washington and the value of working within coalitions of supportive organizations. It describes how even the creative, politically charged mourning rituals gay people created were aimed at reducing the stigma associated with HIV/AIDS.

Using a narrative, journalistic style, the chapter draws from the published literature as well as the first-hand experiences recounted in hundreds of original interviews I conducted across the country as part of my research for *Victory Deferred: How AIDS Changed Gay Life in America* (University of Chicago Press, 1999). These are the people who took great personal risks and suffered tremendous personal losses to bring about extraordinary change at so many levels that we can't accurately say HIV/AIDS changed only gay life in America; in fact, gay America's determined response to the epidemic changed the nation itself, and continues to change the world.

Mobilizing the Community

At the beginning of the AIDS epidemic, gay people were fortunate to have had gay and lesbian doctors and other health care professionals who could advocate within their agencies and organizations for appropriate resources and attention to address the growing health crisis. Prominent gay people, whether politically inclined or not, stepped forward and urged others to rise to the challenges posed by the deadly combination of homophobic prejudice and a mysterious new illness that seemed to be selectively targeting gay men. The outcome was a tremendous outpouring of volunteer time and energy as gay Americans were forced to create a parallel system of health and social service organizations specifically to care for people with HIV/AIDS who could not find compassionate, professional care in the mainstream. They showed the country and the world what people can accomplish when they refuse to bow to the shame society attaches to HIV/AIDS and accept their part in addressing the epidemic – whether it means caring for an ill friend or creating an entire organization to serve friends and strangers alike.

Gay Leaders Step Forward

Larry Kramer had kept a low profile after the uproar over his novel *Faggots* in 1978. Many in the New York gay scene, in which Kramer himself had participated, felt he had betrayed them by daring to expose the spiritual bankruptcy of the frenzied promiscuity that permeated 1970s gay life in New York City. Some condemned Kramer as a self-hating moralist, deriding his book and demanding that no one read it. But in August of 1981, only a month after the first AIDS cases were reported among gay men, Kramer wrote in the *New York Native*, 'This is our disease and we must take care of each other and ourselves' (Kramer, 1989, p. 9).

The same month, Kramer hosted a meeting at his Manhattan apartment of gay men interested in learning what little was then known about the strange diseases that already had killed some of their friends. The following January, Kramer and five other gay men – Nathan Fain, Larry Mass, Paul Popham, Paul Rapoport, and Edmund White – gathered again at Kramer's apartment. From their meeting came an organization they called, straightforwardly, Gay Men's Health Crisis (GMHC), which they created as a means to share information with gay men and raise money for medical research. Many gay people across the country would come to share the view of these men that if 'straight' hospitals and health care providers wouldn't provide compassionate, non-judgmental care for gay men with AIDS then 'we' would take care of 'our people' ourselves.

As with many AIDS organizations that formed in later years, GMHC's first service was a hotline, originally nothing more than the answering service of Rodger McFarlane, Kramer's boyfriend at the time and the first paid director of GMHC. GMHC was initially a kind of ad hoc committee of volunteers who contributed time and created services according to their interests and abilities. Larry Kramer recalled, 'We almost allowed anybody to do anything if they seemed responsible and passionate about it, whether it was doing an epidemiological study, or wanting to start a buddy system, or translating some stuff into Spanish that we would give out in the bars, or designing a brochure, or putting out a newsletter. We didn't have an office; we met in different people's apartments every week' (L Kramer, personal communication, 4 March 1995).

GMHC, the world's first AIDS service organization (ASO), was a model and inspiration for other groups across the country and, literally, around the world. By the late 1980s, hundreds of ASOs had been founded in big cities and small towns experiencing on a smaller scale the impact AIDS was having by then in the big coastal cities, particularly New York, Los Angeles, and San Francisco, all of them home to large numbers of gay men. Besides GMHC the largest, earliest ASOs were AIDS Project Los Angeles, the K.S. Foundation (now the San Francisco AIDS Foundation), the Northwest AIDS Foundation in Seattle, AID Atlanta and the AIDS Action Committee in Boston.

Beginnings of a Gay Health Network and Movement

In addition to the ASOs created specifically to address HIV/AIDS, the gay health care 'infrastructure' at the start of the epidemic included a small, loosely linked national network of STD clinics created in the 1970s to treat the sexual infections running rampant among gay men at the time. These clinics included the Fenway Community Health Center in Boston, the Howard Brown Health Center in Chicago and Whitman-Walker Clinic in Washington, DC. By the time AIDS appeared these agencies already were established in their local gay communities and credibly non-judgmental, so they added HIV/AIDS-related services to their repertoire of 'gay' health issues.

Another important factor in gay America's ability to mount a response to AIDS was the gay men and lesbians employed in the health care professions. Their networking led to the 1976 formation of the National Gay Health Coalition. The coalition was created to provide gay health professionals with a means for sharing data and experience. It also facilitated relationships between the gay and lesbian interest groups that were formed within a number of health-related organizations and with the community-level gay health services, community centers, political organizations and periodicals (Lear, 1984).

Still another cornerstone of gay America's response to AIDS were the ties established in the 1970s between gay physicians working through community clinics with pharmaceutical companies, and government scientists when they collaborated in testing and, in 1978, licensing a vaccine to prevent hepatitis B. In the hepatitis B studies, conducted through gay health centers, gay physicians developed rapport and credibility with government researchers – and vice versa. These relationships proved mutually beneficial in the coming years, providing researchers with at least a basic understanding of gay sexuality and access to community leaders and offering gay people a link to emerging scientific information about AIDS. These relationships also would contribute significantly to bringing gay people into the mainstream of medical research.

A Tremendous Outpouring of Support

By the time of its first anniversary, in 1983, GMHC had grown from its original six founders to more than 300 volunteers. GMHC's board noted in its second newsletter that the group had raised more than US$150 000; distributed 25 000 copies of its first, and 110 000 copies of its second, newsletter; produced 300 000 brochures (in English, Spanish, Creole, and French); fielded almost 5000 hotline calls; formed a network of 'buddies' to provide practical support for people with AIDS; provided legal and financial advisers; organized community forums; trained medical professionals; and served as a source of information about AIDS for the news media. All of its services were provided by volunteers and were offered free. Written by Kramer, the GMHC board statement in the newsletter continued, 'We have never encountered so much love as we have felt at GMHC, and watching this organization grow in response to our community's terrible new needs has been one of the most moving experiences we have ever been privileged to share' (Kramer, 1989, p. 30).

Preventing the Spread of HIV

Creating 'sex-positive' HIV/AIDS prevention education seemed natural to gay men who already were living their lives and embracing their sexual orientation

402

openly and with pride. Even before HIV itself was discovered, in 1984, some gay health leaders already had developed viable guidelines for 'safer' sex to prevent the transmission of whatever 'it' was causing AIDS. They knew, and government scientists confirmed, that the most effective prevention messages used the language and images of their intended audience. 'Targeted and explicit' education became the norm for information about safer sex and HIV/AIDS developed by and for gay men. Despite efforts to suppress or dilute the sometimes very explicit educational campaigns by condemning them as 'obscene,' the programs showed that frank information shared in a respectful way with those who most need it is more effective than moral pronouncements and generic information aimed at raising the general public's awareness. But the programs also found that prevention efforts need to be continually adapted and tailored to young people who may not yet have been sexually active or attuned when earlier prevention messages were created.

Defining 'Safe Sex'

At the Fifth National Lesbian and Gay Health Conference and Second National AIDS Forum, in Denver, in June 1983, San Francisco psychologist Steve Morin was one of the presenters in a workshop on 'Creating Positive Changes in Sexual Mores.' Morin worked with the Bay Area Physicians for Human Rights (BAPHR) to categorize sexual activities into safe, possibly safe, and unsafe practices. As defined by BAPHR, 'safe sex' includes mutual masturbation, social kissing, body massage and hugging, body-to-body rubbing, 'light S&M activities,' and using one's own sex toys. 'Possibly safe' practices include anal intercourse with a condom, 'fellatio interruptus,' mouth-to-mouth kissing, urine contact, vaginal intercourse with a condom, and oral–vaginal contact. 'Unsafe sex' practices include receptive and insertive anal intercourse without a condom, 'manual–anal' intercourse, fellatio, oral–anal contact, and vaginal intercourse without a condom (Peyton, 1989).

In New York, GMHC persisted in telling gay men simply to limit their number of sexual partners and make sure their partners were 'healthy,' a message the K.S. Foundation, in San Francisco, had issued in 1982, before the BAPHR guidelines. GMHC did not want to offend gay men by presuming to tell them anything about specific sexual practices. Sexual freedom had been claimed in the 1970s as the reward for so many years of hatred and repression of gay life, and many, including GMHC, were unwilling to sound like the institutions that had long condemned homosexuals. While San Franciscans had moved on to the soon-to-be-proven assumption that the cause of AIDS was probably an infectious agent, New Yorkers took the attitude that, unless they could present irrefutable evidence, they couldn't expect gay men to listen.

Like the disagreement between the New Yorkers and San Franciscans over what, exactly, was safe sex, the gay community's earliest efforts to translate scientific information about AIDS into educational messages for gay men were pulled in two directions. Some believed that whatever was said had to be couched in 'sex-positive' language, while others believed the only way that gay men would change their behavior was if they were scared enough to do so. In late 1983, the San Francisco AIDS Foundation produced a poster depicting two naked men embracing, with the caption 'You Can Have Fun and Be Safe Too.' Respectful of gay men who had all their lives been told they were 'sick' for loving other men the poster was explicit and positive, yet subtle, in its message and caused an uproar among non-gay San Franciscans (Altman, 1986).

Another group in San Francisco believed a fear-based campaign was needed to discourage gay men from having sex at all. Their materials depicted an hourglass with blood-colored sand pouring into the bottom with the slogan 'Time is Running Out.' One of the earliest AIDS posters in San Francisco was nothing more than a blown-up color photograph of the Kaposi's sarcoma lesions on the foot of early AIDS patient and activist Bobbi Campbell. It was simple and bone chilling in its directness and horror.

Targeted and Explicit Prevention Works Best

When CDC teams in 1984 surveyed AIDS prevention efforts in nine different cities – Atlanta, Chicago, Houston, Los Angeles, Miami, Newark, NJ, New York, San Francisco, and Washington, DC – they found that only San Francisco had the kind of collaboration between the public health department and community-based AIDS groups that was deemed essential if prevention education was to succeed. City leaders, long used to the active participation of its large, visible, politically involved gay community, saw AIDS as San Francisco's problem, not a 'gay' problem. The teams also concluded that the translation of scientific information into usable, understandable prevention messages required graphic language to provide explicit advice about sexual behaviors or needle sharing. They added that to be successful in reaching a particular population, prevention efforts 'must be appropriate for and responsive to the lifestyle, language and environment of the members of that population' (Bailey, 1991).

Despite the recommendations, a 1985 report by the congressional Office of Technology Assessment (OTA) faulted the federal government's inadequate attention to AIDS prevention education. The OTA noted that it had been mostly left to those at greatest risk – gay men and injection drug users – to educate themselves. But of course neither group had the financial nor scientific resources on their own to conduct the kind of massive national prevention campaigns it would take to prevent the spread of HIV. The OTA report said the government had shirked its responsibility at least partly because providing advice on preventive sex practices might be viewed as 'condoning the lifestyles' of homosexuals (US Congress, OTA, 1985).

The CDC was outraged in 1986 when GMHC allegedly used federal funds to produce a safe sex video for gay men. In GMHC's view, this was precisely the kind of 'targeted, explicit' education the CDC teams and the nation's leading medical and public health experts endorsed in no fewer than three major reports in 1986 (Coolfont Report, 1986; Institute of Medicine, 1986, pp. 95–105; Koop, 1986). The video's use of familiar language provided a safe-sex vocabulary that GMHC hoped would prove useful in real-life sexual negotiations. Although GMHC was later vindicated of the charge that it had used federal funds to produce the video, the controversy underscored the government's anti-gay bias.

CDC went even further, prohibiting the development of explicit, 'offensive' materials, and requiring that anyone getting funding to produce HIV prevention materials had to establish local review panels to screen the materials. This requirement was precisely what the Institute of Medicine advised against when it said it was 'concerned about the Centers for Disease Control directive that empanels local review boards to determine whether materials developed for AIDS education are too explicit and in violation of local community standards, what it called, "the dirty words" issue' (Institute of Medicine, 1986, p. 99). It certainly was effective in reminding gay Americans that if they wanted effective HIV prevention education, they would have to provide it themselves.

Prevention Education Worked – for a While

By the beginning of 1987, *US News & World Report* had proclaimed, 'Education has been a dazzling success with homosexuals' (McAuliffe *et al.*, 1987). It seemed that even without much help from the government, gay people had managed to get AIDS under control, gay men had modified their high-risk behavior to avoid transmission of the virus and the community could get back to the business of gay liberation. Riding this wave of optimism, San Francisco's Stop AIDS Project closed its doors in 1987. It seemed gay men 'got it,' that they knew what they needed to do and not do in order to protect themselves and one another. Not only were STD rates down and gay men reporting less risk behavior overall, but they seemed in general to be having less sex. Prevention educators congratulated themselves for stemming the tide of infection and reshaping gay community sexual norms.

But the first of many so-called 'second waves' of the AIDS epidemic was already rolling into shore as gay men outside the major coastal cities ignored the epidemic and partied on. In New Mexico, for example, a 1987 study reported that 20 per cent of a group of 166 gay men were already HIV-positive. Seventy per cent of them reported practicing receptive anal intercourse in the past 12 months, and only 13 per cent used condoms. A history of having sexual partners outside of New Mexico was correlated to an increased risk for seropositivity (Jones *et al.*, 1987).

The intermingling of gay men in the major cities – men from small towns frequently visit or move to cities like New York or San Francisco, and men in those cities often visit their original hometowns – meant it was inevitable that HIV would spread from the coastal cities, where it first appeared, to the heartlands. In the major coastal cities themselves influxes of gay men – many of them becoming sexually active for the first time – meant that community efforts to create social norms that supported safe sex were undermined by the very mobility that brought so many gay men to the cities in the first place. As Daniel Wohlfeiler, the Stop AIDS Project's former education director, put it, 'In 1987, the day the Project shut, there was a community norm that favored safe sex. But that norm is only as durable as the community is static.' As he pointed out, San Francisco is anything but static. In 1987, upwards of a third of the gay men in the city had lived there less than two years. Said Wohlfeiler, 'The norm is obviously not going to withstand that kind of transience' (D Wohlfeiler, personal communication, 15 February 1995).

Clearly it was going to take more than brochures, posters, and workshops to make gay men alter their entrenched sexual habits. Just as clearly, it meant that ongoing prevention efforts needed to be targeted and adapted to new audiences and generations. As had been pointed out early in the epidemic, knowledge alone is not enough to make people change behavior they enjoy, even if they know its potential risks. Jackson Peyton, then director of prevention education for the San Francisco AIDS Foundation, said what he called the 'golden age' of prevention ended with the realization that safe sex had not become quite as 'normal' as educators believed and that the epidemic was not going to end in the foreseeable future. Peyton told me, 'I truly don't believe that anybody thought this was going to be a "rest of our lives" kind of thing until about 1990' (J Peyton, personal communication, 20 February 1995). That's the year the Stop AIDS Project reopened, this time with no set closing date.

Pushing Medicine's Limits

From the beginning of the epidemic, gay men with HIV/AIDS resisted the stigma that the heterosexual mainstream imposed on the deadly new sexually transmitted infection. Just as they had fought the secrecy and shame expected of homosexuals to 'come out' as gay, these men knew it was essential to seize and redefine in positive, hopeful terms even the language associated with HIV/AIDS. Because they were determined to live with HIV and not die from AIDS, people with HIV/AIDS became educated consumers of information related to the virus. They knew that information is power, that being informed could make the difference in the quality of care they received and, literally, between life and death.

People with HIV/AIDS formed 'buyers' clubs' to import, and even smuggle, medications and other substances that might have medicinal value against HIV, from places like China, Israel, and Mexico. The AIDS Coalition to Unleash Power (ACT UP) represented the most visible and organized efforts to share information to achieve powerful results. But some of the most dramatic changes in medical research came about much less dramatically than the protest group's made-for-the-media 'actions'. Gay doctors in San Francisco and New York, working with their HIV-positive patients, showed that medical research and compassionate clinical care do not have to be mutually exclusive and, in fact, can be mutually enforcing – one of the quiet yet profound legacies left by gay Americans that now benefit people with AIDS and other life-challenging illnesses.

People with AIDS – Not Victims

In the spring of 1983, word reached New York that San Francisco nurse Bobbi Campbell, the first person ever to go public about having AIDS, was urging the newly formed AIDS service organizations in various cities to pay the expenses of gay men with AIDS to attend the upcoming Second National AIDS Forum in Denver, where his fellow San Franciscan Steve Morin was presenting information about early prevention efforts in the city. The New Yorkers did not know whether to think Bobbi crazy or courageous for being public about his diagnosis. Michael Callen, one of New York's own first 'out' people with AIDS (PWA), said it had not yet occurred to New York PWAs 'that we could be anything more than passive recipients of the genuine care and concern of those who hadn't (yet) been diagnosed' (Callen and Turner, 1988). But gay San Franciscans were long used to taking an active role in the life of their city, and naturally expected the city to commit its political and financial resources to help save the lives of its residents who were living with AIDS.

In San Francisco on 2 May 1983, a group of gay men smiling at each other, looking vigorous, living with AIDS carried a banner at the first-ever AIDS Candlelight Memorial. 'Fighting for Our Lives', it said. A month later, Bobbi Campbell and Dan Turner, another PWA in San Francisco, took the banner with them to Denver. The people with AIDS at the meeting adopted its message of hopeful determination as their motto.

In Denver, a dozen PWAs met in a hospitality suite at the conference to discuss how they could organize themselves. Bobbi Campbell took charge of the room, helping articulate a plan for a coalition of PWA groups in all cities with large AIDS populations, proposing they all join in forming one national association. The group agreed that they should be known as 'people with AIDS,' or PWAs – not as patients or victims. They drafted the Denver Principles, a bill of rights and recommendations for health care providers, ASOs, and for PWAs themselves. The Denver Principles laid the groundwork for what would become a worldwide movement of self-empowerment among people living with HIV/AIDS.

It is important to note that these first-generation PWAs were out and proud gay men. The fact that they were already living their lives with pride and honesty as gay men was reflected in how they approached having AIDS, and how they believed AIDS should be approached. Early gay PWAs likened the experience of 'coming out' as having AIDS to their coming out as gay men. They knew what it meant to stand up in the face of stigma and discrimination to say, defiantly and yet matter-of-factly, this is who I am and it is good enough. These early people with AIDS were very clear, and showed amply that they were not victims and they were not powerless. That was their vision for being a person living with AIDS, and it reverberates down the years to inform the way we seek today to empower and involve people with AIDS, and people with other illnesses, in their own care and support.

Information is Power

From the earliest organizing among PWAs, there has been a strong emphasis on the sharing and power of information in dealing with HIV/AIDS. Commonly during the AIDS epidemic patients – particularly gay men, because AIDS treatment information has been frequently discussed in the gay press and among friends – have been better informed than their physicians, especially if they are in a part of the country with a low incidence of AIDS. 'This can be daunting for physicians to deal with', said Mervyn Silverman, director of public health in San Francisco at the beginning of the epidemic. 'It speaks to the need for a partnership between the doctor and patient'. He said that gay PWAs benefited from their ties to the gay community, noting, 'This was the first time in history that a community of individuals, linked by various media and socially, were afflicted, so the response was a collective response'. Because gay physicians were both members of the community and typically the first to treat AIDS in their gay patients, Silverman said, 'The doctor looked at himself as a potential patient, so was more willing to work with the patient' (M Silverman, personal communication, 15 February 1995).

In a meeting at the Gay and Lesbian Community Center in New York on 10 March 1987, Larry Kramer told a group of about 250 men and women that Food and Drug Administration (FDA) approval of a new drug could easily take 10 years. 'Ten years', he said. 'Two-thirds of us could be dead in less than five years.' Kramer criticized the speeded-up trials of AZT and plans for the drug's then-imminent approval. He noted that people facing a life-threatening illness like AIDS would lie if they had to in order to get hold of a promising treatment. Cutting to the chase in his inimitable way, Kramer raised a challenge to the FDA: 'We're willing to be guinea pigs, all of us', he thundered. 'Give us the fucking drugs' (Kramer, 1989, pp. 127–39).

The AIDS Coalition to Unleash Power, known as ACT UP, was formed several days later in response to Kramer's rousing challenge. Reiterating Kramer's call for access to potentially beneficial experimental drugs, the group's original slogan was 'Drugs Into Bodies!' Underscoring the group's commitment to speaking openly about AIDS and sharing potentially life-saving information, its best-known slogan was 'Silence = Death'. ACT UP launched into action on 24 March

1987, five days after the FDA approved AZT, the first drug ever approved to treat HIV infection. Despite the excitement that greeted its approval, people with AIDS were shocked at the US$10 000 annual cost of AZT that its manufacturer Burroughs Wellcome said was necessary to recoup its research costs.

At their first 'action,' on Wall Street, ACT UP members handed out copies of a commentary by Larry Kramer that had run in the previous day's *New York Times*, calling the FDA 'the single most incomprehensible bottleneck in American bureaucratic history'. Kramer criticized the kind of double-blind studies tradition-ally used to test new medications. 'Double-blind studies were not created with terminal illnesses in mind', he asserted, calling for the FDA to make experimental AIDS drugs available on a 'compassionate usage' basis (Kramer, 1989, pp. 140–4). Echoing Kramer, ACT UP contended that in the case of a new disease like AIDS, the testing of drugs itself was a form of health care, and that everyone should have the right to receive health care (Crimp and Rolston, 1990).

In San Francisco, a new group called Citizens for Medical Justice rallied thou-sands of people in the Castro area to kick off a 30-mile, two-day march to Burroughs Wellcome's offices in a bid to draw attention to AZT's high price. From the protests emerged an organized effort to circumvent the government's lethargic drug development process by procuring drugs approved in countries outside the US and making them available to people with AIDS who were willing to take them. Under an FDA regulation that allows individuals with life-threaten-ing diseases to import for personal use drugs approved elsewhere, 'buyers' clubs' were formed to buy such drugs in bulk for distribution among PWAs throughout the country.

Buyers' Clubs

Showing what empowered people living with HIV/AIDS could do on their own behalf, Michael Callen and Tom Hannan, another New Yorker with AIDS, announced the launch of a buyers' club, the PWA Health Group, in New York in April 1987. The two had formed a partnership to import a food substance manu-factured in Israel from egg whites, called AL-721, believed to have some efficacy against HIV, based on test tube studies. Callen said, 'If a substance cannot hurt and may help, we will make every effort to see that those PWAs who desire to obtain such a substance may do so' (M Callen, *personal communication*, 24 April 1987).

For Callen and other PWAs, the issue was a matter of self-determination: If they were willing to try an experimental treatment, why should they be denied the opportunity to do so by a paternalistic government's drug regulation system? Callen spoke for many PWAs and everyone else puzzled by the slow pace of treat-ment research when he said, 'Why do PWAs themselves have to take time and energy from their own individual struggles for survival to do the job that others are supposed to be doing?' (M Callen, *personal communication*, 24 April 1987).

John-Manuel Andriote

A New Way of Doing Medical Research – at the Community Level

While ACT UP's protests were the most visible efforts to shake up the drug approval process, others also were creating radical change in how experimental drugs are tested and evaluated, albeit more quietly and mainly out of public view. In San Francisco, physician Don Abrams helped to launch the County-Community Consortium (CCC) in March 1985. A group of Bay Area physicians who originally came together to talk about their AIDS patients and experimental drug protocols, CCC members soon decided to design a clinical drug trial that they could conduct from their own offices. After AZT became available, the group launched a study of aerosol, or inhaled, pentamidine, a drug that had showed promise in preventing *Pneumocystis carinii* pneumonia, the leading killer of people with AIDS at the time. A hundred patients were enrolled at 12 sites throughout the Bay area, with 69 physicians participating in the study. Don Abrams told me the federal government refused to provide funding for the CCC study because 'it was too novel and too community-based' (D Abrams, personal communication, 17 July 1995).

In New York, the PWA Coalition organized its own treatment research program, called the Community Research Initiative, and described by Larry Kramer as 'an historic attempt by the gay community to test drugs on ourselves' (Kramer, 1989, p. 209). Modeled after San Francisco's CCC, the goal of the initiative was to test drugs in a community setting. The CRI was located in rooms adjoining those of the PWA Health Group, on West Twenty-Sixth Street in Manhattan, rather than in an impersonal, intimidating medical research center where medical research was traditionally conducted.

The goal of the CRI's founders PWA activists Michael Callen and Tom Hannan, their physician Joseph Sonnabend, and Mathilde Krim, the founding director of the American Foundation for AIDS Research (AmFAR) was, as Callen described it, 'to conduct rigorous scientific research on promising AIDS therapies in a community-based setting faster and more cheaply than traditional systems do'. In keeping with the Denver Principles, Callen said, 'CRI utilized study designs that are sensitive to the needs of PWAs, because PWAs and physicians who care for us are involved at every level of the decision making process' (Callen, 1990). Ninety New York City physicians and 200 people with AIDS participated in a CRI study of inhaled pentamidine much like the one conducted in San Francisco.

On 1 May 1989, Lymphomed, the drug company that held the patent on pentamidine, presented data from the CCC and CRI studies to the FDA. Physician-researchers from the CCC in San Francisco spoke about the effectiveness of inhaled pentamidine, and speakers from New York's CRI offered additional information about the drug's safety. Based upon the information provided by the CCC and CRI, the FDA committee voted unanimously to approve aerosol pentamidine to prevent pneumocystis pneumonia – the first time a drug had ever been approved based on research conducted at the community level.

By putting research in the hands of the doctors actually caring for people with AIDS and PWAs themselves, community-based trials demonstrated that the need to gather scientific information can be balanced with not merely caring for, but also caring about, patients as human beings, friends, and neighbors. The active involvement of people with AIDS in community-based trials served – like the support groups, coalitions, and buyers' clubs they had formed – to strengthen their own will to survive. As Peter Arno and Karyn Feiden put it, 'Because it empowered patients and fostered strong ties with their physicians, community-based research offered, above all else, something whose value could not be measured: a sense of hope' (Arno and Feiden, 1992). The Presidential Commission on the HIV Epidemic mentioned the CRI in its June 1988 report, urging the federal government to fund similar community-based AIDS research, clearly recognizing that gay people with AIDS and their advocates had created a new way of doing research that was worth replication.

Learning to Do Politics Washington-Style

Until gay people were forced to address HIV/AIDS, they had very limited experience advocating in Washington on their own behalf. By the late 1980s, representatives of the growing AIDS industry and other advocates for people with HIV/AIDS – most of the key players gay men and lesbians – were lobbying government officials and members of Congress to win federal support for HIV/AIDS services then being funded mainly through the generosity of gay people in communities across the country. While ACT UP's high profile 'actions' helped shine the media's spotlight on HIV/AIDS, those working on the inside also achieved impressive results: the Ryan White CARE Act and the provisions of the Americans with Disabilities Act that protect people with HIV/AIDS. They demonstrated that the best way to get things done in Washington was to amplify the power of their advocacy by working within coalitions of organizations with shared interests and similar constituencies.

AIDS and the Gay Movement

'AIDS built the gay movement,' says historian John D'Emilio. 'It shook loose the resources to transform a movement that was small and based almost entirely on volunteer labor into a movement of full-time people who were devoting themselves to this work and getting paid for it.' He added, 'Slowly in time that transition would have happened, but the epidemic compressed all of the change that might have taken a generation basically into a decade' (J D'Emilio, personal communication, 24 May 1996).

411

Before AIDS, gay people had no experience in Washington dealing with federal budgets and appropriations, and certainly not with the Department of Health and Human Services (HHS). The only gay political presence in Washington was Steve Endean's Gay Rights National Lobby and the National Gay Task Force's (now the National Gay and Lesbian Task Force, or NGLTF) efforts to push the federal gay and lesbian civil rights bill, a revision of the 1964 Civil Rights Act, introduced by the late Bella Abzug in 1975 (Vaid, 1995).

Virginia Apuzzo, who became director of the National Gay Task Force in 1982, told me, 'What you have to understand was that the gay and lesbian community in 1980–81 had only one experience with lobbying, that was how to get the gay rights bill through. Every session you'd go in and add two or three more sponsors, get people to write from home. That's where this community's experience was, and it had to turn around on a dime' (V Apuzzo, personal communication, 8 August 1995). Apuzzo testified at the earliest congressional hearings on AIDS, and was perhaps the most visible gay leader speaking publicly about the so-called 'gay plague' in its earliest years. Apuzzo attributes the gay leaders' political education to Tim Westmoreland, then the chief counsel to the House Subcommittee on Health and the Environment and an openly gay man, and some of the staff of the late Representative Ted Weiss, one of whom was Patsy Fleming, President Clinton's second AIDS 'czar'.

At first, said Tim Westmoreland, gay organizations did not want to take on a major public health issue like AIDS. They had their hands full – that is, the very few hands there were in the professional gay civil rights movement at that point – trying to deal with discrimination issues and getting a few more supporters for the (still un-passed) gay rights bill. But there was a collective epiphany. 'They came around quickly to the realization that this was threatening to undermine progress they might make in any other area', said Westmoreland (T Westmoreland, personal communication, 18 July 1995).

Emergence of the AIDS Lobby

The political face of AIDS began to change with the formation of the AIDS Action Council, a lobbying group representing the AIDS service organizations that were being organized throughout the country in the 1980s. AIDS Action began as the 'lobby project' of the Federation of AIDS-Related Organizations (FARO), formed by 38 community-based AIDS organizations at the June 1983 Second National AIDS Forum, in Denver, to provide members with a means to network with one another. The FARO AIDS Action Council, as it was originally called, would be these groups' voice in Washington. Before long, AIDS Action would operate as a fully fledged industry lobbying group as the 'AIDS community' expanded to include service organizations as well as the individuals they served.

Gary MacDonald, AIDS Action's first executive director, was a one-man operation at first. Working out of the second bedroom of his Capitol Hill apartment,

MacDonald spent much time in the early years simply educating people in the government about homosexuals. Because of his own willingness to be open about being gay, MacDonald was invited to join the government's earliest advisory panels on counseling and testing, prevention education and, as he put it, 'really in some sense on the gay community'. He explained, 'There was enormous ignorance in the early days: "Who are these people? How many of you are there? Where do you live?" I'd get calls from people at CDC asking, "What percentage of the population is gay male?" They were doing all this projecting and numbers and statistical models trying to figure out just how bad this really was' (G MacDonald, personal communication, 7 February 1995).

Other AIDS lobbyists, virtually all of them gay, began to appear in Washington in the late 1980s. Besides contributing to AIDS Action Council, large agencies like GMHC in New York, AIDS Project Los Angeles, the San Francisco AIDS Foundation and Seattle's Northwest AIDS Foundation created their own policy departments and hired lobbyists to look out for their particular interests.

The Power of Coalitions

Before this splintering of the AIDS lobby and the intra-community discord it created in the 1990s, AIDS Action spearheaded a political coalition that was effective, powerful and, in fact, accomplished tremendously important political feats on behalf of people with HIV/AIDS. National Organizations Responding to AIDS (known as the NORA coalition) consisted of representatives of 60 organizations, including the national gay groups that had been addressing the epidemic from the beginning. But for the first time the gay groups were no longer the principal spokespeople on AIDS.

NORA depended on what was known as a 'mainstreaming' strategy to make its point that AIDS was more than a gay issue. Tom Sheridan, a lobbyist with AIDS Action Council at the time, explained NORA's inclusiveness. 'We tried to make sure that "the table" looked like the epidemic', he said, 'and that no one was left out and no one was distanced'. The Human Rights Campaign Fund (today the Human Rights Campaign, the largest gay political group in the country) and the National Gay and Lesbian Task Force were NORA members. 'But', said Sheridan, 'the nurses' association had a seat at the table as well. Disability rights groups had a seat at the table. The ACLU had a seat at the table' (T Sheridan, personal communication, 24 February 1995).

NORA succeeded in pushing Congress to pass the Ryan White Comprehensive AIDS Resources Emergency (CARE) Act in 1990. Named after the Indiana teenager who died of AIDS just four months before the bill's passage, the CARE Act provided funding to the cities and states hardest hit by AIDS to pay for services for people living with HIV/AIDS. In its first two years alone, the CARE Act provided more than US$847 million for AIDS services nationwide. Today, the CARE Act annually disburses nearly US$2 billion for AIDS services through programs administered by the HIV/AIDS Bureau of the Health Resources and Services Administration (HRSA).

An even clearer example of NORA's success as a coalition, and the strategic value of working within coalitions more generally, was its victory in making sure that people with HIV/AIDS were included with others whose disabilities would be protected under the Americans with Disabilities Act (ADA), also passed in 1990. The ADA expanded on earlier federal antidiscrimination laws protecting people with disabilities, in such areas as employment and public accommodations. It redefined discrimination to include not only outright discriminatory actions against a disabled person but also the absence of taking certain affirmative steps to accommodate people with disabilities. Under the law, for example, an employer is required to make 'reasonable accommodations' for applicants and employees who are disabled but who are otherwise qualified to do a job (Feldblum, 1993).

People with AIDS are covered under the law because the Supreme Court in 1987 ruled in *School Board of Nassau County v. Gene H. Arline* that contagious diseases, including AIDS – though technically an infectious, not a contagious, disease – are considered a handicap or disability, and are therefore protected under federal disability law (Gianelli, 1987). In its first AIDS-specific decision, the Supreme Court in 1998 ruled that asymptomatic HIV infection also qualifies as a protected disability (Biskupic and Goldstein, 1998).

Within the NORA coalition, disability advocates Curt Decker and Pat Wright were seasoned team players in the Consortium of Citizens with Disabilities. The two showed both the consortium and the NORA coalition how AIDS was relevant to the disability community, and why the AIDS lobby would gain from an alliance with the established disability groups. Decker recalled in an interview that he tried to interest disability organizations in AIDS well before the passage of the ADA. 'I kept pushing the disability community to look at AIDS as a disability before there was a NORA', he said. 'I told them that if they couldn't embrace it, they should realize that a fair amount of their constituency – such as substance abusers and the mentally retarded – might become infected' (C Decker, personal communication, 13 February 1995).

As the ADA made its way through Congress, from its earliest drafts in 1987 to its passage in 1990, there were a number of attempts by hostile members to split apart the disability and AIDS coalition by driving a wedge between the mentally ill and people with AIDS. Fortunately, said Decker, 'The disability community realized what was going on, and said we may not be thrilled about AIDS, but we realized this was trying to slice off unpopular communities, and 20 years ago that was us, with forced sterilizations' (C Decker, personal communication, 13 February 1995).

One attempt to slice off protections for people with HIV/AIDS from the ADA was the so-called Chapman food-handler amendment, which would have prevented HIV-positive food handlers from claiming protection against discrimination. When the amendment passed the House and Senate in the spring of 1990, the disability lobby and NORA joined forces in opposing it, arguing that AIDS is a disability and must be protected under the ADA. Chai Feldblum, recognized by *The American Lawyer* as one of the nation's leading experts on the ADA, said, 'What was key was the disability community as a whole was fighting the amendment. When we went to meetings at the White House there would be 15 people around the table, 10 of them with disabilities, and only two of them whose disability was AIDS. People in wheelchairs, people with cerebral palsy, people who were blind – they were all saying this is a bad amendment' (C Feldblum, personal communication, 12 April 1996).

Although there has been disagreement over the 'mainstreaming' strategy used to win support for HIV/AIDS in Washington by downplaying its impact on gay men and playing up its impact on women and children, the fact is the advocates worked very well with the tools available to them. In the face of blatant homophobia and motivated by the impact of AIDS in their own lives and the life of the gay community, these advocates shrewdly played the game by the rules as they found them. If that meant talking about women and children, that is what had to be done. It was unpleasant business, but the main objective was to win as much support as possible for people with HIV/AIDS of whatever race, age or sexual orientation. By that standard, and as an example of how to work within a political coalition to achieve bigger results than might be achievable alone, the AIDS advocates succeeded beyond their wildest dreams.

The Politics of Mourning

One of the most powerful and visible ways that gay Americans resisted the stigma and shame many people associated with HIV/AIDS was in how we memorialized our friends and lovers who succumbed to AIDS. In memorial services, newspaper obituaries and, particularly, in the AIDS Memorial Quilt, gay people openly and shamelessly named AIDS as the cause of death. They refused to be silent about AIDS, believing that, to paraphrase ACT UP's famous slogan, silence was tantamount to complicity with those who wished us to be dead. Countering stigma by focusing on human beings rather than on statistics is one of the most important lessons gay Americans learned and used to advantage.

A Community in Mourning

On Friday the 13th of March 1987, the morning after ACT UP was officially created, the *Wall Street Journal* reported on page 1, 'AIDS has been cruel to Greenwich Village and its homosexuals'. The Village was being devastated by AIDS. The *Journal* noted that at least 700 of the more than 9000 AIDS cases in New York at that point were reported among the Village's estimated 18 000 homosexuals. One of every 25 gay men in the Village was living with or had already died of AIDS. Life continued in the Village. 'But', noted the *Journal*, 'more

415

young men these days get around with the help of canes or walkers. Wartime metaphors spring to people's lips. And the keeping of lists has become a grotesque commonplace' (Graham and Ricklefs, 1987).

In San Francisco, the heavily gay Castro district was shrouded in gloom thick as the city's famous fog. Men speak today of the 'dark years' in the mid-1980s, when so many gay-owned businesses in the Castro closed – sometimes because the owner had died; other times because the clientele were dead. Thousands would gather for candlelight vigils, then quickly disperse afterward, retreating to the safety of home. The hilarity that had sparkled in the air and sparked the westward migrations of gay men to the city in the 1970s had given way to a stunned, mournful silence.

By the late 1980s, the obituaries of gay men dead from AIDS took up substantial room in the pages of the gay press. In San Francisco's *Bay Area Reporter*, two full pages of obituaries were not uncommon. Gay cultural observer Michael Bronski noted, 'Reading *BAR* is like walking through a graveyard, or viewing the Vietnam Veterans Memorial Wall, the only difference is that you knew these people and may have seen them only a week ago'. Describing his own experience of writing obituaries for Boston's *Gay Community News* in the early and mid-1980s, Bronski said, 'Despite the terrors of writing and reading obits, there is also the satisfaction, however incomplete, that something is being done. Someone's life has been noted. Some attention is being paid. Someone else may read and understand a little more how large, how inclusive and diverse the gay world is.' He added, '[I]n taking action, as well as in remembering and mourning, which are part of each obituary, the pieces ease both the terror and the pity, and they become politically inseparable from the personal' (Bronski, 1988).

Mourning Rituals to De-Stigmatize AIDS

It is precisely this linkage of the personal and political that distinguished many memorial services for gay men who died of AIDS, especially during the 1980s when the fear and stigma associated with the disease reached hysterical proportions. The AIDS dead were commemorated as friends, lovers, sons, neighbors, and co-workers – not simply as people with AIDS. On a political level, as the *New York Times* has noted, the gay community's memorials have been 'platforms for grief and celebration and the politics that surround AIDS. Participants not only cry and reminisce but rail against the government, push for more medical research and raise money to fight on.' At the same time, said the newspaper, 'The friends and colleagues who plan the services make them highly personal, saying that one of their goals is to prevent a friend or relative from turning into one more statistic' (Navarro, 1994).

Gay memorials served to affirm the value of gay lives, and of the deceased individual to the life of the gay community. By insisting that the word AIDS was named openly as the cause of death, gay people sought to remove the sting of what society considered a shameful death. Frequently there was more than one memorial tribute for the same man, generally because the man's family either could not make it to the memorial his friends organized in the place he lived as an adult, or because the family refused to attend a 'gay' event.

The best-known and most impressive AIDS memorial is the AIDS Memorial Quilt, the effort to memorialize the lives of those killed by AIDS in this extraordinary example of public mourning art. It is often compared with the Vietnam War Memorial in Washington, DC, because it represents a collective memorial for many individuals, and because of the way it draws people to publicly share their grief with others who also have lost loved ones. The quilt challenges the taboo of openly mourning our dead, thereby acknowledging the reality of death in life.

Cleve Jones, founder of the NAMES Project AIDS Memorial Quilt, says he got the idea for the quilt when he and others were putting up posters for the annual candlelight memorial march for slain gay city supervisor Harvey Milk. He told me, 'The [San Francisco] *Chronicle* had a headline saying that a thousand San Franciscans had died. I was talking to my friend Joseph saying those thousand, they were all right here: Almost every one of that thousand had died within 10 blocks of where we were standing. But you couldn't see that, couldn't walk down the street and see death everywhere.'

Jones wanted something that would provide a visual image of the toll by showing the lives behind the statistics. During the candlelight march, he asked everyone to carry placards with the name of one person who had died. Using ladders he hid in the shrubbery, Jones and his friends taped the placards of names on the front of the federal building. 'As I was looking at the patchwork of names on the wall,' said Jones, 'I said to myself it looks like a quilt'. The word evoked warm memories for him because his great-grandmother had sewed a series of quilts to pass on to her grandchildren. Jones recalled thinking, 'This is such a warm, comforting, middle-class, middle-American symbol. Every family has a quilt; it makes them think of their grandmothers. That's what we need: We need all these American grandmothers to want us to live, to be willing to say that our lives are worth defending' (C Jones, personal communication, 2 February 1995).

Looking Ahead

In more than two decades of being challenged by HIV/AIDS, gay people have led the way in pushing for compassionate services, realistic prevention, medical care and research that treats patients as partners with the shared goal of good health and effective treatment. Gay Americans' experience of mobilizing at the community and national levels offers important lessons for others who are perhaps only now confronting the epidemic, whether on a personal level, in their community or at the national governmental level.

Beginning early in the HIV/AIDS epidemic gay people, particularly in San Francisco, showed how to provide cost-effective care and support for people living with HIV/AIDS through a 'continuum of care', a network of professional community-based services that combined both professional and volunteer skill and time. AIDS service providers were assisted by activists and community leaders who spoke out about HIV/AIDS, rallied gay people to get involved and castigated elected officials for their lack of leadership in addressing the epidemic. They also discomfited gay and straight alike by insisting on speaking frankly and regularly about the epidemic and the sexual and political behavior that perpetuates it.

Gay America's ability to respond to HIV/AIDS was helped immeasurably by the ability and willingness of gay doctors and health care professionals in the community to be 'out' in their work. Their contacts in the mainstream medical and health fields, the network of gay community health and STD agencies and a fledgling gay and lesbian health movement formed in the 1970s, enabled gay people to mount a viable – if ultimately overwhelmed – response to HIV/AIDS even before there was either public or private philanthropic funding to support their efforts. An important lesson of gay people's experience is that any response to HIV/AIDS must begin by mobilizing networks of influential and visible people to talk openly about it, urge others to be involved and keep the epidemic before the eyes of elected officials.

The prevention efforts mounted by gay Americans from the beginning of the epidemic emphasized 'sex-positive' messages that grew out of gay men's self-acceptance. They correctly believed that preventing the spread of HIV was the supreme challenge – not preventing people from having a fulfilling sex life or dictating whether and with whom they could have sex. From the first guidelines for safer sex, developed in 1982 by the Bay Area Physicians for Human Rights (BAPHR), gay people demonstrated – and the CDC confirmed – that targeted, explicit information, and frank discussion are essential to equipping people at high risk for HIV to make informed choices about their behavior. By the late 1980s, gay people also had realized that prevention efforts must be continually updated and targeted as populations change over time.

Prevention Politics Continue

Although we have known from the earliest years of the epidemic that targeted, explicit prevention works best in reaching those most at risk, prevention – more accurately, government funding for prevention – continues to be a politically charged issue two decades after the CDC in 1984 endorsed the efforts of gay communities. In late 2001, the Bush administration's Secretary of Health and Human Services ordered a national review of prevention programs after a San Francisco AIDS activist, not known for rationality and later convicted of harassing and threatening city health officials, brought the Stop AIDS Project to the attention of a conservative

Republican member of Congress. In a 12 October 2001 report, Health and Human Services Inspector Janet Rehnquist (daughter of conservative Supreme Court Chief Justice William Rehnquist) said the agency's 'Booty Call' and 'Great Sex' workshops could be considered 'obscene' and as 'encouraging, directly ... sexual activity'.

For its part, the Stop AIDS Project said all its educational and promotional materials had been approved by a locally appointed CDC materials review panel. Public health officials defended the programs, pointing out that a variety of messages were needed to reach a varied gay community. Stop AIDS co-executive director Steve Gibson said in a statement, 'Our goal is to ensure that sexually active gay and bisexual men have the tools and the skills necessary to prevent new infections. Period' (Mason, 2001).

After questioning Stop AIDS Project staff over two days, CDC investigators concluded 'that the design and delivery of Stop AIDS prevention activities was based on current accepted behavioral science theories in the area of health promotion', according to the CDC (Delgado, 2003). Despite this vindication, the Bush administration again ordered the Stop AIDS project in June 2003 to immediately halt several of its programs that 'appear to encourage or promote sexual activity'. As much as half a million dollars in federal grants was at stake. The order was prompted by yet another complaint from a conservative Republican legislator. Although Mitchell Katz, director of San Francisco's health department, defended Stop AIDS' workshops, the CDC this time said the local review process was insufficient and would be changed. This of course contradicted the very purpose of the CDC's local prevention planning councils, intended to put decision-making about prevention for communities in the hands of representatives of those communities (Connolly, 2003).

Until there is more than a theoretical commitment within the Republican party to giving power to states, and agreement that preventing the spread of HIV is more important than pushing a conservative moral agenda, projects such as Stop AIDS will continue to be subjected to this kind of hostile parsing of language and images from outside of the communities for which the language and images are intended and relevant. Gay Americans have led the way on HIV prevention for more than 20 years and have managed to mount visible, even effective, prevention efforts without support from the federal government. Perhaps it will be necessary to do so again.

Rethinking Prevention

One of the most novel and exciting developments in prevention efforts aimed at gay men also shows the promise of wider application. Integrating HIV prevention messages into broader efforts to support good health, self-esteem and a sense of community seems to offer a uniquely powerful means of encouraging healthy personal behavior and strengthening communities at the same time.

Seattle's Gay City Health Project was one of the earliest and most dynamic of these efforts. The project used a series of well-attended forums to discuss issues of interest to gay people – such as dating, oral sex, coming-out, drug and alcohol use, and relationships between HIV-positive and HIV-negative men. John Leonard, Gay City's founding director, told me, 'We talk about how you need more than just condoms and practice putting them on a banana to practice safer sex over the long run. You need to address broader social issues, and those have to do with self-esteem and feeling a part of a community that you feel connected to.' Leonard said that in Gay City's follow-up surveys, 'people report that coming to the forums, even if not directly about HIV prevention, has an impact on them that makes them leave the forums feeling more pride and connection to the gay community, and feeling greater motivation to practice safer sex and take care of their health' (J Leonard, personal communication, 2 January 1997). This holistic approach to HIV prevention among gay men has helped inform a broader view of prevention activities – such as the recognition that unsafe sex often happens in the context of power imbalances and may be related to such early life events as childhood sexual abuse which in turn has aided in developing interventions to decrease HIV transmission to women.

Empowering Health Consumers

People with AIDS and their gay advocates also changed the way Americans think about themselves as health care consumers. As Robert M Wachter noted in an editorial in the *New England Journal of Medicine* in the early 1990s, 'Because AIDS activists have demonstrated the degree of influence that a well-organized, highly motivated advocacy group can have, we can be certain that the empowerment of patients will be a major part of the American social landscape of the nineties' (Wachter, 1992). That empowerment has continued beyond the 1990s. Today there is a greater appreciation of the need to be an educated consumer of health care services, armed with the best available information. As people living with HIV/AIDS showed repeatedly, the time invested in doing research and networking with others can pay off in better medical care and even living longer because of it.

The challenges that gay people with HIV/AIDS raised about the pricing of life-saving medications that have been developed through taxpayer-supported research (as was AZT, the first drug approved to treat HIV infection in 1987) continue to reverberate well beyond the gay community. As elderly Americans are forced to cross borders into Canada and Mexico to buy American-made prescription drugs at a fraction of their cost in the US, the experience of people with AIDS in protesting the exorbitant costs of HIV medications continues to be cited as the preeminent example of the ability of empowered consumers to win major victories in the struggle to save lives and provide reasonable profits to drug manufacturers (Harris, 2004).

420

What the Future Holds

As the HIV/AIDS epidemic has stretched on for many more years than anyone expected in the early 1980s when it began, gay people and the activists among them have had to expand their understanding of 'gay health'. Although HIV/AIDS built and brought much-needed resources to gay-focused clinics and services, it became clear in the 1990s that gay people, like all people, have a range of health issues and only a few particular health concerns that might be considered uniquely or primarily 'gay' – such as anal HPV infection in gay men. As Frank Pieri, president of the board of Howard Brown Health Center, in Chicago, put it at the time of our interview in the mid-1990s, 'There are more and more [gay] men who are getting older now who have been essentially "out" since their early twenties, for most of their lives. As they get older, and as they have other health concerns, I think they are going to demand services that are gay-friendly' (F Pieri, personal communication, 3 June 1995).

There are lessons from the gay community's experience with HIV/AIDS that are likely to be helpful in addressing the imminent 'elder boom' as substantial numbers of gay baby boomers move through their middle years to older age. But, points out Ken South, an early director of AID Atlanta and today development director for AIDS Action Council, 'Except for a very few [gay, lesbian, bisexual, transgendered] gerontologists and a handful of social service organizations caring for GLBT elderly, this issue is just not on the community's radar screen'. South suggests that gay elders would benefit if the community adapted the model of integrated, community-based professional and volunteer services created for people with HIV/AIDS. 'The GLBT community did such a remarkable job in establishing the HIV/AIDS industry when the mainstream health care system did not respond in the 80s. Where is the thinking and planning to care for those who have survived the HIV epidemic and will need all the same services like housing, home care, case management, meals on wheels and companionship?' (South, 2004).

One effort to provide a spectrum of gay-friendly health care services was created in the mid-1990s by Chicago's Howard Brown Health Center and nearby Illinois Masonic Hospital. To provide HIV clients a 'continuum of care' that includes a full range of medical and hospital services, the gay clinic and hospital agreed to what amounted to a mutually beneficial affiliation. The health center offered access to HIV and other gay patients, and the hospital guaranteed to provide gay-friendly services. Besides the potential profit, former executive director Eileen Dirkin said at the time of the partnership's formation that the hospital was interested in being perceived as a 'good neighbor' by creating a welcoming environment for the diverse people who live in the Lakeview area of Chicago (E Dirkin, personal communication, 1 June 1995). The expertise that gay community health programs, such as Howard Brown and Fenway Health, gained in expanding services for men who have sex with men has been useful in improving many other health services for lesbians and transgendered populations.

421

Coping with the diversity of human experience and of humans themselves, communities in this country and in the developing world continue to grapple with the stigma and discrimination that prevents people who need it most from being tested for HIV and receiving appropriate care and support if they are positive. Their fear of social opprobrium – and sometimes of literal physical violence against them or their families – keeps them from establishing ties to people and organizations who can show them the acceptance and support they need so they can learn to accept their condition, if HIV-positive, and effectively live with it.

The experience of gay Americans in the 1980s and 1990s in addressing stigma and discrimination will continue to offer powerful examples of how to live with pride and dignity even if one is HIV-positive, even if others disapprove and condemn because of their own fear and ignorance. After the examples of the brave individuals who have lived openly, even defiantly, with HIV/AIDS, the most visible 'face' to the world of gay America's valiant response to the death and devastation in our communities, to the hatred we faced, to the stigma and discrimination associated with HIV/AIDS, is in the many faces of the thousands of individuals remembered in the AIDS Memorial Quilt.

In the Quilt people with AIDS have been shown the honor and respect that too many of them did not receive as they struggled with their final illness. This powerful yet entirely human symbol of the traditional values of love, family, and continuity over time has shown the world that even AIDS can be discussed with compassion rather than hatred, with factual information rather than uninformed prejudice. As represented in the Quilt, respect for the dignity of all human beings, regardless of their sexual orientation or race or the particular cause of their death, will continue to be the greatest legacy of gay Americans to everyone else who must address HIV/AIDS or any other health crisis the future may bring to them as individuals, communities or nations.

References

Altman D (1986) *AIDS in the Mind of America*. New York: Anchor Press/Doubleday, p. 164.

Arno PS, Feiden KL (1992) *Against the Odds: The Story of Drug Development, Politics, and Profits*. New York: HarperCollins, p. 124.

Bailey ME (1991) Community-based organizations and CDC as partners in HIV education and prevention. *Public Health Rep* 106: 702–8.

Biskupic J, Goldstein A (1998) Disability law covers HIV, justices rule. *Washington Post* 26 June, 1.

Bronski M (1988) Death and the erotic imagination; AIDS, art and obits. In: Preston J, ed. *Personal Dispatches: Writers Confront AIDS*. New York: St. Martin's Press, pp. 136, 166.

Callen M (1990) *Surviving AIDS*. New York: HarperCollins, p. 10.

Callen M, Turner D (1988) A history of the people with AIDS self-empowerment movement. In: Shernoff M, Scott WA, eds. *The Sourcebook on Lesbian/Gay Health Care*. Washington, DC: National Lesbian/Gay Health Foundation, pp. 187–92.

CDC (Centers for Disease Control and Prevention) (2002) *Cumulative AIDS Cases Through 31 December 2002*. Available at: www.cdc.gov/hiv/stats.htm

Connolly C (2003) U.S. warns AIDS group on funding. *Washington Post* 16 June.

Coolfont Report (1986) A PHS plan for prevention and control of AIDS and the AIDS virus. *Public Health Rep* 101: 341–8.

Crimp D, Rolston A (1990) *AIDS DemoGraphics*. Seattle: Bay Press, 76–83.

Delgado R (2003) AIDS workshops pass federal test: Tone of S.F. group's safer sex sessions survives legislator's challenge. *San Francisco Chronicle* 20 February.

Feldblum C (1993) Antidiscrimination requirements of the ADA. In: Gostin LO, Bayer HA, eds. *Implementing the Americans with Disabilities Act: Rights and Responsibilities of All Americans*. Baltimore, MD: Paul H. Brookes Publishing, pp. 35–54.

Gianelli DM (1987) High court ruling gives basis for AIDS bias suits. *Am Med News* 13 March, 1.

Graham E, Ricklefs R (1987) AIDS has been cruel to Greenwich Village and its homosexuals. *Wall Street Journal* 13 March, 1.

Harris G (2004) Price of AIDS drug intensifies debate on legal imports. *New York Times* 14 April.

Institute of Medicine/National Academy of Sciences (1986) *Confronting AIDS: Directions for Public Health, Health Care, and Research*. Washington, DC: National Academy Press, pp. 95–105.

Jones CC, Waskin H, Gerety B, Skipper BJ, Hull HF, Mertz GJ (1987) Persistence of high-risk sexual activity among homosexual men in an area of low incidence of the acquired immunodeficiency syndrome. *Sex Transm Dis* 14: 79–82.

Koop CE (1986) *Surgeon General's Report on AIDS*. Rockville, MD: US Government Printing Office, introductory statement.

Kramer L (1989) *Reports from the holocaust: The Making of an AIDS Activist*. New York: St. Martin's Press.

Lear W (1984) The National Gay Health Coalition. *Lesbian & Gay Health* (Newsletter of the National Gay Health Education Foundation), 416. January.

Mason M (2001) Review ordered for HIV programs to see if campaigns too sexy. *Associated Press* 16 November.

McAuliffe K *et al.* (1987) AIDS: At the dawn of fear. *US News & World Report* 12 January, 60–70.

Navarro M (1994) Ritualizing grief, love and politics: AIDS memorial services evolve into a distinctive gay rite. *New York Times* 30 November, B1.

Peyton J (1989) *AIDS Prevention for Gay Men: A Selected History and Analysis of the San Francisco Experience, 1982–1987*. San Francisco: San Francisco AIDS Foundation.

South K (2004) Who cares? *White Crane: A Journal Exploring Gay Men's Spirituality* Spring: 5–6.

US Congress, Office of Technology Assessment (1985) *Review of the Public Health Service Response to AIDS*. Washington, DC: OTA.

Vaid U (1995) *Virtual Equality: The Mainstreaming of Gay and Lesbian Liberation*. New York: Doubleday/Anchor Books, p. 7.

Wachter RM (1992) AIDS activism, and the politics of health. *N Engl J Med* 326: 128–32.

Drug Use

17

Patricia Case
Program in Urban Health, Department of Social Medicine, Harvard Medical School, Boston, USA

Steffanie A Strathdee
Division of International Health and Cross-Cultural Medicine, Department of Family Health Sciences, University of California San Diego School of Medicine, USA

Patricia Case, ScD, MPH is an Assistant Professor in the Department of Social Medicine, Harvard Medical School. She is a behavioral scientist whose work centers on risk at the intersection of policy and behavior, especially among sexual minorities and urban populations. She is the Principal Investigator of a study examining HIV risks and resiliencies among men who have sex with men and use club drugs. Other recent projects include examining the effect of the World Trade Center attack on drug users and rescue workers, the effects of HIV-related laws on the behavior of drug users and men who have sex with men, and an evaluation of the effects of law and enforcement practices on the health of socially vulnerable populations in Russia, Poland and the Ukraine. She received her Masters in Public Health from the University of California, Berkeley and her doctorate from the Harvard School of Public Health.

Steffanie A Strathdee, PhD is an infectious disease epidemiologist, Professor and the Harold Simon Chair and Chief of the Division of International Health and Cross Cultural Medicine in the Department of Family and Preventive Medicine at University of California San Diego. Her work focuses on underserved, marginalized populations in developed and developing countries, most recently on the prevention of blood-borne infections and barriers to care among injection drug using populations, specifically HIV and viral hepatitis. She has published over 150 peer-reviewed publications on HIV prevention and the natural history of HIV infection, and is the principal investigator on several behavioral intervention studies

424

among drug users including the evaluation of needle exchange programs in Canada, the United States and India. Currently, she is engaged in research projects in a number of international settings, including Mexico, Brazil, Canada, Pakistan, India, Tajikistan and Russia.

Long before the advent of the HIV epidemic among injection drug users (IDUs), morbidity and mortality related to the transmission of blood-borne disease between injectors was known to be higher than that of the general population. However, until the HIV epidemic began, prevention efforts among IDUs were largely focused on cessation of drug use rather than the prevention of disease. Drug treatment was generally provided within either a criminal or medical model, with abstinence as the only treatment option and detoxification schemes that were sometimes legally mandated.

In the 1980s, the concept of harm reduction was proposed, with the central notion being that the risk of HIV and other blood-borne infections was a far greater threat to individuals and communities than drug use itself. As a consequence, increased access to sterile syringes for drug users through interventions such as needle exchange programs were introduced in many countries. In this chapter, we review the different approaches to disease prevention among drug using populations before and after the HIV epidemic began, and offer insights into future directions for prevention as the twenty-first century unfolds.

Historical Perspective

Opiates

Before the HIV/AIDS epidemic began, there were examples of disease transmission associated with injection drug use. The first report of an infection associated with injection drug use was a case of tetanus that occurred through needle sharing in 1867 (Berridge and Edwards, 1981). In fact, most tetanus cases occurring in New York City during the 1950s were attributed to injection drug use (Rezza *et al.*, 1996).

As early as 1929, an outbreak of over 100 cases of malaria among IDUs in Cairo, Egypt was reported (Biggam, 1929). Biggam noted that many heroin addicts returned to the practice of sniffing heroin for fear of contracting malaria through injection (Biggam and Arafa, 1930). Outbreaks of malaria were reported in New York City between 1933 and 1934 among IDUs, with 22 fatalities. In the report of this outbreak, Helpern documented one of the first reports of the sharing of contaminated equipment, when he commented that the disease appeared to be transmitted 'as a result of the peculiar practice of sharing unsterilized syringes for the intravenous injection of drugs' (Helpern, 1934). Helpern also noted that New York City addicts did not cease injection as a result of this outbreak, as IDUs did in Cairo.

Interestingly, in these outbreaks of often-fatal malaria, the behavior underlying transmission was observed, as was a change in behavior that reduced harm to injectors (switching from injection to sniffing). Yet no interventions were developed that built on this observational knowledge and outbreaks of malaria continued among IDUs. In this period of time there was not a public health understanding that active IDUs could be engaged in slowing an epidemic outbreak of a fatal disease.

By the time of an outbreak of malaria in California in 1971, public health officials developed strategies that foreshadowed later responses to the HIV epidemic; they completed non-judgmental interviews of injectors and offered two-tiered advice: to avoid sharing syringes and if sharing was unavoidable to clean and attempt to sterilize injection equipment after use by each person (Friedman *et al.*, 1973). Unfortunately, these attempts to reduce the spread of blood-borne infections were small in scale and were not widely applied. Therefore it is not surprising that other blood-borne infections continued to occur among IDU populations.

With time, it became clear that injection drug use is broadly associated with increased morbidity, mortality, health care costs, and economic losses to society. IDUs experience excess morbidity due to a number of bacterial infections, including abscesses, cellulitis, soft tissue infections, wound botulism, tetanus, and endocarditis. Apart from HIV and malaria, other blood-borne viruses acquired through multiperson syringe use include hepatitis B virus (HBV), hepatitis C virus (HCV), and human T-cell lymphotropic viruses I and II (Garfein *et al.*, 1996; Talan and Moran, 1998; Bastos *et al.*, 1999; Merrison *et al.*, 2002). The association between injection drug use and HBV was first described in 1950 (Steigman *et al.*, 1950). Several retrospective studies also revealed that HBV and HCV were transmitted by needle sharing in the 1960s.

Injection drug use also contributes to premature mortality due to drug overdose, suicide, HIV/AIDS, and end-stage liver disease associated with chronic HBV and HCV infections (Davoli *et al.*, 1993; Prins *et al.*, 1997). Mortality among opiate users in Europe is estimated to be 20 times that of non-users. The array of health problems encountered by drug users translates into higher health care costs. Due to poor health care access, many IDUs attend emergency departments to obtain regular health care services (Solomon *et al.*, 1991; Markson *et al.*, 1998; Palepu *et al.*, 1999; French *et al.*, 2000). Low utilization of primary health care services are also costly since IDUs often present with advanced stage illnesses requiring hospital admission (Stein and Sobota, 2001).

Stimulants

Stimulants such as cocaine and methamphetamine were also noted for their deleterious effects on health well before the AIDS epidemic. In 1946, Erich Hesse wrote, 'the repeated sniffing of cocaine leads to the real cocaine intoxication which assumes euphoric nature. It takes a sexual direction, with an intensification of the emotional life and a breakdown of all inhibitions.' He continues, writing, 'A symptom which can regularly be observed in chronic alkaloid addicts is the homosexually toned perversion of their sex life' (Hesse, 1946). In 1967 a study by Ellinwood found an association between 'sexual stimulation' and amphetamine use (Smith *et al.*, 1978). Similarly, Angrist and Gershon found 'disturbances of sexuality were prominent with amphetamine abuse' (Smith *et al.*, 1978). Bell and Trethowan also found a 'tendency toward perversion' among amphetamine users in their 1961 study. Despite the homophobic language of early reports, the association of methamphetamine with high-risk sex among men having sex with men (MSM) was well documented before the epidemic.

Drug Treatment

With the growing acknowledgment that drug addiction was associated with a number of negative health effects to individuals and society, a number of approaches to drug treatment were introduced well before the AIDS epidemic. While these strategies were largely focused on abstinence, there were some alternative treatment strategies that were attempted early on. One early experiment for opiate users was heroin maintenance therapy.

From 1914–1924, morphine and heroin maintenance clinics were in operation in the United States until their termination by the U.S. government (Musto, 1987). Whether these clinics were effective in treating opiate addiction is unknown; scarcity of data has limited evaluation efforts. In the early 1970s, the concept of heroin maintenance treatment was again proposed. The Vera Institute of Justice developed a protocol for a limited experimental trial of heroin maintenance treatment (Bayer, 1976), and the protocol was approved by the State of New York (Lewis, 1998). Despite support from research scientists and policy makers (Koran, 1973; McCarthy, 1974) the Nixon administration strongly opposed the use of heroin in treatment and supported methadone maintenance instead, which effectively ended the possibility of a heroin maintenance trial (Bayer, 1976).

Introduced by Dole and Nyswander in 1963 (Dole and Nyswander, 1965), methadone was first conceptualized as a treatment for heroin addiction that would 'blockade' the effects of heroin and eliminate the effects of withdrawal, thereby allowing opiate addicts to lead a productive life. It was suggested that this would make heroin addiction a treatable medical problem.

Methadone maintenance is an effective treatment for many injectors of opiates. In a seminal paper by Ball and colleagues who evaluated the impact of methadone maintenance in three US cities, 60 per cent of those enrolled ceased injection drug use for at least one year, and more than 80 per cent of those who left treatment programs returned to injecting drugs within 12 months (Ball *et al.*, 1988). These findings were replicated by subsequent studies (Metzger *et al.*,

1993; Booth *et al.*, 1996; McCusker *et al.*, 1996). With the advent of HIV, methadone programs became very important sites of testing, education, and intervention efforts for IDUs.

However, as Rosenbaum has carefully documented, from the introduction of methadone in 1963 there was an increasingly regulatory environment that appeared to be more about the containment of patients in specialized clinics than the treatment of patients. Stringent federal regulations were introduced that countermanded empirical evidence that higher doses worked better, that longer treatment stays were more effective, that fees imposed high barriers to impoverished addicts, and restricted dose levels shortened treatment stays and imposed fees. Furthermore, clinics were swamped with regulations that mandated urine testing, hours, and other elements of each program. Methadone was not seen by the government as benign, rather it became as stigmatized as the drug users. In an echo of the later efforts to increase access to sterile syringes, federal regulations began to hamper the ability of physicians to treat their patients in the absence of scientific evidence. By 1971 there were an estimated 25 000 methadone patients in the United States, but only an estimated 15–20 per cent of IDUs were receiving methadone in North America, in contrast to Europe where estimates were closer to 50 per cent (Rosenbaum, 1997).

The Advent of the AIDS Epidemic

In the very first report in 1981 of pneumocystis pneumonia among five homosexual men in Los Angeles, buried in the details was the information that one of the five reported 'parenteral drug abuse' or the use of injected illegal drugs. This was the first mention of injection drug use in association with symptoms of the new syndrome that later became known as AIDS (Gottlieb *et al.*, 1981).

This report was closely followed by another report of pneumocystis pneumonia cases, among whom there were seven IDUs with no history of sexual contact with men (Masur *et al.*, 1981). By September of 1982, the Centers for Disease Control and Prevention (CDC) had received 593 case reports of AIDS; 13 per cent were injection drug users with no history of homosexual behavior. In 1982, there were still less than 100 cases of AIDS among IDUs in the US (MMWR, 1982). While it would be some time before the HIV virus was definitively identified, the suspicion was that this was a blood-borne disease transmitted by contaminated injection equipment or unprotected sex.

Non-injected drugs have also played a role in the epidemic of HIV. As early as 1982, the use of inhaled nitrites, or 'poppers' among MSM before and during sexual activity was closely associated with unprotected sex and high HIV incidence (Marmor *et al.*, 1982). Using stimulant drugs such as crack cocaine and methamphetamine has also been associated with sexual behaviors that pose a higher risk of HIV infection, including greater numbers of partners, decreased condom use during vaginal and anal intercourse, and involvement in the sex trade (Chaisson *et al.*, 1989; Edlin *et al.* 1994). High rates of the use of inhaled nitrites, methamphetamine, and other so-called club or party drugs that are generally non-injected such as ketamine, MDMA (3,4-methylenedioxymethamphetamine, ecstacy), and GHB (gamma hydroxybutyrate) have been reported among MSM, along with associated high-risk behaviors, underscoring the need to interrupt the HIV transmission chain among MSM who use these drugs.

In the example of methamphetamine, recent studies have found associations between methamphetamine use and sexual behavior that lead to high HIV risk including: social and sexual disinhibition (Frosch *et al.*, 1996; Semple *et al.*, 2002), low rates of condom use (Hando and Hall, 1994; Zule and Desmond, 1999), increased rates of sexually transmitted diseases (Semple *et al.*, 2002), prolonged sexual activities (Smith *et al.*, 1978; Frosch *et al.*, 1996), and increased number of sexual partners (Moliter *et al.*, 1998; Zule and Desmond, 1999). Methamphetamine injectors also report less behavioral change in response to AIDS (Hando and Hall, 1994; Zule and Desmond, 1999).

Worldwide Epidemic

Currently, injection drug use, a risk factor for acquiring HIV infection through the sharing of blood-contaminated injection equipment, is a global phenomenon. By 1992, 80 countries reported injection drug use with 52 (65 per cent) reporting HIV among IDUs (Stimson and Choopanya, 1998). By 1999, the World Health Organization reported 134 countries, regions or territories reporting injecting drug use in 1999, and of these 114 (84 per cent) reported HIV among IDUs (Ball, 2002). This represents approximately a 20 per cent proportionate increase in less than a decade, indicating the potential for rapid diffusion of HIV/AIDS as the prevalence of illicit drug injection grows.

While much is made of the 'epidemic' of injection drug use, there are important regional differences in North America, Western Europe and Australia, injection drug use is a long-standing (Stimson, 1993) 'endemic' behavior that was observed decades before the emergence of HIV/AIDS. Injection drug use can be seen as 'epidemic' in areas where illicit drug markets have emerged rapidly in settings made vulnerable by rapid political, economic, and social changes. In recent years, injection drug use has been documented along drug trafficking routes in places as geographically remote from one another as Eastern Europe, South-East Asia, India, West Africa, and South America (Stimson and Choopanya, 1998; Dehne *et al.*, 1999; Beyrer *et al.*, 2000). Injection drug use has also been reported in at least seven countries in Africa, although its practice is not yet widespread. In parts of South America, such as Brazil, Colombia, and Uruguay, production and trafficking of cocaine, and more recently, heroin, have created local consumption markets with subsequent transitions to drug injection (Stimson and Choopanya, 1998).

Globally, it is estimated that 10 per cent of HIV infections are attributable to injection drug use, but this proportion is increasing. Available figures probably do not reveal the true extent of the impact of injection drug use on the global HIV/AIDS pandemic, however, as they do not account for sexual transmission associated with having a sex partner who injects drugs and perinatal HIV transmission associated with injection drug use. Injection drug use is now the predominant mode of HIV transmission in most of Western and Eastern Europe, North Africa, the Middle East and increasingly, in parts of Asia (Strathdee *et al.*, 1998). The intertwined epidemics of HIV and injection drug use may foreshadow a worsening of the HIV pandemic as epidemics among injectors in certain regions become 'generalized,' reaching well beyond the IDU community.

The paucity of options for the care of drug users changed dramatically with the AIDS epidemic as a remarkable diversity of risk reduction efforts were rapidly developed, primarily focused on (1) risk reduction efforts such as increasing access to sterile syringes through multiple venues, community outreach and education, and syringe disinfection protocols, (2) legal and policy interventions designed to encourage legal and policy changes, and (3) new drug treatment options using formulations of drugs such as buprenorphine. Below, we discuss each of these approaches in turn.

Interventions Targeting Behaviors

Community Outreach and Bleach Syringe-Cleaning Protocols

As the AIDS epidemic took hold among IDUs in the United States, few interventions were offered for IDUs early in the epidemic save the recommendation of not using injection drugs. HIV prevalence among IDUs escalated rapidly; in cities like San Francisco, more than 90 per cent of IDUs reported using another person's syringe in 1986 (Watters *et al.*, 1990). Researchers and interventionists worked to find an emergency intervention that could keep active IDUs safe from HIV infection or transmission. In an environment where waiting lists for drug treatment were long, the law criminalized the possession of syringes and outlawed the purchase of them over the counter, and physicians were reluctant to prescribe sterile syringes to IDUs for disease prevention, there were few options for IDUs who could not or would not discontinue injection.

Early research then showed that ordinary household bleach inactivated HIV *in vitro* and that it was safe, cheap, and easily available (Resnick *et al.*, 1986). As an example of how this intervention was operationalized, researchers and community activists in San Francisco introduced a small bottle of household bleach as a tool to disinfect syringes. Bleach promotion was embedded within an outreach strategy, where street outreach workers would engage IDUs in brief educational discussion and distribute bleach along with condoms and other materials to prevent HIV. The bleach disinfection protocol was rapidly adopted by IDUs in San Francisco and later became a cornerstone of national prevention efforts (Watters, 1994). That the bleach disinfection protocol for IDUs was developed in California was significant; California was one of several states that required a prescription to buy syringes in a pharmacy. As an unintended consequence of the prescription law, needle sharing due to scarcity of syringes was normative where the ability to purchase or obtain sterile syringes was restricted.

Street outreach and the bleach disinfection protocol were successful. This strategy was nationally adopted by the National AIDS Demonstration and Research projects funded by the National Institute of Drug Abuse and implemented in 68 cities. Results of the evaluation of the demonstration projects showed dramatic decreases in HIV risk and sexual behaviors among clients of the projects (Stephens *et al.*, 1993). The outreach model and bleach protocol was elaborated and targeted to neighborhoods and social networks and widely publicized. This emergency strategy was one of the first of many harm reduction efforts for active IDUs in the HIV epidemic.

Unfortunately, the bleach disinfection protocol was imperfect. Later studies found that while many IDUs could perform the basic steps involved in a bleach disinfection protocol, they failed to fill the syringe completely and rinse it according to the protocol (McCoy *et al.*, 1994). Additionally, bleach was not as effective against HIV in the blood as it was against cell-free HIV. While bleach was seen as an important emergency measure, others began to question the validity of teaching a protocol that was secondary to the standard of care in the United States, that is, one sterile syringe for every injection (CDC, 1997). While obstacles to needle exchange had seemed insurmountable earlier in the epidemic, the rising seroprevalence among IDUs and the urgent need to find new interventions found some ready to engage in civil disobedience to enact a new public health effort.

Harm Reduction

This new effort became known as a harm reduction approach. Harm reduction is the term given to a series of strategies and approaches designed to prevent drug-related harm. As noted previously, there have been programs in the United States that fit within a harm reduction conception, but the term harm reduction was not in wide use until the late 1980s. Although it is an emerging paradigm there are a number of common themes to harm reduction programs.

Harm reduction seeks to engage the drug user without judgment; that is, there is a value-neutral stance taken towards drug use and drug users. The user is seen as an active participant, and goal setting is determined by the user. While abstinence from drugs may be a goal the user wishes to work towards, there are many strategies that a user can engage to be healthier and reduce drug-related harm. Thus, a harm reduction program is above all else user-centered, focused on flexible and non-codified choices, and rooted in highly pragmatic approaches.

Concepts of harm reduction vary widely throughout the world and by locality. In the United States, approaches include assisting drug users in making positive changes of their choosing, changes that may have little proximal relationship to their drug use. Increasing access to sterile injection equipment, participating in low-threshold drug treatment programs, increasing access to non-judgmental health care, and otherwise engaging IDUs in the continuum of care available are all examples of a harm reductive approach. Harm reduction relies on having available a diversity of strategies, and indeed, with the advent of the AIDS epidemic among IDUs, a number of strategies described below became part of the armamentarium of prevention efforts in the attempt to slow the spread of HIV among drug users.

Increasing Access – Needle Exchange

Early in 1984, the Junkiebond (Junky Union, a drug users' advocacy group) in Amsterdam expressed concern that the pharmacists of inner-city Amsterdam had decided not to sell syringes to IDUs, even though it was legal to do so. It was feared that restrictions on the purchase of sterile syringes might result in a hepatitis B epidemic. In collaboration with the Municipal Health Service, the Junkiebond began distributing needles and syringes to local IDUs, and the local health department soon adopted the program. At this and other needle exchange programs (NEPs), IDUs exchanged sterile syringes for potentially contaminated ones, usually on a one-for-one basis. In this way NEPs aimed to decrease the circulation of contaminated injection equipment, thereby reducing the spread of blood-borne pathogens in the community.

Results from the Amsterdam NEPs showed excellent results; in 1988, Buning and colleagues from Amsterdam reported declines in needle sharing and injection frequency associated with NEP participation (Buning *et al.*, 1986; Buning, 1991). Activists in North America took note of this important new strategy. Beginning in 1986, syringe distribution occurred as an act of civil disobedience designed to challenge prescription laws in the United States (Lane, 1993). The first organized NEP in the US started in 1988 when Dave Purchase set up a card table on a street corner in Tacoma, Washington (Hagan *et al.*, 1991). This was followed closely by the establishment of the San Francisco NEP, Prevention Point, in late 1988. At the time of the establishment of these NEPs, federal policy prohibited support for NEPs in any context.

Despite efforts to begin introducing NEPs in the US, the initiative was controversial and aroused hot debate. On a national level, several policy statements overtly hindered the implementation of NEPs and in November 1988 a federal ban on US funding for NEPs was enacted, which has been upheld despite the conclusions of several US government-commissioned reports, many of which have specifically called for a lifting of the ban. The reasons for opposition to NEPs in the USA are multifaceted and complex, but are perhaps best viewed in terms of the policy context of 'zero tolerance' towards illicit drug use and the 'war against drugs' that pre-dated the HIV/AIDS epidemic. From this standpoint, drug use is viewed as an immoral or criminal problem that should be punished, rather than a medical problem that requires prevention and treatment.

The first phase of needle exchange in the US stands in contrast to the development of NEPs in Europe, Canada, and Australia. For example in Canada, the federal health minister publicly endorsed NEPs and programs were legally implemented in Toronto, Vancouver, and Montreal in 1988–1989. European and Australian programs, while not free of controversy, were often initiated in the context of municipal health departments, drug treatment programs and the like. In contrast, programs in the United States in the early period were often conducted as activist acts of civil disobedience where providers risked arrest for the act of providing sterile syringes to drug users in time of epidemic (Henman *et al.*, 1998).

Health-Related Services at Needle Exchange

As NEPs became more established, a second important element of some programs emerged – the provision of crucial ancillary services to IDUs, who are typically out of reach of traditional health care services and prevention programs. Many NEPs provide other sterile equipment or paraphernalia that facilitates safer injection (e.g. cottons, cookers, water, bleach), as well as male and female condoms. NEPs have also served as a pivotal entry point for drug treatment and rehabilitation, provided that adequate numbers of treatment slots are available (Heimer, 1998; Strathdee *et al.*, 1999; Shah *et al.*, 2000; MacMaster and Vail, 2002).

In many settings, NEPs tend to attract higher risk IDUs who engage in riskier behaviors compared with IDUs that tend to obtain syringes from other sources (Bruneau *et al.*, 1997; Hahn *et al.*, 1997; Schechter *et al.*, 1999). Some NEPs provide on-site HIV testing and counseling, screening for medical conditions such as sexually transmitted diseases (STDs) and tuberculosis, provision of vaccines against hepatitis B and A, abscess care, overdose prevention materials and multivitamins. The provision of care at NEPs has reduced emergency department utilization by IDUs in some communities (Pollack *et al.*, 2002).

Altice and co-workers recently reported the results of a pilot study to provide highly active antiretroviral therapy (HAART) to 13 IDUs attending mobile NEPs in New Haven, Connecticut (see Chapter 18). The provision of HAART in this context was feasible and an unexpected finding of enhancing HIV care at the NEP was that upon achieving non-detectable viral load, 69 per cent of the pilot study participants chose to enter drug treatment (Altice *et al.*, 2003).

Scientific Evidence for Needle Exchange

The overwhelming majority of studies provide strong evidence of the effectiveness of NEPs in reducing high-risk injection behaviors among HIV-seronegative and HIV-seropositive IDUs. Other studies subsequently reported reductions in incidence of HIV, HBV, and HCV infections (Hagan and Heimer, 1995; Normand *et al.*, 1995; Vlahov *et al.*, 1997; van Ameijden and Coutinho, 1998), decreased needle sharing among HIV-negative and HIV-positive people (Vlahov *et al.*, 1997; Bluthenthal *et al.*, 2000; Vertefeuille *et al.*, 2000), decreases in syringe re-use (Heimer *et al.*, 1998), and increased rates of entry into drug treatment programs (Heimer, 1998; Strathdee *et al.*, 1999; Shah *et al.*, 2000).

Despite variations between programs, an international comparison showed that in 29 cities with established NEPs, HIV prevalence decreased on average by 5.8 per cent per year, but increased on average by 5.9 per cent per year in 51 cities without NEP (Hurley *et al.*, 1997). There appears to be no published evidence that NEPs can cause negative societal effects, such as increases in drug use, discarded needles, crime, or more permissive attitudes towards drugs among youth (Vlahov *et al.*, 1997; Doherty *et al.*, 2000; Marx *et al.*, 2000, 2001).

Needle exchange programs engage IDUs most at risk of HIV and are an important element in a diversified prevention effort. However, they have several important limitations. One is that, at least in the United States, without adequate funding or sufficient hours, NEPs fail to distribute enough syringes so that every IDU has one sterile syringe for every shot. For example, if we assume that a daily injector of drugs injects twice a day, IDUs would need about 730 syringes per year to meet the standard of care for injection, one sterile syringe for every shot. Coverage by inadequately funded and often unsupported or illegal programs is often low.

In a more sophisticated analysis, Lurie estimated that with an estimated 1.5 million IDUs in the United States, NEPs would have to distribute about 1.3 billion syringes a year in order to achieve adequate coverage (Lurie *et al.*, 1998). In 1996, US NEPs reported exchanging a total of 14 million syringes, a number that falls far short of that required (Paone *et al.*, 1999).

Furthermore, to avert HIV infections on a community-wide basis, there would need to be sufficient 'reach' into groups of IDUs to engage them in the NEP. Reach is inadequate in the United States; a 1993 evaluation of 16 North American NEPs reported that these programs seldom reached more than 30 per cent of the IDUs in their communities (Lurie *et al.*, 1993). Finally, while NEPs may reach those at highest risk, other IDUs may not engage with the NEP due to privacy or convenience concerns. Expanding access to sterile syringes through diverse outlets became the next step in ensuring that IDUs have the materials to prevent the spread of infectious disease.

Increasing Access – a Sterile Syringe for Every Injection

In 1997, the CDC, the Health Resources and Services Administration (HRSA), the National Institute on Drug Abuse (NIDA), and the Substance Abuse and Mental Health Services Administration (SAMHSA) issued a joint HIV Prevention Bulletin updating prevention recommendations published in 1993. The bulletin advised health professionals to advise injectors that using a sterile syringe is safer than reusing syringes, even if they have been disinfected with bleach, and advised, in recommendations to drug users who continue to inject, 'Use a new, sterile syringe to prepare and inject drugs' (CDC, 1997).

This seemingly straightforward and clear medical advice to injectors was revolutionary in that it increased the pressure for IDUs to have access to new syringes for health reasons and the prevention of infectious disease and that it stated that the best practice was to not reuse syringes. By recasting the bleach disinfection protocol as a mere emergency measure, and with the recommendation that IDUs adhere to the standard of care even in the injection of illegal drugs, removing barriers and increasing the diversity of outlets for new, sterile syringes became the focus in the prevention of HIV among IDUs. Increasing access to sterile syringes suggested several new strategies in addition to increasing needle exchange services, such as removing legal restrictions on the purchase and possession of sterile syringes, and increasing pharmacy sales of sterile syringes and physician prescription of syringes for prevention of blood-borne disease.

Increasing Legal Access to Sterile Syringes

Currently, 13 states impose some form of prescription requirement for obtaining sterile syringes, however, only five states will not sell syringes at all without a prescription: California, Delaware, Massachusetts, New Jersey, and Pennsylvania. In response to the injection-related HIV epidemic five other states have partially deregulated syringes and now allow non-prescription sale and possession of syringes in limited numbers. The other three states – Nevada, Florida, and Virginia – have very partial prescription requirements. Nevada does not require a prescription for syringes used in the treatment of asthma, diabetes, and other types of medical conditions, and in a fairly tolerant environment, there is fairly good syringe access there. In Florida and Virginia, a prescription is only required for minors (Burris *et al.*, 2003).

Passing the law and establishing improved access to syringes was only half the battle. Early indications were that despite legal status, pharmacists might offer

435

barriers to the purchase of sterile syringes. One purchasing trial study was conducted in the early 1990s in St Louis, where the sale of syringes without a prescription was legal. An African American man and a white man attempted to purchase syringes in local pharmacies and found that the African American man was refused syringes in St Louis pharmacies more often than the white man. Other barriers to purchase, such as asking purchasers to buy a minimum of 100 syringes, were also noted. While the results were suggestive of racial bias, there were a limited number of visits and results were not statistically generalizable (Compton *et al.*, 1992).

A survey of Maine pharmacists conducted three years after the legislature repealed the law requiring a prescription found that only 50 per cent of pharmacists were willing to sell syringes if they suspected that the purchaser was an IDU, and of those willing to sell syringes to a suspected IDU, more than half reported imposing additional requirements, such as asking the customer to provide photographic identification, that were beyond the requirements of the law. In Maine, repealing the law was not enough, as the pharmacists enacted additional barriers to IDUs (Case *et al.*, 1998).

While these studies were either small or relied on pharmacist self-report of practice, other larger purchasing trials and assessment of actual practice have been conducted. In May 2000, the New York State Legislature passed a bill establishing the Expanded Syringe Access Demonstration Program (ESAP), which allowed anyone 18 years of age or older to purchase or obtain syringes from pharmacies and other health care facilities registered with the New York State Department of Health. By March 2002, 49 per cent of pharmacies in New York City had registered with the ESAP program; however, as in Maine there were concerns that drug users might encounter barriers related to stigma or gender, race/ethnicity, or age.

To assess pharmacy practice and the availability of sterile syringes, following the passage of the ESAP law Ruth Finkelstein and her colleagues conducted a large-scale purchasing trial in New York City. They tested purchasing with matched sets of testers who varied on key demographic characteristics such as age, race/ethnicity, and gender. Although significant geographic variability was found throughout the City, purchasers were able to obtain syringes in 69 per cent of attempts with no significant differences in ability to purchase by race/ethnicity or gender (Finkelstein *et al.*, 2002).

Syringe Prescription

It has been widely believed by physicians that prescription of syringes for the purpose of disease prevention in those who injected illegal drugs was prohibited by law and thus, physician prescription of syringes to active IDUs was quite rare. However, in the early 2000, Burris and co-workers found, in a comprehensive legal review in nearly all 50 states, the District of Columbia, and Puerto Rico that (1) physicians may legally prescribe injection equipment to active IDUs for the purposes of disease prevention and (2) pharmacists in most states have a reasonable basis for filling those prescriptions (Burris *et al.*, 2000). In the same year, the American Medical Association endorsed the prescription of syringes to help 'prevent the transmission of contagious disease', (American Medical Association, 2000).

Despite the perception that syringe prescription may be illegal, in 1999, the first syringe prescription program was established in Rhode Island. Physicians provided free medical care, including prescriptions for sterile syringes, for patients who were not ready to stop injecting. Very high-risk injection drug users enrolled in the program; of the 327 actively injecting people enrolled, 63 per cent did not have a primary care physician. This program showed that physician prescription of syringes was feasible and acceptable, with the most important element being open discussion of drug use and disease prevention between physician and patient and the engagement of the patient in care (Rich *et al.*, 2004).

While sales of syringes to IDUs with a prescription are clearly illegal in only three jurisdictions in the United States, the fact that physicians are still reluctant to prescribe speaks to the need to continue working to eliminate legal, regulatory, and cultural barriers to the prescription of syringes for the prevention of disease transmission (Burris *et al.*, 2002). A commitment to funding strategies that increase access to sterile syringes is not only sound from a public health perspective but also fiscally responsible. A national policy of funding NEPs, pharmacy sales, and syringe disposal in the US is estimated to cost US\$34278 per HIV infection averted, which is well below the lifetime costs of treating an individual's HIV infection (Lurie *et al.*, 1998).

Interrupting Sexual Transmission Among MSM Drug Users

Perhaps the most salient development in intervention among drug users is the recognition that the third element – setting – of Zinberg's formulation of 'drug, set, and setting' is critical in designing interventions (Zinberg, 1984). For MSM, concurrent with the timeline of the AIDS epidemic has been the elaboration of two specialized venues – the circuit party and the Internet. Both venues have been associated with increased sexual risk and associated drug use. While it is true that the format and participants of these venues are unique, specialized settings such as crack houses or public sex environments are more similar than different.

In a recent paper by Ross and colleagues (2003), drug use among MSM was significantly associated with both the sensation-seeking and social dimensions of circuit party attendance. Using a greater number of drugs, sexual activity while on drugs, and unsafe sex were more closely associated with the sensation-seeking dimension of attendance at circuit parties. This suggests that interventions which aim to modify sensation-seeking, for example using motivational interviewing techniques, may in turn reduce risky sexual behavior among MSM drug users (Kalichman *et al.*, 1996).

Future interventions should use venue-based interventions to reach high-risk MSM, especially those who attend raves and circuit parties that can function as commercial sex environments. In a recent study, differences between those who frequented these venues and those who did not emerged on several psychosocial factors, including sexual sensation-seeking, depression, and perceived responsibility towards protecting sexual partners from HIV infection (Parsons and Halkitis, 2002).

The Internet has been shown to be a 'virtual venue' for many MSM, who then meet to engage in sex (Benotsch *et al.*, 2002; Lau *et al.*, 2003). The use of the Internet to meet partners has been associated with increased methamphetamine use. In one study of over 600 MSM, one-third reported meeting sex partners online, and those who did reported higher rates of methamphetamine use (Benotsch *et al.*, 2002). MSM who prefer to meet sex partners through the Internet are likely to differ from those who do not. These men may be unwilling to attend more traditional venues for delivering treatment messages because of stigma and fear of being marginalized. A recent study by Lau and colleagues (2003) reported that nearly one-fifth of sexually active Chinese MSM in Hong Kong reported meeting partners on the Internet, and that these men tended to be younger and more likely to engage in anal sex. However, these studies also point out that the Internet has potential as a means of delivering prevention messages or possibly interventions to reach a wide audience of MSM drug users.

Treating HIV-Infected Drug Users

The advent of HAART (Highly Active Antiretroviral Therapy) has offered great hope to HIV-infected individuals and resulted in significant reductions in AIDS mortality (Palella *et al.*,1998; Valdez *et al.*, 2001). For drug users, substance abuse treatment and harm reduction programs take on an important secondary role – that of engaging drug users who are HIV positive in medical care, treatment for HIV disease, and prescription of HAART and support for adherence to HAART regimens.

There are significant adverse consequences associated with poor adherence to HAART to the patient and the community. The patient could develop a drug-resistant strain, limiting choices for treatment, and may transmit the resistant strain to others (Hecht *et al.*, 1998; Wainberg and Friedland, 1998). Generally speaking, drug non-adherence rates among current drug users are comparable to those in patients with other chronic disease (Stein *et al.*, 2000); recent drug use is associated with poor adherence to HIV medication (Palepu *et al.*, 2004). As a result, drug users may not be prescribed HAART and consequently suffer from increased HIV-related morbidity and mortality.

Directly observed therapy (DOT) has been used as a technique around the world to increase adherence to medication for tuberculosis. As with HIV medications, tuberculosis medication must be taken in a highly consistent way in order to avoid developing medication-resistant strains. However, there are key differences between HIV and tuberculosis treatment. Tuberculosis treatment is time-limited, HIV treatment is not; tuberculosis medication regimens often involve fewer medications than HIV regimens; tuberculosis patients can be compelled to take their medication through quarantine, HIV patients cannot. Hoping to find ways to help drug users become more compliant with often challenging HIV medication protocols, DOT has also been tested in the administration of HAART.

When used with HIV medication the practice is variously known as DOT-HAART, (Farmer *et al.*, 2001) MDOT (modified directly observed therapy) (McCance-Katz *et al.*, 2002) and DAART (directly administered antiretroviral therapy) (Altice *et al.*, 2004). All names refer to the use of DOT strategies with HIV medication protocols; each employing variations in flexibility, ancillary services provided, and in the types of observers and venues. DOT-HAART is the practice of observing HIV-infected patients taking at least some of their antiretroviral doses in combination with counseling, supportive cues, and other services to reinforce adherence to medication protocols. For convenience, all DOT strategies in this chapter will be referred to as DOT-HAART strategies.

Adherence to HIV therapy should be supported wherever drug users enter the continuum of care: emergency departments, harm reduction programs, prisons, and substance abuse treatment. In one example of a DOT-HAART program, Altice and colleagues conducted a randomized trial of DOT-HAART versus self-administration located on a medical van associated with the syringe exchange program in New Haven, CT. Those in the DOT-HAART arm received pagers for reminders, a medication bottle that was electronically monitored, and direct observation Monday through Friday of self-administered medication. At baseline participants reported taking a mean of about half the doses of medication required. Under supervision, adherence was increased to taking 76 per cent of doses and 85 per cent had undetectable levels of virus by six months. As an unanticipated consequence of the DOT-HAART program, 69 per cent chose to enter drug treatment after their viral load became undetected. Moving DOT-HAART beyond the walls of a methadone clinic may result in more out-of-treatment HIV-infected persons increasing their adherence; participants in the DOT-HAART trial reported that a methadone clinic was the least acceptable venue for engaging active IDUs in DOT-HAART (Altice *et al.*, 2004).

There is considerably more evidence about DOT-HAART when administered in a methadone clinic. Palepu and colleagues found in a prospective study of HIV-infected patients reporting alcohol and substance abuse that people engaged in substance abuse programs were 1.7 times more likely to receive HAART, but that adherence and viral load were not associated with substance abuse treatment. However, as both poor adherence and higher viral loads were associated with drug or alcohol use in the previous 30 days, engaging individuals in substance abuse treatment with a goal of reducing or stopping drug or alcohol use may greatly assist with adherence (Palepu *et al.*, 2004). In a contrasting cross-sectional study by Clarke, acceptance of and adherence to HAART therapy was associated with regular attendance at a methadone clinic (Clarke *et al.*, 2003). This is supported by health claims reviews that show that consistent participation in a methadone maintenance program was associated with a higher probability of antiretroviral use and, among antiretroviral users, more consistent use of anti-retrovirals (Sambamoorthi *et al.*, 2000).

One disadvantage to methadone patients of HAART is that methadone inter-acts with some antiretroviral medication. In one specific example methadone treatment reduces the bioavailability and absorption of didanosine (ddI) and stavudine (D4T) (Rainey *et al.*, 2000). The dose of antiretrovirals must be increased when a patient is on methadone. In other cases, the efficacy of methadone is reduced and must be increased during treatment. In one small pilot study of DOT-HAART, a mean methadone dose increase of 52 per cent was required (McCance-Katz *et al.*, 2002).

Enrolling methadone patients in DOT programs is efficient as methadone itself is a form of directly observed therapy; methadone is dispensed and administered at specific times under observation by medical providers. Adding HAART to these activities is relatively simple. With medical providers already on site, both HAART medications and methadone levels can be closely monitored and adjusted if necessary. DOT-HAART has also been tested in other structured environments such as prisons (Kirkland *et al.*, 2002), harm reduction programs (Altice *et al.*, 2004), and nursing facilities (Greenberg *et al.*, 1999). In a some-what more labor- and cost-intensive strategy, community or peer health workers have been used for DOT-HAART. Instead of requiring patients to come into a central location, community workers go directly to the patient, in their home or at some other venue to administer medications and provide other services (Mitty *et al.*, 2002).

Harm reduction programs that include syringe exchange also have fairly regu-lar attendance and may have medical personnel associated with the program. NEPs are an excellent venue for reaching out-of-treatment IDUs, and as reported above, have also been used successfully for DOT-HAART (Altice *et al.*, 2004). Whether located in a methadone clinic, in a prison, or at an NEP, these programs are venue-based, that is, patients are asked to come to a central location for DOT-HAART and efficient use is made of the existing practices of the venue.

Cost-effectiveness may be a disadvantage to DOT-HAART programs. Adherence is apparently only increased as long as the patients are observed. Wall found, in an early trial of DOT with AZT, that the effects lasted only as long as the intervention (Wall *et al.*, 1995). This result is found in other studies as well (Altice *et al.*, 2004). With patients who must adhere to HIV medications for a lifetime, DOT-HAART may not be sufficiently cost-effective to use on a large scale. For high-risk non-adherent drug-using populations engaged in structured medical programs, DOT-HAART is likely to significantly reduce morbidity, mortality, and transmission of resistant HIV.

What the Future Holds

Looking ahead, there are many key developments likely to affect the overall health of drug users. Among them are (1) contraction of drug treatment and disease prevention programs, (2) the expansion of the availability of buprenorphine and more diverse venues for treatment of drug addiction, (3) continued work on legal and policy barriers to access to sterile syringes, and (4) new developments in the prevention of sexual transmission of HIV among IDUs and MSM drugs users.

Reductions in funding of state and city health departments nationwide are having dramatic effects on the ability of providers to engage IDUs, and as a result the national drug treatment infrastructure has been profoundly affected. In a sample of 13 484 alcohol and drug treatment facilities, researchers found a further breakdown in the nation's infrastructure of care and addiction counseling. Between October 2001 and February 2003, 15 per cent of the programs had closed, 25 per cent had reorganized under a different administrative structure, more than half of the directors had been in their positions for less than a year, and 20 per cent had other problems with communication services, such as voicemail (McLellan *et al.*, 2003). This erosion of the specialized treatment system in the US supports arguments for drug treatment services to be made available in other settings such as physicians' offices.

In a second, more positive development, one of the great successes of intervention with injection drug use is the establishment of multiple points of entry into a continuum of care, whether to focus solely on preventing the transmission of infectious disease or to also engage a drug user in treatment for drug addiction. One such treatment modality is the use of methadone for detoxification and maintenance. In a recent development, new laws are permitting private physicians to treat patients in the privacy of their medical offices with buprenorphine hydrochloride.

Buprenorphine is easily prescribed and monitored in either a specialty clinic (as in methadone clinics), a general primary care facility, or in the privacy of a physician's office. There appears to be little negative effect of allowing physicians to treat patients for drug abuse in their offices. Gibson and colleagues randomly assigned 115 people seeking treatment for heroin addiction to receive buprenorphine at either a primary care office or a specialist clinic. There were no significant differences found in those retained in treatment in primary care (71 per cent) versus in a specialist clinic (78 per cent) and no significant differences in those retained in maintenance treatment following detoxification between those from primary care (50 per cent) and those from a specialist clinic (61 per cent) (Gibson *et al.*, 2003). With retention in detoxification and maintenance treatment similar between the two venues, some patients may benefit greatly from treatment in physicians' offices.

Buprenorphine treatment is effective and is prescribed either alone or in combination with naloxone in order to mediate cravings. In a randomized, multicenter, placebo-controlled study of 326 opiate-addicted people, Fudala and his colleagues found that two groups receiving buprenorphine were less likely to use opiates than the placebo group; the trial was ended early because of the demonstrated efficacy of buprenorphine (Fudala *et al.*, 2003). Other studies have shown that buprenorphine is just as effective as methadone in reducing opiate cravings (Johnson *et al.*, 2000; Carrieri *et al.*, 2003).

However, as with earlier battles about syringes, methadone, needle exchange, physician prescription of syringes, and other methods of interrupting HIV transmission and engaging IDUs in a continuum of care, regulations surrounding buprenorphine prescription are restricting the ability of patients to access treatment. Under the terms of the law authorizing buprenorphine treatment in the United States, physicians must apply for a waiver to treat and are limited to the treatment of 30 patients. Thus, physicians who are highly experienced with IDUs may not be allowed to apply their skills to their entire patient population. Nevertheless, being able to engage with opiate-dependent patients in the privacy of a physician's office is a major step in the diversification of treatment of IDUs.

In this next period of a worldwide epidemic of HIV and other infectious disease among drug users, one powerful intervention is to firmly address stigma related to drug users. Many resources and efforts have gone into implementing the most straightforward of rational public health recommendations, such as using a sterile syringe for every injection, that more complex and challenging potential interventions have fallen by the wayside. As emergency measures to deal with the AIDS epidemic become more integrated in a continuum of care, opportunities to address the root causes of epidemic transmission among drug users in the global context will open up.

The AIDS epidemic has led to a number of important benefits in other fields of research. For example, the discovery of HIV led to insights about the origin of Kaposi's sarcoma (KS), a malignancy associated with HIV and immunosuppression. It is now known that the main etiologic agent responsible for KS is a novel herpes virus called human herpes virus 8. The rapid analysis of the role of this novel herpes virus is a testament to scientific development and provides a new model for other time-critical investigations. Further, HIV-related studies of virus–host interactions have had a significant impact on our understanding of immunology, virology, molecular biology, and vaccine development and preparedness.

Finally, the need for a concerted response to the HIV pandemic has led to an unprecedented level of multilateral cooperation. Efforts such as the Global Fund to Fight AIDS, Tuberculosis and Malaria have been initiated in an attempt to provide HIV antiretroviral therapies for treatment and prophylaxis of HIV infection to resource-poor countries at a significantly discounted rate. While the mechanism for delivering these therapies has yet to be realized in most developing countries, the prevention and treatment of other scourges, such as tuberculosis and malaria, stand to benefit from these efforts. Additionally, in planning for the delivery of antiretroviral therapies and candidate HIV vaccines, it has been recognized that the infrastructure of health care systems in many countries is under-developed or has been eroded. As steps are made to strengthen these systems, improvements in the health of entire communities should follow. Improving the services available to individuals who use illegal drugs most surely should be a part of the global effort.

References

Altice FL, Springer S, Buitrago M, Hunt DP, Friedland GH (2003) Pilot study to enhance HIV care using needle exchange-based health services for out-of-treatment injecting drug users. *J Urban Health* 80: 416–27.

Altice FL, Mezger JA, Hodges J *et al.* (2004) Developing a directly administered anti-retroviral therapy intervention for HIV-infected drug users: Implications for program replication. *Clin Infect Dis* 38: S376–S387.

American Medical Association (AMA). Access to sterile syringes. Chicago, IL: *AMA*, June 2000.

Ball A (2002) Overview: Policies and interventions to stem HIV-1 epidemics associated with injecting drug use. In: Stimson G, Des Jarlais D, Al B, ed. *Drug Injecting and HIV Infection: Global Dimensions and Local Responses*. London: UCL Press.

Ball JC, Lange WR, Myers CP *et al.* (1988) Reducing the risk of AIDS through methadone maintenance treatment. *J Health Social Behav* 29: 214–26.

Bastos FI, Barcellos C, Lowndes CM, Friedman SR (1999) Co-infection with malaria and HIV in injecting drug users in Brazil: a new challenge to public health? *Addiction* 94: 1165–74.

Bayer R. Heroin maintenance: An historical perspective on the exhaustion of liberal narcotics reform. *Journal of Psychedelic Drugs* 1976, 8: 157–65.

Bell DS, Trethowan WH (1961) Amphetamine addiction. *Journal of Nervous and Mental Disease* 133: 489–96.

Benotsch EG, Kalichman S, Cage M (2002) Men who have met sex partners via the Internet: prevalence, predictors, and implications for HIV prevention. *Arch Sex Behav* 31: 177–83.

Berridge V, Edwards G (1981) *Opium and The People – Opiate Use in Nineteenth Century England*. London: Allen Lane.

Beyrer C, Razak MH, Lisam K, Chen J, Lui W, Yu XF (2000) Overland heroin trafficking routes and HIV-1 spread in south and south-east Asia. *AIDS* 14: 75–83.

Biggam AG (1929) Malignant malaria associated with the administration of heroin intravenously. *Trans R Soc Trop Med Hyg* 23: 147–53.

Biggam AG, Arafa MA (1930) Observations on a series of cases of artificially induced subtertian malaria with special reference to the effect of treatment by plasmoquine compound. *Trans R Soc Trop Med Hyg* 23: 591–607.

Bluthenthal RN, Kral AH, Gee L, Erringer EA, Edlin BR (2000) The effect of syringe exchange use on high-risk injection drug users: a cohort study. *AIDS* 14: 605–11.

443

Booth RE, Crowley T, Zhang Y (1996) Substance abuse treatment entry, retention, and effectiveness: out-of-treatment opiate injection drug users. *Drug Alcohol Depend* 42: 11–20.

Bruneau J, Lamothe F, Franco E *et al.* (1997) High rates of HIV infection among injection drug users participating in needle exchange programs in Montreal: results of a cohort study. *Am J Epidemiol* 146: 994–1002.

Buning EC (1991) Effects of Amsterdam needle and syringe exchange. *Int J Addict* 26: 1303–11.

Buning EC, Coutinho RA, van Brussel GH, van Santen GW, van Zadelhoff AW (1986) Preventing AIDS in drug addicts in Amsterdam. *Lancet* 1: 1435.

Burris S, Lurie P, Abrahamson D, Rich JD (2000) Physician prescribing of sterile injection equipment to prevent HIV infection: time for action. *Ann Intern Med* 133: 218–26.

Burris S, Vernick JS, Ditzler A, Strathdee S (2002) The legality of selling or giving syringes to injection drug users. *J Am Pharm Assoc* 42: S13–S18.

Burris S, Strathdee S, Vernick J (2003) Lethal injections: The law, science and politics of syringe access for injection drug users. *Univ San Francisco Law Rev* 37: 813–83.

Carrieri MP, Rey D, Loundou A *et al.* (2003) Evaluation of buprenorphine maintenance treatment in a French cohort of HIV-infected injecting drug users. *Drug Alcohol Depend* 72: 13–21.

Case P, Beckett GA, Jones TS (1998) Access to sterile syringes in Maine: Pharmacy practice after the 1993 repeal of the syringe prescription law. *J Acquir Immune Defic Syndr Hum Retrovirol* 18: S94–S101.

CDC (Centers for Disease Control) (1997) *HIV Prevention Bulletin: Medical Advice for Persons Who Inject Illicit Drugs.* Atlanta, GA: Centers for Disease Control.

Chaisson RE, Bacchetti P, Osmond D, Brodie B, Sande MA, Moss AR (1989) Cocaine use and HIV infection in intravenous drug users in San Francisco. *JAMA* 261: 561–5.

Clarke S, Delamere S, McCullough L, Hopkins S, Bergin C, Mulcahy F (2003) Assessing limiting factors to the acceptance of antiretroviral therapy in a large cohort of injecting drug users. *HIV Med* 4: 33–7.

Compton WM 3rd, Cottler LB, Decker SH, Mager D, Stringfellow R (1992) Legal Needle Buying in St. Louis. *Am J Pub Health* 82(4): 595–6.

Davoli M, Perucci CA, Forastiere F *et al.* (1993) Risk factors for overdose mortality: a case-control study within a cohort of intravenous drug users. *Int J Epidemiol* 22: 273–7.

Dehne KL, Khodakevich L, Hamers FF, Schwartlander B (1999) The HIV/AIDS epidemic in eastern Europe: Recent patterns and trends and their implications for policy-making. *AIDS* 13: 741–9.

Doherty MC, Junge B, Rathouz P, Garfein RS, Riley E, Vlahov D (2000) The effect of a needle exchange program on numbers of discarded needles: a 2-year follow-up. *Am J Public Health* 90: 936–9.

Dole VP, Nyswander ME (1965) A medical treatment for diaccetyl-morphine (heroin) addiction. *JAMA* 193: 146–50.

Edlin BR, Irwin KL, Faruque S *et al.* (1994) Intersecting epidemics – Crack cocaine use and HIV infection among inner-city young adults. *N Engl J Med* 331: 1422–7.

Farmer P, Leandre F, Mukherjee JS, *et al.* Community-based approaches to HIV treatment in resource-poor settings. *Lancet* 2001, 358: 404–9.

French MT, McGeary KA, Chitwood DD, McCoy CB (2000) Chronic illicit drug use, health services utilization and the cost of medical care. *Social Sci Med* 50: 1703–13.

Finkelstein R, Tiger R, Greenwald R, Mukherjee R (2002) Pharmacy syringe sale practices during the first year of expanded syringe availability in New York City (2001–2002). *J Am Pharm Assoc* 42: S83–S87.

Friedman CTH, Dover AS, Roberto RR, Kearns OA (1973) A malaria epidemic among heroin users. *Am J Trop Med Hyg* 22: 302–7.

Frosch D, Shoptaw S, Huber A, Rawson RA, Ling W (1996) Sexual HIV risk among gay and bisexual male methamphetamine abusers. *J Subst Abuse Treat* 13: 483–6.

Fudala PJ, Bridge TP, Herbert S *et al.* (2003) Office-based treatment of opiate addiction with a sublingual-tablet formulation of buprenorphine and naloxone. *N Engl J Med* 349: 949–58.

Garfein RS, Vlahov D, Galai N *et al.* (1996) Viral infections in short-term injection drug users; the prevalence of the hepatitis C, hepatitis B, human immunodeficiency virus, and human T-lymphotropic virus. *Am J Public Health* 86: 655–61.

Gibson AE, Doran CM, Bell JR, Ryan A, Lintzeris N (2003) A comparison of buprenorphine treatment in clinic and primary care settings: a randomised trial. *Med J Austr* 179: 38–42.

Gottlieb MS, Schanker HM, Fan PT, Saxon A, Weisman JD, Pozalski I (1981) Pneumocystis pneumonia – Los Angeles. *MMWR Morb Mortal Wkly Rev* 30: 1–3.

Greenberg B, Berkman A, Thomas R *et al.* (1999) Evaluating supervised HAART in late-stage HIV among drug users: a preliminary report. *J Urban Health* 76: 468–80.

Hagan H, Heimer R (1995) Hepatitis C virus infection and drug injection. Paper presented at the 5th North American Syringe Exchange Convention, San Juan, Puerto Rico.

Hagan H, Des Jarlais DC, Purchase D, Reid T, Friedman SR (1991) The Tacoma Syringe Exchange. *J Addict Dis* 10: 81–8.

Hahn JA, Vranizan KM, Moss AR (1997) Who uses needle exchange? A study of injection users in treatment in San Francisco, 1989–1990. *J. Acquired Immune Defic Synd Human Retrovir* 15(2): 157–64.

Hando J, Hall W. (1994) HIV risk-taking behavior among amphetamine users in Sydney, Australia. *Addiction* 89: 79–85.

Hecht FM, Grant RM, Petropoulous CJ *et al.* (1998) Sexual transmission of an HIV-1 variant resistant to multiple reverse-transcriptase and protease inhibitors. *N Engl J Med* 339: 307–11.

Heimer R (1998) Can syringe exchange serve as a conduit to substance abuse treatment? *J Subst Abuse Treat* 15: 183–91.

Heimer R, Khoshnood K, Bigg D, Guydish J, Junge B (1998) Syringe use and reuse: effects of syringe exchange programs in four cities. *J Acquir Immune Defic Syndr Hum Retrovirol* 18: S37–S44.

Helpern M (1934) Epidemic of fatal estivo-autumnal malaria among drug addicts in New York City transmitted by common use of hypodermic syringe. *Am J Surg* XXVI: 111–21.

Henman AR, Paone D, Des Jarlais DC, Kochems LM, Friedman SR (1998) From ideology to logistics: the organizational aspects of syringe exchange in a period of institutional consolidation. *Subst Use Misuse* 33: 1213–30.

Hesse E (1946) *Narcotics and Drug Addiction*. New York: Philosophical Library.

Hurley SF, Jolley DJ, Kaldor JM (1997) Effectiveness of needle-exchange programs for prevention of HIV infection. *Lancet* 349: 1797–800.

Johnson RE, Chutuape MA, Strain EC, Walsh SL, Stitzer ML, Bigelow GE (2000) A comparison of levomethadyl acetate, buprenorphine, and methadone for opioid dependence. *N Engl J Med* 343: 1290–7.

Kalichman SC, Heckman T, Kelly JA (1996) Sensation seeking as an explanation for the association between substance use and HIV-related risky sexual behavior. *Arch Sex Behav* 25: 141–54.

Kirkland LR, Fischl MA, Tashima KT *et al.* (2002) Response to lamivudine-zidovudine plus abacavir twice daily in antiretroviral-naïve, incarcerated patients with HIV infection taking directly observed treatment. *Clin Infect Dis* 34: 511–18.

Koran LM (1973) Heroin maintenance for heroin addicts: Issues and evidence. *N Engl J Med* 288: 654–60.

Lane SD (1993) A brief history. In: Stryker J, Smith MD, eds. *Dimensions of HIV Prevention: Needle Exchange*. Menlo Park, CA: Henry J. Kaiser Family Foundation, pp. 1–9.

Lau JT, Kim JH, Lau M, Tsui HY (2003) Prevalence and risk behaviors of Chinese men who seek same-sex partners via the Internet in Hong Kong. *AIDS Educ Prev* 15: 516–28.

Lewis DC. "Commentator Panel." Presented at: The First International Conference on Heroin Maintenance. New York Academy of Medicine, New York, NY. June 6, 1998.

Lurie P, Reingold AL, Bowser BP *et al.* (1993) *The Public Health Impact Of Needle Exchange Programs In The United States And Abroad: Summary, Conclusions And Recommendations*. Berkeley, CA: School of Public Health, University of California.

Lurie P, Gorsky R, Jones TS, Shomphe L (1998) An economic analysis of needle exchange and pharmacy-based programs to increase sterile syringe availability for injection drug users. *J Acquir Immune Defic Syndr Hum Retrovirol* 18: S126–S132.

MacMaster SA, Vail KA (2002) Demystifying the injection drug user: willingness to participate in traditional drug treatment services among participants in a needle exchange program. *J Psychoactive Drugs* 34: 289–94.

Markson LE, Houchens R, Fanning TR, Turner BJ (1998) Repeated emergency department use by HIV-infected persons: effect of clinic accessibility and expertise in HIV care. *J Acquir Immune Defic Syndr Hum Retrovirol* 17: 35–41.

Marmor M, Friedman-Kien AE, Laubenstein L *et al.* (1982) Risk factors for Kaposi's sarcoma in homosexual men. *Lancet* 1: 1083–7.

Marx MA, Crape B, Brookmeyer RS *et al.* (2000) Trends in crime and the introduction of a needle exchange program. *Am J Public Health* 90: 1933–6.

Marx MA, Brahmbhatt H, Beilenson P *et al.* (2001) Impact of needle exchange programs on adolescent perceptions about illicit drug use. *AIDS Behav* 5: 379–86.

Masur H, Michelis MA, Greene JB *et al.* (1981) An outbreak of community-acquired Pneumocystis carinii pneumonia: Initial manifestation of cellular immune dysfunction. *N Engl J Med* 305: 1431–8.

McCance-Katz EF, Gourevitch MN, Arnsten J, Sarlo J, Rainey P, Jatlow P (2002) Modified directly observed therapy (MDOT) for injection drug users with HIV disease. *Am J Addict* 11: 271–8.

McCarty F (1974) A case for heroin maintenance (Editorial) *Clin Toxicol* 7: 337–42.

McCoy CB, Rivers JE, McCoy HV *et al.* (1994) Compliance to bleach disinfection protocols among injecting drug users in Miami. *J Acquir Immune Defic Syndr* 7: 773–6.

McCusker J, Stoddard AM, Hindin RN, Garfield FB, Frost R (1996) Changes in HIV risk behavior following alternative residential programs of drug abuse treatment and AIDS education. *Ann Epidemiol* 6: 119–25.

McLellan AT, Carise D, Kleber HD (2003) Can the national addiction treatment infrastructure support the public's demand for quality care? *J Subst Abuse Treat* 25: 117–21.

Merrison AF, Chidley KE, Dunnett J, Sieradzan KA (2002) Wound botulism associated with subcutaneous drug use. *BMJ* 325: 1020–1.

Metzger DS, Woody GE, McLellan AT *et al.* (1993) Human immunodeficiency virus seroconversion among in- and out-of-treatment intravenous drug users: an 18-month prospective follow-up. *J Acquir Immune Defic Syndr* 6: 1049–56.

Mitty JA, Stone VE, Sands M *et al.* (2002) Directly observed therapy for the treatment of people with human immunodeficiency virus infection: a work in progress. *Clin Infect Dis* 34: 984–90.

Moliter F, Traux S, Ruiz J, Sun R (1998) Association of methamphetamine use during sex with risky sexual behaviors and HIV infection among non-injection drug users. *West J Med* 168: 93–7.

MMWR (1982) Current trends update on acquired immune deficiency syndrome (AIDS) – United States. *MMWR Morb Mortal Wkly Rep* 31: 507–8, 513–14.

Musto D (1987) *The American Disease*. New York: Oxford University Press.

Normand J, Vlahov D, Moses LE (eds) (1995) *Preventing HIV Transmission: The Role of Sterile Needles and Bleach*. Washington: National Academy Press.

Palella FJ, Delaney K, Moorman A *et al*. (1998) Declining morbidity and mortality among patients with advanced HIV infection. HIV Outpatient Study Investigators. *N Engl J Med* 338: 853–60.

Palepu A, Strathdee SA, Hogg RS *et al*. (1999) The social determinants of emergency department and hospital use by injection drug users in Canada. *J Urban Health* 76: 409–18.

Palepu A, Horton N, Tibbetts N, Meli S, Samet J (2004) Uptake and adherence to highly active antiretroviral therapy among HIV-infected people with alcohol and other substance use problems: the impact of substance abuse treatment. *Addiction* 99: 361–8.

Paone D, Clark J, Shi Q, Purchase D, Des Jarlais DC (1999) Syringe exchange in the United States, 1996: A national profile. *Am J Public Health* 89: 43–6.

Parsons JT, Halkitis PN (2002) Sexual and drug-using practices of HIV-positive men who frequent public and commercial sex environments. *AIDS Care* 14: 815–26.

Pollack HA, Khoshnood K, Blankenship KM, Altice FL (2002) The impact of needle exchange-based health services on emergency department use. *J Gen Intern Med* 17: 341–8.

Prins M, Hernandez Aguado IH, Brettle RP *et al*. (1997) Pre-AIDS mortality from natural causes associated with HIV disease progression: evidence from the European Seroconverter Study among injecting drug users. *AIDS* 11: 1747–56.

Rainey PM, Friedland G, McCance-Katz EF *et al*. (2000) Interaction of methadone with didanosine and stavudine. *J Acquir Immune Defic Syndr* 24: 241–8.

Resnick L, Veren K, Salahuddin SZ, Tondreau S, Markham PD (1986) Stability and inactivation of HTLV-III/LAV under clinical and laboratory environments. *JAMA* 255: 1887–91.

Rezza G, Pizzuti R, De Campora E, De Masi S, Vlahov D (1996) Tetanus and injections drug use: rediscovery of a neglected problem? *Eur J Epidemiol* 12: 655–6.

Rich JD, McKenzie M, Macalino GE *et al*. (2004) A syringe prescription program to prevent infectious disease and improve health of injection drug users. *J Urban Health* 81: 122–34.

Rosenbaum M (1997) The de-medicalization of methadone maintenance. In: Erickson PG, Riley DM, Cheung YW, O'Hare PA, eds. *Harm Reduction: A New Direction for Drug Policies and Programs*. Toronto: University of Toronto Press, pp. 69–79.

Ross MW, Mattison AM, Franklin DR Jr (2003) Club drugs and sex on drugs are associated with different motivations for gay circuit party attendance. *Men. Subst Use Misuse* 38(8): 1173–83.

Sambamoorthi U, Warner LA, Crystal S, Walkup J (2000) Drug abuse, methadone treatment, and health services use among injection drug users with AIDS. *Drug Alcohol Depend* 60: 77–89.

Schechter MT, Strathdee SA, Cornelisse PG *et al*. (1999) Do needle exchange programmes increase the spread of HIV among injection drug users?: An investigation of the Vancouver outbreak. *AIDS* 13: F45–51.

Semple S, Patterson T, Grant I (2002) Binge use of methamphetamine among HIV-positive men who have sex with men: Pilot data and HIV prevention implications. *AIDS Educ Prev* 15: 133–47.

Shah N, Celentano DD, Vlahov D *et al*. (2000) Correlates of enrollment in methadone maintenance programs differ by HIV-serostatus. *AIDS* 14: 2035–43.

Smith D *et al*. (1978) *Amphetamine Use, Misuse, and Abuse: Proceedings of the National Amphetamine Conference*. Boston, MA: GK Hall Medical.

Solomon L, Frank R, Vlahov D, Astemborski J (1991) Utilization of health services in a cohort of intravenous drug users with known HIV-1 serostatus. *Am J Public Health* 81: 1285–90.

Steigman F, Hyman S, Goldbloom R (1950) Infectious hepatitis (homoogous serum type) in drug addicts. *Gastroenterology* 15: 642–6.

Stein MD, Sobota M (2001) Injection drug users: hospital care and charges. *Drug Alcohol Depend* 64: 117–20.

Stein MD, Rich JD, Maksad J, Chen MH, Hu P, Sobota M *et al.* (2000) Adherence to anti-retroviral therapy among HIV-infected methadone patients: effect of ongoing illicit drug use. *Am J Drug Alcohol Abuse* 26: 195–205.

Stephens R, Simpson D, Coyle S *et al.* (1993) Comparative effectiveness of NADR interventions. In: Brown B, Beschner G, eds. *Handbook of Risk of AIDS: Injection Drug Users and Sexual Partners*. Westport, CT: Greenwood Press.

Stimson GV. The global diffusion of injecting drug use: implications for Human Immunodeficiency Virus infection. *United Nations Office on Drugs and Crime Bulletin on Narcotics* 1993, 1: 3–17.

Stimson GV, Choopanya K (1998) Global perspectives on drug injecting. In: Stimson GV, Des Jarlais DC, Ball AL, eds. *Drug Injecting And HIV Infection: Global Dimensions And Local Responses*. London: UCL Press, pp. 1–21.

Strathdee SA, van Ameijden E, Mesquita F, Wodak A, Rana S, Vlahov D (1998) Can HIV epidemics among injection drug users be prevented? *AIDS* 12: S71–79.

Strathdee SA, Celentano DD, Shah N *et al.* (1999) Needle-exchange attendance and health care utilization promote entry into detoxification. *J Urban Health* 76: 448–60.

Talan DA, Moran GJ (1998) Tetanus among injecting-drug users – California, 1997. *Ann Emerg Med* 32: 385–6.

Valdez H, Chowdhry T, Asaad R *et al.* (2001) Changing spectrum of mortality due to HIV: analysis of 260 deaths during 1995–1999. *Clin Infect Dis* 32: 1487–93.

van Ameijden EJ, Coutinho RA (1998) Maximum impact of HIV prevention measures targeted at injecting drug users. *AIDS* 12: 625–33.

Vertefeuille J, Marx MA, Tun W, Huettner S, Strathdee SA, Vlahov D (2000) Decline in self-reported high risk injection-related behaviors among HIV seropositive participants in the Baltimore Needle Exchange Program. *AIDS Behav* 4: 381–8.

Vlahov D, Junge B, Brookmeyer R *et al.* (1997) Reductions in high-risk drug use behaviors among participants in the Baltimore needle exchange program. *J Acquir Immune Defic Syndr Hum Retrovirol* 16: 400–6.

Wainberg MA, Friedland G (1998) Public health implications of antiretroviral therapy and drug resistance. *JAMA* 279: 1977–83.

Watters JK (1994) Historical perspective on the use of bleach in HIV/AIDS prevention. *J Acquir Immune Defic Syndr* 7: 743–6.

Watters JK, Downing M, Case P, Lorvick J, Cheng YT, Fergusson B (1990) AIDS prevention for intravenous drug users in the community: street-based education and risk behavior. *Am J Community Psychol* 18: 587–96.

Wall TL, Sorensen JL, Batki SL, Delucchi KL, London JA, Chesney MA (1995) Adherence to zidovudine (AZT) among HIV-infected methadone patients: a pilot study of supervised therapy and dispensing compared to usual care. *Drug Alcohol Depend* 37: 261–9.

Zinberg NE (1984) Drug, Set, and Setting: The Basis For Controlled Intoxicant Use. Yale University Press.

Zule WA, Desmond DP (1999) An ethnographic comparison of HIV risk behaviors among heroin and methamphetamine injectors. *Am J Drug Alcohol Abuse* 25: 1–23.

Management of HIV/AIDS in Correctional Settings

18

Frederick L Altice
Associate Professor and Director of Clinical Research, AIDS Program, Section of Infectious Diseases, Yale University School of Medicine, New Haven, USA

Sandra A Springer
Clinical Instructor, AIDS Program, Section of Infectious Diseases, Yale University School of Medicine, New Haven, USA

Frederick L Altice, MD is Associate Professor of Medicine and Director of the HIV in Prisons Program and the Community Health Care Van at the AIDS Program, Section of Infectious Diseases, at Yale University School of Medicine. He received his medical degree from Emory University and completed his post-doctoral training at Yale University. He has published extensively in the areas of health care delivery for HIV-infected drug users, prisoners and other marginalized populations. He is a clinical epidemiologist and health outcomes researcher and has been the principal investigator on several grants from NIDA, SAMHSA, CDC, HRSF and private foundations. He is currently the recipient of a career development award from the National Institute on Drug Abuse where he is developing and evaluating interventions for HIV-infected drug users – specifically the integration of buprenorphine into HIV clinical care and directly administered antiretroviral therapy.

Sandra A Springer, MD recently completed her Post-doctoral Fellowship in Infectious Diseases and is currently a Clinical Instructor at the AIDS Program, Section of Infectious Diseases, at Yale University School of Medicine. During her post-doctoral training, she was the recipient of the Bristol-Myers Squibb HIV Virology Fellowship Award as well as supplemental funding from the National Institutes on Drug Abuse for her research on prisoners with HIV infection. She is currently interested in developing novel interventions at the interface of HIV/AIDS, substance abuse treatment and mental illness.

449

The overlapping epidemics of incarceration, illicit drug use, and HIV infection continue to grow in the United States, with each epidemic compounding and negatively impacting the other. Prisoners are at exceptional risk for HIV infection because of the association between injection drug use and incarceration. Women prisoners are at additional risk for HIV as a consequence of being more likely to be drug users than men and to have engaged in commercial sex work that puts them at increased sexual risk. This chapter reviews the following issues associated with HIV infection in prisoners: epidemiology, prevalence, and transmission; the growing complications from managing co-morbid conditions; institutional constraints, including prison policies and practices, confidentiality, informed consent, and medical research; the extensive involvement of the legal system in the area of HIV in prisoners; prevention and the role of educational programs and issues surrounding the transition of prisoners to community settings.

Epidemiology and Background

As of 31 December 2001, 6 million people in the United States lived under the jurisdiction of the criminal justice system, and 2.1 million were in jail or prison. The United States imprisons its population at the highest known rate in the world at 686 per 100 000. In 1998, 11.5 million people were released from jails and prisons to communities in the United States. These figures, which increase daily, indicate the country's devotion to a formidable social policy of imprisonment, and the huge public health impact of prisoners' health on the community at large. Prison populations have multiplied in recent decades, primarily because incarceration has been the central tactic of the 'war on drugs' in the United States. The millions of intermittently incarcerated people in America, many of whom are illicit drug users, are among the most difficult people to reach with critical health information. The National Commission on AIDS stated in its 1991 report: 'By choosing mass imprisonment as the federal and state governments' response to the use of drugs, we have created a de facto policy of incarcerating more and more individuals with HIV infections. Fifty-seven per cent of federal prisoners were incarcerated for drug offenses in 2001 (US National Commission on AIDS, 1991; US Bureau of Justice Statistics, 2000; Maruschak, 2001; Harrison and Beck, 2002).

The prevalence of HIV is fives times higher (Spauldin, *et al.*, 2002) and that of AIDS four times (Maruschak, 2002) higher in state and federal prisons than in the general US population. Twenty-six per cent of people living with HIV/AIDS in the United States have spent time in the correctional system (Hammett *et al.*, 2002). No precise prevalence is available of HIV cases in prisons and jails; brief incarceration, limited access to health care, and inadequate health services prevent identification and diagnosis of inmates with HIV infection. Arrestees may choose not to declare their HIV status. In addition, there is no national system for reporting prison cases in the United States; the Centers for Disease Control and Prevention (CDC) surveillance information does not include patients' custody status. Independent surveys and many regional studies in the United States and internationally, however, have been performed.

In 1999, the US National Institute of Justice survey of 50 state prison systems, the federal prison system, and 3365 local jail systems reported 9723 current CDC-defined AIDS cases (Maruschak, 2001). State prisons in New York, Texas, Florida, and California reported more than half of the confirmed AIDS cases in all 50 state prisons.

The prevalence of reported HIV cases in 2000 was 2.2 per cent in the 50 state prison systems and 0.8 per cent in the federal prison system (Maruschak, 2002). The 30 June 1999 census of jails found 1.7 per cent of local jail inmates were HIV-infected. Jails in the south and north-east accounted for 80 per cent of all known HIV-infected inmates. The highest reported prevalence of HIV cases was found in jails in the north-east corridor – Washington, DC (7.6 per cent), New York (4.3 per cent), and Massachusetts (4.0) per cent.

Although women account for only 5–10 per cent of the prison population and have represented a smaller percentage of total CDC-defined AIDS cases, women prisoners have a higher HIV prevalence than male prisoners (3.0 per cent compared with 2.0 per cent, respectively). This discrepancy exists in most state prison systems, and cumulatively in each of the four US regions identified by the Department of Justice: Northeast, Midwest, South, and West. In three prison systems – Nevada, District of Columbia, and New York – more than 20 per cent of all female inmates were known to be HIV-infected. In all states, fewer than 10 per cent of male inmates were reported to be HIV-infected (Singleton *et al.*, 1990; Vlahov *et al.*, 1991; US Bureau of Justice Statistics, 1995; Maruschak, 2001).

The incidence of CDC-defined AIDS in US prison inmates parallels the uneven geographic distribution of CDC-defined AIDS in injection drug users (IDUs), and regional patterns of incarceration and case finding. Through March 1994, 93 per cent of CDC-defined AIDS patients in New York's prisons were inmates with histories of injection drug use. A comparison of prison AIDS cases with total US AIDS cases in 1994–1996 found that 61 per cent of prison cases had injected drugs compared with 27 per cent of total cases (Dean-Gaitor and Fleming, 1999). By 1996, the AIDS case rate per 100 000 for incarcerated persons was 199, six times higher than the national rate of 31 cases per 100 000 US population. AIDS case rates per 100 000 for women (287) were higher than for men (185) and higher for blacks (253) and Hispanics (313) than for whites (100). Though New York has the highest absolute number of AIDS cases, Connecticut had the highest AIDS case rate among incarcerated persons (1348 per 100 000). This rate is 43-fold greater than found in the general population in Connecticut (Dean-Gaitor and Fleming, 1999).

The disproportionate burden of HIV infection among racial minorities is more pronounced in prison than in the community. Racial statistics are not routinely collected in seroprevalence studies. The comparison of prison and total AIDS cases cited above found that African Americans comprise 58 per cent of prison

451

cases versus 39 per cent of total cases. A report from Maryland of 888 AIDS cases identified in the state's prisons noted that 91 per cent were African American, versus 75 per cent statewide (Kassira *et al.*, 2001).

Improved HIV identification and treatment in the late 1990s resulted in a precipitous drop in AIDS deaths in custody as well as in the community. In 1999, 242 state prisoners died from AIDS, down from 1010 in 1995. HIV seroprevalence in state prisons nationwide has dropped slightly from 4.0 per cent to 3.4 per cent in female prisoners and from 2.3 per cent to 2.1 per cent in male prisoners, although the absolute numbers have risen with the increasing rates of incarceration (Maruschak, 2001).

The New York State Commission of Correction published the first extensive report on state prison cases of HIV infection. By the end of 1999, 25 per cent of all US inmates known to be HIV-infected were in New York State's prisons. New York State had recorded 2186 prison deaths from CDC-defined AIDS through September 1996. New York's early experience with markedly high numbers of prisoners with HIV offered a view into the future for other prison systems. Most recent seroprevalence information from New York State was reported in 2000: 4.7 per cent of men and 13.9 per cent of women were HIV-infected upon entry to the state prison (Gido and Gaunay, 1990; Mikl *et al.*, 1993; Lyons *et al.*, 1994; Bureau of HIV/AIDS Epidemiology, 1996; Maruschak, 2001; Wang *et al.*, 2002).

Prisons in other nations first reported AIDS cases several years after the United States. The rate of increase in cases in these countries, however, has been steep. No comprehensive surveys have been reported, but countries with particularly high seroprevalence identified among prisoners include Brazil (15 per cent in 2001 [0.6 per cent in community]), Côte d'Ivoire (27.5 per cent in 2001 [10.8 per cent in community]), South Africa (15 per cent in 2001 [19.9 per cent in community]), Zambia (26.7 per cent), Nigeria (9.0 per cent), Honduras (6.8 per cent), Russian Federation (3.1 per cent), the Netherlands (3.1 per cent), France (4.1 per cent), and Spain (16.4 per cent in 2000) (Harding, 1990; Harding and Schaller, 1992; Thomas and Moerings, 1994; Hernandez *et al.*, 1996; Hammett, 2002; Menoyo *et al.*, 2002).

Survival Experience

In 2002, AIDS deaths among New York inmates became increasingly rare. In the 1980s, however, the time from AIDS diagnosis until death among NY state prison inmates was significantly lower than that in matched New York City unincarcerated people with AIDS (Smith *et al.*, 1991). The survival time for female inmates in New York State was significantly shorter than that for male inmates (Mikl *et al.*, 1991). In addition, HIV-infected inmates with a first case of *Pneumocystis jiroveci* pneumonia (PCP) had a 22 per cent mortality rate, compared with a rate of 8 per cent among patients with HIV and PCP in the community at large in 1989

(Sharp, 1989). A remarkable statistic from New York in 1988 was that more than 25 per cent of CDC-defined AIDS diagnoses in prison were first made at autopsy (Correction Association of New York, 1988). Some diagnoses of tuberculosis (TB) in inmates have been made only at autopsy. In 1997, AIDS diagnoses of New York State inmates were still often established only at autopsy, delaying statistical monitoring by at least eight months pending autopsy completion. Although New York State held one-third of all US prisoners known to be HIV-infected, a 2001 report showed that the number of AIDS deaths in 1999 among New York State prisoners was 26, down from an annual peak of 258 in 1994, and the lowest it had been in 16 years (Maruschak, 2001). The availability of prophylaxis for opportunistic infections and provision of highly active antiretroviral therapy (HAART) to prisoners, as well as the slightly lower rate of HIV sero-prevalence in inmates are all believed to contribute to this reduced mortality (CDC, 1999; Maruschak, 2001).

A report from Spain describes a parallel improvement in case identification and survival. A review of the delay between time of discovery of HIV infection until AIDS diagnosis revealed that in 1984, 100 per cent of prisoners' HIV infections were diagnosed in the same month as AIDS, whereas in 2000 only 4 per cent of HIV and AIDS diagnoses were made contemporaneously (Guerrero *et al.*, 2002).

HIV Transmission in Prisons

Numerous studies have identified high-risk behaviors for HIV transmission in correctional settings, including injection drug use (Clarke *et al.*, 2001; Calzavara *et al.*, 2003; O'Sullivan *et al.*, 2003) and unprotected sex (Douglas *et al.*, 1989; Wolfe *et al.*, 2001). Despite the high prevalence of HIV risk behaviors within prison, there are few data demonstrating widespread intra-prison transmission of HIV. Several studies have identified transmission of HIV in prison, based on serial serological testing for HIV antibody, some identifying seroconversion in inmates after more than five years of continuous incarceration (Brewer *et al.*, 1988; Horsburgh *et al.*, 1990; Castro *et al.*, 1991; Mutter *et al.*, 1994). Molecular analysis of 14 HIV-infected inmates in Glenochil prison in Scotland in 1993 found sequencing similarities and clinical histories in 13 of the 14, indicating that transmission had occurred at the institution (Yirrell *et al.*, 1996).

No confirmed cases of HIV infection among US prison staff have been attributed to contact with inmates. There is a report from Australia of seroconversion of a correctional officer who was injected by an infected inmate with a syringe full of his own blood (Hammett, 1991).

Sexual activity between male inmates is not uncommon in prisons and jails. A Federal Bureau of Prisons study in 1982 reported that 30 per cent of federal prison inmates engaged in homosexual activity while incarcerated (Nacci and Kane, 1982). In a 1984 study of Tennessee inmates, 17 per cent reported homosexual activity in prison (Decker *et al.*, 1984). Former prisoners surveyed in New York reported use of makeshift devices for safer sex, such as fingers of latex gloves, when condoms were not available (Mahon, 1996).

The frequency of homosexual rape in jails and prisons is extremely difficult to estimate. The victim who reports rape in prison faces a probability of further suffering and worse injury. The Federal Bureau of Prisons study reported that 9–20 per cent of federal inmates, especially new or homosexual inmates, were victims of rape (Nacci and Kane, 1982). The text of the *Prison Rape Reduction Act of 2002* states that the best expert estimate of the number of individuals sexually attacked at least once during their incarceration is a national median of 13.6 per cent. (The act establishes standards for identifying, investigating, and eliminating prison rape in the United States; S. 2619, HR. 4943.)

Other incidents of interpersonal violence (including fights involving lacerations, bites, and bleeding in two or more participants) present some risks for HIV transmission. These risk activities in prisons and jails do not involve consenting participants, and condoms or educational programs are not likely to prevent HIV transmission in these situations. Prison authorities prevent violence among prisoners with adequate staffing, supervision, programming, and housing. Housing more than one inmate per cell, common now in crowded institutions, is a major contributing factor to incidents of violence and sexual assault.

British investigators interviewed 452 released prisoners about activities before, during, and after prison stays and found that people engaged in fewer incidents of HIV risk behavior in prison compared with in the community, but that activities in prison were associated with increased risk. Those who reported engaging in penetrative sex while in prison also reported doing so with greater frequency outside, although they only used condoms outside. Compared with outside the correctional setting, increased sharing of syringes and less effective methods of syringe cleaning were reported during the period of incarceration (Turnbull *et al.*, 1992). In another report from the United Kingdom, IDUs who were former prisoners reported a high prevalence of injection and sexual risk behaviors while in prison; 33 of 50 had injected drugs, and 5 of 50 had had sex with 2–16 men (Carvell and Hart, 1990).

Although imprisoned IDUs do not use drugs with the same frequency they use them in the community setting, they do share injection equipment more and sterilize it less because of scarce resources within the correctional setting. A handmade syringe may be fashioned from (among other things) parts of pens and light bulbs. Prisoners may also share toothbrushes, another potential source of HIV infection, in facilities where they are not issued, where inmates are unable to purchase their own, or where infection control precautions are not understood.

Tattooing is widely practiced in prisons and is usually performed without fresh or sterile instruments. It involves multiple skin punctures with recycled, sharpened, and altered implements such as staples, paper clips, guitar wire, and the plastic ink tubes from ballpoint pens. Prison wisdom holds that tattooing that causes blood to flow results in the best quality image and is least likely to become infected. Homemade pigment is delivered intradermally (at a sharp angle) rather than through direct puncture. Metal points connected to a battery or other electrical source are capable of producing vibration, increasing the number of skin punctures exponentially, thereby creating a better tattoo, but also increasing the probability of HIV transmission. Body piercing is becoming more popular in prison as in the outside community, and clean instruments for this practice are similarly unavailable.

Some sites have adopted approaches to reduce the likelihood of HIV transmission in correctional settings. Unfortunately, these policies are minimally available in the US and when implemented, are done so such that they are likely to have minimal effect on HIV transmission. Presently, only seven US correctional systems have made condoms available within correctional settings. These include two state prison systems (Vermont and Mississippi) and five county/jail systems (District of Columbia, Los Angeles, New York City, Philadelphia and San Francisco) (Hammett, 1999). While theoretically these policies are developed to reduce HIV transmission, logistical constraints have impaired their effectiveness. For instance, limiting access to condoms, requiring multiple counseling sessions before providing condoms, and self-identifying oneself as a 'homosexual' have reduced the effectiveness of such programs.

To date, no programs in the US provide clean syringes or bleach for cleaning paraphernalia for those who inject while incarcerated. Pilot programs making bleach available in Canadian (Jurgens, 2002) and New Zealand (Dolan *et al.*, 1998) prisons have demonstrated some initial successes. The attitudes about HIV prevention among correctional staff, however, may be pivotal in ensuring effective programs (Godin *et al.*, 2001). Accessible clean injection equipment, through syringe exchange programs, has been initiated in several European correctional settings, including Switzerland. After the introduction of syringe exchange, methadone maintenance, and bleach into prison settings in Switzerland, no new cases of transmission of hepatitis viruses B and C or HIV were detected (Anonymous, 1996).

Interventions that may reduce transmission of HIV and other infections have been poorly studied and almost completely ignored in correctional settings. The primary reason for ignoring this very important public health issue has been a political one. Correctional facilities are politicized, particularly in the US, and are outside the jurisdiction of public health authorities. To acknowledge that HIV risk behaviors occur in correctional settings is to acknowledge that the correctional setting is not enforcing their zero tolerance policy toward sexual and drug use activities. Moreover, correctional systems indicate that condoms may provide a method to store contraband and that injecting equipment may be used as a weapon. Notwithstanding these concerns, the research and correctional communities have been almost silent on this issue and a thorough evaluation is merited after more than two and a half decades of HIV/AIDS.

HIV and Co-morbid Conditions

HIV-infected prison inmates have a disproportionate number of multiple other co-morbid conditions including other infectious diseases such as tuberculosis and viral hepatitis, as well as mental illness, obstetric and gynecologic issues, and untreated drug and alcohol dependency or abuse.

An evaluation of infectious diseases among inmates of and releasees from US correctional facilities found that although about only 3 per cent of the US population spent time in a correctional facility that year, a disproportionate number had other infectious diseases in addition to HIV/AIDS. This study found that during 1997 alone, over 40 per cent of all those infected with hepatitis C and 40 per cent of all those with tuberculosis had passed through a correctional facility that year (Hammett *et al.*, 2002).

HIV and Tuberculosis

Tuberculosis has had a significant impact on the correctional system long before HIV became a problem. In particular, its higher prevalence and incidence among individuals who are incarcerated (e.g. injection drug users, homeless, inner city poor, people of color) compared with the community at large and the ease and frequency of airborne transmission of tuberculosis bacilli in the crowded conditions make prisons a volatile place for tuberculosis outbreaks (Snider and Hutton, 1989). Furthermore, prisoners released to the community have a much higher percentage of active tuberculosis cases (35 per cent) (National Commission on Correctional Health Care, 2003). In the presence of HIV infection, latent tuberculosis is more likely to become active. Moreover, in the setting of a high prevalence of inmates with HIV infection with a compromised immune system, tuberculosis is more likely to be silently transmitted to HIV-infected inmates as well as progress into active disease. Tuberculosis among the immunocompromised is also more likely to clinically present in an atypical fashion and obscure and delay its diagnosis – often allowing many individuals to become infected in the crowded correctional setting. Moreover, the inconsistent treatment that often characterizes prisoners' medical care can permit the development of multidrug-resistant strains of tuberculosis (MDR-TB) – a medical travesty reported in the New York and California state prisons. In 1991 in New York, seven inmates and one immune-suppressed correctional officer died with rapidly fatal, untreatable tuberculosis, and drug-resistant tuberculosis became epidemic in the New York City – New Jersey metropolitan area (MMWR, 1991).

The clinical history of a California prison inmate treated for active tuberculosis and later for MDR-TB over 3.5 years illustrates the full range of problems in prison management of tuberculosis: poor record keeping at initial screening, delay in diagnosis of symptomatic disease, lack of isolation of the patient at the time of diagnosis, lack of supervision or observation of medication ingestion, lack of follow-up after completion of initial treatment, infirmary treatment in a setting with susceptible HIV patients, inadequate ventilation of patients' rooms, transfers of this patient during treatment for MDR-TB among three different prisons, and inadequate screening and testing of most prison staff to ascertain their response to this exposure (MMWR, 1993). Illustrating the dangers of tuberculosis to HIV-infected prisoners, a 1999 CDC report describes multiple purified protein derivative (PPD) conversions in 1995–1996 among California prisoners, staff, and community contacts despite tuberculosis control practices. Two HIV-infected inmates, one with a documented negative PPD, the other, previously treated for positive PPD, with *Mycobacterium tuberculosis*-negative sputum smears and cultures, proved to be infected with tuberculosis after initial placement in the dedicated prison HIV housing unit. Similarly in an HIV housing unit in South Carolina from 1999–2000, 31 HIV-infected prison contacts of an inmate with unsuccessfully treated latent tuberculosis were subsequently diagnosed with active tuberculosis – a magnitude greater than would have been expected if this had occurred in a non-HIV housing unit. Therefore, one of the negative consequences of segregating HIV housing is the resultant rapid spread of tuberculosis when a single case goes undetected (MMWR, 1999, 2000).

Reports described a six-fold increase in the incidence of tuberculosis among New York State inmates from 1976 to 1986, by which time more than 50 per cent of inmates with tuberculosis were also infected with HIV (Braun *et al.*, 1989). An analysis of tuberculosis cases reported in New York City from 1985 to 1992 demonstrated an association between incarceration and subsequent diagnosis of tuberculosis; one year of time in jail increased the risk of tuberculosis to 2.2 times the risk of the general population (Bellin *et al.*, 1993). Although reports from Maryland and the UK failed to find a similar association, the New York figures underscore the need for routine, thorough screening, and prophylactic treatment of all HIV-infected prisoners as well as others at risk for tuberculosis (Darbyshire, 1989; MMWR, 1989a; Salive *et al.*, 1990). This screening should minimally include chest X-rays, medical history, and examination.

In jails, many inmates are not incarcerated long enough to permit diagnosis or treatment. Clinical investigation for suggestive signs and symptoms is critical. To detect active pulmonary disease in the setting of rapid inmate turnover, the Los Angeles County Jail performs 'mini chest films' – single-view, low-dose screening radiographs – at much greater cost than the widely practiced skin test, but with fairly immediate results. Although they will not detect all cases of tuberculosis, these radiographic images identify people with communicable disease who require immediate treatment and isolation (Hammett and Harrold, 1994).

In addition to intake screening for tuberculosis, subsequent routine follow-up and surveillance programs are essential for inmates and prison staff. The CDC published recommendations for prevention and control of tuberculosis in correctional institutions in 1989 and 1996 (MMWR, 1989b, 1996). Despite these recommendations, tuberculosis screening and treatment policies in prisons and jails are not uniformly adopted and will likely contribute to further tuberculosis outbreaks that are fueled by the high prevalence of HIV.

Hepatitis C Virus

Hepatitis C virus (A review of HCV infection and treatment in correctional settings has recently been published, Altice and Bruce,2004) is primarily transmitted parenterally, yet sexual transmission does occur. Unlike HIV, HCV is more efficiently transmitted and is more prevalent among IDUs and appears to be transmitted within the first five years after initiation of injection (Garfein *et al.*, 1998). Because HCV is associated with injection drug use, its prevalence is higher in the North-East than in other geographical sites in the US. It is therefore not surprising that there is a significant number of inmates who are co-infected with HIV and HCV. It is estimated that the prevalence of HCV in state and federal correctional facilities is between 16 and 41 per cent, significantly greater than that found within the general US population (1.8 per cent) (Allen *et al.*, 2003), and in other countries (Allwright *et al.*, 2000; Long *et al.*, 2001). This high HCV prevalence in correctional facilities is responsible for approximately 30 per cent of released prisoners being infected with HCV. The prevalence of HCV among female prisoners, similar to the increased HIV prevalence among incarcerated women, ranges from 35 to almost 50 per cent. Unlike the case for HIV, the prevalence of HCV among African American prisoners is lower than that found among white prisoners in one prison system in Texas (Baillargeon *et al.*, 2003).

Co-infection with HCV has important implications for the management of HIV. While chronic HCV infection results in progression to cirrhosis in about 10 per cent per decade of infection among individuals not infected with HIV, patients co-infected with both viruses are likely to progress to end-stage liver disease and death as rapidly as within seven years (Mathews and Bhagani, 2003; Mohsen *et al.*, 2003). End-stage liver disease due to HCV is now recognized as the leading cause of death in HIV-infected persons in the general community as well as in many custody-related deaths (Allen, 2003a). Therefore it is now recommended to actively assess all HIV-infected persons for HCV infection and treat if appropriate. Moreover, all HCV infected prisoners should be vaccinated against HAV and HBV if susceptible to infection. A recent published recommendation by the CDC on the prevention and control of hepatitis viral infections in the correctional setting (CDC, 2003) resulted in a sudden increase of interest by correctional administrators and physicians to determine how to better manage HCV in the correctional environment (Allen, 2003b). Unfortunately, this has not translated to significant increases in treatment in correctional settings due to the lack of expertise and resources to pay for treatment.

Screening for liver disease due to HCV infection and determining who should undergo treatment, although recommended by the CDC, has not been adopted by all correctional systems in the US. Virginia has implemented a management strategy and actively offers HCV antibody testing for all inmates, followed by HCV RNA confirmation of infection and liver biopsy. Only patients with stage 2–4 liver disease are offered treatment and, according to official estimates, limiting treatment to more advanced fibrosis scores saves almost US$125 000 per 100 patients (Allen, 2003b). Liver biopsies are recommended for all genotype 1 HCV-infected patients. Because genotypes 2 and 3 have a higher rate of response and often require a shorter duration of treatment, treatment is often offered without liver biopsy. However all inmates with HIV should be actively screened for HCV and assessed for treatment by obtaining genotype with HCV RNA followed by liver biopsy.

Although HIV infection is not a contraindication for treatment of HCV, the use of pegylated interferon and ribavirin (PEG/RBV) may complicate treatment with antiretroviral therapy (ART), with adverse events such as transamititis with fulminate hepatic failure, anemia, thrombocytopenia, neutropenia, and weight loss. Furthermore, interferon can exacerbate co-morbid psychiatric diseases including depression – a common co-occurring disorder among HIV-infected prisoners. This can cause difficulty with adherence to both therapies and potentially worsen morbidity if there is not a rigorously controlled program instituted in each correctional facility to provide appropriate screening and follow-up care of co-infected inmates. In correctional systems that offer mental health treatment, however, coordination of treatment of HCV-infected persons with mental health problems should be carefully integrated.

Few data are available for the treatment of HCV in correctional settings. In the Rhode Island Department of Corrections, 90 HCV mono-infected patients were treated with directly observed standard interferon alpha-2b (3 MU three times a week) and ribavirin (dosage based on weight) from 1997–2001 (Allen *et al.*, 2003). Only 17 (19 per cent) had the more susceptible genotypes 2 or 3. Efficacy was determined by measurement of HCV RNA six months into treatment. Fifty-five per cent (50/90) of the patients completed treatment; 72 per cent of these (39/50) had an undetectable HCV RNA level at end of treatment; and 34 per cent (17/50) had an undetectable HCV RNA level at one year after the end of treatment. The current accepted treatment of hepatitis C in mono- and co-infected adults in the community is PEG/RBV for 6–12 months of therapy (Fried *et al.*, 2002). Unfortunately, consensus on duration of treatment for HIV and HCV co-infected patients is still forthcoming and there are no current data on the use of PEG/RBV in correctional settings.

The major reason that HCV infection has not been treated systematically in correctional settings has been the concern about the lack of available expertise in the correctional setting, costs for treatment, and potential toxicity of treatment of co-infected patients among a group already with significant co-morbidity from HIV and mental illness – both of which may result in increased complications with therapy and decreased benefit. It is incumbent on the leaders in the area of correctional health care to develop appropriate guidelines and expertise for the treatment of HIV/HCV-infected patients in this structured setting where patients are often free from active drug use and have universal access to medical and mental health services.

Hepatitis B Virus

Hepatitis B virus (HBV) can be transmitted both parenterally and sexually. Compared with HCV and HIV, it is efficiently acquired by both modes of transmission. It is possible for a prisoner to obtain all three of these viruses from blood exposure via injection drug use. Compared with HCV, HBV is less likely to develop into chronic liver disease; it is, however, more likely to develop into hepatocellular carcinoma if infection becomes chronic. Furthermore, unlike HCV or HIV infection, HBV infection can be prevented through vaccination. Therefore it is essential for all HIV-infected inmates to be screened for active or prior infection and vaccinated if not previously infected. For prisoners with longer sentences, a three-part vaccination may be provided over six months. For jail inmates who remain incarcerated for shorter periods, an accelerated vaccination schedule should be considered. The high rates of completion of two vaccinations within one month support the use of an accelerated HBV vaccination schedule (immunizations at 0, 7, and 21 days) for IDUs as recommended in 2000 (Yirrell *et al.*, 1996). The high rate of completion of two doses, coupled with known benefit from one to two doses of vaccine (Mutter *et al.*, 1994; Yirrell *et al.*, 1996), suggests that accelerated, high-dose vaccination (0, 1 month and 2 months) schedules (Hammett, 1991) may greatly benefit this population, including those in correctional settings. Even if the vaccination series is not continued in the community after release, an incomplete series can still have considerable benefit: the first dose confers immunity in 50 per cent of patients; the second dose confers 85 per cent immunity (National Commission on Correctional Health Care, 2003). Correctional inmates are considered a group at high risk for development of future HBV. In recognition of this, the CDC now recommends either (1) routine vaccination against HBV for all new prison and jail inmates or (2) screening all new inmates for the infection (National Commission on Correctional Health Care, 2003). Routine vaccination is not appropriate as many inmates should be screened for active infection and may actually have had prior HBV infection, which obviates the need for vaccination. In both cases, vaccination would have not benefited the patient and lack of detection of active infection may result in a missed opportunity for treatment.

Overall there is a paucity of accurate data on HBV prevalence in correctional settings. Inconsistencies in serologic testing used in different prison systems have contributed to the lack of detail. In one study of 35 000 inmates and 155 000 released prisoners in 1996, an estimated 2 per cent of prison and jail inmates and 12–15 per cent of released prisoners had current or chronic hepatitis B infection evidenced by a positive HBV surface antigen (National Commission on Correctional Health Care, 2003).

Co-infection with HBV and HIV complicates ART. Patients with co-infection who initiate ART that does not include antiviral agents that treat both infections (lamivudine, tenofovir, and adefovir) may result in impressive increases in hepatic transaminases when the immune system is restored (Lascar *et al.*, 2003). While these agents result in cure rates for HBV of approximately 30–40 per cent of patients, such agents will reduce the likelihood of elevated transaminases that might otherwise be interpreted as hepatotoxicity caused by antiretroviral medications.

Sexually Transmitted Diseases: Syphilis, Gonorrhea, and Chlamydia

Sexually transmitted diseases (STDs) other than HIV that are most common in the incarcerated setting include syphilis, gonorrhea, and chlamydia infections. In 1997, there were at least 200 000 inmates in prisons or jails who were released to the community who had a documented STD (National Commission on Correctional Health Care, 2003). The most common STD was syphilis. Prevalence rates among inmates with STDS were as follows: syphilis in prisons and jails (2.6–4.3 per cent); gonorrhea (1.0 per cent); and chlamydia (2.4 per cent) (National Commission on Correctional Health Care, 2003). Syphilis is on the rise in the general population as well and has been linked to increased transmission risk of HIV infection (Funnye and Akhtar, 2003). Syphilis may also have a more rapid course with development of tertiary syphilis in immunocompromised patients with HIV (Singh and Romanowski, 1999). Therefore it is important to routinely screen for and treat STDs in all incarcerated people to decrease the fueling of sexual transmission of HIV. The structured correctional setting is one such place where routine screening and treatment programs can positively impact the community at large.

Despite recommendations for routine screening for STDs, correctional facilities seldom succeed with this recommendation. Reasons for lack of adherence with recommendations includes the cost for testing, the costs for treatment and the logistical problems associated with the high turnover rate of individuals who are incarcerated in jail settings where the median stay may be as short as a few days. Rapid testing assays, though more expensive, may prove to be an effective screening strategy among jail detainees where turnover is high.

Mental Illness

The correctional system has become the repository for the mentally ill who have fallen through community safety nets after deinstitutionalization of the mentally ill in the 1960s. Though an underestimate of true prevalence, approximately 16–28 per cent of state prisoners have self-reported having some mental illness (Beck and Marushchak, 2000). In 2000, 191 000 inmates were being treated for mentally illness. National estimates of the most common Axis I psychiatric disorders among prison and jail inmates in 1995 were as follows when compared to total US population prevalence: schizophrenia (1.0 per cent vs. 0.4 per cent); major depression (8–15 per cent vs. 8 per cent); and bipolar disorder (3–4 per cent vs. 2 per cent) (National Commission on Correctional Health Care, 2003). In terms of gender differences, men are more likely to suffer from psychotic disorders such as schizophrenia (3.0 per cent vs. 1.8 per cent) and anxiety disorders (11.6 per cent vs. 3.5 per cent), while women suffer more from affective disorders including major depression (13.7 per cent vs. 3.4 per cent), bipolar disorder (2.2 per cent vs. 1.2 per cent), and post-traumatic stress disorder (22.3 per cent vs. N/A) (Veysey and Bichler-Robertson, 2002).

Despite the disproportionate number of incarcerated people suffering from co-morbid serious psychiatric disorders, only 1.6 per cent of all inmates or 10 per cent of those identified as mentally ill were receiving any form of treatment for their psychiatric disorder. Furthermore, only 10 per cent of all inmates or 79 per cent of those identified as mentally ill were receiving psychotropic medications (Beck and Marushchak, 2000). Although prisons offer a stable population and appropriate setting for observed treatment of mental illness, 92 per cent of state prisons do not provide inpatient care within the facility (Veysey and Bichler-Robertson, 2002).

In addition to complicating treatment for HIV, depression and other mental illnesses increase one's risk for acquiring HIV infection (Stein *et al.*, 2003). One report of male prisoners in Connecticut showed a three-fold risk of acquiring HIV among patients with a history of mental illness (Altice *et al.*, 1998). Furthermore, social instability, depression, as well as other mental illnesses including anxiety disorders have been associated with difficulty adhering to antiretrovirals (Bouhnik *et al.*, 2002; Carrieri *et al.*, 2003; Tucker *et al.*, 2003; Turner *et al.*, 2003). Non-adherence to antiretroviral treatment increases the potential for developing multidrug-resistant virus. More importantly from a public health perspective if such people are partaking in high-risk behavior such as unprotected sexual intercourse or sharing needles, then there is a high risk of transmitting multidrug-resistant virus to HIV-negative people in the community. A recent presentation from a cohort of HIV-infected patients in a clinical setting identified poor mental health as the only independent factor associated with transmitting multidrug-resistant virus (Kozal *et al.*, 2004).

The concentration of HIV and mental illness in correctional settings magnifies the problems associated with either condition alone. Many individuals with either condition remain either undiagnosed or under-treated. Because many inmates with HIV and mental illness also suffer from substance abuse disorder, release to the community without adequate treatment poses a major public health emergency for communities struggling to control the HIV epidemic. This is particularly true for individuals with triple diagnosis who remain outside of our medical and mental health care system and therefore result in poor clinical outcomes (Douaihy *et al.*, 2003a, b; Bruce and Altice, 2003). Furthermore, those with co-morbid mental illness are potentially more likely to transmit multidrug resistant HIV infection to the general population via sexual intercourse and injection drug use, making this a major public health concern. It is therefore vital to improve our services to detect and treat mental illness in every newly admitted inmate and ensure that appropriate follow-up for their mental illness as well as their HIV infection is arranged prior to release to the community.

Obstetric and Gynecologic Issues

Compared with male prisoners, female prisoners are more likely to be incarcerated for drug-related and public disorder offenses – including commercial sex work; men are more likely to be incarcerated for violent offenses. Incarcerated women are therefore at increased risk for other STDs associated with unprotected sex such as syphilis, herpes, gonorrhea, and chlamydia infections. Pelvic inflammatory disease is a potential result of gonorrhea and chlamydia infection, especially if undiagnosed or inadequately treated. In addition, HIV-infected women have high rates of cervical dysplasia, resulting in Infectious Diseases Society of America (IDSA) and Department of Health and Human Services (DHHS) guidelines recommend pap smears every six months for HIV-infected women.

Approximately 4–6 per cent of all women are pregnant upon incarceration. The high rate of undiagnosed HIV infection among prisoners requires enhanced HIV testing for pregnant women. Other issues for female prisoners include pregnancy and prompt treatment of HIV infection during the peripartum and post-partum period to the baby (Hammett *et al.*, 2002). All pregnant women should be screened for HIV infection especially in a high-risk group such as inmates. Due to recent advances in ART, several studies have shown that treatment of the mother peripartum and the infant post-partum decreases risk of transmission of HIV infection to the infant significantly. A cost-effectiveness analysis supported the use of routine screening of pregnant women or mandatory newborn screening for incarcerated pregnant women (Resch *et al.*, 2004). Therefore rapid diagnosis, perhaps using rapid HIV testing assays, and initiation of appropriate ART should be addressed in all incarcerated pregnant women.

Illicit Drug Use and Prisoners

Compared with the overall US population of people living with HIV/AIDS, HIV-infected prisoners are more likely to be IDUs (Maruschak, 2001), most of whom have derived less benefit from ART compared to other populations. The high prevalence of IDUs, homeless people, people of lower education and socioeconomic status, and those with mental illness has resulted in the markedly high rates of HIV in the US correctional system. It is reported that over 60 per cent of HIV-infected people utilize mental health or substance abuse services, with African

American people, those with lower educational level, and those living in the North-East as well as those with higher CD4 lymphocyte counts being more likely to access substance abuse treatment (Burnam *et al.*, 2001). Previous evaluations of vulnerable HIV-infected persons have shown that factors associated with being less likely to have HAART prescribed by community physicians were: active illicit drug and alcohol use (Turner *et al.*, 2001), being homeless, African American race, lower educational background, female gender, or uninsured (Andersen *et al.*, 2000; Cunningham *et al.*, 2000). HIV-infected prisoners are more likely to belong to such vulnerable groups and are likely to benefit from the HIV care provided by the highly structured setting of prison.

Treatment of Opiate Addiction

Although injection drug use is the most common mode of HIV acquisition among prisoners in the North-East and drug-related offenses are the most common causes of crimes, especially among female prisoners, opiate dependence and abuse is rarely treated with pharmacotherapy in the US correctional system. In one study, 64–70 per cent of inmates reported using drugs regularly during the month immediately preceding incarceration (Hammett *et al.*, 2002). Drug-related crimes also confer high rates of recidivism. Given the high frequency of inmates with opiate dependence, it is crucial to use community standards of care for treating a medically diagnosed condition of substance abuse or dependence – including the use of opiate substitution therapy.

Very few programs have been instituted to initiate treatment of opiate dependence in correctional facilities. Only 32 per cent of state prisoners and 36 per cent of federal prisoners with substance abuse problems receive any form of treatment while in prison (Mumola, 1997). Yet inmates in one survey study stated they would be interested in opiate treatment while in prison if treatment was offered (Brooke *et al.*, 1998).

Currently there are three evidence-based pharmacological treatments for supervised opiate withdrawal and maintenance. These include: methadone, naltrexone, and buprenorphine. A fourth agent, LAAM, is no longer available because of resultant prolongation of the QTC interval that results in life threatening cardiac arrythmias – specifically torsades de pointes.

Methadone

Methadone is a full mu-receptor agonist and has been shown in numerous studies to be effective in decreasing relapse to opiate use and improving retention rates in drug treatment programs. Furthermore, methadone treatment has decreased crime and HIV risk behaviors. Several studies of methadone maintenance programs have been evaluated and have been successful in incarcerated settings in Canada (Sibbald,

2002), Australia (Dolan *et al.*, 1996), and the United States (Tomasino *et al.*, 2001). The only program in the United States is within the jail setting in New York's Rikers Island. In Project KEEP (Key Extended Entry Program), inmates entering the prison already on methadone are maintained. The program also offers methadone initiation or supervised opiate withdrawal for opiate-dependent patients who are not receiving pharmacological treatment. Upon release, patients may be between continued on methadone treatment. Injection drug behaviors six months after release were reduced among Project KEEP participants who were main-tained on methadone compared with those who were tapered off methadone (85 per cent vs. 37 per cent). Retention in drug treatment six months after release, unfortunately, was modest with 27 per cent of methadone maintained vs. only 9 per cent of those tapered off methadone remaining in treatment. The low retention was likely due to the suboptimal dose of methadone provided to maintained patients (Magura *et al.*, 1993). One limitation to use of methadone in the treat-ment of HIV has been the drug interactions between these two treatments (Khalsa *et al.*, 2002), some of which may precipitate opiate withdrawal (Altice *et al.*, 1999).

Naltrexone

Naltrexone is a full mu-receptor (opiate-receptor) antagonist and extremely safe. It has been viewed as a favorable treatment of 691 work-release inmates in Nassau County, New York in a non-randomized uncontrolled cohort design (Brahen *et al.*, 1984) which was later followed up as a supervised treatment method using historical controls (Cornish *et al.*, 1997). Retention in treatment and opiate positive urine tests in this later study were improved in the subjects with supervised naltrexone treatment. Naltrexone has been found to be less effect-ive in unmotivated patients who were not under the coercive supervision of the correctional system, making it an unviable option for many released prisoners who are not on probation or parole.

Buprenorphine

Buprenorphine, a partial mu-receptor agonist, can be prescribed by community and correctional physicians who complete an 8-hour training program. This treat-ment for opiate dependence does not require the stringent regulations of a federally licensed methadone clinic. As a partial opiate receptor agonist, buprenorphine does not produce serious adverse side-effects such as respiratory depression that can result in lethal overdose. The potential for abuse exists, however efforts in this regard have been thwarted through the co-formulation of buprenorphine with naloxone that when crushed and injected, results in marked opiate withdrawal symp-toms. Buprenorphine has been shown to be equivalent to methadone with respect to relapse to drug use (Schottenfeld *et al.*, 1997; Mattick *et al.*, 2002). It should not be co-administered in patients with benzodiazepine abuse or dependence.

Buprenorphine, with its safety profile and its relative lack of federally legislated constraints, opens up new possibilities for the supervised withdrawal and maintenance of prisoners with opiate dependence or abuse (Rohrberg-Smith *et al.*, 2004).

While corrections-based buprenorphine programs have yet to be implemented in the US, the French have provided buprenorphine to opiate-dependent inmates since 1996 (Durand, 2001; Levasseur *et al.*, 2002). In a retrospective cohort study, 3600 medical files of French prisoners were analyzed to determine the comparative effectiveness of methadone, buprenorphine, and abstinence treatment following the legalization of prison-administered buprenorphine (Levasseur *et al.*, 2002). Compared with abstinence-based treatment, both buprenorphine and methadone maintenance treatment within prison resulted in reduced recidivism rates. The early successes of the French experience with buprenorphine highlight the need to apply and evaluate buprenorphine within the US correctional system.

The use of buprenorphine and methadone as pharmacologic treatment strategies to maintain opiate-dependent people are evidence – based and the community standard of care. Such studies have demonstrated decreases in relapse to drug use, decreases in recidivism rates, and improved adherence to ART. Applying these models of treatment to correctional and prison-release programs should be carefully considered for those with HIV infection in order to reduce recidivism to prison, reduce HIV risk behaviors and to enhance adherence to ART. It is crucial that the correctional system addresses this unmet need if they are to stem the tide of new HIV infections.

Medical Treatment of HIV-infected Prisoners

Prisons and jails, designed to confine and punish people (many of whom are generally poor and without influential outside advocates), frequently fail to provide the level of health services required by patients with HIV infection. As with other chronic illnesses, HIV treatment requires provision of health services that are expensive in terms of staff effort, laboratory testing, and medication. Prisons have often escaped outside attention to serious failures of care. The prisoner infected with HIV faces obstacles to care that do not exist in the general community. HIV has placed an enormous fiscal burden on prisons, which are already financially stressed. The cost of HIV care in the twenty-first century in prisons is now rivaled by the costs and controversies surrounding management of hepatitis C, which affects 30 per cent of prison inmates and the cost of current psychotropic agents for the large number of individuals with mental illness who are imprisoned in the United States (Reindollar, 1999).

Prisons are increasingly recognizing the need for consultation and treatment of HIV by medical specialists, and several states provide care in conjunction with outside university-based clinic systems. Participation by HIV specialists, however, is by no means the rule. Treatment with potent ART is the standard of care for HIV and AIDS in prison, as in the community. The increased availability of anti-retroviral medications and appropriate use of ART has resulted in improved outcomes among people living with HIV/AIDS in community and correctional settings. It has long been demonstrated that care within prisons is often inadequate compared with care provided in community settings and inconsistent with federal guidelines for care.

A survey of treatment regimens of the 3563 prisoners supplied through Stadtlander Pharmacy's Corrections Division in February 1999 found that only 45 per cent of patients were receiving drug regimens recommended by existing DHHS guidelines. Seven per cent were on regimens categorized as 'alternative', 28 per cent were on 'not generally recommended' regimens, 8 per cent were receiving 'not recommended' regimens, and 12 per cent were reported as 'unclassified' regimens (Gajewski-Verbanac *et al.*, 1999). In a small retrospective study of 81 HIV-infected prisoners in London, investigators reported that less than 50 per cent of prisoners who were eligible for treatment according to British HIV Association guidelines were actually prescribed ART (Edwards *et al.*, 2001). A larger retrospective study of the prescribing patterns in the Texas Prison System evaluated 2360 HIV-infected inmates from January 1998 to December 1999; one-third of the inmates who met the 1997 US DHHS criteria for initiation of HAART were not prescribed it (Baillargeon *et al.*, 2000).

Not all prisons report such dismal adherence with federal treatment guidelines. In a study of 1844 Connecticut prisoners prescribed HAART from 1997 to 2002, over 99 per cent of patients were prescribed recommended or alternative anti-retroviral regimens. Among patients who were prescribed six or more months of ART, 59 per cent of patients achieved an HIV-1 RNA level below the limits of detection at the time of release to the community (Springer *et al.*, 2004).

One would presume that prisons would be the ideal place to provide HIV care. They are structured institutions that can control appropriate prescription of medication, can monitor laboratory values, schedule appointments, and supervise medication dispensation to enhance health outcomes. Unfortunately, the difference in adherence to treatment guidelines scratches the surface of the difference in care provided from system to system. Prison medication dispensation conditions can undermine the consistent dosing schedules essential to the long-term effectiveness of ART. Dispensation can occur at suboptimal hours, have exaggeratedly long lines, and not coincide with food that may be important for proper absorption of medications. Gaps in treatment occur due to frequent transfers of inmates among correctional institutions. Confiscation of all medications from prisoners is also a common practice of prison staff in the course of searches for contraband. Court appearances, transfers between facilities, punitive detentions, and release from custody are all part of the prisoner's life, and provisions must be made to continue therapy through these events without interruption. Prison

467

pharmacies may not be responsive to timely refill needs, resulting in lapses in treatment.

Every jurisdiction is responsible for providing health care to its prisoners. No required or generally accepted standards of care exist, although several organizations have developed voluntary health care standards for correctional facilities. The American Correctional Association, the American Public Health Association (APHA), and the National Commission on Correctional Health Care (NCCHC) have published standards for health care in jails and prisons. The NCCHC also provides accreditation for subscribing institutions that meet its standards. The World Health Organization (WHO) published guidelines for management of HIV in prisons in 1987 and 1993 (WHO, 1993), and the APHA included guidelines in its book of standards in 1986, updated in 1996 (Dubler, 1986). Medical personnel, public health advisers, prison administrators, legislators, courts, and the electorate have developed policies for management of HIV in prisons.

Among 19 countries in an international survey prepared for the WHO, the United States was one of four that did not have a national policy for HIV management in prisons (Harding and Schaller, 1992). The National Commission on AIDS, in its March 1991 report, proposed that the US Public Health Service develop guidelines for the prevention and treatment of HIV in all US correctional facilities (US National Commission on AIDS, 1991).

In the fall of 1987, the WHO Special Programme on AIDS held a consultation on the prevention and control of HIV in prisons, and specialists from 26 nations attended. This group's consensus statement recognized the risks of HIV transmission in prisons and recommended the following general approaches:

- Treatment of prisoners in a manner similar to other members of the community
- Consideration of compassionate release for prisoners with AIDS
- Non-discriminatory practices relating to HIV infection
- Provision of information on HIV to staff as well as prisoners
- Informed consent and confidentiality in the event of HIV antibody testing
- Devotion of additional human and financial resources to HIV management in prisons, but not at the expense of other health services and activities.

A subsequent WHO conference held in Geneva in 1992 drafted more extensive and specific guidelines outlining applications of the principles above (WHO, 1993).

Adherence to ART and Dispensing Medications Within Prison

Two main options exist for dispensing medications for HIV to prisoners: (1) self-administered therapy (SAT), where physicians prescribe antiretrovirals and the inmates are responsible for taking their own medications, and (2) directly observed therapy (DOT), where patients must obtain their medications in a medication line under supervision. SAT has the potential problem of confidentiality breach as inmates may have their medications stolen, but does not impinge on inmates' autonomy and tends to be preferred by the inmates (Wohl *et al.*, 2003). DOT in prisons has been demonstrated to improve adherence to ART and thereby improve morbidity and mortality. Several problems exist for DOT, however, including confidentiality issues imposed by the medication line (other inmates may view the medications) and furthermore requires more nursing time to do the observations and keep records (Altice *et al.*, 2002).

In many prisons, ART is administered under direct observation to prisoners. Among a group of HIV-infected patients who were enrolled in five randomized controlled clinical trials, patients in the community setting self-administered their medications while prisoners received their study medications as DOT. After 80 weeks of therapy, 95 per cent of the DOT patients in the prison had an HIV-1 RNA level below the limits of detection compared with 75 per cent of the group in the community who self-administered their medications (Fischl *et al.*, 2001). Though impressive, these findings were found among highly motivated individuals who volunteered for a clinical trial. Impressive findings in other prisons, however, demonstrate impressive outcomes from DOT. Patients in Italian prisons who received DOT were statistically more likely to achieve an HIV-1 RNA level below the limits of detection (62 per cent vs. 34 per cent) and increase their CD4 count above 200 cells/ml (95 per cent vs. 68 per cent) than those who self-administered their medications (Babudieri *et al.*, 2000). Observers have reported that adherence to ART has apparently been good among prisoners; at Rikers Island in New York City, patients' CD4 counts rose in a pattern almost identical to that found in clinical trials (Shuter, 2002). Among 170 prisoners in Wisconsin who self-administered medications, improvements in CD4 and viral measures were comparable with those found in community patients (Sosman *et al.*, 2002). A 1996 survey of 205 HIV-infected prisoners eligible for potent ART that found an acceptance rate of 80 per cent and an adherence rate of 84 per cent also found that adherence was 82 per cent in those who received DOT, and 85 per cent in those who self-administered medications (Altice *et al.*, 2001).

The discrepancies in outcomes found in systems using DOT and SAT is likely explained by the variety of approaches used to define DOT. For instance, in some settings, correctional officers observe therapy. This will result in widespread non-adherence by HIV-infected individuals who do not want to disclose their HIV status. Other systems provide DOT only to those who can get free from their housing units to attend the DOT window that may be remote and difficult to reach. Until correctional systems make a commitment to DOT, it is likely that discrepancies will persist and health outcomes will vary.

Due to the highly unstructured lives that prisoners tend to lead in the community and the degree of co-morbid illness that they suffer from, DOT provides a potentially effective way to improve morbidity and mortality in HIV-infected inmates. DOT can offer a bridge to SAT in the community by assisting them with reminding them to take their medications and identifying their medications. DOT should be considered a valuable mode of improving adherence in HIV-infected inmates who are considered to be non-adherent.

HIV Testing and Housing Policies

HIV in prisons raises a number of issues that do not exist for the general community; one of these is mandatory HIV antibody testing. In fact, early public policy debates on HIV in prisons focused not on care and prevention but on whether to mandate testing to control the HIV epidemic in the correctional setting. In 1999, 19 state prison systems and the Federal Bureau of Prisons had mandatory mass HIV screening policies for their inmates. Studies suggest that mandatory testing is less productive and probably less effective in educating prisoners and changing their behavior than voluntary testing and broad education programs (Andrus *et al.*, 1989; Maruschak, 2001). Such policies may, however, result in improved health outcomes as long as the correctional systems are obligated to educate and treat those identified with HIV infection.

Prisoners cannot give true, free informed consent. In every area of life, inmates bargain for privileges, better conditions, and, ultimately, release. Where HIV testing is not mandatory, prisoners require more information than others to make informed decisions about taking the test or participating in HIV-related studies. To give informed consent, prisoners must understand the institutional consequences of a positive HIV antibody test result, such as segregation and loss of access to activity programs, visitation, and jobs. Even this information may not permit prisoners to make a free choice about testing, as many prisons have policies of segregating prisoners who refuse testing with the policy that they can join the general population only after they have been 'medically cleared.'

Antibody testing has benefited inmates in institutions that offer ART and prophylaxis against opportunistic infections. Voluntary testing has become increasingly available to prisoners since early medical intervention has been available. A review of HIV infections identified through voluntary counseling and testing programs for prisoners in 48 US project areas between 1992 and 1998 found a steady increase in the use of testing services. There were 16 797 reactive tests (3.4 per cent), 56 per cent of these were in individuals who had been unaware of their serostatus at the time of testing (Sabin *et al.*, 2001). Acceptance rates for seroprevalence testing by new inmates in Maryland and Wisconsin have been reported at 47–83 per cent (Shuter, 2002). In the future, correctional systems should examine routine HIV testing policies to increase detection of HIV, introduce risk reduction programs and initiate and manage HIV infection in the prison and upon transition to the community after release.

Confidentiality

Confidentiality of medical information in the prison setting is virtually impossible to maintain. Where quarantines exist, confidentiality cannot. People other than medical staff may handle medical records, and staff members may not be meticulous about protecting privacy. Once information is released in a prison, it travels rapidly. Many people in the prison setting believe they have a particular 'need to know' who in the institution is infected with HIV. It has been argued that prisoners have a greater need for privacy than those outside because they live in a closed community where violence is common.

Prison policies regarding disclosure of test results vary. Fear of disclosure and its consequences may discourage voluntary testing. Prison officials use HIV antibody test results to make decisions about housing and segregation, work assignments, and visiting privileges, among others. It has been common practice to ban inmates with HIV (or AIDS) from kitchen work and to serve them food only on paper plates. In some jurisdictions, results of HIV tests go directly to prison staff. In 1988, California voters passed Proposition 96, an initiative authored by the sheriff of Los Angeles County requiring prison and jail physicians to give lists of known or suspected HIV-infected prisoners to prison staff. Such policies reflect the fear and misinformation prevalent in many prisons, reinforce the misinformation, and undermine the message and practice of universal precautions.

Education

Prisons historically have approached prevention of HIV transmission in two very different and often contradictory ways: either quarantine and segregation, or education.

In 2000, Alabama, Mississippi, and South Carolina still tested and placed all those identified as HIV infected in segregated housing. The trend over time has been away from such segregation and toward case-by-case determination of housing placement.

In its report on HIV in correctional facilities, the National Commission on AIDS stated that 'resources expended for screening would likely be better spent on prevention activities, such as education' (US National Commission on AIDS, 1991). For the purpose of HIV infection control in prison, the educational message is that no risk activity is safe, and exposure to semen and bloody body fluids should be avoided. Prisoners represent a crucial and huge target population for HIV education programs; prisons concentrate people at risk who are not easily reached in the community by such efforts. As many as 50 per cent of US prisoners are functionally illiterate, and many are not native English speakers; to be effective, educational programs must be modified to reach them. The generally available literature on HIV infection and AIDS either cannot be understood by most inmates or fails to address many of their particular needs.

471

Although the primary goal of HIV education in prisons is prevention, other critical objectives include promoting an understanding that engenders rational and humane treatment of affected inmates. Because of the dynamics of the correctional setting, information that comes from people who are not prisoners, from general facts to specific medical advice, is often not trusted. Recommendations to begin ART, for instance, have not been as readily accepted in prisons as in the general community. Therefore, HIV education in prisons must transmit information in a manner that recognizes and bridges not only language, cultural, and literacy gaps, but also the distrust of people on the other side of the bars.

Coupling educational programs with voluntary testing and counseling services has been effective in identifying individuals with previously unknown infection, promoting acceptance of and adherence to treatment interventions and post-release follow-up, and reducing risk behavior in custody and after release (Sabin *et al.*, 2001). An analysis of the cost-effectiveness of HIV counseling and testing in US prisons identified cost benefits from reduction of HIV transmission among otherwise unidentified and uninformed people (Varghese and Peterman, 2001).

Individual counseling, peer counseling, support groups, and special programs for women, designed for and by prisoners, have been successful in a number of institutions and seem to be the best educational tools. Several gripping and effective videotapes have been made by and for prisoners.

Two HIV/AIDS hotlines have been available in New York State to prisoners who use toll-free telephone services designed to be culturally sensitive. English- and Spanish-speaking counselors, mostly former prisoners, provide general details, information about treatment, prevention, and discharge-planning referrals. In 1995 as in 2001, the Prison Hotline NY (+212 233 5560) logged 2500 calls, and the Osborne Association Prison AIDS Hotline (+718 842 0500) reported 350–450 calls monthly in 2001 (Nesselroth and Lopez, 1996).

Accurate and adequate information for staff and inmates can reduce fears and ultimately affect institutional policies in ways that can profoundly alter prisoners' lives. All people entering prison must be informed in clear, simple terms, and in their own language about how to avoid transmission of HIV and other communicable diseases. Educational programs can reduce fears about HIV and its transmission among the majority of staff and inmates.

A Quebec City study of probation agency staffs from halfway houses and prisons found that correctional officers were the least informed about HIV transmission and prevention and expressed the most negative attitudes about HIV-infected people (Allard *et al.*, 1992). A Pennsylvania prison study reported that prisoners, staff, community groups, and legal authorities believe the 'quality of life for HIV-infected inmates was most influenced by education of prison staff. Effective education for staff and inmates was live and interactive, targeted to the perceived risk of distrustful audiences, delivered by a trusted source, accurate, and aimed at reducing risk-perception' (Stewart, 1992).

Other Prevention Measures

Increasing staff-to-prisoner ratios, classifying and housing inmates properly, decreasing overcrowding, and providing activities for inmates prevents transmission through non-consensual behavior (i.e. violence, including rape). Preventing violence is the ongoing responsibility of prison staff.

Condom availability in prison is one of the many issues over which legal and public health interests conflict. Most prison administrators have not permitted the distribution of condoms to inmates. Statutes in many jurisdictions make sexual activity in prison a punishable crime. It is argued that condom distribution would condone and promote this behavior. In Britain, where homosexual acts in private are not an offense if both parties have consented and are 21 or older, prison cells are not regarded as places of privacy, so sex between prisoners is illegal (Stewart, 1992). Another objection to condoms in institutions is that they are considered contraband – a container for hiding drugs or other illegal things that inmates may swallow and later retrieve.

Condoms are now available to inmates living in a dormitory for homosexual men in the New York City jail on Rikers Island, to all inmates in the state prison of Vermont, and to all those in San Francisco County jails through the medical staff (where distribution is accompanied by counseling). Philadelphia jail inmates receive condoms on arrival. In Mississippi, condoms are sold from vending machines at institutional canteens (Hammett *et al.*, 1994). Los Angeles County Jail has recently introduced condoms to inmates who identify as being homosexual and undergo counseling. Condoms have been available to inmates of Canadian federal prisons since January 1992. Eleven of 17 European countries reported that condoms were available to their prisoners (Harding and Schaller, 1992). A 1998 report of a survey of prison systems in 20 European countries found that 'condom availability is becoming widely accepted' (Laporte and Bolinni, 1998). In Canada, 10 per cent of the staff reported that condoms were a problem, primarily because of the nuisance of their use as water balloons.

The distribution of sterile syringes to inmates has also been discussed as a means of preventing HIV transmission but does not occur in any US prison. Several European prisons have made sterile syringes available to their inmates. The Swiss Hindelbank pilot project performed a one-year study of the effects of a needle exchange program, and observed that there was no increase in drug use, needles were not used as weapons, and that fewer abscesses occurred among inmates (Nelles *et al.*, 1998). One Danish prison reports dispensing a sterile syringe at the time of release to inmates who had syringes confiscated on arrival. Safer injecting practice information is included in the education and counseling programs of many correctional systems, whereas only two US jails provided bleach for cleaning syringes. Half of the 20 European countries' prison systems surveyed above provided disinfectant for injection materials in 1998 (Laporte and Bolinni, 1998).

Discharge Planning

Discharge Planning and Community Linkages

With the recognition of the importance of prisons in the AIDS epidemic, the disproportionate number of prisoners affected, and the potential for public health and educational interventions in prisons to reduce the disease's devastation in the larger community, prisons and jails are gradually making efforts to assure continuity of care and follow-up of AIDS patients after their release from custody. The transition for prisoners from custody to community is often chaotic and difficult, and health care concerns often take a lower priority than the search for jobs and housing, rebuilding personal relationships, and a myriad of other chores. Many policies exist on paper but not in practice. The planning that does occur ranges from giving inmates information about outside resources, to making appointments, to accompanying released inmates and assisting with enrollment for housing, health care, drug rehabilitation, financial benefits, HIV counseling, and psychosocial support. Several states provide case management services, establishing contact with prisoners and beginning to plan several months before scheduled release dates.

All inmates need more and better services to help them make successful transitions to the community, resist relapse to substance use, and avoid a return to high-risk behavior and criminal activity. This is especially true for inmates with HIV disease, who might benefit from a range of services including continuity of health care, stable housing, effective drug treatment, assistance gaining eligibility for benefits, and job training and placement services.

Results of the 1996–1997 CDC/National Institute on Justice survey show that 92 per cent of state/federal prison systems and 76 per cent of the largest city/county jail systems were providing at least some discharge planning for inmates with HIV/AIDS (National Institute on Justice, 2004). However, further analysis of the survey data reveals that while large percentages of systems were making passive referrals for HIV medications (82 per cent of state/federal systems and 66 per cent of city/county systems), drug treatment (75 per cent and 63 per cent), and for Medicaid and related benefits (78 per cent and 56 per cent), much smaller percentages were actually making concrete appointments for inmates to receive these services in the community (31 per cent of state/federal systems and 27 per cent of city/county systems for HIV medications, 22 per cent and 24 per cent for drug treatment, and 35 per cent and 29 per cent for benefits). Making a referral can involve simply giving an individual a list of agencies where they might apply for services with no further assistance in actually accessing the services. Making an appointment for a soon-to-be-released inmate with a specific service provider by no means guarantees that the person will show up and receive the services, but it represents an additional step in the process.

Geography can be a significant obstacle to achieving a successful transition. Exemplary programs in small geographic locations in Rhode Island (Vigilante *et al.*,

1999) and Hampden County, Massachusetts (Conklin *et al.*, 1998) successfully provide continuity of services by having local clinicians provide care both within and outside of the correctional facility. Successful models in moderate-sized geographic areas, such as in Connecticut (Altice and Khoshnood, 1997), have adopted a transitional case management model to overcome problems associated with geography. Such programs are beginning to demonstrate salutary effects on clinical outcomes as well as on recidivism rates of inmates participating in them. Most of these model programs have not been rigorously evaluated and have been limited only to those who were retained in the program. In a study evaluating recidivism and health outcomes among prisoners in Connecticut, recidivism among released HIV-infected prisoners was 27 per cent per year. Among these 293 individuals, CD4 counts decreased by 82 cells/ml and HIV-1 RNA levels increased by 1.12 $\log_{10}$ after three months in the community. This suggests that adherence to ART was diminished or discontinued completely (Springer *et al.*, 2004). These findings suggest that the current case management programs in place for released prisoners are not working adequately to treat HIV infection nor link them with appropriate long-term services. Drug treatment appears to be the missing link in such programs. Because drug treatment is not considered to be an active issue upon release, it often requires relapse to drug use in order to initiate effective treatment. Programs in the future should consider relapse prevention as a central component for discharge programs and institute effective treatment, for example buprenorphine or methadone maintenance, for opiate-dependent patients. This important result suggests that more action is required to effectively link potential releasees to effective HIV treatment programs as well as drug treatment (Rohrberg-Smith *et al.*, 2004).

AIDS Research

The Nuremberg Code, developed after World War II as the result of hearings regarding Nazi treatment of prisoners, stated that 'the voluntary consent of the human subject is absolutely essential' for medical research. Many countries subsequently outlawed all research on prisoners. The pharmaceutical industry regularly performed medical research involving prisoners in the United States until banned by federal prisons and several states in the 1970s. Prisoners who participated often lived in separate and superior housing units, ate better food, earned more money than was available for other prison work, and were offered hope of parole.

The issue of medical experimentation and research on prisoners arose in a new context, as HIV and related conditions were treated in the community with experimental drugs that the Food and Drug Administration had not yet approved and that were not generally available to prisoners. There is a clear distinction between experimental drug treatments used primarily for the benefit of the imprisoned HIV-infected patients and those used to test the hypotheses of drug developers or others (Dubler and Sidel, 1989). A comprehensive review has examined clinical trials within the prison context and found that there are few legal restrictions but cautions that correctional systems must demonstrate an acceptable standard of care for HIV and other conditions to avoid coercion in favor of experimental therapies (Lazzarini and Altice, 2000). In 1994, 15 of the 51 state or federal systems surveyed reported offering experimental therapies to inmates with HIV disease. Only 3 of 29 large city or county jail systems surveyed offered such experimental therapies (Hammett *et al.*, 1994). It is unclear whether any inmates in these settings actually had experimental HIV therapies available to them. In 1995, a telephone survey of medical directors of 32 state prisons found that inmates were likely to be allowed to enroll in clinical studies in states where AIDS incidence and death rates were high. Relatively few inmates, however, had enrolled in studies (Collins *et al.*, 1995). A study of Connecticut prisoners found that 50 per cent were willing to participate in clinical trials within the prison, whereas 66 per cent were willing to do so 'outside' (Mostashari *et al.*, 1998). Other studies of HIV treatment have been conducted within the correctional system, including the use of ARTs (Kirkland *et al.*, 2002) and DOT for HIV medications (Wohl *et al.*, 2003). Notwithstanding the unsavory history of experimentation on prisoners, rational and well-controlled non-placebo controlled trials for the treatment of HIV should be considered to provide options for prisoners similar to the ones that they might otherwise receive in non-correctional settings. A systematic review of the legal and ethical issues for the conduct of HIV-related clinical research has addressed the many issues confronting correctional systems (Lazzarini and Altice, 2000).

Legal Issues in US Prisons

Prisoners have a constitutional right to health care that people 'on the outside' do not have. Under the Eighth Amendment, inmates are entitled to a 'safe and humane environment'. In an important US Supreme Court decision, this right was further defined as prohibiting 'deliberate indifference to serious medical need' (*Estelle v. Gamble*, 429 US 97 [1976]). In 1991, the US Supreme Court ruled that to show 'deliberate indifference', plaintiffs must demonstrate that correctional officials actually intended to cause the alleged inadequate treatment (*Wilson v. Seiter*, 111 SCt 2321 [1991]). This narrowed standard is much more difficult for prisoners to prove (Gostin and Porter, 1991).

Since the mid-1970s, prison health services have improved extensively, as civil rights advocates and attorneys advocating prisoners' rights have challenged conditions of confinement. Prisoners do not vote, and legislators have generally not granted resources for their health care. Litigation, or fear of it, has compelled state and local governments and prison administrations to provide a level of care closer to that available in the general community. Case law regarding HIV in prison has involved a wide range of issues and has contributed to policy development.

Historically, the US courts have been reluctant to scrutinize or challenge prison and jail conditions, assuming that the complexities and peculiarities of those institutions were best left to the prison authorities. Since the critical *Estelle v. Gamble* decision (429 US 97 [1976]), courts have still generally supported existing institutional policies when these were challenged by prisoner plaintiffs. In the area of HIV management and care, courts have also generally deferred to prison managers despite their lack of medical or public health credentials. In at least nine separate decisions, courts have upheld policies of segregation of HIV-infected persons as well as policies of no segregation. In 1990, for the first time, a court overturned one state's mandatory HIV testing policy for prisoners. The Ninth Circuit Court of Appeals declared that the state of Nevada failed to show that its policy 'was reasonably related to legitimate penological interests'. In addition, several settlements modified strict policies of segregation of HIV-infected inmates by prisons, including those in Connecticut and California. In contrast, a federal court upheld mandatory testing and segregation in the Alabama state prison in 1990 and stated that prisoners who requested AZT treatment were not entitled to 'state of the art' treatment, but only reasonable care according to the community standard (Gostin *et al.*, 1990; Gostin and Porter, 1991). In January 2000, the US Supreme Court refused to consider an appeal by Alabama inmates who challenged their segregation in that state's prisons, and let stand a lower court decision. This decision was later reversed in 2003.

Other prison HIV issues that have been challenged in the courts include breaches of confidentiality, conspicuous special handling of HIV-infected inmates in court and other public places, inadequate medical and psychological care, HIV antibody testing without consent, lack of mandatory HIV testing, incorrect HIV diagnosis, and lack of HIV education. In addition, prisoners have been tried for aggravated assault, assault with a deadly weapon, and attempted murder for alleged biting, spitting, or spilling blood in altercations with guards. A Texas prisoner serving a two-year term was sentenced to life in prison for allegedly spitting at a prison guard (Greenspan, 1990). In August of 1997, a former inmate of the Illinois state prison system sued prison staff, claiming prison gang members infected him with HIV as a result of ongoing sexual abuse while his requests for help from staff were ignored. He had a documented seroconversion while in custody. His claim was disputed and ultimately was rejected after two trials (*Blucker v. Washington*, 95c50110, US District Court [ND Ill]).

Incarceration has also been used as a means of punishing and controlling people who are believed to be knowingly infecting others. Many statutes have created criminal sanctions against HIV-infected people believed to be spreading the virus through irresponsible behavior. These statutes fall into the following seven areas (Vermeullen, 1988):

1. Mandatory HIV antibody testing of people either charged with sex-related offenses or suspected of being IDUs
2. Mandatory testing of people convicted of sex-related offenses or injection drug use

3. Intentional transmission of HIV
4. Enhancement of charges and sentences for certain sex-related crimes if the defendant knowingly exposed someone else to HIV
5. Mandatory HIV testing as a condition of probation or parole
6. Laws aimed at HIV risk in special populations, such as mental patients, military personnel, prisoners, and people in the county youth authority
7. Quasi-criminal quarantine laws to segregate persons who are seropositive and considered 'non-compliant'.

Prison health reform is unlikely to be effective using the court system in the future. Federal legislation has limited the duration of class action suits, irrespective of whether the correctional system has responded to the challenges in the original suit. Moreover, this legislation has limited the payment to litigators who may otherwise incur great costs in bringing a case against the correctional system and their reimbursement is not included in the compensation. Thus, new approaches to prison reform are needed in the future.

Prison Hospice

Although AIDS-related deaths have decreased by 80 per cent in state prisons in 2000 (174 deaths) as compared to 1995 (1010) (Maruschak, 2002), the number of deaths from natural causes, excluding AIDS, and average age of prisoners has been steadily increasing (Linder *et al.*, 2002). Given that the prisoners are in fact older adults, health concerns such as terminal illnesses other than AIDS are an increasing concern in correctional facilities. By law all patients, including prisoners, should be entitled to receive palliative care in their end-stages of life. Palliative care in the prison system should include people inside and outside of the prison such as: specific family members, friends, community-based hospice volunteers, nurses, physicians, clergy, social work services, and ancillary services as needed (Altice *et al.*, 2002). The focus of the palliative care interdisciplinary team is on patient comfort and on the relief of any suffering.

State and federal prisons vary widely in the degree of palliative care that is offered to their inmates. The first prisons to offer a formal end-of-life program for inmates were the Medical Center for Federal Prisoners in Springfield, Missouri and the California Medical Facility in Vacaville, California approximately 15 years ago (Shimkus, 2002). It was not until the late 1990s when the GRACE Project started, a Volunteers of America initiative that promoted high-quality end-of-life care for terminally ill inmates predominantly dying from AIDS, that hospices became an issue for inmates (Shimkus, 2002). Since 2001, 19 states have one formal hospice program and 14 more have programs under development.

Oregon State Penitentiary (OSP) is one prison that stands out more than the others in terms of providing prison-based hospice care (Shimkus, 2002). This program stated in April of 1999 and comprises an interdisciplinary model including one inmate volunteer who is trained by a respected community hospice trainer. The hospice trainer meets with the volunteers initially for education and then monthly for more updated education. A nurse meets with the volunteer weekly to discuss specific patient-comfort knowledge and a third type of meeting occurs in the prison's chapel where the inmate volunteers are assisted in working through bereavement issues with the chaplain or a social services professional. This program is innovative in that the inmates serve as hospice caregivers rather than staff or community members. The volunteers must meet specific criteria and cannot be convicted of sexual or drug-related crimes. Other aspects of the program that are unique to OPS are that the terminally ill inmates live in their cells as long as possible where the volunteer visits them. When the inmates are in their last stages of life, they can be moved to a more private room with furnishings, CD player and video player to ensure more comfort for them. The hospice team meet weekly to discuss patient treatment plans.

Prison hospices should be an active issue of development in state and federal prisons and efforts should be made to provide the same care as OSP as described above. Incorporation of hospice teams that utilize inmate volunteers are likely to be most effective. Given that inmates are living longer and are therefore dying of diseases related to older age such as terminal malignancies, it is vital for all correctional facilities to adopt a palliative care program.

What the Future Holds

Correctional systems cannot be expected to take full responsibility for addressing the serious public health problem or exploiting the important public health opportunity represented by the related epidemics of infectious diseases in correctional facilities. Public health departments, community-based organizations such as AIDS service organizations and community-based substance abuse treatment agencies, and other community-based providers have critical roles to play as well. There is increasing collaboration among these entities, but there remain far more opportunities and needs for working together. There are differences in philosophy and priority among these organizations, to be sure, but there are also growing examples of overcoming the barriers and forging successful collaborations to provide needed services to inmates and releasees as well as to benefit the public health and serve the interests of society at large (Hammett, 1998).

Acknowledgements

This research was made possible through funding from the National Institute on Drug Abuse (K24-DA 017072 and R01-DA13805) and the Substance Abuse and Mental Health Services Agency (H79 TI 15767).

Frederick L Altice and Sandra A Springer

References

Allard F, April N, Martin G *et al.* (1992) Knowledge and attitudes of correctional facilities staff towards HIV and HBV infections. In: *Program and Abstracts of the VIII International Conference on AIDS*, Amsterdam, abstract PUD 9003.

Allen SA (2003a) Hepatitis C: The RI experience. In: *Proceedings of the Management of Hepatitis C in Prisons Conference*, 25–26 January, San Antonio, Texas.

Allen S (2003b) Developing a systematic approach to hepatitis C for correctional systems: Controversies and emerging consensus. *HIV and Hepatitis Education Prison Project* 6(4). www.hivcorrections.org

Allen SA, Spaulding AC, Osei AM *et al.* (2003) Treatment of chronic hepatitis C in a state correctional facility. *Ann Intern Med* 138: 187–90.

Allwright S, Bradley F, Long J *et al.* (2000) Prevalence of antibodies to hepatitis B, hepatitis C and HIV and risk factors in Irish prisoners: results of a national cross sectional survey. *BMJ* 321: 78–82.

Altice FL, Khoshnood K (1997) Transitional case management as a strategy for linking HIV-infected prisoners to community health and social services (Project TLC) [monograph]. Connecticut Department of Public Health.

Altice FL, Mostashari F, Selwyn PA *et al.* (1998) Predictors of HIV infection among newly sentenced male prisoners. *J Acquir Immune Defic Syndr* 18: 444–53.

Altice FL, Friedland GH, Cooney EL (1999) Nevirapine induced opiate withdrawal among injection drug users with HIV infection receiving methadone. *AIDS* 13: 957–62.

Altice FL, Mostashari F, Friedland GH (2001) Trust and the acceptance of and adherence to antiretroviral therapy. *J Acquir Immune Defic Syndr* 28: 47–58.

Altice FL, Selwyn P, Watson R (2002) Reaching in, reaching out: Treating HIV/AIDS in the correctional community. National Commission on Correctional Health Care, Chicago.

Altice FL, Bruce RD (2004) Hepatitis C virus infection in United States correctional institutions. Current Hepatitis Reports 3: 112–118.

Andersen R, Bozzette S, Shapiro M *et al.* (2000) Access of vulnerable groups to antiretroviral therapy among persons in care for HIV disease in the United States. HCSUS Consortium. HIV Cost and Services Utilization Study. *Health Serv Res* 35: 389–416.

Andrus JK, Fleming DW, Knox C *et al.* (1989) HIV testing in prisoners: is mandatory testing mandatory? *Am J Public Health* 79: 840–2.

Anonymous (1996) Needle exchange ends HIV transmission in Swiss jail. *AIDS Policy Law* 11: 9.

Babudieri S, Aceti A, D'Offizi GP, Carbonara S, Starnini G (2000) Directly observed therapy to treat HIV infection in prisoners. *JAMA* 284: 179–80.

Baillargeon J, Borucki MJ, Zepeda S *et al.* (2000) Antiretroviral prescribing patterns in the Texas prison system. *Clin Infect Dis* 31: 1476–81.

Baillargeon J, Wu H, Kelley MJ *et al.* (2003) Hepatitis C seroprevalence among newly incarcerated inmates in the Texas correctional system. *Public Health* 117: 43–8.

Beck AJ, Marushchak LM (2000) Mental health treatment in state prisoners, 2000. Bureau of Justice Special Report. NCJ 188215.

Bellin EY, Fletcher DD, Safyer SM (1993) Association of tuberculosis infection with increased time in or admission to the New York City jail system. *JAMA* 269: 2228–31.

Bouhnik AD, Chesney M, Carrieri P *et al.* (2002) Nonadherence among HIV-infected injecting drug users: The impact of social instability. *J Acquir Immune Defic Syndr* 31: S149–S153.

Brahen LS, Henderson RK, Capone T, Kordal N (1984) Naltrexone treatment in a jail work-release program. *J Clin Psychiatry* 45: 49–52.

480

Braun MM, Truman BI, Maguire B *et al.* (1989) Increasing incidence of tuberculosis in a prison inmate population. Association with HIV infection. *JAMA* 261: 393–7.

Brewer TF, Vlahov D, Taylor E, Hall D, Munoz A, Polk BF (1988) Transmission of HIV-1 within a statewide prison system. *AIDS* 2: 363–7.

Brooke D, Taylor C, Gunn J, Maden A (1998) Substance misusers remanded to prison – a treatment opportunity? *Addiction* 93: 1851–6.

Bruce RD, Altice FL (2003) Editorial comment: why treat three conditions when it is one patient? *AIDS Read* 13: 378–9.

Bureau of HIV/AIDS Epidemiology (1996) *AIDS Surveillance Quarterly Update.* Albany, NY: Bureau of HIV/AIDS Epidemiology, New York State Department of Health, September.

Burnam MA, Bing EG, Morton SC *et al.* (2001) Use of mental health and substance abuse treatment services among adults with HIV in the United States. *Arch Gen Psychiatry* 58: 729–36.

Calzavara LM, Burchell AN, Schlossberg J *et al.* (2003) Prior opiate injection and incarceration history predict injection drug use among inmates. *Addiction* 98: 1257–65.

Carrieri MP, Chesney MA, Spire B *et al.* (2003) Failure to maintain adherence to HAART in a cohort of French HIV-positive injecting drug users. *Int J Behav Med* 10: 1–14.

Carvell AL, Hart GJ (1990) Risk behaviours for HIV infection among drug users in prison. *BMJ* 300: 1383–4.

Castro K, Shansky R, Scardino V *et al.* (1991) HIV transmission in correctional facilities. In: *Program and Abstracts of the VII International Conference on AIDS*, Florence, Italy, abstract MC 3067.

CDC (Centers for Disease Control and Prevention) (1999) Decrease in AIDS-related mortality in a state correctional system: New York, 1995–1998. *MMWR Morb Mortal Wkly Rep* 47: 1115–17.

CDC (2003) Prevention and control of infections with hepatitis viruses in correctional settings. *MMWR Morb Mortal Wkly Rep* 52 (RR-1).

Clarke JG, Stein MD, Hanna L, Sobota M, Rich JD (2001) Active and former injection drug users report of HIV risk behaviors during periods of incarceration. *Subst Abus* 22: 209–16.

Collins A, Baumgartner D, Henry K (1995) U.S. prisoners' access to experimental HIV therapies. *Minn Med* 78: 45–8.

Conklin TJ, Lincoln T, Flanigan TP (1998) A public health model to connect correctional health care with communities. *Am J Public Health* 88: 1249–50.

Cornish JW, Metzger D, Woody GE *et al.* (1997) Naltrexone pharmacotherapy for opioid dependent federal probationers. *J Subst Abuse Treat* 14: 529–34.

Correctional Association of New York (1988) *AIDS in Prison Report.* June.

Cunningham WE, Markson LE, Andersen RM *et al.* (2000) Prevalence and predictors of highly active antiretroviral therapy use in patients with HIV infection in the united states. HCSUS Consortium. HIV Cost and Services Utilization. *J Acquir Immune Defic Syndr* 25: 115–23.

Darbyshire JH (1989) Tuberculosis in prisons. *BMJ* 299: 874.

Dean-Gaitor HD, Fleming PL (1999) Epidemiology of AIDS in incarcerated persons in the United States, 1994–1996. *AIDS* 13: 2429–35.

Decker MD, Vaughn WK, Brodie JS, Hutcheson RH Jr, Schaffner W (1984) Seroepidemiology of hepatitis B in Tennessee prisoners. *J Infect Dis* 150: 450–9.

Dolan K, Hall W, Wodak AD (1996) Methadone maintenance reduces injecting in prison. *BMJ* 312: 1162.

Dolan KA, Wodak AD, Hall WD (1998) A bleach program for inmates in NSW: an HIV prevention strategy. *Aust N Z J Public Health* 22: 838–40.

Douaihy AB, Jou RJ, Gorske T, Salloum IM (2003a) Triple diagnosis: dual diagnosis and HIV disease, part 1. *AIDS Read* 13: 331–2, 339–41.

Douaihy AB, Jou RJ, Gorske T, Salloum IM (2003b) Triple diagnosis: dual diagnosis and HIV disease, part 2. *AIDS Read* 13: 375–82.

Douglas RM, Gaughwin MD, Ali RL, Davies LM, Mylvaganam A, Liew CY (1989) Risk of transmission of the human immunodeficiency virus in the prison setting. *Med J Aust* 150: 722.

Dubler N, ed. (1986) *Standards for Health Services in Correctional Institutions.* Washington, DC: American Public Health Association.

Dubler NN, Sidel VW (1989) On research on HIV infection and AIDS in correctional institutions. *Milbank Q* 67: 171–207.

Durand E (2001) Changes in high-dose buprenorphine maintenance therapy at the Fleury-Merogis (France) prison since 1996. *Ann Med Interne (Paris)* 152 (Suppl 7): 9–14.

Edwards S, Tenant-Flowers M, Buggy J *et al.* (2001) Issues in the management of prisoners infected with HIV: the King's College Hospital HIV prison service retrospective cohort study. *BMJ* 322: 398–9.

Fischl M, Castro J, Mondoig R *et al.* (2001) Impact of directly observed therapy on long-term outcomes in HIV clinical trials. In: *Program and Abstracts of the 8th Conference on Retroviruses and Opportunistic Infections (Chicago)*. Alexandria, VA: Foundation for Retrovirology and Human Health, abstract 528, p. 202.

Fried MW, Shiffman ML, Reddy KR *et al.* (2002) Peginterferon alfa-2a plus Ribavirin for chronic patients with hepatitis C virus infection. *NEJM* 347: 975–82.

Funnye AS, Akhtar AJ (2003) Syphilis and human immunodeficiency virus co-infection. *J Natl Med Assoc* 95: 363–82.

Gajewski-Verbanac L, Lewis SM *et al.* (1999) Retrospective analysis of antiretroviral treatment guidelines in a national correctional base. In: *Program and Abstracts for the 39th Interscience Conference on Antimicrobial Agents and Chemotherapy*, September 1999, San Francisco, abstract 600, p. 482.

Garfein RS, Doherty MC, Monterroso ER, Thomas DL, Nelson KE, Vlahov D (1998) Prevalence and incidence of hepatitis C virus infection among young adult injection drug users. *J Acquir Immune Defic Syndr Hum Retrovirol* 18 (Suppl 1): S11–S19.

Gido RL, Gaunay W (1990) *Acquired Immune Deficiency Syndrome: A Demographic Profile of New York State Inmate Mortalities*, 4th edn. Albany, NY: New York State Commission of Correction.

Godin G, Gagnon H, Alary M, Noel L, Morissette MR (2001) Correctional officers' intention of accepting or refusing to make HIV preventive tools accessible to inmates. *AIDS Educ Prev* 13: 462–73.

Gostin L, Porter L (1991) *AIDS Litigation Project II: A National Survey of Federal, State and Local Cases before Courts and Human Rights Commissions. Objective Description of Trends in AIDS Litigation*. Washington, DC: Department of Health and Human Services, Public Health Service, National AIDS Program Office.

Gostin L, Porter L, Sandomire H (1990) *AIDS Litigation Project: A National Survey of Federal, State and Local Cases before Courts and Human Rights Commissions*. Washington, DC: Department of Health and Human Services, Public Health Service, Office of the Assistant Secretary for Health, Office of Public Health Service HIV/AIDS Coordination.

Greenspan J (1990) Transmission laws: the repression of HIV positive persons. In: *The Exchange*, Vol 13. San Francisco: National Lawyers Guild, pp. 3–5.

Guerrero RA *et al.* (2002) Diagnostic delay related to HIV infection in patients with prison history. In: *Program and Abstracts of the XIV International AIDS Conference*, July, Barcelona.

Hammett TM (1991) *1990 Update: AIDS in Correctional Facilities*. Washington, DC: US Department of Justice.

Hammett TM (1998) *Public Health/Corrections Collaborations: Prevention and Treatment of HIV/AIDS, STDs, and TB*. Washington, DC: National Institute of Justice and Centers for Disease Control and Prevention. Available online at www.ncjrs.org

Hammett TM (1999) Prevention and treatment of HIV/AIDS and other infectious diseases in correctional settings: An opportunity not yet sized. *HIV Education Prison Project News* 2.

Hammett TM (2002) The burden of HIV among prisoners. In: *Program and Abstracts of the XIV International AIDS Conference*, July, Barcelona.

Hammett TM, Harrold L (1994) *Tuberculosis in Correctional Facilities*. Washington, DC: US Department of Justice.

Hammett TM, Widom R, Epstein J *et al.* (1995) *1994 Update: HIV/AIDS and STDs in Correctional Facilities*. Washington, DC: US Dept of Justice, National Institute of Justice, and Centers for Disease Control and Prevention.

Hammett TM, Harmon P, Rhodes W (2002) The burden of infectious disease among inmates and releasees from correctional facilities. In: *The Health Status of Soon-to-be-Released Inmates*. Report to Congress, National Commission on Correctional Health Care, March, Chicago.

Harding TW (1990) *HIV/AIDS and Prisons*. Report for WHO Global Programme on AIDS. Geneva: World Health Organization.

Harding TW, Schaller G (1992) *HIV/AIDS and Prisons: Updating and Policy Review. A Survey Covering 55 Prison Systems in 31 Countries*. Geneva: University Institute of Legal Medicine for the WHO Global Programme on AIDS.

Harrison PM, Beck AJ (2002) *Prisoners in 2001*. Washington, DC: US Department of Justice, Bureau of Justice Statistics.

Hernandez R *et al.* (1996) Drug addiction and AIDS in prison populations. In: *Program and Abstracts of the XI International Conference on AIDS*, 7–12 July, Vancouver, British Columbia, abstract D.1411.

Horsburgh CR Jr, Jarvis JQ, McArther T, Ignacio T, Stock P (1990) Seroconversion to human immunodeficiency virus in prison inmates. *Am J Public Health* 80: 209–10.

Jurgens R (2002) HIV/AIDS in prisons: recent developments. *Can HIV/AIDS Policy Law Rev* 7: 13–20.

Kassira EN, Bauserman RL, Tomoyasu N, Caldeira E, Swetz A, Solomon L (2001) HIV and AIDS surveillance among inmates in Maryland prisons. *J Urban Health* 78: 256–63.

Khalsa J, Genser S, Vocci F, Francis H, Bean P (2002) The challenging interactions between antiretroviral agents and addiction drugs. *Am Clin Lab* 21: 10–13.

Kirkland LR, Fischl MA, Tashima KT *et al.* (2002) Response to lamivudine-zidovudine plus abacavir twice daily in antiretroviral-naive, incarcerated patients with HIV infection taking directly observed treatment. *Clin Infect Dis* 34: 511–8.

Kozal M, Amico R, Chiarella J *et al.* (2004) Continuing high-risk sexual behavior and increasing antiretroviral resistance among HIV+ patients in care helps explain the rising prevalence of resistance among new HIV infections. In: *Program and Abstracts of the 11th Conference on Retroviruses and Opportunistic Infections* 8–11 February, San Francisco, CA, abstract 35 LB.

Laporte J, Bolinni P (1998) Management of HIV/AIDS-related problems: situation in European prisons. In: *Program and Abstracts of the XII World AIDS Conference*, Geneva, abstract 44193.

Lascar RM, Gilson RJ, Lopes AR, Bertoletti A, Maini MK (2003) Reconstitution of hepatitis B virus (HBV)-specific T cell responses with treatment of human immunodeficiency virus/HBV coinfection. *J Infect Dis* 188: 1815–19.

Lazzarini Z, Altice FL (2000) A review of the legal and ethical issues for the conduct of HIV-related research in prisons. *AIDS Public Policy J* 15: 105–35.

Levasseur L, Marzo JN, Ross N, Blatier C (2002) Frequency of re-incarcerations in the same detention center: role of substitution therapy. A preliminary retrospective analysis. *Ann Med Interne* 153 (3 Suppl): 1S14–19.

Linder JF, Enders SR, Craig E *et al.* (2002) Hospice care for the incarcerated in the United States: an introduction. *J Palliat Med* 5: 549–52.

Long J, Allwright S, Barry J *et al.* (2001) Prevalence of antibodies to hepatitis B, hepatitis C, and HIV and risk factors in entrants to Irish prisons: a national cross sectional survey. *BMJ* 24: 1–6.

Lyons JA, Greifinger RA, Flannery T (1994) *Deaths of New York State Inmates 1978–1992*. Albany, NY: New York State Department of Correctional Services.

Magura S, Rosenblum A, Lewis C, Joseph H (1993) The effectiveness of in-jail methadone maintenance. *J Drug Issues* 23: 75–99.

Mahon N (1996) New York inmates' HIV risk behaviors: the implications for prevention policy and programs. *Am J Public Health* 86: 1211–15.

Maruschak L (2001) HIV in prisons and jails, 1999. *Bureau of Justice Statistics Bulletin*, Document NCJ 187456. Available at: http://www.ojp.usdoj.gov/bjs/pubalp2.htm (accessed 28 August 2003).

Maruschak L (2002) HIV in prisons, 2000. *Bureau of Justice Statistics Bulletin*. October.

Mathews G, Bhagani S (2003) The epidemiology and natural history of HIV/HBV and HIV/HCV co-infections. *J HIV Ther* 8: 77–84.

Mattick RP, Ali R, White JM *et al.* (2002) Buprenorphine versus methadone maintenance therapy: a randomized double-blind trial with 405 opoid-dependent patients. *Addiction* 98: 441–52.

Menoyo C, Suarez M, Lopez JA (2002) Needle exchange programmes in prison are feasible. In: *Program and Abstracts of the XIV International AIDS Conference*, July, Barcelona.

Mikl J, Kelley KF, Smith PF *et al.* (1991) Survival among NY State prison inmates with AIDS. In: *Program and Abstracts of the VII International Conference on AIDS*, Florence, Italy, abstract MC 3124.

Mikl J, Smith PF, Greifinger RB (1993) HIV seroprevalence among New York State (NYS) prison entrants. In: *Program and Abstracts of the IX International Conference on AIDS*, Berlin, abstract POC21-3108.

MMWR (1989a) Tuberculosis and human immunodeficiency virus infection: recommendations of the Advisory Committee for the Elimination of Tuberculosis (ACET). *MMWR Morb Mortal Wkly Rep* 38: 236–8, 243–50.

MMWR (1989b) Prevention and control of tuberculosis in correctional institutions: recommendations of the Advisory Committee for the Elimination of Tuberculosis. *MMWR Morb Mortal Wkly Rep* 38: 313–20, 325.

MMWR (1992) Transmission of multidrug-resistant tuberculosis among immunocompromised persons in a correctional system – New York, 1991. *MMWR Morb Mortal Wkly Rep* 41: 507–9.

MMWR (1993) Probable transmission of multidrug-resistant tuberculosis in a correctional facility – California. *MMWR Morb Mortal Wkly Rep* 42: 48–51.

MMWR (1996) Prevention and control of tuberculosis in correctional institutions: recommendations of the Advisory Committee for the Elimination of Tuberculosis. *MMWR Morb Mortal Wkly Rep* 45: RR-8.

MMWR (1999) Tuberculosis outbreaks in prison housing units for HIV-infected inmates – California, 1995–1996. *MMWR Morb Mortal Wkly Rep* 48: 79–82.

MMWR (2000) Drug-susceptible tuberculosis outbreak in a state correctional facility housing HIV-infected inmates – South Carolina, 1999–2000. *MMWR Morb Mortal Wkly Rep* 49: 1041–4.

Mohsen AH, Easterbrook PJ, Taylor C *et al.* (2003) Impact of human immunodeficiency virus (HIV) infection on the progression of liver fibrosis in hepatitis C virus infected patients. *Gut* 52: 1035–40.

Mostashari F, Riley E, Selwyn PA, Altice FL (1998) Acceptance and adherence with anti-retroviral therapy among HIV-infected women in a correctional facility. *J Acquir Immune Defic Syndr Hum Retrovirol* 18: 341–8.

Mumola C (1997) Substance abuse and treatment, state and federal prisoners. Document NCJ 172871. US Department of Justice.

Mutter RC, Grimes RM, Labarthe D (1994) Evidence of intraprison spread of HIV infection. *Arch Intern Med* 154: 793–5.

Nacci P, Kane T (1982) Sex and sexual aggression in federal prisons. Washington, DC: Federal Bureau of Prisons.

National Commission on Correctional Health Care: A Report to Congress (2003) Prevalence of communicable disease, chronic disease, and mental illness among the inmate population. http://www.ncchc.org (accessed 23 March 2003).

National Institute on Justice (2004) Executive summary: Issues and practices: 1996–1997 Update: HIV/AIDS, STDs, and TB in correctional facilities. http://www.abtassoc.com/reports/ES-176344.pdf (accessed 6 May 2004).

Nelles J, Fuhrer A, Hirsbrunner H, Harding T (1998) Provision of syringes: the cutting edge of harm reduction in prison? *BMJ* 317: 270–3.

Nesselroth SL, Lopez W (1996) AIDS/HIV hotline for prisoners: education, counseling and services to an underserved population. In: *Program and Abstracts of the XI International Conference on AIDS*, Vancouver, British Columbia, abstract We.D.3668.

O'Sullivan BG, Levy MH, Dolan KA *et al.* (2003) Hepatitis C transmission and HIV post-exposure prophylaxis after needle- and syringe-sharing in Australian prisons. *Med J Aust* 178: 546–9.

Reindollar RW (1999) Hepatitis C and the correctional population. *Am J Med* 107: 100S–103S.

Resch S, Paltiel AD, Altice FL (2005) Cost-effectiveness of HIV screening for incarcerated pregnant women. *J Acquir Immun Defic Syndr* 38(1).

Rohrberg-Smith D, Bruce RD, Altice FL (2004) Review of corrections-based therapy for opiate-dependent patients: implications for buprenorphine treatment among correctional populations. *J Drug Issues* 34(2) 451–480.

Sabin KM, Frey RL Jr, Horsley R, Greby SM (2001) Characteristics and trends of newly identified HIV infections among incarcerated populations: CDC HIV voluntary counseling, testing, and referral system, 1992–1998. *J Urban Health* 78: 241–55.

Salive ME, Vlahov D, Brewer TF (1990) Coinfection with tuberculosis and HIV-1 in male prison inmates. *Public Health Rep* 105: 307–10.

Schottenfeld RS, Pakes JR, Oliveto A *et al.* (1997) Buprenorphine vs methadone maintenance treatment for concurrent opioid dependence and cocaine abuse. *Arch Gen Psychiatry* 54: 713–20.

Sharp V (1989) Comparison of first episode of PCP in community patients and inmates. In: *Program and Abstracts of the IV International Conference on AIDS*, Montreal, Quebec, abstract T. B. P. 18.

Shimkus J (2002) Prison hospice comforts the dying, touches the living. National Commission on Correctional Health Care Website. http://www.ncchc.org/pubs/cc/hospice.html

Shuter J (2002) Communicable diseases in inmates; public health opportunities. In: *The Health Status of Soon-to-be-Released Inmates*. Report to Congress, National Commission on Correctional Health Care, March, Chicago.

Sibbald B (2002) Methadone maintenance expands inside federal prisons. *Can Med Assoc J* 167: 1154.

Singh AE, Romanowski B (1999) Syphilis: review with emphasis on clinical, epidemiologic, and some biologic features. *Clin Microbiol Rev* 12: 187–209.

Singleton JA, Perkins CI, Trachtenberg AI, Hughes MJ, Kizer KW, Ascher M (1990) HIV antibody seroprevalence among prisoners entering the California correctional system. *West J Med* 153: 394–9.

Smith PF, Mikl J, Hyde S, Morse DL (1991) The AIDS epidemic in New York State. *Am J Public Health* 81 (Suppl): 54–60.

Snider DE Jr, Hutton MD (1989) Tuberculosis in correctional institutions. *JAMA* 261: 436–7.

Sosman JM, Baker J, Catz SL *et al.* (2002) Clinical and immune recovery during antiretroviral therapy among HIV-infected prisoners. In: *Program and Abstracts for the XIV International AIDS Conference*, Barcelona.

Spaulding A, Stephenson B, Macalino G, Ruby W, Clarke JG, Flanigan T (2002) Human immunodeficiency virus in correctional facilities: a review. *Clin Infect Dis* 35: 305–12.

Springer SA, Pesanti E, Hodges J, Macura T, Altice FL (2004) Effectiveness of antiretroviral therapy among HIV-infected prisoners: reincarceration and the lack of sustained benefit after release to the community. *Clin Infect Dis* 38: 1754–60.

Stein MD, Solomon DA, Herman DS *et al.* (2003) Depression severity and drug injection HIV risk behaviors. *Am J Psychiatry* 160: 1659–62.

Stewart L (1992) The relationship between AIDS education, risk perception and quality of life for HIV-infected inmates in Pennsylvania prisons. In: *Program and Abstracts of the VIII International Conference on AIDS*, Amsterdam. abstract POD 5070.

Thomas PA, Moerings M (1994) *AIDS in Prison*. Aldershot, England: Dartmouth Publishing.

Tomasino V, Swanson AJ, Nolan J, Shuman HI (2001) The Key Extended Entry Program (KEEP): A methadone treatment program for opiate-dependent inmates. *Mt Sinai J Med* 68: 14–20.

Tucker JS, Burnam A, Sherbourne CD *et al.* (2003) Substance use and mental health correlates of nonadherence to antiretroviral medications in a sample of patients with human immunodeficiency virus infection. *Am J Med* 114: 573–80.

Turnbull PJ, Dolan KA, Stimson GV *et al.* (1992) Prison decreases the prevalence of behaviours but increases the risks. In: *Program and Abstracts of the VIII International Conference on AIDS*, Amsterdam, abstract POC 4321.

Turner BJ, Fleishman JA, Wenger N *et al.* (2001) Effects of drug abuse and mental disorders on use and type of antiretroviral therapy in HIV-infected persons. *J Gen Intern Med* 16: 625–33

Turner BJ, Laine C, Cosler L, Hauck WW (2003) Relationship of gender, depression, and health care delivery with antiretroviral adherence in HIV-infected drug users. *J Gen Intern Med* 18: 248–57.

US Bureau of Justice Statistics (1995) *Sourcebook of Criminal Justice Statistics*. Washington, DC: US Department of Justice, Bureau of Justice Statistics, p. 601.

US Bureau of Justice Statistics (2001) *Sourcebook of Criminal Justice Statistics 2000*. Washington, DC: US Department of Justice, Bureau of Justice Statistics.

US National Commission on AIDS (1991) *HIV Disease in Correctional Facilities*. Washington, DC: US National Commission on AIDS.

Varghese B, Peterman TA (2001) Cost-effectiveness of HIV counseling and testing in US prisons. *J Urban Health* 78: 304–12.

Vermeullen M (1988) The criminalization of the AIDS epidemic. In: *The Exchange*. San Francisco: National Lawyers Guild, p. 8.

Veysey BM, Bichler-Robertson G (2002) Prevalence estimates of psychiatric disorders in correctional settings. In: *The Health Status of Soon-to-be Released Inmates*. Report to Congress, Vol 2. National Commission on Correctional Health Care. March, Chicago.

Vigilante KC, Flynn MM, Affleck PC *et al.* (1999) Reduction in recidivism of incarcerated women through primary care, peer counseling, and discharge planning. *J Women's Health* 8: 409–15.

Vlahov D, Brewer TF, Castro KG *et al.* (1991) Prevalence of antibody to HIV-1 among entrants to US correctional facilities. *JAMA* 265: 1129–32.

Wang L, Sabin K, Wright LN *et al.* (2002) HIV seroprevalence among inmates entering NY State Department of Correctional Services. In: *Program and Abstracts of the 9th Conference on Retroviruses and Opportunistic Infections*, February, Seattle.

WHO (World Health Organization) (1993) *Guidelines on HIV Infection and AIDS in Prisons*. Geneva: World Health Organization.

Wohl DA, Stephenson BL, Golin CE *et al.* (2003) Adherence to directly observed antiretroviral therapy among human innumnodeficiency virus-infected prison inmates. *Clin Infect Dis* 36: 1572–6.

Wolfe MI, Xu F, Patel P *et al.* (2001) An outbreak of syphilis in Alabama prisons: correctional health policy and communicable disease control. *Am J Public Health* 91: 1220–5.

Yirrell DL *et al.* (1996) Molecular investigation confirming an outbreak of HIV in a Scottish prison. In: *Program and Abstracts of the XI International Conference on AIDS*, Vancouver, Canada, abstract Mo.C.1532.

Medical Ethics and the Law

19

Zita Lazzarini
Director, Division of Medical Humanities, University of Connecticut Health Center, Farmington, Connecticut, USA

Jonathan E Von Kohorn
Halloran & Sage LLP, Westport, Connecticut, USA

Zita Lazzarini, JD, MPH teaches health law and bioethics at the University of Connecticut Health Center and the Harvard School of Public Health, and directs the Division of Medical Humanities at the University of Connecticut. She serves as a Special Consultant for the Center for Law and the Public's Health at Johns Hopkins University, the Georgetown-Johns Hopkins program on Law and Public Health and for the Centers for Disease Control and Prevention. She has worked with the WHO. Her research focuses on public health law, including privacy and confidentiality, human subjects regulations, HIV prevention among pregnant women and injection drug users, health and human rights, and the relationship between law, policy and behavioral health outcomes. Ms. Lazzarini has co-authored *Human Rights and Public Health in the AIDS Pandemic* (Oxford University Press, 1997), as well as numerous articles in a variety of medical and legal journals.

Jonathan E, Von Kohorn JD is an Associate with the law firm of Halloran & Sage, LLP. He graduated from the University of Rochester in 2001 and the University of Connecticut School of Law in 2004. He has provided research assistance on various treatises and publications in law reviews and journals including An Introduction to International Law 4th Ed., The Journal of Law, Medicine & Ethics and the Yale Human Rights and Development Law Journal. While at the University of Connecticut he was a member of the Student Health Law Organization.

From the very beginning in 1981, the HIV/AIDS epidemic has had enormous impact on medical ethics and the law. From the outset, advocates for the 'vulnerable' and public health professionals joined in making unprecedented demands for privacy protection. These spokespersons argued vigorously that socially ostracized individuals, like sexually active gay men and injection drug users, would not participate in education, testing, or treatment efforts unless their privacy was protected. Despite these efforts, many people with HIV/AIDS and those at risk experienced discrimination in insurance, housing, and employment. Establishing legal mechanisms to protect confidentiality and prevent or mitigate discrimination became important priorities for many AIDS advocates. With the advent of effective antiretroviral combination therapy for infected adults and the demonstration that even monotherapy could greatly reduce perinatal transmission, there has been increased pressure to increase mandatory reporting of HIV infection to state health departments and to promote universal testing of pregnant women followed by antiretroviral therapy for mothers and newborns.

In the area of medical ethics HIV/AIDS forced individuals, families, clinicians, and staff to confront some of the long-held assumptions about who constitutes the 'family' of a dying patient. It is rare now, although it was not in 1983, to have a patient's birth family assume they can exclude a patient's chosen partner from care and decision-making at the end of life. The increased use of medical advanced directives and appointments of durable powers of attorney or health care proxies have also provided a legal means for patients to ensure that they can choose their decision-maker.

Although HIV/AIDS may now be seen as a chronic and treatable disease in much of the developed world, it remains a deadly presence in the developing world. About 14 000 new infections occurred per day in 2003. More than 95 per cent of these infections occurred in low and middle-income countries (UNAIDS, 2003). This chapter cannot hope to address all the legal issues that arise globally, however, we will discuss some of the innovative changes in international and domestic law and practices related to access to pharmaceuticals. The areas of US domestic law covered include public health HIV testing, reporting, and confidentiality provisions, antidiscrimination law, and criminal law.

The Right to Privacy

Concerns over privacy and confidentiality arise in many contexts related to HIV/AIDS. Decisional privacy (whether or not to be tested) and informational privacy (control over who has access to HIV test results or diagnoses as well as sexual and social histories) are both key areas of privacy doctrine in which the law has been active. Additionally, since HIV/AIDS has been associated with various stigmatized behaviors (homosexual sex, drug use, and sex work) identification as someone with, or at risk for HIV can subject an individual to discrimination as a member of that group, independent from discrimination directly related to HIV. The law provides only limited protection from discrimination based purely on these grounds. While a complete review of privacy law is beyond the scope of this section and chapter, the following should provide a basic foundation of the right to privacy and how the development of that right was impacted by HIV/AIDS. As is most evident in the instance of perinatal HIV transmission, new technologies and treatments can constantly upset the factual basis of the equation, thereby upsetting the balance of privacy rights against state and federal interests. The result is that the current state of HIV-related privacy rights is in flux.

The ethical principle of respect for people, from which we derive the notion of autonomy and its legal corollary, informed consent, grounds both the right to decisional and informational privacy (Beauchamp and Childress, 2001). As far back as 1914, Justice Benjamin Cardozo stated 'Every human being of adult years and sound mind has a right to determine what shall be done with his own body' (*Schloendorff* v. *Society of New York Hospital*, 211 N.Y. 125, 105 N.E. 92). It follows that individuals ought to be able to refuse or accept medical interventions, including testing under most circumstances. From an ethical perspective it is not difficult to extrapolate that a right to control actual medical interventions ought to extend to control of information gained as a result of those interventions. Thus, generally, medical ethics supports maintaining patient control over who receives information about his or her diagnosis, prognosis, and treatment (Beauchamp and Childress, 2001). Of course, medical ethics also recognizes the potential for conflicting duties in the area of privacy. For example, what is a physician's duty to protect a patient's confidential medical information, when that patient appears to place a third party at risk? Codes of medical ethics and the courts have found an exception to the normal duty to protect private information when doing so will place an identifiable third party at risk. In fact, absent some legal provision providing immunity, a physician may have a duty to warn an individual put at risk by a patient (*Tarasoff* v. *Regents of the University of California*, 17 Cal.3d 425, 1976).

The legal bases for a 'right to privacy' are less clear. While there remains significant debate about the existence or nature of a 'right to privacy' under the US federal constitution, courts have recognized a right to privacy in a number of cases: *NAACP* v. *Alabama*, 357 U.S. 449 (1958), *Griswold* v. *Connecticut*, 381 U.S. 479 (1965), *Katz* v. *United States*, 389 U.S. 347 (1967) and *Stanley* v. *Georgia*, 394 U.S. 557 (1969). Congress recognized the right to privacy in the Privacy Act of 1974 and Amendments (5 U.S.C. § 552(a)), which addresses the potential for government's violation of privacy through its collection of personal information (American Library Association, 2002). Recently the Health Insurance Portability and Accountability Act (HIPAA) also recognized the need for uniform federal protection of personally identifiable health information. This has led to the promulgation of privacy regulations that have a far-reaching impact on handling HIV and other information within the health care setting.

Privacy protection also exists on the state level. Eleven state constitutions guarantee a right of privacy or bar unreasonable intrusions into citizens' privacy (American Library Association, 2002). For example, the constitution of the state of Alaska provides that the 'right of the people to privacy is recognized and shall not be infringed' (Art. 1, § 22). Although somewhat weaker than a fundamental right, the US Supreme Court has consistently recognized that individuals have an interest in protecting the privacy of sensitive medical information from disclosures that might cause them harm (*Whalen* v. *Roe*, 429 U.S. 589, 605, 1977). Thus, although the state's police power clearly supports state efforts to mandate reporting of sensitive medical information including communicable disease diagnoses, prescriptions for controlled substances, and certain behaviors, the government also has a duty to protect that information and prevent misuse (*Whalen* v. *Roe*, 429 U.S. 589, 605, 1977).

In addition to constitutional and ethical sources, notions of a right to privacy involving medical decision-making and information can also be found in statutory and common law. From a practical perspective, however, the greatest scope of privacy protections for persons with HIV infection have come in the form of state laws governing testing, reporting, and confidentiality of information related to HIV/AIDS (Gostin *et al.*, 1999). At least 37 states have statutes specifically dealing with HIV testing, consent, and confidentiality that are generally applicable to all people seeking testing (Lazzarini and Rosales, 2002). Additionally, 17 states have laws specific to testing pregnant women and children, and many more have specific provisions related to testing prisoners, applicants to certain jobs, and donors of blood, organs, sperm, and ova. General HIV testing statutes may require pre- and/or post-test counseling, a separate written, informed consent for testing, documentation of specific consent, either oral or written, or permit HIV testing based on general consent, or without consent in limited circumstances (Lazzarini and Rosales, 2002). The majority of HIV provisions require specific informed consent in some form. These provisions also usually protect confidentiality, enumerate or limit permitted disclosures, and often provide some kind of penalty for improper disclosure. Maine enforces a typical HIV testing statute, which provides: 'Pre-test counseling' must include '[f]ace-to-face counseling that includes, at a minimum, a discussion of: (1) the nature and reliability of the test being proposed; (2) the person to whom the results of the test may be disclosed; (3) the purpose for which the test results may be used; (4) any reasonably foreseeable risks and benefits resulting from the test' (Me. Rev. Stat. Ann. tit 5, § 19204-A (West, 2002)).

State laws have required laboratories or physicians to report diagnoses of AIDS since early in the epidemic. However, although HIV testing became widely available in the mid-1980s, most states did not immediately mandate reporting of positive HIV tests. The debate over HIV reporting has evolved in relation to other advances in public health and clinical medicine (Gostin *et al.*, 1997). In recent years the Centers for Disease Control and Prevention (CDC) has strongly supported moving to a system of named reporting at the state level as the best way to accurately track the epidemic, facilitate prevention activities, and forecast needs for treatment. Currently at least 35 states, districts, or territories mandate reporting

491

of HIV diagnoses by name or unique identifier to the state and more require reporting anonymously, or only for pediatric cases (HIV Criminal Law and Policy Project, 2001).

The debate over whether reporting should be by name or unique identifier raises many of the same concerns common throughout the AIDS epidemic whether: public health departments will adequately protect such confidential information; state governments will try to use the information for non-health related uses; or individuals will be deterred from testing. Public health departments have a generally excellent record of protecting communicable disease data from improper disclosure. However, state legislatures and to a lesser degree health departments have been tempted to and tried to use AIDS and HIV registries for non-health purposes. A recent example includes an amendment to the South Dakota HIV testing and confidentiality statute that would allow the Secretary of Health, based on her own discretion, to disclose confidential HIV testing results to local prosecutors for possible prosecution under the state's felony HIV exposure/transmission law (South Dakota Statutes § 22-18-31; Goodman *et al.*, 2003). This represents a significant change in the role of the health department and one that could have negative long-term consequences if health departments become identified with law enforcement so closely that individuals at risk for HIV fail to get tested, or refuse to disclose the names of their past or current contacts. Although the 'names debate' over whether or not states should endorse reporting by name, unique identifier, or at all, seems to have been resolved largely in favor of reporting by name, those concerned about privacy have a whole new range of possible legislative initiatives to consider.

Despite the prevalence of general HIV testing statutes, these provisions have sparked scant litigation on privacy grounds. A recent case, *Sierakowski* v. *Ryan*, 223 F.3d 440 (7th Cir., 2000) arose over the Illinois AIDS Confidentiality Act (410 Ill. Comp. Stat. 305, 2002) which grants physicians discretion to test without patient consent. The facts in Sierakowski involved a plaintiff who attempted to refuse an HIV test during a routine hospital visit. He was tested, nonetheless, and notified of the negative results at his next appointment. Sierakowski alleged that the test, relying on the Illinois statute referred to above, violated his rights under the Fourth and Fourteenth Amendments. The District Court for the Northern District of Illinois dismissed the suit, and the Seventh Circuit affirmed the dismissal. According to the Seventh Circuit, not only were the alleged injuries abstract and conjectural, but also 'there [was] nothing in the proposed amended complaint or the record below to suggest that future injury [was] likely and that Sierakowski faced an immediate threat of harm.' In other words, because the test results were negative and he would not be forced to return to that hospital, he was in no risk of being targeted by the statute. By deciding the case on the narrowest possible grounds (applying the findings only to Sierakowski), the court overlooked the possibility that other patients could be harmed and provided no guidance to other health care providers and patients on when non-consensual testing is permitted.

A few other cases challenging HIV testing statutes have been brought on indirect statutory grounds. In *Doe* v. *High Tech Institute, Inc.*, 972 P.2d 1060 (Colo. Ct. App., 1998), for example, although the court held that a Colorado statute allows for testing without consent under certain circumstances, the plaintiff's situation did not fall within any statutory exceptions. Where the plaintiff was told that his blood sample was obtained only for rubella testing, and there was no other demonstrable reason for taking the plaintiff's blood, then there was no legitimate reason for testing the sample for HIV. The court held that 'a person has a privacy interest in his or her blood sample and in the medical information that may be obtained from it', and that 'an additional, unauthorized test ... can be sufficient to state a claim for relief for intrusion upon seclusion' (*Doe* v. *High Tech Institute, Inc.*, 972 P.2d 1068 (Colo. Ct. App., 1998) 'Intrusion upon seclusion' is a variant of the tort of invasion of privacy).

In other words, it is illegal to obtain a blood sample for non-HIV testing purposes and then subject the same sample to HIV testing without medical justification. There is a continuing privacy interest in blood samples taken such that others must adhere to those privacy rights that exist.

Plaintiffs can also challenge how AIDS or HIV diagnoses results are protected. In, *Estate of William Behringer, M.D.* v. *The Medical Center at Princeton, et al.*, 249 N.J. Super. 597; 592 A.2d. 1251 (April 25, 1991), the plaintiff's estate claimed that the hospital improperly disclosed Dr Behringer's HIV status to staff, patients, and others after the doctor was diagnosed and treated for AIDS. Although Behringer's larger claim that he should not have been barred from practice failed, the court did find that the defendant hospital did breach the plaintiff doctor's confidentiality with potential substantial harm from the non-consensual disclosure. Within days of undergoing an HIV test at the hospital, the doctor received multiple well-wishing phone calls related to the results of the supposedly confidential test. Although courts have not always found for plaintiffs claiming violations of state HIV confidentiality provisions, general HIV testing and confidentiality statutes represent significant specific protections for both decisional privacy and informational privacy. Named HIV reporting statutes represent a significant expansion of use of HIV information and may provide opportunities for acceptance of non-health uses which could threaten the relationship between public health officials and persons seeking testing.

Compare the above to the controversy over mandatory partner notification. Both advantages and disadvantages exist concerning the decision to require notification of previous sexual partners. Whether or not to apply the limited resources of the public health system to locating and contacting casual and anonymous partners is a contentious issue and one without clear answers. Mandatory partner notification has been used for certain sexually transmitted diseases (STDs) in San Francisco, which between 1998 and 2002 experienced a spike in the number of reported syphilis cases. Public health officials have been frustrated by high numbers of anonymous sexual partners (92 per cent) among those reporting. Of course the term 'mandatory' is somewhat misleading in situations where health workers are dependent on the index case to disclose his or her contacts because the index case can refuse to disclose, fail to provide names, or provide inaccurate information. This is not an issue where health workers know the names and identities of the index case's partner(s) or spouse.

An alternative approach, currently being tested by the San Francisco Department of Public Health, is known as 'venue notification'. This approach includes issuing warnings of possible STD transmission for those who were exposed at certain locations. While this may encourage more honest disclosure of unprotected sex by the index case, the warnings may not reach those who were actually exposed, or provide the sense of urgency that a face to face notification might create. The efficacy of venue notification is unknown and will likely be substantially limited compared to the traditional partner notification approach (San Francisco Department of Public Health, 2002).

HIV Prevention and Consent

Without treatment, women with HIV infection have a 25–35 per cent chance of transmitting HIV to their babies (Lazzarini and Rosales, 2002). That risk is higher if the woman breast feeds, has concurrent sexually transmitted infections, or has advanced AIDS. The United Nations Joint Programme on AIDS (UNAIDS) estimated in 2002 that approximately 2.5 million women with HIV/AIDS become pregnant each year (UNAIDS, 2002). These pregnancies result in an estimated 800 000 infants with HIV (Steinbrook, 2002). This largely reflects the enormous burden of HIV on families in the developing world. In the US and other developed countries the numbers of new perinatal infections have fallen precipitously since the discovery in the mid-1990s of interventions that significantly reduce the risk of HIV transmission from mother to child.

In 1994 the Pediatric AIDS Clinical Trial Group 076 (PACTG 076) released early results that demonstrated that maternal and neonatal zidovudine (ZDV) treatment reduced perinatal HIV transmission by 66 per cent (Connor *et al.*, 1994). The ZDV treatment allowed a transmission rate between infected pregnant mother and infant of only 8 per cent. Since then the introduction of combination antiretroviral therapy and some use of cesarean delivery have reduced overall transmission rates in US studies to less than 2 per cent (Mofenson, 2000). The US numbers show just how successful perinatal intervention can be. Reported cases of perinatal HIV transmission have decreased every year since 1992, from 901 new cases in 1992, to approximately 144 newly infected infants in 1999 (CDC, 2001).

Advances in treating pregnant women to reduce transmission of HIV led to a reconsideration of laws, policies, and practices for counseling and testing pregnant women. At Congress's request, between 1997 and 1999 the Institute of Medicine

(IOM) reviewed state efforts to reduce perinatal HIV infection (Stoto *et al.*, 1999). The IOM report, issued in 1999, concluded that although states were actively trying to address the issue, the level of new perinatal HIV infections was higher than necessary, given the advances in antiretroviral treatment. The primary problem identified by the IOM was that not all pregnant women were being tested for HIV and therefore not all were receiving appropriate treatment. The IOM noted that some health care professionals were not offering their patients testing because of the patients' perceived 'low risk' of infection, while others failed to promote testing because they found the pre-test counseling and informed consent procedures too burdensome or time consuming. The solution, according to the IOM report, was to move to a policy of universal HIV testing of pregnant women. As stated in the Executive Summary of the IOM Report:

> [T]he committee's central recommendation is for the adoption of a national policy of universal HIV testing, with patient notification, as a routine component of prenatal care. There are two key elements to the committee's recommendation. The first is that HIV screening should be *routine with notification*. This means that the test for HIV would be integrated into the standard battery of prenatal tests and women would be informed that the HIV test is being conducted and of their right to refuse it. ... The second key element to the recommendation is that screening should be *universal*, meaning that it applies to all pregnant women, regardless of their risk factors and of prevalence rates where they live. (p. 19)

In 2001, the CDC issued revisions of its recommendations for HIV counseling and testing of pregnant women. The revised guidelines differed from the previous 1995 guidelines as they emphasized HIV testing as a routine part of prenatal care. It is important to note, however, that HIV testing remains, technically, voluntary under these regulations. To achieve the goal of testing all pregnant women for HIV, the CDC recommended that the test process be simplified so that pretest counseling would no longer be a barrier; that various types of informed consent be allowed; that health care providers explore and address a woman's reasons for refusing testing; and that HIV testing and treatment be offered to women who had not received prenatal testing and antiretroviral drugs.

In 2002, the CDC (re-)issued comprehensive recommendations and reiterated its policy of advocating the use of antiretroviral drugs during pregnancy after universal early testing and treatment of pregnant women in order to prevent HIV transmission to their fetuses (CDC, 2002).

While no professional organization has, as yet, advocated mandatory testing of pregnant women, some tension remains between whether HIV/AIDS testing of pregnant women should follow an 'opt-out' or an 'opt-in' scheme. The American College of Obstetricians and Gynecologists (ACOG) has endorsed the more aggressive approach, the opt-out. The ACOG recommends that all pregnant women in the US be tested for HIV as a routine part of prenatal care with patient notification and the right to refuse (American College of Obstetricians and Gynecologists, 2000).

Other professional organizations also endorse routine HIV counseling and testing for pregnant women, but insist that testing be of the opt-in variety. For example, the American College of Nurse Midwives (ACNM) opposes mandatory testing as a condition of prenatal care. Instead, the ACNM recommends, 'All women should be counseled on HIV risk behaviors and risk reduction strategies. Following counseling, all women should be offered HIV testing with informed consent' (American College of Nurse Midwives, 1999). Reiterating the importance of identifying HIV-positive pregnant women, the American Academy of Pediatrics (AAP) recommends 'documented, routine HIV education, and routine testing with consent, for all pregnant women in the United States' and 'utilization of consent procedures that facilitate rapid incorporation of HIV education and testing into the routine medical care setting' (American Academy of Pediatrics, 1995).

The consensus among principal professional organizations involved with the delivery of care for pregnant women is for routine testing with consent. These organizations have rejected mandatory testing even to prevent perinatal HIV transmission. While the ACOG recommends that women be given the right to refuse testing, the ACNM, the AAP, the AMA, and the APHA have been more resolute in their protection of the pregnant women's rights by recommending they be counseled and afforded an opportunity to consent prior to testing. Thus, although the public health justification for HIV testing of pregnant women is very strong, it appears that most professionals would not override a pregnant woman's ethical right to participate in the testing decision.

Currently at least 17 state laws specifically address the issue of perinatal HIV testing. While the majority of these laws (11) require informed consent for pregnant women under all circumstances, some states have modified their maternal or neonatal testing provisions to reflect the IOM's recommendations. After contentious public debate, New York adopted a policy of mandatory testing of newborns for HIV. This reflects the belief that some infected women who had not been tested for HIV were still giving birth and that health care professionals were missing crucial opportunities to either administer post-birth prophylaxis to the babies, or provide early diagnosis and treatment for exposed or infected babies (New York State Department of Health, 1999). Connecticut adopted a new maternal and perinatal testing provision in 1999 that has three distinct phases. First, the state law now requires that women be offered HIV counseling and testing with full informed consent at least two times during pregnancy, preferably in the first and third trimesters. Second, if a woman in labor has no record of a recent HIV test in her medical chart, she will be tested 'routinely' during labor, unless she refuses in writing (an opt-out type law). Finally, for women who have no test results and or have refused testing during labor, her newborn will be tested at birth. This testing is mandatory, unless she refuses on religious grounds (Conn. Gen. Stat. Ann. § 19a-55(b) (West, 2002)).

496

Although privacy concerns obviously still apply to pregnant women, advances in perinatal prevention have shifted the terms of the debate. The public health justification for identification of infection among pregnant women, in order to prevent transmission to infants, has led some advocates and legislators to back provisions that decrease women's autonomy in testing decisions regarding themselves and their children. To the degree that such measures promote healthy babies, most people, especially mothers, support efforts to increase testing. However, the net result may be the elimination of most procedures related to informed consent for pregnant women and the loss of crucial opportunities to educate women about their risk of HIV and its consequences for this or future pregnancies. The focus on pregnant women also suggests that HIV prevention among women for their own sake is less important.

Impact on Research Ethics

The original ACTG 076 protocol for treating pregnant women and their infants required identifying women in their second trimester of pregnancy and initiating treatment with antiretrovirals for up to six months of pregnancy, intravenously during labor, and for the baby orally for six weeks after birth. Diagnosis, treatment, and monitoring of this regimen are time and effort intensive and far too expensive to be feasible in developing countries. In the late 1990s, a flurry of studies sought to identify interventions that could be effective in reducing mother to child transmission of HIV, yet could also be delivered safely in low-income, low-resource environments. Although studies rapidly demonstrated that alternative therapies were possible (shorter courses of ZDV, nevarapine in labor and after birth), the studies themselves provoked an enormous controversy in research ethics that remains active. The key issue was whether it was ethical to design trials to be conducted in developing countries that compared short-course antiretroviral therapy to placebo in terms of their efficacy on perinatal transmission (Angell, 1997). On the one hand clinicians in developing countries and researchers designing 15 of the 16 studies in that year argued that the new treatments should be compared to placebo, because that was the only way the treatment's actual efficacy in those countries could be judged (Varmus and Satcher, 1997). On the other hand, some ethicists, clinicians, and developed country academics argued that it is never ethical to design a study using a placebo group where an effective treatment is known and that to do so in this case needlessly exposed mothers and babies in the placebo groups to preventable risk of transmission (Lurie and Wolfe, 1997).

The debate over use of placebos, and more generally about the definition of the 'standard of care' that must be provided in research studies continued and has influenced the re-drafting of the World Medical Association's Declaration of Helsinki. The newest draft (issued 2000, updated by clarification 2002) states: 'The

497

benefits, risks, burdens and effectiveness of a new method should be tested against those of the best current prophylactic, diagnostic, and therapeutic methods. This does not exclude the use of placebo, or no treatment, in studies where no proven prophylactic, diagnostic or therapeutic method exists' (paragraph 29).

This paragraph sets a very high standard and would have invalidated most of the perinatal HIV trials and many other research efforts in developing countries that lack the resources or infrastructure to deliver 'the best current prophylactic, diagnostic, and therapeutic methods'. In 2002, however, the drafters added the following clarification, which appears to add an exception to paragraph 29 that would allow use of placebos in limited circumstances where an effective treatment is known.

> The WMA hereby reaffirms its position that extreme care must be taken in making use of a placebo-controlled trial and that in general this methodology should only be used in the absence of existing proven therapy. However, a placebo-controlled trial may be ethically acceptable, even if proven therapy is available, under the following circumstances: – Where for compelling and scientifically sound methodological reasons its use is necessary to determine the efficacy or safety of a prophylactic, diagnostic or therapeutic method (World Medical Association, Declaration of Helsinki, 2002).

Antidiscrimination Law

The American's with Disabilities Act (ADA) was signed into law on 26 July 1990 with the purpose of creating a more accessible American society for those with disabilities (42 U.S.C.A § 12101(b)). The statute is divided into five titles or subject areas. These are Employment, Public Services, Public Accommodations, Telecommunications and Miscellaneous. The Employment title generally provides that businesses must provide reasonable accommodations to protect the rights of individuals with disabilities and highly regulates medical examinations of employees. The Public Services title includes state and local governments along with commuting authorities (i.e. trains, subways, and buses). The Public Accommodations title includes all new construction and modifications to facilities like hotels, restaurants, stores, hospitals, health care professionals' offices, and other sites. Existing facilities must be made accessible, if this is readily achievable. The Telecommunications title generally mandates that telephone companies make TTY or similar relay devices available. The Miscellaneous title provides for prohibitions against threatening, coercing and/or retaliating against the disabled who may assert their rights under the ADA.

The ADA was written to provide relief from discrimination to the approximate and increasing minority population of 43 000 000 American citizens with disabilities. What actually constitutes a disability under the ADA can sometimes be a difficult question to answer. The Equal Opportunity Commission (EEOC) and the

Department of Justice (DOJ) were each granted limited authority by Congress to interpret and regulate the provisions of the ADA.

The ADA applies to disabled individuals who are defined as such when they meet any one of the following statutory criteria:

1. He or she has a physical or mental impairment that substantially limits one or more of his/her major life activities;
2. He or she has a record of such an impairment; or
3. He or she is regarded as having such impairment.

Discrimination by association is likewise prohibited. This could include discrimination against a parent with a disabled child. The ADA does not apply to all companies, however, it is sufficiently broad to have had a major impact on the daily lives of those living with disabilities.

Currently, HIV/AIDS is considered a disability nearly 100 per cent of the time by case law and under the regulations. This recognition allows for qualified individuals to seek protection from many of the primary forms of discrimination. However, the continued recognition of HIV/AIDS as a disability under the ADA is not a certainty and the scope of protection offered by the ADA to the disabled in general has been narrowed by recent cases.

Courts are free to depart from the regulations when they are in conflict with the statutory language of the ADA as enacted by Congress. Additionally, courts have refused to label certain conditions and diseases as being indicative of a disability under the ADA *per se* and have been traditionally reluctant to find a disability based on a 'third prong' of the statutory test for disability: whether or not the person is generally regarded by society as suffering from a disability. Thus, the classification of HIV/AIDS as a disability *per se* is not possible and there remains no universal alternate theory for the designation of HIV/AIDS as a disability under the ADA. This section reviews some of the most recent antidiscrimination decisions important to people with HIV infection.

The Supreme Court in *Randon Bragdon* v. *Sidney Abbott, et al.*, 524 U.S. 624, 118 S. Ct. 2196, 141 L. Ed. 2d 540 (25 June 1998) answered the question of whether or not HIV/AIDS qualifies as a disability under the ADA in the affirmative. The petitioner, Randon Bragdon, was a dentist, who refused to treat a cavity of the respondent, Sidney Abbott, in his dental offices. Bragdon offered to perform the work at a hospital without additional cost; however, the patient would have had to pay a hospital use fee out of her own pocket. She declined his offer and brought suit against the dentist under § 12182 of the ADA. The Supreme Court held that an HIV infection impaired the host from the time of infection and that infection would substantially limit the host's ability to reproduce, which was a major life activity.

Following *Bragdon* v. *Abbott* HIV has generally been considered a disability for the purposes of the ADA. However, the question of whether or not HIV/AIDS continues to be defined as a disability became unclear given the Court's own interpretation of their *Bragdon* ruling in *Sutton* v. *United Airlines*, 527 U.S. 471 (1999):

> Thus, whether a person has a disability under the ADA is an individualized inquiry. See Bragdon v. Abbott, [citations omitted] (declining to consider whether HIV infection is a per se disability under the ADA); 29 CFR pt. 1630, App. § 1630.2(j) ('The determination of whether an individual has a disability is not necessarily based on the name or diagnosis of the impairment the person has, but rather on the effect of that impairment on the life of the individual').

The *Sutton* Court went on to note that inquiries should be individualized such that the disability is determined in its corrected or medicated state.

This raises a 'Catch-22' for the infected individual, in that protection under the ADA may cease depending on the effectiveness of their treatment. Someone whose vision can be perfectly corrected with glasses will lose protection otherwise established by poor eyesight. However, if the person with glasses is subsequently and irrationally regarded as having a disability, protection may reattach. In the case of HIV/AIDS the impact of evaluating the impairment 'as treated', particularly in the early stages of infection, might be to negate a finding either of significant impairment in the ability to reproduce or of any other life activities. As with hypertension, or near-sightedness, medication (or glasses) can greatly reduce the degree of daily impairment. If successful treatment (that reduces impact but does *not* cure the disease), makes the ADA inapplicable, then people are caught in a paradox, where adherence to physician's advice to begin treatment might render them unprotected by the ADA and thus vulnerable to loss of a job, educational opportunities, or public services.

Most recently, courts have revisited this topic and held that there can never be, by statutory interpretation, *per se* disabilities under the ADA:

> People afflicted with Hepatitis C, an infectious disease, may well find that their ability to procreate or have sexual intercourse is limited by that condition. However, we will not treat Hepatitis C as if it were a per se disability ('There are no per se rules as to what is or what is not a disability'.). A per se approach would contravene the applicable standard articulated by the Supreme Court. In recent years, the Supreme Court has consistently held that 'the existence of a disability [must] be determined in ... a case-by-case manner'. ('Whether a person has a disability under the ADA is an individualized inquiry.'); ('ADA imposes a "statutory obligation" to determine the existence of disabilities on a case-by-case basis.') Therefore, 'the determination of whether an individual is disabled under the ADA is made on an individualized, case-by-case basis' (*Sussle* v. *Sirina Prot. Sys. Corp.*, 269 F. Supp. 2d 285, 305 (2003) citations and references omitted).

Bragdon v. *Abbot* is a remarkable ruling, in retrospect, for several reasons. First, Abbot was asymptomatic as her HIV infection was at an early stage. Most recognized disabilities covered by the ADA are symptomatic (i.e. blindness, paralysis, etc.). Secondly, as discussed, courts have been reluctant to define conditions as disabilities *per se* in favor of making individual inquiry into the particular symptoms of the condition (i.e. how blind, degree of paralysis, etc.). This has caused confusion because if the inquiry into a condition is individualized, then how can an asymptomatic 'disability' be defined as a disability at all? The answer in *Bragdon* came from recognizing that while the virus may not be compromising the plaintiffs well-being at that time, it had caused a disruption to her major life activities. HIV, as a disability, was narrowly tied by the majority opinion to the major life activity of reproduction.

Connecting HIV to a major life activity, in this case, of reproduction, is a necessity for protection under the ADA. However, it also represented a departure from traditional interpretations of the ADA. Major life activities have usually been described by regulations to include activities like working, speaking, seeing, and listening, all often considered activities of daily life. To include reproduction as a major life activity was surprising because while reproduction is clearly an important life activity, it is not daily.

In fact, many people may never pursue reproduction, may have completed their reproductive years, or currently might not be considering reproduction. Relying on reproduction made the holding in *Bragdon* somewhat narrow and was criticized by some legal scholars.

For people with HIV infection, continued protection from discrimination under the ADA may now depend solely on the impact the virus actually has on their reproductive options and viability. While Justice Ginsburg's concurrence to the majority opinion indicates that the court may be willing to accept alternative theories of HIV/AIDS as a disability under the ADA, a new court may have to consider that question and the status of HIV as a disability as these theories remains unclear. There are two primary causes of concern for the loss of HIV/AIDS as a recognized disability. First, since antiretroviral treatment of pregnant women and their babies can effectively reduce the risk of transmission of HIV to less than 2 per cent, the degree of impact the virus has on reproductive choices has been lessened since *Bragdon* went to trial and the Supreme Court reviewed the case. Secondly, the efficacy of combination therapy for those with HIV infection has lessened the possible impact the virus may have on other major life activities that could serve as alternate theories under the ADA.

Advances in the treatment of HIV/AIDS may ultimately cause courts to change their position on whether or not the ADA can continue to protect this class of people. This concern is not without precedent. Indeed, cases released since *Bragdon* have limited and confined the scope of ADA coverage for HIV/AIDS.

In *Luciano Montalvo* v. *James P. Radcliffe*, 167 F.3d 873 (4th Cir. 1999), Montalvo was a 12-year-old boy with AIDS who was denied admission to a martial arts school because of his HIV-positive status. The court's holding can be interpreted to allow any program involving controlled fighting, sparring, or possibly aggressive exercise to exclude HIV-positive applicants. Another case involved segregation of HIV-infected prisoners. In *Lydia Kay Onishea, et al.* v. *Joe S. Hopper, Commissioner of the Alabama Department of Correction, et al.*, 171 F.3d 1289 (11th Cir. 1999), inmates were screened for HIV infection and those infected were segregated into HIV-positive 'units' away from the general population. The case was decided on grounds that would directly implicate the rights of those covered under the ADA. The court found that the cost of accommodating the HIV-infected prisoners to reduce the discrimination of segregated units would pose an undue hardship on the state, as it would necessitate the hiring of more guards where the prison was already operating with an insufficient number of guards. The *Vickie Lesley* v. *Hee Man Chie, M.D.*, 250 F.3d 47 (1st Cir. 2001) case resulted in a holding that is difficult to harmonize with *Bragdon*; a woman was refused treatment by her obstetrician-gynecologist after she tested positive for HIV. The doctor referred her to another hospital that was better qualified, in his judgment, to deal with her. The doctor's testimony was given deferential weight and the court held there was no violation. *Lesley* and *Onishea* both involved alleged violations of the Rehabilitation Act (29 U.S.C.S. § 794(a)) which directly implicates the decisions under the ADA.

The finding that HIV/AIDS is a disability for the limited reason of the impact the disease has on the reproductive choices of the infected person means that advances in perinatal treatments described above may invalidate this legal 'hook'. If this were to happen, a court would either need to adopt a theory similar to Justice Ginsburg's concurrence, finding that HIV impairs a wide range of potential major life activities, or find other statutory criteria with which to justify the continued classification of HIV/AIDS as a disability. A possible, although rarely used, statutory approach under the ADA would be to include HIV/AIDS as a disability under the 'regarded as' language of the statute. Courts have disfavored this approach because of its broad implications, possibly extending the ADA beyond what Congress originally contemplated. The failure of courts to consider HIV/AIDS a disability would deal a severe blow to the protections and independence that currently benefit persons with HIV/AIDS. Many of those who test positive for the disease can enjoy a lifetime of productivity and are fully qualified employees and consumers of necessary services. It would be ironic indeed if asymptomatic HIV were no longer considered a disability, thus depriving persons with HIV of protection from discrimination and only providing protection when persons become so ill with advanced AIDS that they may not be able to benefit from the protections that the ADA can provide.

Another way that recent cases have limited the scope of the ADA has been in the court's decisions related to suits against state entities. These cases have held that state employees cannot sue states for discrimination under the employment title of the ADA. Depending on the outcome of the current Supreme Court case, the prohibition against discrimination in public services may also be revoked. Although these cases do not apply specifically to people with HIV, they would clearly limit the scope of protection offered to the many people with HIV infection who are state employees, use state services, or use state-owned public accommodations.

Criminal Law

A crime at common law is considered an act with both *actus reus* and *mens rea*. These Latin terms translate respectively as 'guilty act' and 'guilty mind'. Punishable offenses traditionally needed to include both of these elements. Thus, prosecution for a crime usually requires proof of both a prohibited act and a specific state of mind, or 'intent'. The goals of criminal law include punishment, retribution, and sometimes, rehabilitation. Public health, by contrast aims to detect and control disease; prevent disease through public health interventions; promote healthy behavior; and educate the public about health risks and benefits. Although their goals differ, law enforcement and public health may have similar interests in some cases.

Criminal law has been used since early in the HIV/AIDS epidemic as one of many tools to try to control the spread of HIV or punish apparently risky behavior. Prosecutors have used traditional criminal statutes, including attempted murder and assault; HIV-specific provisions criminalizing knowing or intentional exposure or transmission; and public health provisions imposing penalties for exposure to communicable or sexually transmitted diseases. All states have traditional criminal laws that can be used to prosecute individuals who knowingly expose or infect others under certain circumstances. Twenty-four states have enacted laws that criminalize exposure or transmission of HIV by certain behaviors, including exchanging bodily fluids, sexual contact, sharing injection equipment, donating blood or organs, or other activities. Some of these statutes clearly define the prohibited activity, others are quite vague, permitting prosecution for exposure to bodily fluids that can include biting or spitting or other very low-risk activities. Most statutes are also unclear about the role of condoms and safe sex. Only two laws distinguish between protected and unprotected sex. The role of disclosure and consent is also not clearly defined in each law. While 11 states laws make consent of the other person an affirmative defense, eight related to sexual exposure and four related to needles define exposure without disclosure as the criminal act, the rest do not specify an impact of disclosure. Finally, no statute distinguishes between types of sexual exposure, even though these entail significantly different risks of infection. Thus, prosecution may be equally possible for insertive or receptive anal, vaginal, or oral sex, or even masturbation. Theoretically, in some states *any* sex between a person with HIV infection and one without could be a crime.

Additionally, 15 states have HIV-specific enhancements to other crimes, including rape, prostitution, assaulting a police, corrections or emergency response officer, which impose additional penalties when the perpetrator knows he or she has HIV infection. In three of these states, the HIV-specific enhancement is their only HIV-related criminal law.

Twenty-two states make their HIV-specific provisions a felony, while one has both felony and misdemeanor provisions, and one makes actual infection a more

503

severe penalty. Twenty-five states have provisions in their public health codes that punish exposure of another person to a communicable or sexually transmitted disease. In contrast to the HIV-specific provisions, 20 of these 25 are misdemeanors. These laws have been used in over 300 cases to prosecute behavior that may have placed others at risk of HIV infection, and occasionally, led to documented infection (Lazzarini *et al.*, 2002). Of 316 cases of prosecution identified between 1986 and 2001, 211 involved sexual exposure, of which 84 were consensual sex, 41 prostitution or solicitation of a prostitute, and 95 non-consensual or unclear consent; 75 involved spitting biting or scratching; 12 injection with a contaminated syringe or threat of injection; 5 selling blood; and 14 unknown or other mode of exposure. Overall, more than 80 per cent of defendants were convicted (for those where results were known). Of those convicted, seven received life sentences, and two were sentenced to 20 years to life. Of the non-life sentences, the average minimum sentence was 14.3 years, the median was 6 years, and the range was 0.15–125 years. Thirteen defendants received probation.

Well-publicized cases of exposure or transmission, such as that which occurred in New York State in 1997 (in which more than 40 women were identified as having been sexually exposed to HIV by the defendant, 13 infected), have sparked intense legislative debates and led to the introduction of bills to criminalize exposure (failed to pass), to make HIV reporting by name mandatory (enacted into law), and to tighten partner notification provisions (also adopted) (Gottfried, 1998; CDC, 1999). In theory, criminal law could influence HIV risk behavior in at least three ways. First, criminalization (followed by prosecution and imprisonment) could *incapacitate* individuals who continue to undertake risky behavior by imprisonment. Second, the threat of prosecution could *deter* individuals from prohibited behavior, through fear of punishment. Finally, the adoption of criminal provisions could *establish norms of conduct* that reflect or shape the norms in the community through defining what people find right or wrong.

In practice, there is limited evidence that any of these theoretical effects is taking place. The limited number of prosecutions over 15 years suggests that these laws are being used selectively. In terms of incapacitation, the actual number of individuals incarcerated (142) could not have had a significant impact on actual transmissions. Due to the very low probability that any single act of exposure will be punished, it is not clear whether or not these prosecutions could be deterring risky behavior. Finally, due to the substantial empirical evidence that many people with HIV continue to engage in some of these prohibited activities it is difficult to conclude that these laws set norms that HIV-positive people feel are necessary to abide by (Marks and Crepaz, 2001). In spite of this lack of empirical evidence of their efficacy, both prosecutions and the adoption of laws that facilitate prosecution remain politically popular, with states continuing to adopt HIV-specific criminal provisions. South Dakota enacted this law in 2000 criminalizing knowing exposure as a felony punishable by up to 15 years in jail.

Incarceration is a Public Health Issue

Quite independently of HIV exposure and transmission provisions, the criminal justice system is experiencing changes that directly implicate the public health. The US incarcerates a higher percentage of its own population than any other western-style democracy. More than 6.5 million Americans on average spend their day under the care, custody, or control of federal, state, or local criminal justice authorities (US Department of Justice, Bureau of Justice Statistics, 2002). This represents more than 2.8 per cent of the adult US population. Drug-related offenses have primarily contributed to a doubling and sometimes quadrupling of certain prison and jail populations. These prisoners generally have more health problems compared with the rest of the population. In addition to HIV, rates of tuberculosis, hepatitis, and mental illness are many times higher among incarcerated people than among the non-incarcerated.

According to the Bureau of Justice Statistics, on 31 December 2001, 2.0 per cent of state prison inmates were known to be HIV-positive while 1.2 per cent of federal inmates were as well. Women prisoners are significantly more likely to be infected with HIV than their male counterparts, making HIV clinical care, prenatal screening and treatment, education and prevention even more crucial for women's institutions.

Overall medical care for those in prisons often falls far below that available to the general population. In fact, inadequate medical care has spawned many lawsuits against prison systems on US Constitutional grounds for 'cruel and unusual punishment' (Eighth Amendment violation). As recently as 1993, 11 states and 32 other jurisdictions had all or some of their correctional facilities operating under a kind of judicial surveillance (called a Consent Decree) (Lazzarini and Altice, 2001).

Indeed, while antiretroviral therapy is readily available (albeit for a price) to the general population in the United States, statistics seem to show that the same may not be true for the prison population. The rate of confirmed AIDS cases among prison inmates is three times that among the general population. The percentage of AIDS-related deaths among prisoners is twice as high as the rate among the general population. These figures seem to imply that prisoners are receiving below-average care.

Prisoners are wholly within the control of the government during their terms, and do not have the ability, the funding, or even the right to seek outside treatment for HIV/AIDS, TB, diabetes, heart disease, cancer, or other chronic or communicable diseases. Given this, government has a clear responsibility to ensure that prisoners receive treatment for HIV that meets a community standard of care and does not expose prisoners to preventable decline and death through lack of access to clinical care.

Access to Pharmaceuticals

The role of economics in the AIDS crisis became apparent in the later half of the 1990s. In 1995, researchers unveiled what became commonly known as 'combination therapy'. By taking a combination of three or four different drugs at the same time, an infected individual could restore, partially at least, his or her immune system and reduce the virus to undetectable levels in the blood. Most importantly, the drugs could prevent the progression of HIV to AIDS, or even reverse it where such progression had already occurred (Gulick *et al.*, 1997).

But the promise of a more normal life came at a high price. Combination therapy cost approximately US$16 000 per year (Stansell *et al.*, 2000). An extremely expensive treatment even for the typical US citizen, this price tag made combination therapy virtually unreachable for millions of infected individuals in poorer countries.

International law and policy can either encourage or hinder access to HIV/AIDS therapies. Poor countries' reliance on loans from international financial institutions for economic sustenance forces such countries to accept loan terms which, while intended to strengthen the currency or ensure repayment of debts, ultimately forces the countries to cut funding to social welfare programs. Likewise, international legislative bodies such as the World Trade Organization (WTO) create treaties meant to protect and promote commerce at the international level. Such treaties, while clearly beneficial to the international business community, can have a drastic economic impact on poorer countries. For example, a treaty requiring member nations to honor pharmaceutical patents prevents these countries from producing generic forms of the drugs, often making the drugs too expensive to obtain (Weissman, 1996).

The Trade-Related Aspects of Intellectual Property Agreement (TRIPS), enacted by the WTO in 1994, created such a restriction on international generic production of protected pharmaceuticals (see also Chapter 12). Participating countries have agreed to 'protect all products and processes against use, sale, import, or manufacture without the permission of the patent holder, except under very specific circumstances' (Lazzarini, 2003).

It does seem, however, that exceptions built into the TRIPS agreement may allow developing countries to obtain needed drugs at an affordable price. Brazil is one example of a country that has managed to find a way to provide generic forms of patented drugs to its people without violating the terms of the treaty. In the early 1990s, faced with the likelihood that its country would have 1.2 million HIV-positive individuals by the year 2000, the Brazilian government became determined to fight back. The country's success in this battle can be largely attributed to its decision to guarantee free antiretroviral treatment to all infected citizens. Indeed, between 1997 and 2002, the number of people in Brazil receiving antiretroviral treatment increased from 25 000 to 100 000 (Piot, 2002). As a result, Brazil entered 2000 with only 540 000 individuals infected, less than half of the 1994 projection of 1.2 million.

But how did Brazil manage to fund such extensive free access to antiretroviral therapy? Clearly they could not afford to pay market price for the drugs, and their membership in the WTO held them to the TRIPS requirements. It seems that these two factors should have created a barrier to availability for antiretroviral therapy in Brazil.

Brazil, however, has managed to exploit exceptions in the TRIPS agreement and the desire of international pharmaceutical companies to avoid compulsory licensing in order to develop affordable and legal (albeit highly contested) methods of obtaining drugs. First, TRIPS only applied to pharmaceuticals patented after 1994, freeing Brazil to generically produce any of the drugs that were created before 1994. Next, Brazil had specified in its patent-protection laws that in order to be protected, at least a part of the manufacturing of a drug would have to take place in Brazil. This allowed for local licensing and production of several of the post-1994 antiretroviral drugs.

Brazil's final measure for attaining affordable AIDS drugs is the one that has been highly criticized by pharmaceutical companies and wealthier nations, although it seems to be allowable under TRIPS. Namely, the President of Brazil issued a decree allowing for 'compulsory licensing in cases of national emergency, including situations in which there is an impending public health crisis'. Compulsory licensing allows the government to issue a license to provide a generic version of an otherwise patented drug within a country, based on necessity, in exchange for paying the patent holder a reasonable licensing fee (Weissman, 1996). Although Brazil has yet to actually impose such compulsory licensing, the mere threat of such action has been sufficient to persuade drug companies to offer discounts to Brazil on specific drugs.

Brazil's success in increasing access to HIV treatment among its population is certainly commendable, and its procedure for doing so may serve as a model for developing countries facing a plight similar to that of Brazil in the early 1990s. Factors to consider in determining the adaptability of Brazil's model to other countries include the eventual obsolescence of pre-1994 AIDS drugs and the long-term effect that the threat of compulsory licensing may have on a pharmaceutical companies' willingness to remain in a country and the need for considerable political will, on the part of the developing country's government, to adopt and maintain such a policy in the face of threats from powerful multinational companies, the US, and other governments. At the same time, wealthier countries currently opposed to Brazil's efforts to obtain affordable pharmaceuticals should look closely at whether their own actions of threatening trade sanctions, insisting on maintaining high market prices, and discouraging developing countries from utilizing compulsory licensing, might actually have a net detrimental affect on the international economy. For example, by considering the increased demand for international assistance to countries such as Brazil that would become necessary if these countries were forced to halt the generic production of patented drugs.

In December of 2003, the World Health Organization (WHO) unveiled the '3 by 5 Initiative', a plan to provide antiretroviral treatment for 3 million people living with HIV/AIDS in developing countries by the year 2005. The cost of this initiative was estimated at US$5.5 billion, and the WHO noted that the program's success relied heavily on international funding and an effort by pharmaceutical companies to reduce the cost of treatment.

Of particular importance to the success of the project was the US$15 billion in funding promised by the United States under President Bush's HIV/AIDS Initiatives. Recent actions by the US presidential administration, however, seem to indicate that this promise of funds may have been misinterpreted, and that the President's plan may not result in any increase in funding by the US.

The International AIDS Conference in July 2004 was dedicated to the theme 'Access for All'. For such a theme to prove accurate, however, an enormous international commitment of money, time, and resources is essential.

While each of these areas of international law has the potential significantly to effect health and access to pharmaceuticals, our current approach has not reconciled the conflicts between them.

What the Future Holds

The impact of HIV/AIDS on national and international law has been both profound and pervasive. Controversies over personal privacy rights and discrimination have been resolved by the US Supreme Court against the backdrop of rapidly changing fact patterns concerning the treatment and spread of the virus. The status of HIV as a disability and the scope of individuals protected will continue to be negotiated in the federal courts. Another area of probable legal activity includes the trend toward HIV case surveillance, with the dominant form being name-based reporting. Although public health-related uses of HIV surveillance data may cause some controversy (e.g. mandatory partner notification provisions), non-health uses may pose the greatest danger to the public's sense of trust in public health authorities. Legislatures have also widely adopted HIV-specific criminal exposure or transmission laws. It is possible that these laws will be enforced more frequently or public health data will be sought for prosecution. Although many people with HIV in the US have access to combination antiretroviral therapy, some groups, including prisoners and the un- or under-insured, often lack access to effective HIV treatment and the necessary monitoring and health care that goes along with it.

On the international front legal and ethical issues are likely to arise in several contexts. One is whether or not the significant public and private monies which have been promised by the US and other developed countries will actually be released to fight the spread and human devastation of HIV/AIDS. These monies, intended to support research, prevention, and care, could turn the tide of the epidemic in some countries and alleviate much suffering in others. However, failure to meet these commitments will pose grave public health risks at a time when global public health faces other infectious disease threats. In recent years, activist groups have mounted unprecedented challenges to international patent and trade law. These efforts have focused on making critical pharmaceuticals more affordable and building the capacity of developing countries to manufacture, purchase, and administer them. Legal questions for the future include whether these challenges will continue to expand access to HIV and other medications. International cooperation in increasing access to pharmaceuticals and funding global prevention and treatment programs remains questionable in an era in which the 'war on terrorism' has taken center stage.

Internationally, injection drug use drives the epidemic in many countries or regions. Laws, policies, and law enforcement practices that limit access to sterile syringes, incarcerate large numbers of drug users, or promote risky activity among drug users and their partners may represent a key area for legal and policy intervention. Understanding the role of laws and law enforcement in countries with newer epidemics of HIV and drug use is vital to future efforts to reduce these risks.

References

American Academy of Pediatrics (1995) Perinatal human immunodeficiency virus testing. *Pediatrics* 95: 303–6. Available at: http://www.aap.org/policy/re9507.html

American College of Nurse Midwives (1999) Reducing perinatal transmission of HIV/AIDS: a tip sheet for ACNM state legislative contacts, November.

American College of Obstetricians and Gynecologists (2000) Press release: HIV tests urged for all pregnant women: Ob-Gyns launch campaign for universal HIV screening. Available at: http://www.acog.org/from_home/publications/press_releases/nr05-23-00-2.cfm (accessed 23 May 2000).

American Library Association (2002) *Privacy: An Interpretation of the Library Bill of Rights*, 19 June. Available at: http://www.ala.org

Angell M (1997) The ethics of clinical research in the Third World. *N Engl J Med* 337: 847–9.

Beauchamp TL, Childress JF (2001) *Principles of Biomedical Ethics*, 5th edn. New York: Oxford University Press.

CDC (Centers for Disease Control and Prevention) (1999) Cluster of HIV-positive young women – New York. 1997–1998. *MMWR Morb Mortal Wkly Rep* 48: 413–16.

CDC (2001) HIV and AIDS – United States, 1981–2000. *MMWR Morb Mortal Wkly Rep* 50: 430–3.

CDC (2002) US Public Health Service Task Force recommendations for use of antiretroviral drugs in pregnant HIV-1-infected women for maternal health and interventions to reduce perinatal HIV-1 transmission in the United States. *MMWR Morb Mortal Wkly Rep* 51: 1.

Connor EM, Sperling RS, Gelber R *et al.* (1994) Reduction of maternal – infant transmission of human immunodeficiency virus type 1 with zidovudine treatment. *N Engl J Med* 331: 1173–80.

Goodman RA, Munson JW, Dammers K, Lazzarini Z, Barkley JP (2003) Forensic epidemiology: law at the intersection of public health and criminal investigations. *J Law Med Ethics* 31: 684–700.

Gostin LO, Ward JW, Baker AC (1997) National HIV case reporting for the United States: a defining moment in the history of the epidemic. *N Engl J Med* 337: 1162–6.

Gostin L, Burris S, Lazzarini Z (1999) The law and the public's health: a study of infectious disease law in the United States. *Columbia Law Rev* 59: 101.

Gottfried RN (1998) Lessons from Chautauqua County. *Albany Law Rev* 61: 1079–90.

Gulick RM, Mellors JW, Havlir D *et al.* (1997) Treatment with indinavir, zidovudine, and lamivudine in adults with human immunodeficiency virus infection and prior antiretroviral therapy. *N Engl J Med* 337: 734–9.

HIV Criminal Law and Policy Project (2001) *HIV Reporting*. Available at: http://www.hivcriminallaw.org/laws/reporting.cfm

Lazzarini Z (2003) Making access to pharmaceuticals a reality: legal options under TRIPS and the case of Brazil. *Yale Hum Rights Devel Law J* 6: 103–9.

Lazzarini Z, Altice F (2001) A review of the legal and ethical issues for the conduct of HIV-related research in prisons. *AIDS Public Policy* 15: 104–31.

Lazzarini Z, Rosales L (2002) Legal issues concerning public health efforts to reduce perinatal HIV transmission. *Yale J Health Policy Law Ethics* 3: 67–98.

Lazzarini Z, Bray S, Burris S (2002) Evaluating the impact of criminal laws on HIV risk behavior. *J Law Med Ethics* 30: 239–53.

Lurie P, Wolfe SM (1997) Unethical trials of interventions to reduce perinatal transmission of the human immunodeficiency virus in developing countries. *N Engl J Med* 337: 853–6.

Marks G, Crepaz N (2001) HIV-positive men's sexual practices in the context of self-disclosure of HIV status. *J Acquir Immune Defic Syndr* 27: 79–85.

Mofenson LM (2000) Perinatal exposure to zidovudine B – benefits and risks. *N Engl J Med* 343: 803–5.

New York State Department of Health (1999) Changes in the state's newborn HIV screening program. Available at: http://www.health.state.ny.us/nysdoh/aids/pindex.htm

Piot P (2002) Efforts to combat overseas HIV/AIDS. Hearings before Senate Foreign Relations Committee, 107th Congress, 13 February (statement of Peter Piot, Executive Director, UNAIDS).

San Francisco Department of Public Health (2002) Minutes of Joint Conference Committee Meeting for Population Health and Prevention, Tuesday 25 June. AIDS Programs Office, 25 Van Ness, Suite #500, San Francisco, CA 94102, USA. See comments by Jeff Klausner, M.D. Available at: http://www.dph.sf.ca.us/Meetings/PHP/Minutes/JCCPHPM062502.htm (accessed 2 April 2004).

Stansell J, Gary D, Slacker *et al.* (2000) Trends in comorbidities, utilization and cost of care in HIV+ patients 1996–1999. Paper presented at the International Conference on AIDS, 9–14 July, abstract no. TuPeC3371.

Steinbrook R (2002) Preventing HIV infection in children. *N Engl J Med* 346: 1842.

Stoto MA *et al.* eds. (1999) *Reducing the Odds: Preventing Perinatal Transmission of HIV in the United States*. Institute of Medicine. Available at: http://nap.edu/readingroom/books/rto/index.html (accessed 27 February 2002).

UNAIDS (Joint United Nations Programme on HIV/AIDS) (2002) *Report on the Global HIV/AIDS Epidemic*. Available at: http://www.unaids.org/epidemic_update/report_july02/

UNAIDS (2003) *AIDS Epidemic Update*, December. Available at: http://www.unaids.org/wad/2003/Epiupdate2003_en/EpiUpdate2003_en.pdf

US Department of Justice, Office of Justice Programs, Bureau of Justice Statistics (2002) *Bureau of Justice Statistics 2002: At a Glance*. Available at: http://www.ojp.usdoj.gov/bjs/pub/pdf/bjsg02.pdf. See also http://www.ojp.usdoj.gov/bjs/pub/pdf/hivp01.pdf

Varmus H, Satcher D (1997) Ethical complexities of conducting research in developing countries. *N Engl J Med* 337: 1003–5.

Weissman R (1996) A long, strange TRIPS: the pharmaceutical industry drive to harmonize global intellectual property rules, and the remaining WTO legal alternatives available to third world countries. *Univ Pennsylvania J Int Econ Law* 17: 1069.

World Medical Association (2000) *Declaration of Helsinki: Ethical Principles for Medical Research Involving Human Subjects*. Available at: http://www.wma.net/e/policy/b3.htm

Index